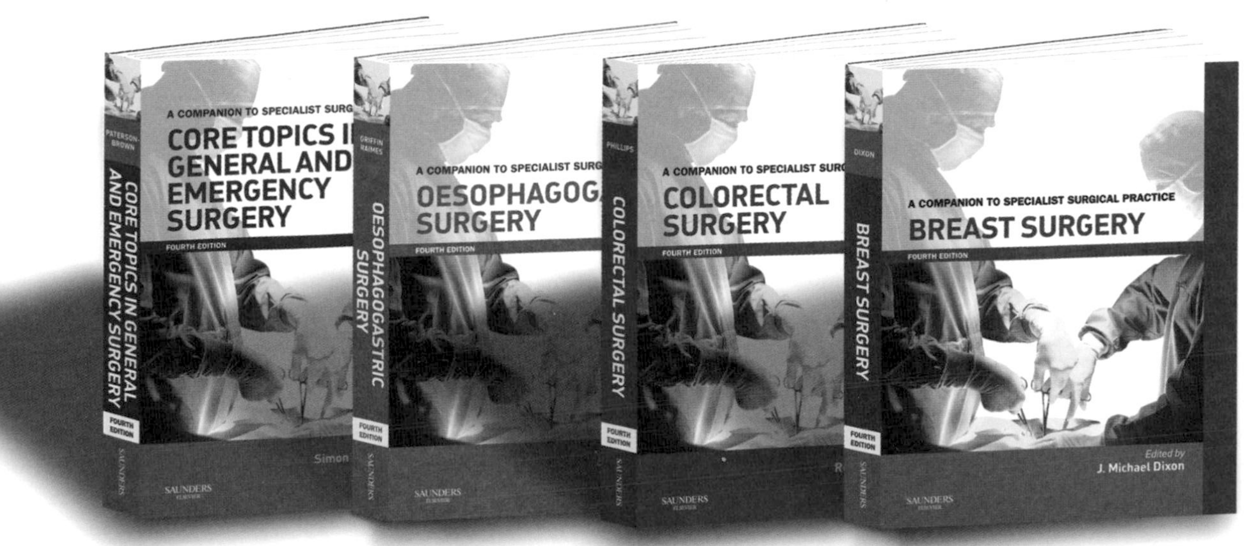


## A COMPANION TO SPECIALIST SURGICAL PRACTICE

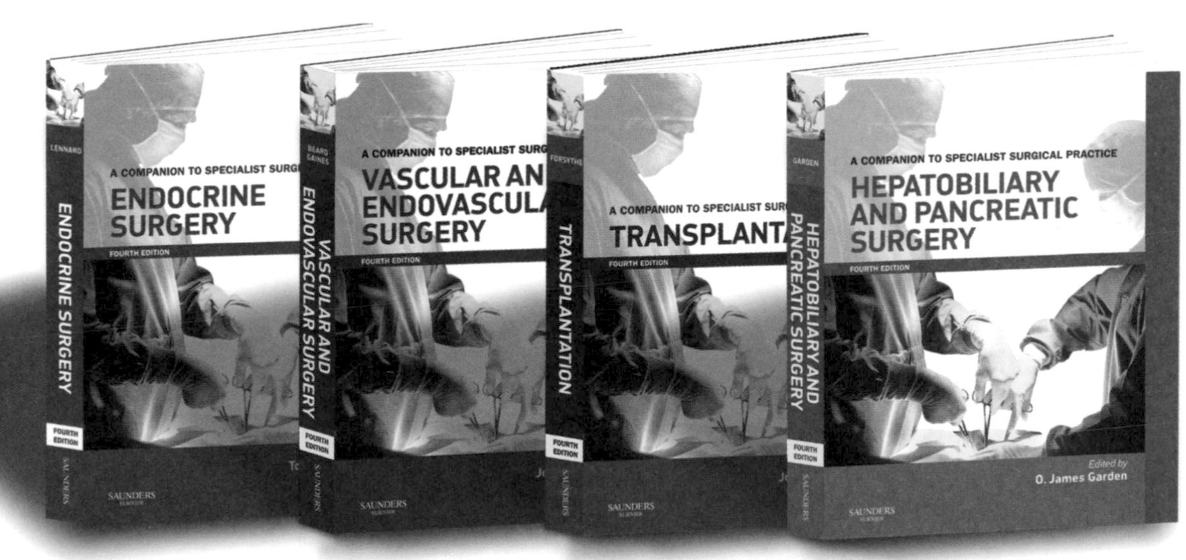

A Companion to Specialist Surgical Practice

**Series Editors**
O. James Garden
Simon Paterson-Brown

# VASCULAR AND ENDOVASCULAR SURGERY

**FOURTH EDITION**

**Edited by**


Jonathan D. Beard
ChM MEd FRCS
Consultant Vascular Surgeon
The Sheffield Vascular Institute;
Professor of Surgical Education
The University of Sheffield, UK

Peter A. Gaines
FRCP FRCR
Consultant Vascular Radiologist
The Sheffield Vascular Institute;
Professor of Radiology
Sheffield Hallam University, UK


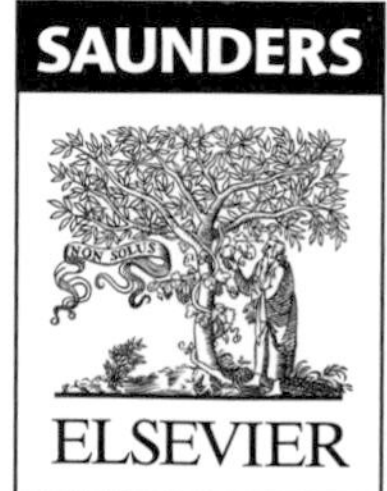



Edinburgh London New York Oxford Philadelphia St Louis Sydney Toronto 2009

SAUNDERS
ELSEVIER



First edition 1997
Second edition 2001
Third edition 2005
Fourth edition 2009

ISBN 9780702030116

**British Library Cataloguing in Publication Data**
A catalogue record for this book is available from the British Library

**Library of Congress Cataloging in Publication Data**
A catalog record for this book is available from the Library of Congress

**Notice**
Knowledge and best practice in this field are constantly changing. As new research and experience broaden our knowledge, changes in practice, treatment and drug therapy may become necessary or appropriate. Readers are advised to check the most current information provided (i) on procedures featured or (ii) by the manufacturer of each product to be administered, to verify the recommended dose or formula, the method and duration of administration, and contraindications. It is the responsibility of the practitioner, relying on their own experience and knowledge of the patient, to make diagnoses, to determine dosages and the best treatment for each individual patient, and to take all appropriate safety precautions. To the fullest extent of the law, neither the Publisher nor the Editors assumes any liability for any injury and/or damage to persons or property arising out of or related to any use of the material contained in this book.

*The Publisher*



Printed in China

*Commissioning Editor:* Laurence Hunter
*Development Editor:* Elisabeth Lawrence
*Project Manager:* Andrew Palfreyman
*Text Design:* Charlotte Murray
*Cover Design:* Kirsteen Wright
*Illustration Manager:* Gillian Richards
*Illustrators:* Martin Woodward and Richard Prime

# Contents

# Contributors

**Ajmad Alomari, MD**
Instructor in Radiology
Division of Vascular and Interventional Radiology
Department of Radiology
The Children's HospitaL Boston
Harvard Medical School
Boston, MA, USA

**Gillian Atkinson, MCSP**
Senior Physiotherapist
Mobility and Specialised Rehabilitation Centre
Northern General Hospital
Sheffield, UK

**Faisal Aziz, MD**
Vascular Resident
Jobst Vascular Center
The Toledo Hospital
Toledo, OH, USA

**Arun Balakrishnan, AFRCS**
Senior Clinical Fellow in Vascular Surgery
Northern Vascular Centre
Department of Vascular Surgery
Freeman Hospital
Newcastle upon Tyne, UK

**Jonathan D. Beard, BSc, ChM, MEd, FRCS**
Consultant Vascular Surgeon
The Sheffield Vascular Institute;
Professor of Surgical Education
The University of Sheffield
Sheffield, UK

**Jill J.F. Belch, MB, ChB, MD, FRCP(Glasg), FRCP(Ed) FRCP**
Director
The Institute of Cardiovascular Research
University of Dundee;
Honorary Consultant Physician
Ninewells Hospital and Medical School
Dundee, UK

**Sherab G. Bhutia, MS, FRCS**
Specialist Registrar in Vascular Surgery
Department of Vascular Surgery
North Tees Hospital
Cleveland, UK

**John Bottomley MB, ChB, FRANZCR**
Sheffield Vascular Institute
Northern General Hospital Sheffield, UK

**Andrew J.M. Boulton, MD, FRCP**
Professor of Medicine
University of Manchester;
Consultant Physician
Manchester Royal Infirmary
Manchester, UK

**Andrew W. Bradbury, BSc, MB, ChB, MD, MBA, FRCS(Ed)**
Education Dean and Sampson Gamgee
Professor of Vascular Surgery
University of Birmingham;
Consultant Vascular and Endovascular Surgeon
Heart of England NHS Foundation Trust
Birmingham, UK

**Peter W.G. Brown, BSc, MB, ChB, FRCS(Ed), FRCR**
Consultant Radiologist
Department of Diagnostic Imaging
Northern General Hospital
Sheffield, UK

**Jan Brunkwall, MD, PhD**
Professor and Chairman
Department of Vascular Surgery
University Clinics
University of Cologne
Cologne, Germany

**Patricia Burrows, MD**
Vascular Surgeon
Center for Endovascular Surgery
Roosevelt Hospital
New York, NY, USA

**Nicholas Cheshire MB, ChB, FRCSS, MD, FRCS (Gen)**
Professor of Vascular Surgery
Department of Vascular Surgery
St Mary's NHS Trust
London, UK

**Trevor Cleveland, BMedSci, BM, BS, FRCS, FRCR**
Consultant Vascular Radiologist
Sheffield Vascular Institute
Sheffield Teaching Hospitals NHS Trust
Sheffield, UK

**Anthony J. Comerota, MD, FACS, FACC, RVT**
Director, Jobst Vascular Center
The Toledo Hospital
Toledo, OH;

Adjunct Professor of Surgery
University Of Michigan
Department of Surgery
Ann Arbor, MI, USA

**Dipak Datta, MB, BS, FRCS(Ed), FRCS(Glasg), FRCP**
Consultant in Rehabilitation Medicine
Mobility and Specialised Rehabilitation Centre
Northern General Hospital;
Honorary Senior Clinical Lecturer
University of Sheffield
Sheffield, UK

**Philip Davey, MD, FRCS**
Specialist Registrar in Vascular Surgery
Northern Vascular Centre
Freeman Hospital
Newcastle upon Tyne, UK

**Michael Dialynas, MS, FRCS**
Department of Vascular Surgery
Broomfield Hospital
Chelmsford, UK

**Brian Dillon, MD**
Fellow
Division of Vascular and Interventional Radiology
Department of Radiology
The Children's Hospital Boston
Harvard Medical School
Boston, MA, USA

**Richard Donnelly, MB, ChB(Hons), MD, PhD, FRCP, FRACP**
Professor of Vascular Medicine
University of Nottingham;
Honorary Consultant Physician
Derby City General Hospital
Derby, UK

**Jonothan J. Earnshaw, MB, BS, DM, FRCS**
Consultant Surgeon
Gloucestershire Royal Hospital
Gloucester, UK

**Peter A. Gaines, FRCP, FRCR**
Consultant Vascular Radiologist
The Sheffield Vascular Institute;
Professor of Radiology
Sheffield Hallam University
Sheffield, UK

**Christopher P. Gibbons, MA, DPhil, MCh, FRCS**
Consultant Vascular Surgeon
Morriston Hospital
Swansea, Wales

**Edward B. Jude, MB, BS, MD, MRCP**
Consultant Physician
Tameside General Hospital
Ashton-under-Lyme, UK

**Philip Kalra, MA, MB, BChir, FRCP, MD**
Consultant Nephrologist
Hope Hospital
Salford, UK

**Timothy A. Lees, MB, ChB, MD, FRCS**
Consultant Vascular Surgeon
Northern Vascular Centre
Freeman Hospital
Newcastle upon Tyne, UK

**Sumaira MacDonald MB, ChB, FRCP, FRCR, FRCS (US,IR), PhD**
Consultant Vascular Radiologist
Radiology Department
Freeman Hospital
Newcastle upon Tyne, UK

**Etienne Marchand, MD**
Fellow in Vascular Surgery
Vascular Surgery Service
University Hospital Jean Bernard
Poitiers, France

**Jacobus van Marle, MB, ChB, MMed(Surg), FCS(SA)**
Professor of Vascular Surgery
Vascular Society of Southern Africa
Centurion, South Africa

**Rob Morgan, MRCP, FRCR**
Consultant Interventional Radiologist
Radiology Department
St George's Vascular Institute
St George's Healthcare NHS Trust
London, UK

**Jonathan G. Moss, MB, ChB, FRCS(Ed), FRCR**
Consultant Interventional Radiologist
Department of Radiology
Gartnavel General Hospital
Glasgow, UK

**A. Ross Naylor MB, ChB, MD, FRCS**
Professor of Vascular Surgery
University of Leicester;
Consultant Vascular Surgeon
Leicester Royal Infirmary
Leicester, UK

**Andre Nevelsteen MD, PhD, FRCS**
Professor of Vascular Surgery
Department of Vascular Surgery
University Hospital Gasthuisberg
Leuven, Belgium

**Anthony Nicholson, BSc, MSc, MB, ChB, FRCR**
Consultant Interventional Radiologist
Department of Radiology
Leeds Teaching Hospital NHS Trust
Leeds, UK

**Janet T. Powell, MD, PhD, FRCPath**
Professor of Vascular Biology
Department of Vascular Surgery
Imperial College
London, UK

**Nicholas F.W. Redwood, MB, BS, FRCS**
Consultant Vascular and General Surgeon
The Queen Elizabeth Hospital
King's Lynn, UK

**Jean-Baptiste Ricco, MD, PhD**
Fellow in Vascular Surgery
Vascular Surgery Service
University Hospital Jean Bernard
University of Poitiers
Poitiers, France

**Celia Riga, MB, BS, BSc, MRCS(Eng)**
Clinical Research Fellow in Vascular Surgery
Department of Biosurgery and Surgical Technology
Division of Surgery, Oncology, Reproductive
Biology and Anaesthetics
Imperial College
London, UK

**John Rose, FRCR**
Consultant Interventional Radiologist
Department of Clinical Radiology
Freeman Hospital
Newcastle upon Tyne, UK

**Dirk A. le Roux, MB, ChB, FCS(SA), CVS(SA)**
Consultant Vascular Surgeon
Johannesburg General Hospital;
Lecturer in Vascular Surgery
University of the Witwatersrand
Johannesburg, South Africa

**Julian Scott, MD, MB, ChB, FRCS, FRCSEd, FEBVS**
Professor of Vascular Surgery
Surgery Division of Cardiovascular
and Diabetes Research
Leeds Institute of Genetics, Health
and Therapeutics
University of Leeds
Leeds, UK

**Cliff Shearman, BSc, MB, BS, FRCS, MS**
Professor of Vascular Surgery
Department of Vascular Surgery
Southampton General Hospital
Southampton, UK

**Matthew Thompson, MA, MB, BS, MD, FRCS**
Professor of Vascular Surgery
University of London;
Consultant Vascular Surgeon
St George's Vascular Institute
St George's Healthcare NHS Trust
London, UK

**Michael Wyatt, MD, FRCS**
Consultant Vascular Surgeon
Department of Vascular Surgery
Freeman Hospital
Newcastle upon Tyne, UK

# Series preface

Since the publication of the first edition in 1997, the *Companion to Specialist Surgical Practice* series has aspired to meet the needs of surgeons in higher training and practising consultants who wish contemporary, evidence-based information on the subspecialist areas relevant to their general surgical practice. We have accepted that the series will not necessarily be as comprehensive as some of the larger reference surgical textbooks which, by their very size, may not always be completely up to date at the time of publication. This Fourth Edition aims to bring relevant state-of-the-art specialist information that we and the individual volume editors consider important for the practising subspecialist general surgeon. Where possible, all contributors have attempted to identify evidence-based references to support key recommendations within each chapter.

We remain grateful to the volume editors and all the contributors of this Fourth Edition. Their enthusiasm, commitment and hard work has ensured that a short turnover has been maintained between each of the editions, thereby ensuring as accurate and up-to-date content as possible. We remain grateful for the support and encouragement of Laurence Hunter and Elisabeth Lawrence at Elsevier Ltd. We trust that our aim of providing up-to-date and affordable surgical texts has been met and that all readers, whether in training or in consultant practice, will find this fourth edition an invaluable resource.

**O. James Garden** MB, ChB, MD, FRCS(Glas), FRCS(Ed), FRCP(Ed), FRACS(Hon), FRCSC(Hon)

Regius Professor of Clinical Surgery, Clinical and Surgical Sciences (Surgery), University of Edinburgh, and Honorary Consultant Surgeon, Royal Infirmary of Edinburgh

**Simon Paterson-Brown** MB, BS, MPhil, MS, FRCS(Ed), FRCS

Honorary Senior Lecturer, Clinical and Surgical Sciences (Surgery), University of Edinburgh, and Consultant General and Upper Gastrointestinal Surgeon, Royal Infirmary of Edinburgh

# Editors' preface

*Vascular and Endovascular Surgery* is designed to be a comprehensive and affordable textbook for all those involved with the management of patients with vascular disease, whether they be trainees, vascular or non-vascular specialists, or other healthcare professionals. A modern vascular service encompasses many disciplines, and success depends upon a team approach. Whilst the vascular surgeon often remains in overall charge of the patient, management may involve clinical nurse specialists, angiologists and interventional radiologists. Other clinicians are frequently involved with the management of many of our patients, including diabetologists, neurologists, rheumatologists and haematologists. Physiotherapists and other rehabilitation specialists are also vital for successful patient outcomes. Our choice of authors for this Fourth Edition reflects this diversity.

Many of the chapters from the Third Edition have been retained, although all of them have been extensively revised and updated in line with recently published evidence, such as the Trans-Atlantic Inter-Society Consensus (TASC) II guidelines. The continued move towards non-invasive imaging, medical therapy and endovascular techniques is reflected in the content of this book. In response to the reviews of the Third Edition, the technical chapters on grafts and stents have been removed. The space created has allowed us to add a new chapter on the medical treatment of chronic lower limb ischaemia. Vascular surgeons and radiologists are increasingly undertaking access procedures and therefore we have also added a chapter on central and peripheral access. To reflect the problem-orientated nature of the book, the titles of the chapters dealing with venous insufficiency have been focused on the management of the acutely swollen leg and the chronically swollen leg. Another feature of this new edition is the use of colour illustrations throughout the book. The unique use of symbols to denote levels of evidence has been retained.

To reflect the collaborative nature of a modern vascular service, many of the chapters are co-authored by a vascular surgeon and a vascular radiologist. We have continued to expand our authorship to include more experts from Europe and North America, with an emphasis on global practice. We are grateful to all our authors for the hard work that they have put into their respective chapters.

**Jonathan D. Beard**
**Peter A. Gaines**
**Sheffield**

# Evidence-based practice in surgery

Critical appraisal for developing evidence-based practice can be obtained from a number of sources, the most reliable being randomised controlled clinical trials, systematic literature reviews, meta-analyses and observational studies. For practical purposes three grades of evidence can be used, analogous to the levels of 'proof' required in a court of law:

1. **Beyond all reasonable doubt.** Such evidence is likely to have arisen from high-quality randomised controlled trials, systematic reviews or high-quality synthesised evidence such as decision analysis, cost-effectiveness analysis or large observational datasets. The studies need to be directly applicable to the population of concern and have clear results. The grade is analogous to burden of proof within a criminal court and may be thought of as corresponding to the usual standard of 'proof' within the medical literature (i.e. $P < 0.05$).
2. **On the balance of probabilities.** In many cases a high-quality review of literature may fail to reach firm conclusions due to conflicting or inconclusive results, trials of poor methodological quality or the lack of evidence in the population to which the guidelines apply. In such cases it may still be possible to make a statement as to the best treatment on the 'balance of probabilities'. This is analogous to the decision in a civil court where all the available evidence will be weighed up and the verdict will depend upon the balance of probabilities.
3. **Not proven.** Insufficient evidence upon which to base a decision, or contradictory evidence.

Depending on the information available, three grades of recommendation can be used:

a. Strong recommendation, which should be followed unless there are compelling reasons to act otherwise.
b. A recommendation based on evidence of effectiveness, but where there may be other factors to take into account in decision-making, for example the user of the guidelines may be expected to take into account patient preferences, local facilities, local audit results or available resources.
c. A recommendation made where there is no adequate evidence as to the most effective practice, although there may be reasons for making a recommendation in order to minimise cost or reduce the chance of error through a locally agreed protocol.

## Strong recommendation 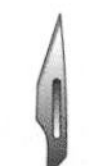

Evidence where a conclusion can be reached **'beyond all reasonable doubt'** and therefore where a **strong recommendation** can be given.

This will normally be based on evidence levels:

- Ia. Meta-analysis of randomised controlled trials
- Ib. Evidence from at least one randomised controlled trial
- IIa. Evidence from at least one controlled study without randomisation
- IIb. Evidence from at least one other type of quasi-experimental study.

## Expert opinion 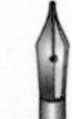

Evidence where a conclusion might be reached **'on the balance of probabilities'** and where there may be other factors involved which influence the recommendation given. This will normally be based on less conclusive evidence than that represented by scalpel icons:

- III. Evidence from non-experimental descriptive studies, such as comparative studies and case–control studies
- IV. Evidence from expert committee reports or opinions or clinical experience of respected authorities, or both.

Evidence in each chapter of this volume which is associated with either a strong recommendation or expert opinion is annotated in the text by either a **scalpel** or **pen-nib** icon as shown above. References associated with **scalpel** evidence will be highlighted in the reference lists, along with a short summary of the paper's conclusions where applicable.

# Further reading

The compact format of this book means that it cannot cover every detail of vascular and endovascular surgery, diagnostic imaging and vascular medicine. The books listed below will provide more detail when required.

## General

**Vascular surgery, 6th edn**
Rutherford RB (ed.). WB Saunders, 2005.
The 'bible' of vascular surgery. Encyclopaedic but expensive, with a strong American influence.

**Comprehensive vascular and endovascular surgery, 2nd edn**
Hallet JW, Mills JL, Earnshaw JJ, Reekers JA, Rooke (eds.). Mosby, 2009.
A more affordable, comprehensive textbook with a transatlantic flavour. Excellent colour illustrations and diagrams.

**Pathways of care in vascular surgery**
Beard JD, Murray S (eds.). TFM Publishing, 2002.
A useful book produced by the Joint Vascular Research Group. Evidence-based, multidisciplinary approach to the management of common vascular conditions.

**ABC of arterial and venous disease**
Donnelly R, London NJM (eds.). BMJ Books, 2000.
An inexpensive, well-illustrated, soft-cover book suitable for junior doctors, students and nurses.

## Specialist

**Abrams' angiography: interventional radiology, 2nd edn**
Baum S, Pentecost MJ (eds.). Lippincott, Williams & Wilkins, 2005.

**Connective tissue diseases**
Belch JJF, Zurier RB (eds.). Chapman & Hall, 1995.

**The vein book**
Bergan JJ (ed.). Elsevier, 2007.

**The foot in diabetes, 3rd edn**
Boulton AJM, Connor H, Cavanagh PRC (eds.). John Wiley, 2000.

**Atlas of vascular disease, 2nd edn**
Creager MA, Braunwald E (eds.). Philadelphia, PA: Current Medicine, 2003.

**Interventional radiology explained**
Francis I, Watkinson A (eds.). Remedica Series for Clinicians. Remedica, 2000. ISBN 1–90134602–1.

**An introduction to vascular biology, 2nd edn**
Halliday AW, Hunt BJ, Poston L, Schachter M (eds.). Cambridge University Press, 2002.

**Interventional radiology: a survival guide, 2nd edn**
Kessel D, Robertson I. Elsevier, 2005.

**Peripheral arterial disease**
Mohler E, Jaff M (eds.). ACP, 2008.
Good coverage of epidemiology of peripheral arterial disease.

**Amputation surgery and lower limb prosthetics**
Murdoch G (ed.). Blackwell, 1988.

**Atlas of vascular surgery: operative procedures**
Ouriel K, Rutherford RB (eds.). WB Saunders, 1998.
Clear line diagrams of vascular surgical techniques and exposures.

**CT and MR angiography: comprehensive vascular assessment**
Rubin GD, Rofsky NM (eds.). Lippincott, Williams & Wilkins, 2008.

**Recent advances in thrombosis and haemostasis**
Tanaka K, Davie EW (eds.). Springer, 2008.

**Atlas of vascular anatomy: an angiographic approach**
Uflacker R (ed.). Lippincott, Williams & Wilkins, 2006.

**Interventional radiology: a practical guide**
Watkinson AF, Adam A (eds.). Radcliffe Medical Press, 1996. ISBN 1–85775031–4.

**Endovascular therapies: current evidence**
Wyatt MG, Watkinson AF (eds.). TFM Publishing, 2006. ISBN 1–90337846-X.

**Introduction to vascular sonography, 5th edn**
Zweibel W (ed.). WB Saunders, 2005.

## Websites

Books can become outdated, which is why *Vascular and Endovascular Surgery* is published frequently in an affordable format. Websites and journals provide up-to-the-minute information on recent trials and technological developments, as well as news of meetings and courses. A few of the more useful websites are listed below.

American Board of Surgery: http://home.absurgery.org/default.jsp?index
American Venous Forum: http://www.venous-info.com
British Society of Interventional Radiology: http://www.bsir.org
Cardiovascular and Interventional Radiological Society of Europe: http://www.cirse.org
European Board of Vascular Surgery: http://www.uemsvascular.com
European Journal of Vascular and Endovascular Surgery: http://www.sciencedirect.com/esvs
European Society for Vascular Surgery: http://www.esvs.org
European Venous Forum: http://www.european-venousforum.org
Society for Vascular Surgery (North America): http://www.vascularweb.org
Vascular Society of Great Britain and Ireland: http://www.vascularsociety.org.uk

# 1

# Epidemiology and risk factor management of peripheral arterial disease

Richard Donnelly
Janet T. Powell

## Introduction

Atherosclerotic peripheral arterial disease (PAD) involving one or more major vessels of the lower limb is common, especially in older patients, due to complex genetic and environmental interactions which result in structural and functional vascular abnormalities and reduced blood flow. PAD may be asymptomatic in the early stages, but is always associated with shortened survival due to the invariable association with atherosclerosis in other arterial territories, especially the coronary, carotid and cerebral circulation. This is highlighted by observational studies showing that reduced ankle–brachial pressure index (ABPI, a marker of disease severity in PAD) is associated with an increased risk of cardiovascular mortality (Table 1.1).[1] However, calcification and sclerosis lead to incompressible arteries, with false elevation of ABPI even in the presence of major distal atherosclerosis. The Strong Heart Study has identified associations between low (<0.90) and high (>1.40) ABPI and increased risk of all-cause and cardiovascular (CV) disease mortality, reporting a U-shaped relationship between a non-invasive measure of PAD and reduced life expectancy (**Fig. 1.1**).[2] For example, adjusted risk estimates for all-cause mortality were 1.69 for low and 1.77 for high ABPI, while the corresponding estimates for CV disease mortality were 2.52 and 2.09.[2]

This chapter considers the epidemiology of PAD, the observational studies identifying reversible and irreversible risk factors for disease progression, and the evidence from randomised controlled trials which underpins clinical use of disease-modifying therapies as part of multiple risk factor intervention.

Table 1.1 • Adjusted relative risk for mortality for levels of ankle–brachial pressure index (ABPI)

| ABPI | Relative risk | 95% CI | *P* value |
|---|---|---|---|
| <0.4 | 3.35 | 2.16–5.20 | <0.001 |
| 0.4–0.85 | 2.02 | 1.34–3.02 | <0.001 |
| >0.85 | 1.00 | Reference | |

From McKenna M, Wolfson S, Kuller L. The ratio of ankle and arm arterial pressure as an independent predictor of mortality. Atherosclerosis 1991; 87:119–28. With permission from Elsevier.

## Epidemiology of PAD

Obtaining accurate figures for the prevalence and incidence of PAD has not been straightforward. For example, several epidemiological studies have focused on specific groups, e.g. in the workplace setting or referrals to hospital, which may not be truly representative of the wider population. Thus, workplace screening studies for PAD have excluded those who have retired and those who may be unfit for work. Similarly, epidemiological studies based on inpatient or outpatient referrals tend to underestimate the prevalence of PAD in the community. One of the largest and most reliable sources of information about the overall prevalence of symptomatic and asymptomatic PAD is the Edinburgh Artery Study, which screened large random samples of the

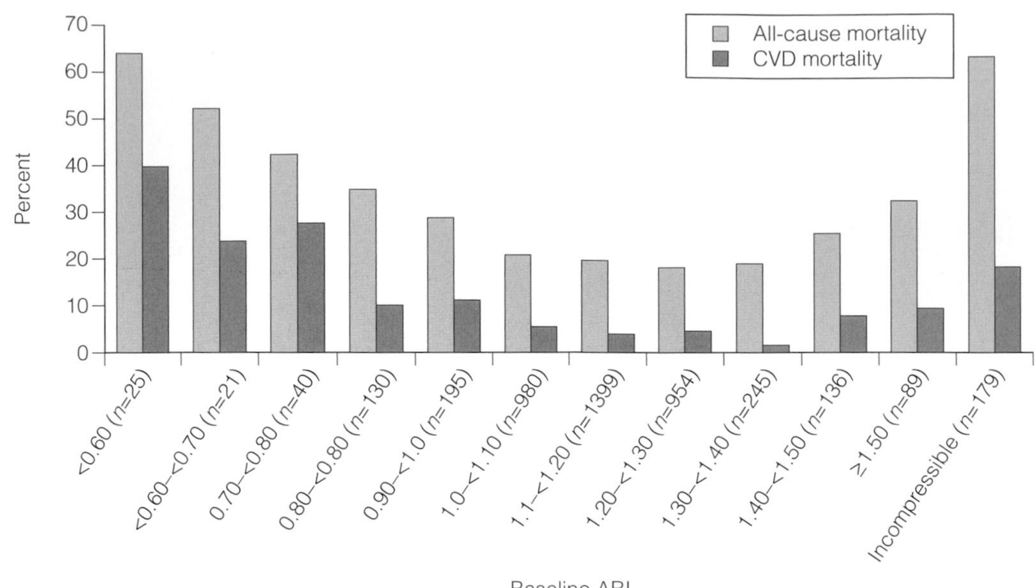


**Figure 1.1** • Relationship between ABPI (ankle–brachial pressure index) and survival in patients in the Strong Heart Study.[2] There is a U-shaped relationship such that both low (<0.9) and high (>1.4) ABPI is associated with increased risk of CV and all-cause mortality.

general population using age/sex registers from general practices.[3,4]

## Investigative techniques for epidemiological screening

Clearly, the technique used to establish the presence or absence of PAD will also affect the results of epidemiological surveys. Questionnaires have often been used to establish the nature and severity of symptomatic PAD, e.g. the WHO/Rose questionnaire designed in 1962. The original questionnaire developed by Rose was shown to be highly sensitive but only moderately specific, and therefore in 1985 the tool was modified in a way that increased the specificity, albeit at the expense of a small decrease in sensitivity.[5] The Edinburgh Artery Questionnaire is designed to be self-administered and has a sensitivity of 91% and a specificity of 99% for symptoms of PAD.[6] In general, all questionnaires appear to underestimate the true prevalence of intermittent claudication and the Transatlantic Inter-Society Consensus (TASC) group recommend great caution in interpreting epidemiological studies of symptomatic PAD based solely on questionnaires.

Physical examination to establish the presence or absence of peripheral pulses has also been used in epidemiological surveys to confirm a history of intermittent claudication. However, the absence of a peripheral pulse is not necessarily due to PAD, and at least one pulse may be undetectable in up to 10% of the adult population even though only 3% have symptomatic arterial disease.[7]

Establishing the prevalence of asymptomatic PAD in the general population is equally important. The most useful non-invasive test for this purpose is the ABPI, which is quick and painless and has excellent sensitivity and specificity. An ABPI <0.9 is 95% sensitive and 100% specific for detecting angiogram-positive disease.[8] At the more severe end of the spectrum, most of the data on the prevalence of critical limb ischaemia has been obtained from inpatient records, and only rarely from population-based studies or using ABPI criteria.

## Prevalence and incidence of PAD

Evidence from epidemiological studies using ABPI suggests that the prevalence of asymptomatic PAD in the middle-aged and elderly population is around 7–15%.[3,9] However, in the British Regional Heart Study, direct assessment of the femoral artery with ultrasound found that 64% of people aged 56–77 years had significant femoral atherosclerosis and only 10% of these were symptomatic.[10] Autopsy studies have found similar results suggesting that the true incidence of asymptomatic PAD may be much higher than previously recognised.

Population studies have varied widely in reporting the incidence of intermittent claudication. Most of these are based on questionnaire surveys and therefore prone to some degree of over-reporting. Nevertheless, it is clear that the incidence of intermittent claudication increases steeply with age. The Scottish Heart Study, for example, found a prevalence of 1.1% in subjects aged 40–59 years;[1] in the Limburg study (subjects aged 40–79 years) the reported prevalence varied between 1.4% and 6.1%[12] depending on the criteria used and the Edinburgh Artery Study indicated a higher prevalence of 4.5%, but in a group (55–74 years) with older mean age.[3]

Information about the prevalence of PAD in the USA has emerged from the National Health and Nutrition Examination Survey (NHANES, 1999–2000).[13] By analysing data from 2174 participants, Selvin and Erlinger found that, among adults aged 40 years and over, the prevalence of PAD was 4.3% (PAD was defined as ABPI <0.90 in either leg). This equates to approximately 5 million people in the USA with PAD. Among those over 70 years old, the prevalence was 14.5%[13] (**Fig. 1.2**).

The incidence of critical limb ischaemia has been estimated to be around 400 cases per million population per year, which equates to a prevalence of 1 in 2500 of the population annually.[14] For every 100 patients with intermittent claudication, approximately one new patient per year will develop critical ischaemia.[8]

# Natural history of PAD: cardiovascular and lower limb outcomes

It is important in discussing the natural history of PAD to consider both the progression of the disease in the legs and the fate of the patient as a whole in terms of systemic cardiovascular complications.

## Asymptomatic disease

The Edinburgh Artery Study is one of the few studies to have examined the pattern of progression among asymptomatic patients with abnormal

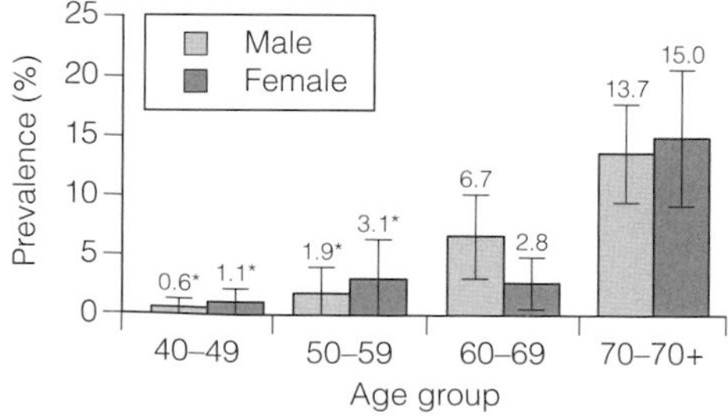


**Figure 1.2** • Recent information about the prevalence of PAD from the US National Health and Nutrition Survey, confirming a steep age-related prevalence.[13]

ABPIs and the rate of development of symptoms; 7–15% of subjects with asymptomatic PAD developed intermittent claudication over a 5-year period, depending on the initial severity of the disease.[4] A more recent study from the Netherlands reported similar conversion rates, with 27 of 177 asymptomatic patients (15%) developing lower limb symptoms during a 7-year follow-up period.[15]

Information about longitudinal changes in ABPI, and risk factors for declining ABPI, has emerged from the Cardiovascular Health Study.[16] Among 5000 patients with normal ABPI at baseline, 9.5% had a significant decrease in ABPI during 6-year follow-up. Independent predictors of ABPI decline included age (odds ratio (OR) 1.96 for the 75–84 age group and 3.79 for those >85 years), current cigarette use (OR 1.74), hypertension (OR 1.64), diabetes (OR 1.77) and raised low-density lipoprotein (LDL) cholesterol.[16] Reduced ABPI has also been associated with rising serum creatinine,[17] indicating that even asymptomatic PAD may affect renal outcomes.

There is good evidence that subjects with asymptomatic PAD have a much higher risk of systemic CV complications. The risk of death or disability from cardiac or cerebral events may be much higher than the risk of lower limb symptoms (claudication or acute limb ischaemia). The Edinburgh Artery Study showed that asymptomatic PAD patients have an increased risk of acute myocardial infarction and stroke; in fact, they have almost the same increased risk of CV events and death as that reported among patients with claudication.[3] The reverse also applies, e.g. in men with asymptomatic carotid stenosis ABPI was the strongest predictor of stroke risk.[18]

## Intermittent claudication

Large population follow-up studies suggest that up to 50% of patients with intermittent claudication will remain relatively stable (i.e. no deterioration in walking distance) or experience some spontaneous improvement in symptoms during a 5-year period; only 25% of claudicants will develop significant deterioration in walking distance.[19,20] The Basle study[20] is typical of several observational follow-ups in showing that, although two-thirds of patients surviving at 5 years reported no limiting intermittent claudication (i.e. their symptoms had resolved), 63% actually had angiographic progression of the disease. This suggests that although PAD is pathologically progressive, other factors contribute to symptomatology, e.g. collateral vessel formation or physiological and psychological adaptation. Although one-quarter of patients with intermittent claudication have symptoms that worsen over time, only 5% deteriorate sufficiently to merit revascularisation and only 1–2% will require a major amputation.[8]

Although lower limb outcomes are mostly very good for patients with uncomplicated intermittent claudication, the major concern for these patients relates to a heightened risk of CV complications due to silent or symptomatic atherosclerosis in other vascular territories. Patients with intermittent claudication have a 2–4% risk of undergoing a non-fatal CV event within the first year of diagnosis and a 1–3% yearly incidence thereafter.[8] For most patients, however, absolute coronary heart disease (CHD) risk is greater than 30% over 10 years, and all-cause mortality rates are similar to those associated with many forms of cancer. In the CASS study, patients with PAD had a 25% greater likelihood of mortality than patients without PAD.[21]

## Critical limb ischaemia

A national survey conducted in 1993 by the Vascular Surgical Society of Great Britain and Ireland found that around 70% of patients with critical ischaemia were offered some form of revascularisation procedure, with a 75% chance of limb salvage. The overall amputation rate, however, was still 21.5% and the mortality rate was 13.5%.[14] Thus, the overall long-term prognosis for these patients is very poor.

## The Reduction of Atherothrombosis for Continued Health (REACH) registry

This large multinational registry is providing useful observational data about the spectrum of disease progression, CV outcomes and patterns of treatment in the 21st century. A total of 67 888 patients, aged 45 years or more, from 44 countries were registered in the database if they had either established CV disease or if they were asymptomatic with more than three risk factors ($n$ = 12 389). Among the symptomatic group, patients were enrolled on the basis of coronary artery disease (CAD; $n$ = 40 248), cerebrovascular disease (CVD; $n$ = 18 843) or PAD ($n$ = 8273);[22] 16% of this group had polyvascular disease.

One-year outcome data for the REACH cohort have been published.[23] Among patients with established CV disease, CV death, myocardial infarction (MI) or stroke rates were 4.52% for patients with CAD, 6.47% for patients with CVD and 5.35% for patients with PAD. Correspondingly, the incidences for the composite end-point of CV death, MI or stroke, or hospitalisation for atherothrombotic events were 15.20% for CAD, 14.53% for CVD and 21.14% for PAD.

The number of vascular territories affected by atherosclerosis was an important determinant of outcome, so those patients with polyvascular disease had the highest rates of major CV events in the first year (**Fig. 1.3**).[23]

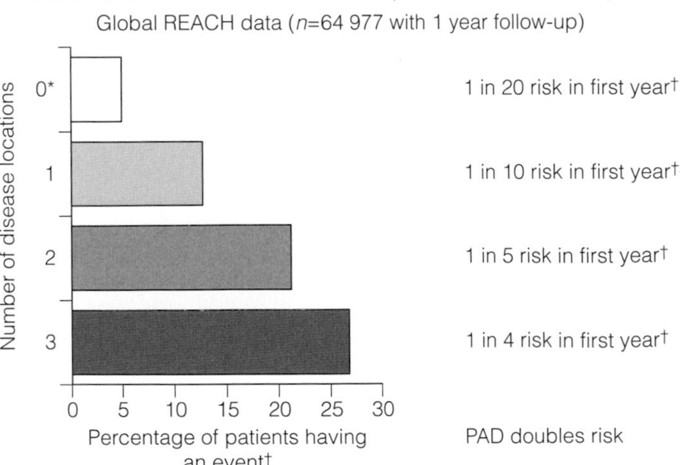


**Figure 1.3** • The REACH registry confirmed that patients with atherosclerotic disease affecting several arterial territories had proportionately higher risk of a major CV event.[23] *Points with three risk factors but no symptoms are counted as 0, even in the presence of asymptomatic carotid plaque or reduced ABI. †CV death, MI, stroke or hospitalisation for an atherothrombotic event (transient ischaemic attack, unstable angina, other ischaemic arterial event including worsening of peripheral arterial disease). ‡Figures vary marginally by disease location – this figure refers to stroke alone.

# Epidemiological risk factors for PAD and randomised trials of disease-modifying therapy for secondary prevention

## CV risk factors in general

There are numerous CV risk factors associated with atherosclerotic disease progression (**Fig. 1.4**). However, it is important to emphasise the distinction between a CV risk factor and the evidence that intervention to modify that risk factor improves clinical outcomes (i.e. symptoms or survival). Factors such as high serum homocysteine[24] or fibrinogen concentrations may be weak risk factors for PAD, but for clinicians in practice this is largely meaningless without evidence from randomised prospective trials that lowering of homocysteine or fibrinogen affects disease outcome. Indeed, the point is well illustrated by a recent placebo-controlled trial of folic acid and vitamin B ($B_6$ and $B_{12}$) supplements which achieved their aim of producing a sustained reduction in plasma homocysteine levels in patients with established CV disease, but the intervention had no effect on clinical endpoints such as mortality or non-fatal CV events.[25]

## Risk factors for PAD

In the NHANES study, using age- and gender-adjusted logistic regression analyses, the following risk factors (and odds ratios) were significantly associated with PAD: black race/ethnicity (OR 2.83), current smoking (OR 4.46), diabetes (OR 2.71), hypertension (OR 1.75), hypercholesterolaemia (OR 1.68) and poor kidney function (OR 2.00). Elevated fibrinogen and C-reactive protein levels also were associated with PAD.[13] A similar profile of risk factors for PAD has been defined for patients with diabetes using the Atherosclerosis Risk in Communities (ARIC) study database.[26]

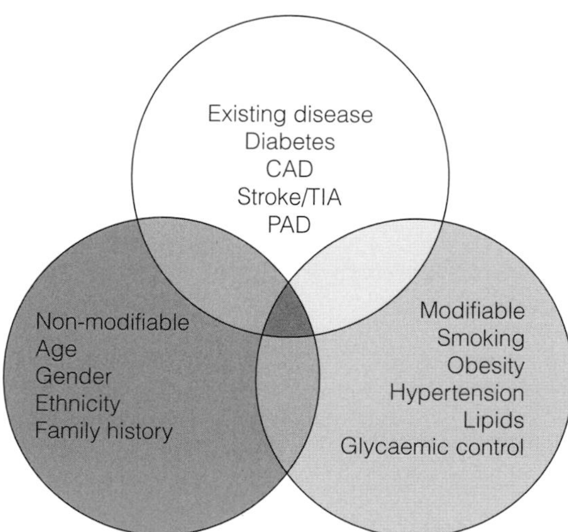


**Figure 1.4** • Major CV risk factors can be grouped into: existing disease; non-modifiable risk factors; and modifiable risk factors, where placebo-controlled trials have shown the benefits of intervention.

## Age and gender

There is clear evidence from several studies that increasing age is associated with an increased risk of PAD in both men and women[3,27] (Fig. 1.2). The evidence for a gender difference is slightly less clear. Several studies, including the Framingham Heart Study, have suggested that men have nearly double the risk of developing intermittent claudication compared with women,[27] but the Edinburgh Artery Study failed to show any significant difference between the sexes,[3] and a follow-up to the Limburg study suggested that the incidence of both symptomatic and asymptomatic PAD was greater in women.[15] Family history is an independent risk factor for premature CHD, but studies have failed to show the same (presumably genetic) association for PAD.

## Cigarette smoking

Cigarette smoking is associated with excess premature deaths from CV, respiratory and cancer-related diseases. Smoking is undoubtedly the most important modifiable risk factor for PAD. The relationship between smoking and lower limb arterial disease was first identified in 1911 by clinicians who reported a threefold increase in the incidence of claudication among smokers. Smoking not only affects the development of PAD but also affects the clinical outcome in those patients with PAD who continue to smoke. Smokers with PAD are much more likely to progress to critical ischaemia, and more likely to require an amputation or vascular intervention.[28] Furthermore, smoking increases the overall mortality rate among claudicants by a factor of 1.5–3.0.[6]

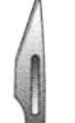

In women, smoking cessation reduces overall CV risk to the level of non-smokers within 2–4 years.[29]

However, the excess cancer risk associated with smoking often takes 10 years to subside after smoking cessation. In men, the benefits take longer, about 5 years, to take effect. Nevertheless, smoking cessation for CV prevention is highly cost-effective; the benefits appear relatively quickly.

Nicotine is addictive and spontaneous smoking cessation rates are very low (<10%), even among genuinely motivated patients. In terms of helping motivated patients to quit smoking, several approaches are available.

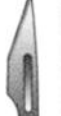

The antidepressant bupropion, nicotine replacement therapy (NRT) and the new agent varenicline are all considered to be first-line options; nortriptyline is occasionally used but only as second-line treatment.[30]

A meta-analysis of more than 100 randomised trials shows that all forms of NRT are equally effective in aiding long-term smoking cessation[31] (Table 1.2). In randomised trials, quit rates after 1 year, on average, are nearly double those following placebo (OR 1.77).[31] Combination NRT (e.g. patch + gum) can also be effective in those patients who have found a single form of NRT insufficient to control nicotine withdrawal symptoms.

Varenicline, a partial agonist at the $\alpha_4\beta_2$ acetylcholine nicotinic receptor, has recently been licensed for smoking cessation.

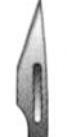

Varenicline appears to be more effective than NRT,[32] and a meta-analysis of randomised trials showed that quit rates are threefold higher than with placebo and superior to those after use of bupropion (OR 3.22).[33]

## Diabetes

Diabetes mellitus is well recognised as an important risk factor for cardiovascular disease and, apart from smoking, is probably the single most important risk factor in the development of PAD. Lower limb arterial disease tends to be more diffuse and distal in diabetics, with both ischaemic and neuropathic ulceration being common. The Edinburgh Artery Study and the Health Professionals Follow-up Study showed that people with diabetes have a 1.5- to 2.5-fold increased risk of symptomatic and asymptomatic PAD compared with non-diabetics, and the lifetime risk of a lower limb amputation is increased 10–16 fold.[34,35] Duration of diabetes is also important, e.g. in the Health Professionals Follow-up Study patients were grouped according to diabetes duration and the relative risks of PAD were 3.63 (diabetes duration 6–10 years), 2.55 (11–25 years) and 4.53 (duration >25 years) compared with patients diagnosed less than 5 years.[35]

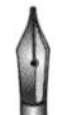

Diabetics with critical ischaemia fare less well than their non-diabetic counterparts, e.g. higher amputation rates and less success following revascularisation procedures.[36]

The risks of lower limb ulceration are exacerbated by coexistent microvascular disease and peripheral neuropathy.

Several studies in both type 1 and type 2 diabetes have identified the glucose level as an independent risk factor for PAD.[37,38]

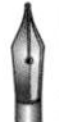

The UK Prospective Diabetes Study (UKPDS) identified a strong association between HbA1c and risk of PAD: each 1% increase in HbA1c was associated with a 28% increased risk of PAD.[38]

However, other important features of the 'metabolic syndrome' of type 2 diabetes include insulin resistance, hypertension, obesity and dyslipidaemia (typically low high-density lipoprotein (HDL) cholesterol and high triglycerides). Epidemiological data have suggested that both insulin resistance and hyperinsulinaemia are independent risk factors for PAD in diabetic and non-diabetic individuals.[39]

Hypertension plays a significant role in the development of PAD in diabetic subjects.

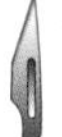

In the UKPDS, for every 10 mmHg reduction in systolic blood pressure there was a 12% reduction in overall CV risk, but more specifically a 16% reduction in risk of lower limb amputation or peripheral vascular disease-related mortality.[40]

**Table 1.2** • A summary of more than 100 randomised trials of NRT for smoking cessation

| Comparison | Trials (*n*) | Participants (*n*) | Pooled OR | 95% CI |
|---|---|---|---|---|
| Gum | 52 | 17783 | 1.66 | 1.52–1.81 |
| Patch | 37 | 16691 | 1.81 | 1.63–2.02 |
| Nasal spray | 4 | 887 | 2.35 | 1.63–3.38 |
| Inhaler | 4 | 976 | 2.14 | 1.44–3.18 |
| Tablets/lozenges | 4 | 2739 | 2.05 | 1.62–2.59 |
| Combination vs. single type | 7 | 3202 | 1.42 | 1.14–1.76 |
| Any NRT vs. control | 103 | 39503 | 1.77 | 1.66–1.88 |

The pooled odds ratios show that overall, for different forms of therapy, NRT has a quit rate 1.77-fold higher than placebo at 1 year.[31]

The Hypertension Optimal Treatment (HOT) trial showed that vigorous blood pressure control had a greater effect in reducing CV events in those patients with diabetes than those without,[41] and effective control of hypertension may limit vascular events even more effectively than tight glycaemic control.[42] The major benefits of glycaemic control appear to be in microvascular protection and prevention of neuropathy and secondary foot complications such as ulceration and infection.

The association of traditional and non-traditional risk factors with PAD incidence in a population of patients with diabetes has been investigated in the ARIC study.[26] This analysis showed that patients with diabetes were more likely to develop PAD if they were smokers (relative risk (RR) 1.87), had CHD at baseline (RR 2.27) and high triglycerides (RR 1.75). Patients taking insulin therapy were also at higher risk.[26]

## Blood pressure (BP)

The Framingham and other studies have provided good evidence that hypertension is a powerful predisposing risk factor in the development of intermittent claudication. A BP >160/95 mmHg increased the risk by 2.5-fold in men and fourfold in women during 26 years of follow-up.[27] Hypertension is a major associated CV risk factor, present in up to 55% of patients with PAD.[43] Hypertension also increases the risk of CV complications and mortality in patients with established PAD. Up to 5% of hypertensive patients have been reported to have clinical evidence of PAD at presentation, with a marked age-related increase in hypertension-associated PAD.[44] Isolated or predominantly systolic hypertension is common in PAD patients.

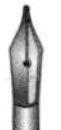

In the Rotterdam Study investigating determinants of PAD, after multivariate analysis each 10 mmHg increase in systolic BP conferred an increased risk of PAD (OR 1.3, 95% CI 1.2–1.5).[45]

Effective antihypertensive therapy is likely to ameliorate the progression of PAD as well as reducing the mortality from stroke and CHD.[46,47] However, there are few randomised trials which have addressed the efficacy of different types of antihypertensive drugs specifically in patients with PAD; rather patients with PAD have represented small subgroups of much larger studies. Furthermore, BP management in patients with PAD tends to be poor. Systolic hypertension is especially difficult to treat in patients with calcified arteries which have lost their elasticity. In PARTNERS,[48] for example, hypertension was less often treated in new (84%) and previous (88%) patients with PAD as compared to patients with CHD. So what treatments and what guidelines for treatment of hypertension in PAD patients should be recommended?

The treatment of hypertension in patients with PAD has been reviewed recently.[49] There are to date no specific national guidelines for choice of antihypertensive therapy in PAD patients.

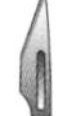

The latest joint British Hypertension Society/National Institute for Health and Clinical Excellence (NICE) guideline[50] states that persistent raised BP with existing cardiovascular disease should be treated if, after measurement on two separate visits, systolic BP, diastolic BP or both are above 140/90 mmHg.

The aim should be to reduce BP to an optimum target of below 140/85 mmHg among treated hypertensives. It has become clear that small differences in BP translate into relatively large differences in clinical outcome, and that patients achieve worthwhile benefits from antihypertensive therapy even if BP control does not meet the stringent target of <140/85 mmHg.

For patients with PAD there is a significant risk of renal artery stenosis as a causative factor in hypertension.[51] This must be considered before selecting antihypertensive therapy, since angiotensin-converting enzyme (ACE) inhibitors (and other drugs targeting the renin–angiotensin axis) are contraindicated in the presence of significant renal artery stenosis. Ethnic status and comorbidities also must be considered before recommending treatment.

The British Hypertension Society has recommended an 'ABCD' algorithm for drug selection and drug sequencing in hypertension (**Fig. 1.5**). More recently, however, beta-blockers have been removed as a first-line treatment recommendation in younger patients, and in practice most hypertensive patients require two or three drugs (ACE inhibitor, calcium channel blocker and diuretic) to achieve BP targets.[52]

## Renin–angiotensin–aldosterone system blockade

The importance of the renin–angiotensin–aldosterone system (RAAS) in cardiovascular pathophysiology is a continued focus of intense research. There has been considerable interest in whether drugs which block the RAAS confer useful therapeutic and disease-modifying effects, over and above those attributable to BP reduction, in the secondary prevention of CV disease.[53] It is well established that ACE inhibitors and angiotensin receptor blockers (ARBs) improve left ventricular (LV) function in heart failure patients and retard the decline in glomerular

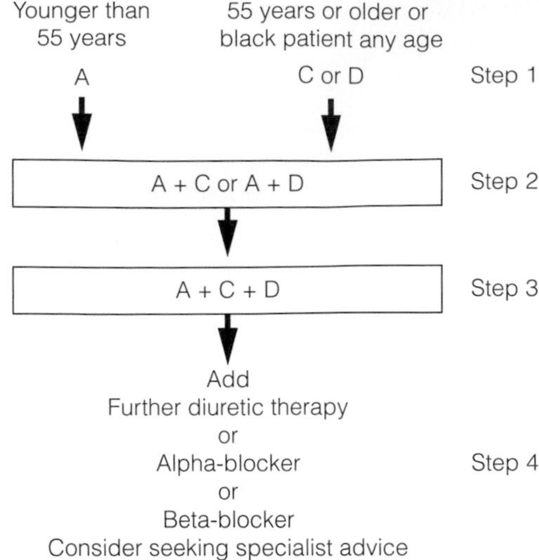


**Figure 1.5** • Drug selection and drug sequencing for patients with hypertension. Algorithm published by the British Heart Foundation and endorsed by NICE. Beta-blockers are no longer recommended in step 1, but may be added at step 4. A, ACE inhibitor (consider angiotensin II receptor antagonist if ACE intolerant); C, calcium-channel blocker; D, thiazide-type diuretic. Black patients are those of African or Caribbean descent and not mixed-race, Asian or Chinese patients.

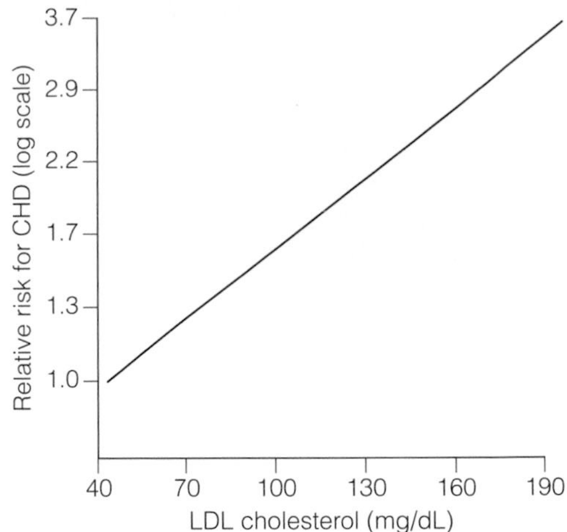


**Figure 1.6** • A log-linear relationship between LDL cholesterol levels and the relative risk of CHD. The relationship is steep. For every 30 mg/dL (0.8 mmol/L) change in LDL cholesterol the relative risk of CHD changes in proportion by 30% (divide by 38.46 to convert mg/dL to mmol/L).

filtration rate in patients with chronic renal disease. These drugs also improve CV outcomes in patients with atherosclerotic disease (in the absence of LV or renal dysfunction) but whether this is mediated solely via BP lowering, or whether RAAS blockade confers additional (BP-independent) benefits on the blood vessel wall, has been hotly debated.

A new mode of RAAS inhibition is now available with the development of aliskiren, an orally active non-peptide renin inhibitor which is licensed for use as antihypertensive therapy. Aliskiren may be used alone or in combination with other BP-lowering drugs, including ARBs, and may be especially effective in patients with coexistent renal disease.[54]

## Serum lipids

The epidemiological evidence relating serum cholesterol levels to CV mortality is well established (**Fig. 1.6**). In terms of PAD, the Framingham Study showed that a fasting cholesterol >7 mmol/L doubled the risk of intermittent claudication,[55] but not all observational studies have reached the same conclusion. Low HDL cholesterol, or an increased LDL:HDL ratio, appear to be independent risk factors for PAD,[3] and there are further independent associations between PAD and circulating levels of apolipoproteins A and B (proteins contained within LDL particles).[56,57]

Circulating cholesterol is derived from two sources (**Fig. 1.7**): (1) endogenous synthesis in the liver, cholesterol is then transported in the blood stream via lipoprotein particles and some is secreted into bile; and (2) gastrointestinal absorption of dietary cholesterol and (reabsorption of) bile acids. Statins (drugs that inhibit the rate-limiting enzyme in cholesterol biosynthesis in the liver, hydroxymethylglutaryl (HMG)-CoA reductase) have become the mainstay of clinical practice for lowering cholesterol levels, but a cholesterol absorption inhibitor, ezetimibe, is now available for adjunctive use with statins. Ezetimibe is not systemically absorbed, but effectively blocks cholesterol transport in the gut, which in turn increases faecal loss of cholesterol and lowers serum cholesterol levels.

The large intervention trials using statins (mostly in CHD and stroke patients) have included only small numbers of patients with coexistent PAD. For instance, patients with PAD contributed only ≈20% of the total patients in the Heart Protection Study; nevertheless, in this subgroup treatment with simvastatin was associated with a substantial reduction in major cardiovascular events (27.6% vs. 34.3% in the placebo group) (**Fig. 1.8**).[58]

PAD is now considered a CHD risk equivalent,[59] and unless contraindicated statins should be recommended for all patients with symptomatic PAD.

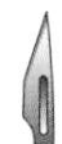

A target LDL cholesterol concentration of <2.6 mmol/L is included in most international guidelines,[60] mainly because of two observations: (1) a retrospective pooled analysis of the achieved LDL cholesterol levels in the placebo and active therapy arms of the major statin trials has shown

Exogenous
Dietary cholesterol
(~300–700 mg/day)
Intestine
Faecal bile acids
and neutral sterols
Biliary cholesterol
(~1000 mg/day)
~700 mg/day
Extrahepatic
tissues
Liver synthesis
(~800 mg/day)
Endogenous

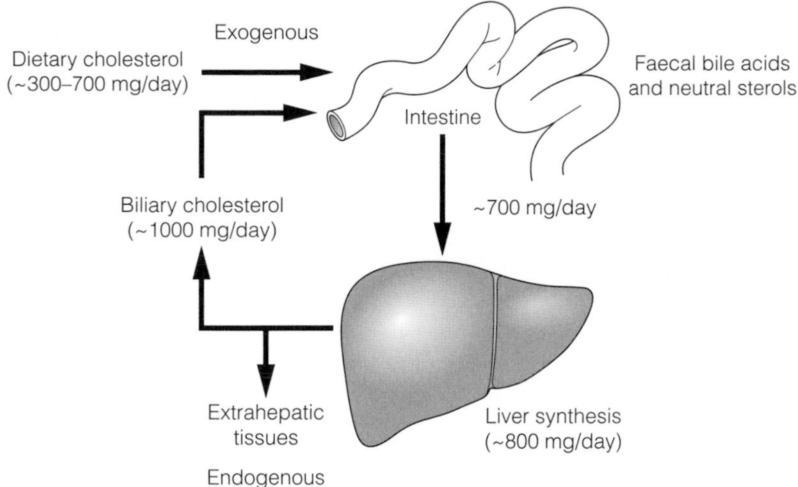

**Figure 1.7** • Circulating cholesterol is derived from endogenous synthesis in the liver and exogenous sources (dietary intake and bile acids) absorbed through the gut. Statins block synthesis, ezetimibe blocks gut absorption. The drugs have additive effects on serum cholesterol.

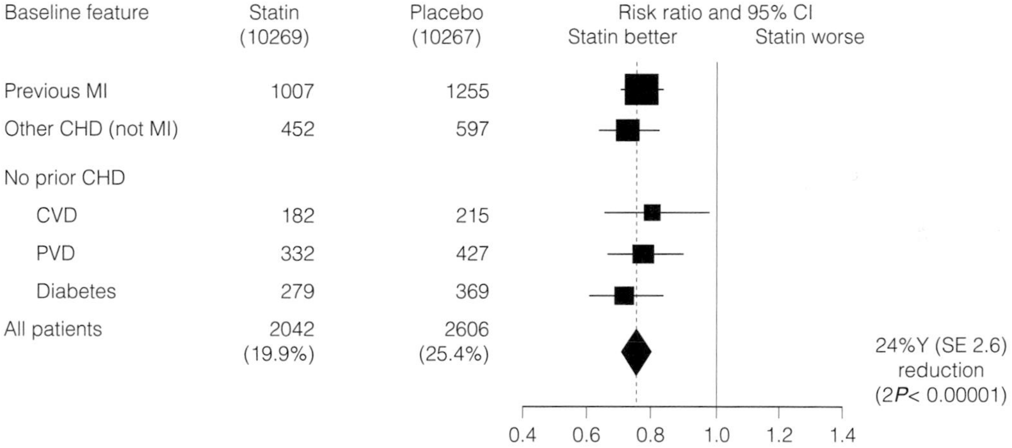

Baseline feature
Statin
(10269)
Placebo
(10267)
Risk ratio and 95% CI
Statin better
Statin worse
Previous MI 1007 1255
Other CHD (not MI) 452 597
No prior CHD
CVD 182 215
PVD 332 427
Diabetes 279 369
All patients 2042 (19.9%) 2606 (25.4%)
24%Y (SE 2.6)
reduction
(2P< 0.00001)
0.4
0.6
0.8
1.0
1.2
1.4

**Figure 1.8** • In the Heart Protection Study, the benefits of simvastatin 40 mg were evident in those patients with peripheral vascular disease (PVD) at baseline and were independent of age, BP status and baseline cholesterol. Data from the Heart Protection Study Collaborative Group. MRC/BHF Heart Protection Study of cholesterol-lowering with simvastatin in 20,536 high-risk individuals. Lancet 2002; 360:7–22.

that the lower the achieved cholesterol level, the lower the risk of major CV events (**Fig. 1.9**); and (2) prospective trials comparing low-dose versus high-dose statin therapy in patients with established CV disease have shown that more intensive cholesterol-lowering (e.g. atorvastatin 80 mg) confers a mortality advantage compared with less intensive cholesterol lowering (e.g. atorvastatin 10 mg) (**Fig. 1.10**).

Achieving a target LDL cholesterol level <2.6 mmol/L is very difficult using standard doses of first-generation statins. For example, <35% of patients will reach this target using simvastatin 40 mg daily. Thus, clinicians may need to switch to one of the second-generation statins which are more potent, e.g. atorvastatin or rosuvastatin.

A Cochrane review of studies of lipid-lowering therapy in patients with PAD concluded that

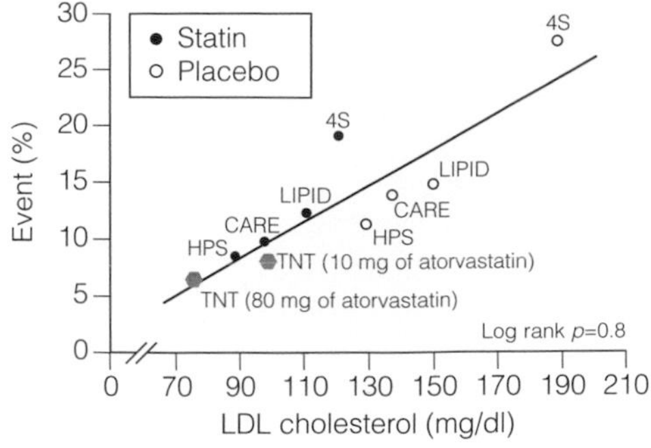


**Figure 1.9** • A pooled analysis of achieved LDL cholesterol levels in the placebo group and the active therapy group for each of the major placebo-controlled statin trials. The lower the LDL cholesterol level, the lower the CV event rate (divide by 38.46 to convert mg/dL to mmol/L). Reproduced from LaRosa JC, Grundy SM, Waters DD et al. Intensive lipid lowering with atorvastatin in patients with stable coronary disease. N Engl J Med 2005; 352:1425–35. 

'lipid-lowering therapy may be useful in preventing the deterioration of underlying disease and alleviating symptoms' and found a marked, although non-significant, reduction in mortality.[61]

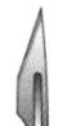

There are several trials that have been published since this initial Cochrane review which report that statins are associated with functional improvement in PAD. The largest of these studies showed that atorvastatin (versus placebo) was associated with an increase in pain-free walking distance and quality of life at 12 months.[62] Similar findings were also reported in smaller trials (**Fig. 1.11**).[60]

Patients with PAD benefit from statin therapy, irrespective of the baseline cholesterol concentration. This viewpoint has been confirmed by a recent meta-analysis of trials.[63] Each 1 mmol/L reduction in LDL cholesterol results in about a one-third reduction in mortality from CHD, independent of age, BP and initial cholesterol concentration.

## Evidence for dietary control or supplementation

Dietary control is rarely considered for patients with PAD, despite there being at least four important reasons to consider dietary management:

- claudication distance decreases with increasing body weight;[64]
- glucose intolerance increases with increasing body weight;
- increased plasma lipid concentrations are associated with increased atherosclerotic burden;
- reducing salt intake can reduce blood pressure.

Apart from cholesterol and triglycerides, several other dietary components have been associated with effects on atherosclerosis and PAD: these include the polyunsaturated fatty acids, niacin, folate, vitamins B, C and E.

A recent WHO report recommends regular consumption of fish to provide 200–500 mg of eicosapentaenoic acid and docosahexaenoic acid per week, replacement of saturated fat by monounsaturated fat and increased consumption of fruit and vegetables to achieve proper vitamin, antioxidant and fibre status.[65] Increased dietary fish intake is associated with diminished progression of CHD and another randomised trial has shown that supplementation with 1.65 g/day of polyunsaturated fatty acids reduces the age-dependent increase in carotid artery intima media thickness.

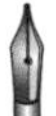

There has been only one trial of polyunsaturated fatty acid supplementation in patients with PAD: although there was no significant effect on walking distance, after 2 years BP was lower and there were fewer coronary events in those taking the active supplements.

Diets which limit the daily energy intake from fats to 30% or less are effective in reducing plasma lipid and lipoprotein concentrations by 5–20% and can affect weight reduction in those with above average body mass index.

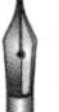

A portfolio of dietary changes including reduction of dietary fat, use of soy protein, sterols and almonds can facilitate larger reductions in plasma lipids, similar to those that can be achieved by the first-generation statins, but such diets are very difficult to adhere to.

Therefore, although dietary control is very useful in managing patients with borderline hyperlipidaemia, it cannot replace statins and other drug therapies for the management of hyperlipidaemia.

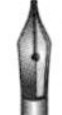

In contrast, moderate intake of alcohol (1–2 units/day) reduces the risk of developing intermittent claudication,[66] and has the beneficial effect of increasing HDL cholesterol concentrations.

There is no consistent evidence for the role of vitamin C or E supplementation on coronary events or other clinical markers of atherosclerosis, although both may have beneficial effects on endothelial function and arterial stiffness in early

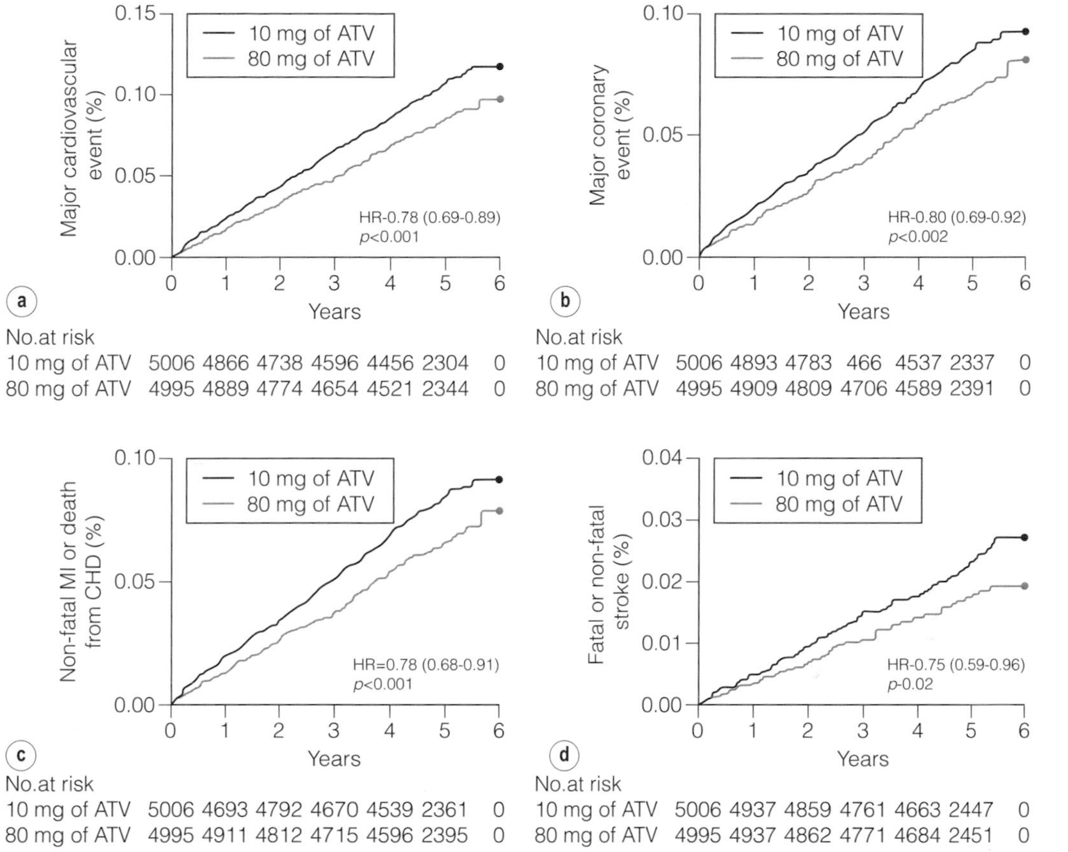

0.15 0.10 0.05 0.00
Major cardiovascular event (%)
— 10 mg of ATV
— 80 mg of ATV
HR-0.78 (0.69-0.89)
$p$<0.001
0 1 2 3 4 5 6
Years
(a)

| No.at risk | | | | | | | |
|---|---|---|---|---|---|---|---|
| 10 mg of ATV | 5006 | 4866 | 4738 | 4596 | 4456 | 2304 | 0 |
| 80 mg of ATV | 4995 | 4889 | 4774 | 4654 | 4521 | 2344 | 0 |

0.10 0.05 0.00
Major coronary event (%)
— 10 mg of ATV
— 80 mg of ATV
HR-0.80 (0.69-0.92)
$p$<0.002
0 1 2 3 4 5 6
Years
(b)

| No.at risk | | | | | | | |
|---|---|---|---|---|---|---|---|
| 10 mg of ATV | 5006 | 4893 | 4783 | 466 | 4537 | 2337 | 0 |
| 80 mg of ATV | 4995 | 4909 | 4809 | 4706 | 4589 | 2391 | 0 |

0.10 0.05 0.00
Non-fatal MI or death from CHD (%)
— 10 mg of ATV
— 80 mg of ATV
HR=0.78 (0.68-0.91)
$p$<0.001
0 1 2 3 4 5 6
Years
(c)

| No.at risk | | | | | | | |
|---|---|---|---|---|---|---|---|
| 10 mg of ATV | 5006 | 4693 | 4792 | 4670 | 4539 | 2361 | 0 |
| 80 mg of ATV | 4995 | 4911 | 4812 | 4715 | 4596 | 2395 | 0 |

0.04 0.03 0.02 0.01 0.00
Fatal or non-fatal stroke (%)
— 10 mg of ATV
— 80 mg of ATV
HR-0.75 (0.59-0.96)
$p$-0.02
0 1 2 3 4 5 6
Years
(d)

| No.at risk | | | | | | | |
|---|---|---|---|---|---|---|---|
| 10 mg of ATV | 5006 | 4937 | 4859 | 4761 | 4663 | 2447 | 0 |
| 80 mg of ATV | 4995 | 4937 | 4862 | 4771 | 4684 | 2451 | 0 |

**Figure 1.10** • The 'Treating to New Targets' study randomised 10 000 patients with CHD to atorvastatin 80 mg vs. atorvastatin 10 mg once daily. Mean LDL cholesterol levels were 2.0 and 2.6 mmol/L in the two groups respectively. This difference translated into big differences in CV outcomes. Reproduced from LaRosa JC, Grundy SM, Waters DD et al. Intensive lipid lowering with atorvastatin in patients with stable coronary disease. N Engl J Med 2005; 352:1425–35. Copyright © 2005 Massachusetts Medical Society. All rights reserved.

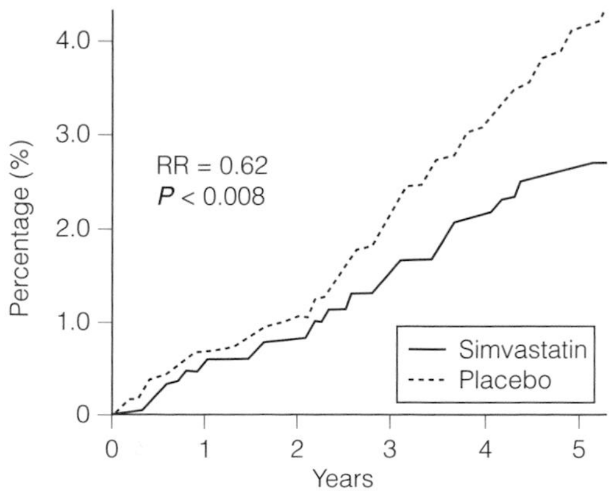


**Figure 1.11** • Incidence of new or worsening claudication among 4000 participants in the 4S study of simvastatin vs. placebo in post-MI patients. Reproduced from Pedersen TR, Kjekshus J, Pyörälä K et al. Effect of simvastatin on ischemic signs and symptoms in the Scandinavian Simvastatin Survival Study (4S). Am J Cardiol 1998; 81:333–5. With permission from Elsevier.

disease. Similarly, dietary supplementation with folic acid and B vitamins (to lower plasma homocysteine concentrations) has no consistent effect on clinical end-points.[25]

Another diet which merits consideration is the DASH diet (Dietary Approaches to Stop Hypertension).[67] The DASH diet includes increased intake of fruit, vegetables and dietary fibre, together with increased potassium, calcium, magnesium and non-red meat protein, similar to the WHO recommendations. Long-term reduction in dietary salt intake (by 30–40 mmol/day) can also reduce both BP and coronary events in those with marginal hypertension.[68]

## Antiplatelet therapy and warfarin

There is some evidence that PAD is associated with a hypercoagulable state. For example, it has been suggested that patients with intermittent claudication have a higher haematocrit and blood viscosity than the general population, but the Framingham

Study found no association between haematocrit and symptomatic PAD. Several studies, however, have confirmed the association of high plasma fibrinogen levels with PAD, and that fibrinogen is a marker of thrombotic risk.

There have been numerous large randomised trials of antiplatelet therapy in patients with cardiovascular disease.

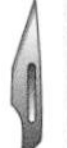

A meta-analysis by the Antiplatelet Trialists' Collaboration showed that antiplatelet therapy, mainly with low-dose aspirin, reduced the risk of non-fatal MI, non-fatal stroke and vascular death in high-risk patients, including those with intermittent claudication.[69]

Aspirin has no effect on symptoms of claudication, but some trials have shown that aspirin alone or in combination with dipyridamole delays the angiographic progression of PAD and reduces surgical intervention rates. The standard dose of aspirin for secondary prevention, 75–150 mg daily, is effective in inhibiting platelet function but does not cause the excessive number of gastro-intestinal side-effects associated with higher doses.

The CAPRIE trial evaluated the efficacy and safety of clopidogrel compared to aspirin for secondary prevention in 19 185 patients with CV disease.[70] It showed a relative reduction in the risk of MI, ischaemic stroke and vascular death of 8.7% ($P$ = 0.04) in favour of clopidogrel after a mean follow-up of 1.9 years, and an absolute risk reduction of 0.51% (number needed to treat = 196 to avoid one ischaemic event during 1.9 years). Although a subgroup analysis in PAD patients suggested that the clinical benefit of clopidogrel was greater than 8.7%, it should be noted that many hypotheses raised by subgroup analyses are subsequently refuted in trials specifically designed to test them. As yet there are no prospective studies to test whether patients with PAD benefit more from clopidogrel than from aspirin.

The combination of clopidogrel and aspirin is superior to aspirin alone in patients with acute coronary syndromes (unstable angina or acute MI), i.e. when there is evidence of unstable plaque, and these benefits are especially evident in patients who require percutaneous coronary intervention or bypass surgery. More recently the CHARISMA trial was performed to assess the effects of dual antiplatelet therapy (clopidogrel + aspirin) in patients with more stable atherosclerotic disease.[71] Overall, there were some safety concerns with dual therapy and no convincing benefit compared with aspirin alone.

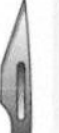

Guidelines for the use of antiplatelet therapy in PAD have been published.[72]

Recently a major trial has compared antiplatelet therapy + anticoagulation with antiplatelet therapy alone in patients with PAD; warfarin + aspirin was not more effective than aspirin alone in preventing major CV events in this setting.[73]

However, anticoagulation with warfarin is superior to aspirin in patients with PAD who are in atrial fibrillation, especially for reducing the risks of embolic stroke and acute limb ischaemia.[74]

## Conclusions

Occlusive arterial disease of the lower limbs is common and disabling; the prevalence increases steeply with age. Although lower limb symptoms and outcomes are variable and generally benign, the associated excess risks of cardiovascular disease (i.e. MI, stroke or sudden death) among patients with PAD are considerable and merit aggressive secondary prevention with atherosclerotic disease-modifying medical therapies. PAD is a CHD risk equivalent, and indeed recent results from the REACH registry indicate that the CV risks associated with PAD have been underestimated.

Epidemiological studies have identified numerous risk factors which, in longitudinal follow-up studies in large populations, are associated with a higher incidence and more rapid progression of PAD. Identifying a risk factor in a population, however, does not necessarily imply that intervention in individuals to lower that risk factor will necessarily improve clinical outcomes. Such evidence only comes from randomised placebo-controlled trials and there are very few that have focused only on patients with PAD. Most of the recommendations derive from studies of patients with other forms of cardiovascular disease.

The major modifiable risk factors are smoking, hyperlipidaemia, hypertension and diabetes. All patients with PAD merit secondary prevention with disease-modifying therapies to lower BP and cholesterol levels, assist with smoking cessation, reduce platelet function and improve glycaemic control.

## Key points

- Among adults aged 40 years and over, the prevalence of PAD is 4.3% (PAD defined as ABPI <0.90 in either leg). This equates to approximately 5 million people in the USA with PAD. Among those over 70 years old, the prevalence was 14.5%.
- There is a U-shaped relationship between ABPI and reduced life expectancy. Adjusted risk estimates for all-cause mortality were 1.69 for low ABPI (<0.9) and 1.77 for high ABPI (>1.4), while the corresponding estimates for CV mortality were 2.52 and 2.09.
- The incidence of PAD increases steeply with increasing age and may be slightly more common in men.
- Although lower limb outcomes are relatively good in most patients with PAD, these patients are at very high risk of premature death from other CV events, as illustrated recently by the REACH registry.
- Risk factors for the development of PAD are similar to those for atherosclerotic disease in general, but smoking and diabetes may have a more significant impact in the lower limbs.
- Smoking cessation reduces the excess CV risk within a relatively short period, and treatments to alleviate nicotine withdrawal symptoms include NRT, varenicline or bupropion. NRT doubles quit rates at 1 year, relative to placebo, but the newer agent, varenicline, appears to be superior to NRT and bupropion.
- Other lifestyle modifications including diet and exercise have been underused.
- Glycaemic control for those with diabetes is important in the prevention of microvascular complications, but other factors in the diabetes syndrome, such as hypertension and dyslipidaemia, may be more important in the development of PAD.
- Lipid-lowering (statin) therapy increases walking distance and survival among patients with CV disease, and all PAD patients should be treated.
- Antiplatelet therapy with low-dose aspirin (or clopidogrel if aspirin is not tolerated) is indicated in all patients with PAD.

## References


1. McKenna M, Wolfson S, Kuller L. The ratio of ankle and arm arterial pressure as an independent predictor of mortality. Atherosclerosis 1991; 87:119–28.
2. Resnick HE, Lindsay RS, McGrae M et al. Relationship of high and low ankle brachial index to all-cause and cardiovascular disease mortality: the Strong Heart Study. Circulation 2004; 109:733–9.
3. Fowkes F. Edinburgh Artery Study: prevalence of asymptomatic and symptomatic peripheral arterial disease in the general population. Int J Epidemiol 1991; 20:384–92.
4. Leng GC. Incidence, natural history and cardiovascular events in symptomatic and asymptomatic peripheral arterial disease in the general population. Int J Epidemiol 1996; 25:1172–81.
5. Criqui MH. The sensitivity, specificity, and predictive value of traditional clinical evaluation of peripheral arterial disease: results from noninvasive testing in a defined population. Circulation 1985; 71:516–22.
6. Leng GC, Fowkes FG. The Edinburgh Claudication Questionnaire: an improved version of the WHO/Rose Questionnaire for use in epidemiological surveys. J Clin Epidemiol 1992; 45:1101–9.
7. Schroll M, Munck O. Estimation of peripheral arteriosclerotic disease by ankle blood pressure measurements in a population study of 60-year-old men and women. J Chronic Dis 1981; 34:261–9.
8. Transatlantic Inter-Society Consensus (TASC) Document. Management of peripheral arterial disease. J Vasc Surg 2000; 31:S5–35.
9. Newman AB. Ankle–arm index as a marker of atherosclerosis in the Cardiovascular Health Study. Cardiovascular Heart Study (CHS) Collaborative Research Group. Circulation 1993; 88:837–45.
10. Leng GC. Femoral atherosclerosis in an older British population: prevalence and risk factors. Atherosclerosis 2000; 152:167–74.
11. Smith W, Woodward M, Tunstall-Pedoe H. Intermittent claudication in Scotland. In: Fowkes FGR (ed.) Epidemiology of peripheral vascular disease. London: Springer-Verlag, 1991; pp. 109–15.
12. Stoffers HE. The prevalence of asymptomatic and unrecognized peripheral arterial occlusive disease. Int J Epidemiol 1996; 25:282–90.
13. Selvin E, Erlinger TP. Prevalence of and risk factors for peripheral arterial disease in the United States: results from the National Health and Nutrition

Examination Survey (1999–2000). Circulation 2004; 110:738–43.

Recent information about the prevalence of PAD in the USA.

14. Critical limb ischaemia: management and outcome. A report of a national survey by The Vascular Surgical Society of Great Britain and Ireland. Eur J Vasc Endovasc Surg 1995; 10:108–13.
15. Hooi JD. Incidence of and risk factors for asymptomatic peripheral arterial occlusive disease: a longitudinal study. Am J Epidemiol 2001; 153:666–72.
16. Kennedy M, Solomon C, Manolio TA et al. Risk factors for declining ankle–brachial index in men and women 65 years or older. Arch Intern Med 2005; 165:1896–902.
17. O'Hare AM, Rodriguez RA, Bacchetti P. Low ankle–brachial index associated with rise in creatinine level over time. Arch Intern Med 2005; 165:1481–5.
18. Ogren M. Ten year cerebrovascular morbidity and mortality in 68 year old men with asymptomatic carotid stenosis. Br Med J 1995; 310:1294–8.
19. Bloor K. Natural history of arteriosclerosis of the lower extremities. Ann R Coll Surg Engl 1961; 28:36–51.
20. Da Silva A. The Basle longitudinal study: report on the relation of initial glucose level to baseline ECG abnormalities, peripheral artery disease, and subsequent mortality. J Chronic Dis 1979; 32:797–803.
21. Eagle KA. Long-term survival in patients with coronary artery disease: importance of peripheral vascular disease. The Coronary Artery Surgery Study (CASS) Investigators. J Am Coll Cardiol 1994; 23:1091–5.
22. Bhatt DL, Steg PG, Ohman EM et al. International prevalence, recognition and treatment of cardiovascular risk factors in outpatients with atherothrombosis. JAMA 2006; 295:180–9.

    The REACH registry is a large multinational observational study of >67 000 patients with CV disease, including those with PAD. The registry documents clinical outcomes, patterns of disease and treatment in a 21st century setting.

23. Steg PG, Bhatt DL, Wilson PWF et al. One-year cardiovascular event rates in outpatients with atherothrombosis. JAMA 2007; 297:1197–206.

    The first outcome data showing what has happened to the 67 000 patients in the registry highlights that PAD confers a substantial risk of MI and stroke.

24. Boers G. Moderate hyperhomocysteinaemia and vascular disease: evidence, relevance and the effect of treatment. Eur J Pediatr 1998; 157(Suppl 2):S127–30.
25. Bonaa KH, Njolstad I, Ueland PM et al. Homocysteine lowering and cardiovascular events after acute myocardial infarction. N Engl J Med 2006; 354:1578–88.

    Although serum homocysteine is a risk factor for CV disease in population studies, this intervention trial shows no clinical benefit of homocysteine-lowering therapy (folic A + B vitamins).

26. Wattanakit K, Folsom AR, Selvin E et al. Risk factors for peripheral arterial disease incidence in persons with diabetes: the Atherosclerosis Risk in Communities (ARIC) study. Atherosclerosis 2005; 180:389–97.
27. Murabito JM et al. Intermittent claudication. A risk profile from The Framingham Heart Study. Circulation 1997; 96:44–9.
28. Jonason T, Ringqvist I. Factors of prognostic importance for subsequent rest pain in patients with intermittent claudication. Acta Med Scand 1985; 218:27–33.
29. Rosenberg L, Palmer JR, Shapiro S. Decline in the risk of myocardial infarction among women who stop smoking. N Engl J Med 1990; 322:213–17.

    Data illustrating the health outcomes following smoking cessation.

30. Aveyard P, West R. Managing smoking cessation. Br Med J 2007; 335:37–41.

    Modern clinical services to aid smoking cessation using NRT, varenicline and bupropion. Summarises the evidence for smoking cessation and the clinical practicalities.

31. Silagy C, Lancaster T, Stead L et al. Nicotine replacement therapy for smoking cessation. Cochrane Database Syst Rev 2004; 3:CD000146.

    Systematic review of NRT.

32. Wu P, Wilson K, Dimoulas P et al. Effectiveness of smoking cessation therapies: a systematic review and meta-analysis. BMC Public Health 2006; 6:300.
33. Cahill K, Stead LF, Lancaster T. Nicotine receptor partial agonists for smoking cessation. Cochrane Database Syst Rev 2007; i:CD006103.

    The evidence for smoking cessation treatments.

34. MacGregor AS, Price JF, Hau CM et al. Role of systolic blood pressure and plasma triglycerides in diabetic peripheral arterial disease. The Edinburgh Artery Study. Diabetes Care 1999; 22:453–8.
35. Al-Delaimy WK, Merchant AT, Rimm EB et al. Effect of type 2 diabetes and its duration on the risk of peripheral arterial disease among men. Am J Med 2004; 116:236–40.
36. da Silva A. The management and outcome of critical limb ischaemia in diabetic patients: results of a national survey. Audit committee of the vascular surgical society of Great Britain and Ireland. Diabetic Med 1996; 13:726–8.
37. Beks P. Peripheral arterial disease in relation to glycaemic level in an elderly Caucasian population: the Hoorn study. Diabetologia 1995; 38:86–96.
38. Adler A. UKPDS 59: hyperglycaemia and other potentially modifiable risk factors for peripheral arterial disease in type 2 diabetes. Diabetes Care 2002; 25:894–9.

A large study conducted in the UK which showed a strong association between glycaemic control and PAD.

39. Price J, Lee A, Fowkes F. Hyperinsulinaemia: a risk factor for peripheral arterial disease in the non-diabetic population. J Cardiovasc Risk 1996; 3:501–5.

40. Adler A. Association of systolic blood pressure with macrovascular and microvascular complications of type 2 diabetes (UKPDS 36): prospective observational study. Br Med J 2000; 321:412–19.

Pooled analysis of UKPDS data with respect to achieved BP and outcomes, including lower limb events.

41. Hansson L. Effects of intensive blood-pressure lowering and low-dose aspirin in patients with hypertension: principal results of the Hypertension Optimal Treatment (HOT) randomised trial. HOT Study Group. Lancet 1998; 351:1755–62.

42. Beckman J, Creager M, Libby P. Diabetes and atherosclerosis: Epidemiology, pathophysiology and management. JAMA 2002; 287:2570–81.

43. Lip GY, Makin AJ. Treatment of hypertension in peripheral arterial disease. Cochrane Database Syst Rev 2003; 4:CD003075.

44. The sixth report of the Joint National Committee on prevention, detection, evaluation, and treatment of high blood pressure. Arch Intern Med 1997; 157:2413–46.

45. Meijer WT, Grobbee DE, Hunink MG et al. Determinants of peripheral arterial disease in the elderly: the Rotterdam study. Arch Intern Med 2000; 160:2934–8.

46. Feringa HH, van Waning VH, Bax JJ et al. Cardioprotective medication is associated with improved survival in patients with peripheral arterial disease. J Am Coll Cardiol 2006; 47:1182–7.

47. Ostergren J, Sleight P, Dagenais G et al. HOPE study investigators. Impact of ramipril in patients with evidence of clinical or subclinical peripheral arterial disease. Eur Heart J 2004; 25:17–24.

48. Hirsch AT, Criqui MH, Treat-Jacobson D et al. Peripheral arterial disease detection, awareness, and treatment in primary care. JAMA 2001; 286:1317–24.

49. Singer DJ, Kite A. Management of hypertension in peripheral arterial disease: does the choice of drugs matter. Eur J Vasc Endovasc Surg 2008; 35:701-8.

50. British Hypertension Society and National Institute for Healthcare Excellence. Hypertension: Management in adults in primary care: pharmacological update, July 2007; www.nice.org.uk. Joint NICE and BHS guidance for BP management.

51. Missouris CG, Buckenham T, Cappuccio FP et al. Renal artery stenosis: a common and important problem in patients with peripheral vascular disease. Am J Med 1994; 96:10–14.

52. Williams B, Poulter NR, Brown MJ et al. British Hypertension Society. Guidelines for management of hypertension: report of the fourth working party of the British Hypertension Society, 2004-BHS IV. J Hum Hypertens 2004; 18:139–85.

53. Donnelly R, Manning G. Angiotensin converting enzyme inhibitors and coronary heart disease prevention. JRAAS 2007; 8:13–22.

54. Staessen JA, Li Y, Richart T. Oral renin inhibitors. Lancet 2006; 368:1449–56.

55. Kannel WB. Intermittent claudication. Incidence in the Framingham Study. Circulation 1970; 41:875–83.

56. Cheng SW, Ting AC, Wong J. Lipoprotein (a) and its relationship to risk factors and severity of atherosclerotic peripheral vascular disease. Eur J Vasc Endovasc Surg 1997; 14:17–23.

57. Pilger E. Risk factors for peripheral atherosclerosis. Retrospective evaluation by stepwise discriminant analysis. Arteriosclerosis 1983; 3:57–63.

58. Heart Protection Study Collaborative Group. MRC/BHF Heart Protection Study of cholesterol-lowering with simvastatin in 20,536 high-risk individuals. Lancet 2002; 360:7–22.

59. Hirsch AT, Haskal ZJ, Hertzer NR et al. ACC/AHA guidelines for the management of patients with peripheral arterial disease. Circulation 2006; 113:463–5.

Updated US guidelines for management of PAD.

60. Erez G, Leitersdorf E. The rationale for using HMG-CoA reductase inhibitors (Statins) in peripheral arterial disease. Eur J Vasc Endovasc Surg 2007; 33:192–201.

Effects of statins on PAD.

61. Leng GC, Price JF, Jepson RG. Lipid-lowering for lower limb atherosclerosis. Cochrane Database Syst Rev 2000; 2:CD000123.

Analysis of currently available data suggests that lipid lowering therapy is of benefit for PAD patients to reduce morbidity and possibly mortality.

62. Mohler ER, Hiatt WR, Creager MA. Cholesterol reduction with atorvastatin improves walking distance in patients with peripheral arterial disease. Circulation 2003; 108:1481–6.

Effects of statin therapy on functional status in PAD.

63. Prospective studies collaboration. Blood cholesterol and vascular mortality by age, sex and blood pressure: a meta-analysis of individual data from 61 prospective studies with 55 000 vascular deaths. Lancet 2007; 370:1829–39.

Overview of the large statin trials, quantifies the benefits of cholesterol reduction.

64. Wyatt MG, Scott PM, Poskitt K et al. Effect of weight on claudication distance. Br J Surg 1991; 78:1386–8.

65. WHO Study Group. Diet, nutrition and prevention of chronic diseases. Technical report series no. 916. Geneva: World Health Organisation, 2003.

66. Djousse L, Levy D, Murabito JM et al. Alcohol consumption and risk of intermittent claudication in the Framingham Heart Study. Circulation 2000; 102:3092–7.

**Relationship between alcohol intake and PAD in observational follow-up studies.**

67. Sacks FM, Svetkey LP, Vollmer WM et al. Effects on blood pressure of reduced dietary sodium and the Dietary Approaches to Stop Hypertension (DASH) diet. N Engl J Med 2001; 344:3–10.

68. Cook NR, Cutler JA, Obarzanek E et al. Long term effects of dietary sodium reduction on cardiovascular disease outcomes: observational follow-up of the trials of hypertension prevention (TOHP). Br Med J 2007; 334:885.

69. Collaborative meta-analysis of randomised trials of antiplatelet therapy for prevention of death, myocardial infarction, and stroke in high risk patients. Br Med J 2002; 324:71–86.

**Meta-analysis of the effects of antiplatelet therapy in CV disease.**

70. CAPRIE Steering Committee. A randomised, blinded trial of clopidogrel versus aspirin in patients at risk of ischaemic events (CAPRIE). Lancet 1996; 348:1329–39.

71. Bhatt DL, Fox KAA, Hacke W et al. Clopidogrel and aspirin versus aspirin alone for the prevention of atherothrombotic events (CHARISMA). New Engl J Med 2006; 354:1706–17.

72. Peripheral Arterial Disease Antiplatelet Consensus Group. Antiplatelet therapy in peripheral arterial disease: Consensus statement. Eur J Vasc Endovasc Surg 2003; 26:1–16.

**Recent, evidence-based consensus guidelines for use of antiplatelet therapy in different clinical scenarios related to PAD.**

73. The Warfarin Antiplatelet Vascular Evaluation Trial Investigators. Oral anticoagulant and antiplatelet therapy and peripheral arterial disease. N Engl J Med 2007; 357:217–27.

74. Stroke Prevention in Atrial Fibrillation II Study. Warfarin versus aspirin for prevention of thromboembolism in atrial fibrillation. Lancet 1994; 343:687–91.

**Rationale and superiority of warfarin for patients with chronic atrial fibrillation.**

# 2

# Assessment of chronic lower limb ischaemia

Jan Brunkwall
John Bottomley

## Introduction

Atherosclerosis is a generalised disease involving the arterial tree with preponderance for the arteries supplying the lower limbs. The reasons for this are unknown. The most commonly affected site is the superficial femoral artery in the thigh. This usually causes intermittent claudication. Other typical sites for peripheral arterial disease (PAD) are the aortic and common femoral artery bifurcations. The tibial arteries are commonly affected by calcification in patients with diabetes and those of advanced age. More generalised disease involving proximal and distal arteries, or long occlusions in locations with poor collaterals, may result in critical ischaemia with rest pain, ulceration or gangrene involving the toes or forefoot. This chapter deals with the assessment of patients with chronic lower limb ischaemia and the principles of vascular imaging.

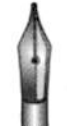

There are several classifications based on the severity of PAD. The simplest is the Fontaine classification (Table 2.1). The Rutherford classification (Table 2.2) is more detailed, useful for reporting standards, but rarely used in clinical practice.

## Intermittent claudication (IC)

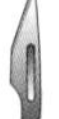

IC is a frequent symptom in the elderly, occurring in 14% of men over the age of 65 years, increasing to 21% in those over the age of 85 years (see Chapter 1).

The classic features of IC are that the pain on walking develops in the muscle groups distal to the occlusion, i.e. usually in the calf, but in proximal occlusions also in the thigh or buttock. This pain is not felt at rest or when the first few steps are taken but develops progressively on walking and is described as an ache, cramp or tightening in the muscle that usually forces the patient to stop. Occasionally, mild claudication may be felt only while walking uphill or quickly. The symptoms are rapidly relieved by rest and reappear after walking a similar distance.

The differential diagnosis includes osteoarthritis of the hip or knee and lumbar nerve route irritation. Patients with spinal stenosis may have symptoms that are very similar to intermittent (vascular) claudication.[1] Whereas patients with vascular claudication get pain relief by just standing still, patients with spinal stenosis need to relieve the pressure in the spinal canal, which they do by sitting or lying down. A history of pain on standing as well as walking therefore suggests neurogenic claudication due to spinal stenosis. Patients with osteoarthritis of the hip with referred pain down the leg and a history similar to claudication usually experience some pain in the buttock or groin when turning their body, even in a sitting or supine position. The pain is not relieved by just standing still, as the patient needs to lessen the burden on the joint. Although the diagnosis can usually be established by history and examination alone, minimally invasive investigations, including an exercise test to exclude arterial disease, may be reassuring.

Lumbar nerve route irritation may also cause aching in the calf or down the back of the leg from

Table 2.1 • Fontaine classification of the severity of PAD

| Fontaine stage | | Description |
|---|---|---|
| I | Asymptomatic | PAD present but no symptoms |
| II | Intermittent claudication | Cramping pain in leg muscles precipitated by walking and rapidly relieved by rest |
| III | Rest pain | Constant pain in feet (often worse at night) |
| IV | Tissue loss | Ischaemic ulceration or gangrene |

Table 2.2 • Rutherford classification of the severity of PAD

| Grade | Category | Description |
|---|---|---|
| 0 | 0 | Asymptomatic |
| I | 1 | Mild claudication |
| I | 2 | Moderate claudication |
| I | 3 | Severe claudication |
| II | 4 | Ischaemic rest pain |
| II | 5 | Minor tissue loss |
| III | 6 | Major tissue loss |

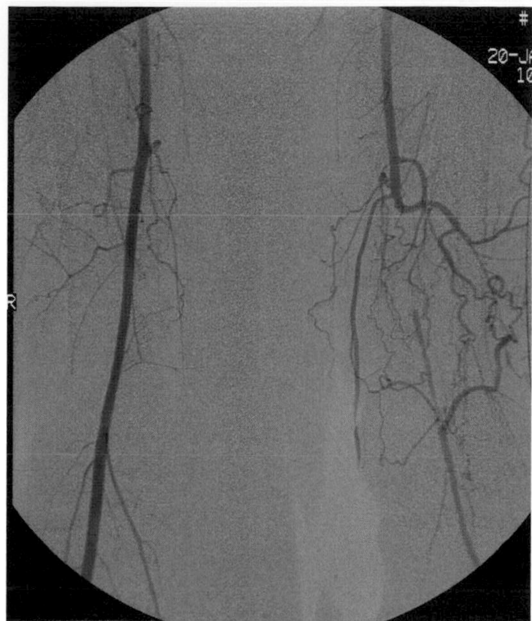

**Figure 2.1** • Arteriogram showing well-collateralised occlusion of left superficial femoral artery. The patient had palpable foot pulses and almost normal resting ABPIs. These fell after exercise.

buttock to ankle. The sensation appears to be very similar to that of claudication, particularly when confined to the calf. Direct enquiry for these symptoms is helpful, but the key feature is again the need to sit or lie to obtain relief. Spinal flexion may release the involved nerve roots, whereas a straight leg raise will often precipitate the pain. When both sciatic nerve irritation or spinal stenosis and PAD coexist in the same patient, it can be extremely difficult to identify which is contributing most to the patient's symptoms. Sometimes empirical revascularisation is required, after warning the patient that symptomatic relief cannot be guaranteed.

The cornerstones in the assessment of chronic lower limb ischaemia are a careful history, palpation of pulses, auscultation for bruits and ankle–brachial pressure index (ABPI) measurement. The important point is to verify that the clinical findings correlate well with the patient's symptoms. As the patients get older so does the arterial tree. The mere presence of PAD does not mean that it is the cause of the symptoms. The history should include the duration of symptoms and the mode of onset. Most patients gradually become aware of pain on walking, which is typical in progressive PAD. The patient experiences pain when the arterial supply to the leg muscles is insufficient to meet the metabolic needs during exercise.

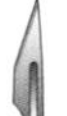

The blood supply required by resting muscles is relatively small (130–150 mL/min) and may be increased five- to tenfold during exercise.[2]

Arterial occlusions can be well tolerated when collaterals can develop, as is the case when the occlusion is surrounded by muscle. This can result in the same volume flow at rest as in normal individuals.[3] Examples include the thigh muscles around the superficial femoral artery at the adductor canal, which is well collateralised by the profunda femoris artery and occlusions of the iliac arteries, where collaterals through the pelvis and buttock may result in normal resting pressures and even a palpable foot pulse (**Fig. 2.1**). Significant PAD is usually associated with an ABPI of <0.9 (see later), but in such cases an exercise challenge will result in a fall in ankle pressures and disappearance of the distal pulses.

## Critical ischaemia

Ischaemic rest pain, ischaemic ulceration or gangrene of the feet requires urgent investigation and revascularisation in order to avoid limb loss due to progressive tissue necrosis and/or infection. Untreated, the prognosis is poor both for the patient and the leg, and recognition of critical ischaemia is therefore vitally important. There have been several attempts at a consensus for the definition of critical limb ischaemia (CLI).

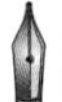

The European Consensus defines CLI as rest pain for more than 2 weeks, or ulceration/gangrene, and an ankle pressure of <50 mmHg or a toe pressure of <30 mmHg.[4]

However, this definition has been criticised because the pressures required for healing in the presence of ulceration or gangrene may be higher and ankle pressures are often falsely elevated in patients with diabetes (see later).[5] The Trans-Atlantic Inter-Society Consensus (TASC) II suggests that an ankle pressure of <70 mmHg or a toe pressure of <50 mmHg is more realistic in the presence of ulceration or gangrene.

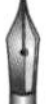

The precise definition is more relevant for reporting standards than for clinical use and the consensus document recommends that the term critical limb ischaemia should be used for all patients with chronic ischaemic rest pain, ulcers or gangrene attributable to objectively proven arterial occlusive disease.[6]

CLI in its very mild form may start with numbness in the forefoot at night sufficient to disturb the patient's sleep.

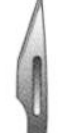

This progresses to pain, mostly at night, when the feet are in the supine position in bed. The reason for this is that cardiac output and blood pressure are decreased during the night.[7]

When the patient hangs the leg out of the bed or if they stand up and walk, thereby increasing the blood flow to the foot, the pain is relieved. If the patient constantly hangs their feet out of bed at night, or even sleeps sitting in a chair, the limb swells due to dependency oedema. This can lead to a vicious circle with more tissue damage and the key is to use strong painkillers (usually opiates) so that the limb can be kept in the supine position overnight to relieve the oedema prior to arterial reconstruction.

To the experienced eye the diagnosis of CLI seems obvious, but it is easy to miss a small ischaemic lesion on the heel or between the toes. When established necrosis or gangrene is present with absent limb pulses there is no doubt about the diagnosis. The stage when critical ischaemia without necrosis or gangrene is present (Rutherford II 4) is characterised by pallor when the leg is elevated compared to the heart and by redness when hanging down (Buerger's or Ratshow's test positive). The sunset red colour is caused by the dilated capillaries of the foot (**Fig. 2.2**). Normally, only one-third are open at any time but in the state of critical ischaemia autoregulation is paralysed and, as a consequence, all capillaries are open.[8] It may take a while for pallor on elevation to occur but capillary refill will be abolished immediately.

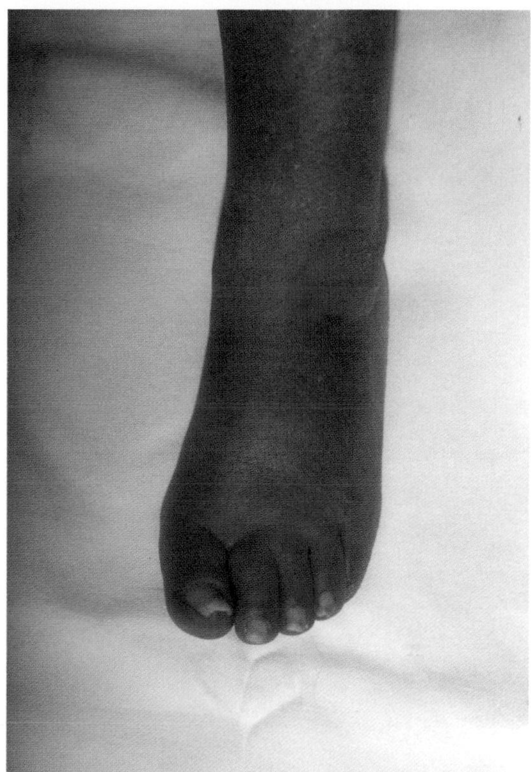

**Figure 2.2** • Sunset red foot due to dilated capillaries caused by critical (limb-threatening) ischaemia. Elevation of the foot will result in pallor (Buerger's or Ratshow's test positive).

## Rare causes of ischaemia

The vast majority of cases of chronic lower limb ischaemia are caused by atherosclerotic PAD, but some rarer conditions exist that tend to affect a younger age group. A good history of IC in a young patient should be taken seriously, as some of these conditions may progress rapidly to CLI. Resting ABPIs should be measured in all patients with leg pain on exercise, especially if foot pulses are absent. Those with a good history of IC and palpable foot pulses should also undergo an exercise test and post-exercise ABPIs.

## Persistent sciatic artery

In this congenital anomaly, the embryonic axial limb artery, the sciatic artery, does not obliterate and remains continuous with the popliteal artery, providing the major blood supply to the lower limb. The anomaly is bilateral in 22% of cases and is commonly associated with failure of the iliofemoral vessels to develop properly. The presenting symptoms include pain and a pulsatile mass in the buttock due to aneurysmal degeneration of the artery as it emerges from the sciatic foramen. Thrombosis or distal embolism may lead to acute ischaemia.[9] Although pedal pulses may be present, the femoral pulse will be reduced or absent if the iliofemoral vessels are hypoplastic (Cowie's sign) and IC will result if neither system has developed properly (**Fig. 2.3**). Symptomatic patients can be treated by combined bypass grafting and endovascular exclusion of the aneurysm.[9] Asymptomatic patients should be monitored for aneurysm development.

## Cystic adventitial disease (CAD)

CAD, caused by a cystic abnormality of the adventitia of the popliteal artery, occasionally presents with IC. The contents resemble that of a ganglion and the cysts may be connected to the synovium of the knee joint. IC may be severe and of rapid onset. The condition should be particularly suspected in young patients without significant risk factors for PAD. Pedal pulses sometimes disappear on knee flexion. Arteriography may show an unusually smooth 'hourglass' or eccentric stenosis (**Fig. 2.4**). Duplex will demonstrate the cystic abnormality, as will computed tomography (CT) or magnetic resonance (MR) scanning. Angioplasty should not be attempted as the cyst contents may embolise distally. The affected segment of artery requires resection and repair with an interposition vein graft via a posterior approach.[10]

## Popliteal artery entrapment

Popliteal artery entrapment is more common than previously recognised. The condition can be anatomical or functional. In the anatomical variant, the artery courses around the medial head of gastrocnemius rather than between the two heads or, more rarely, passes deep to the popliteus muscle. Compression of the artery occurs during flexion, resulting in IC, classically in athletes. Aneurysmal degeneration and/or thrombosis may develop. Two-thirds of cases are bilateral and the popliteal vein is involved in 10%.[11] Examination may reveal reduction or obliteration of pedal

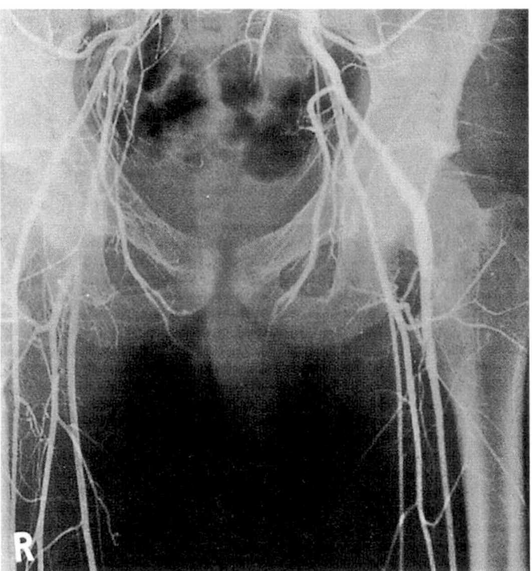


**Figure 2.3** • Persistent bilateral sciatic arteries arising from the common iliac arteries with dilatation and intimal irregularity of the left sciatic artery at the level of the acetabulum.

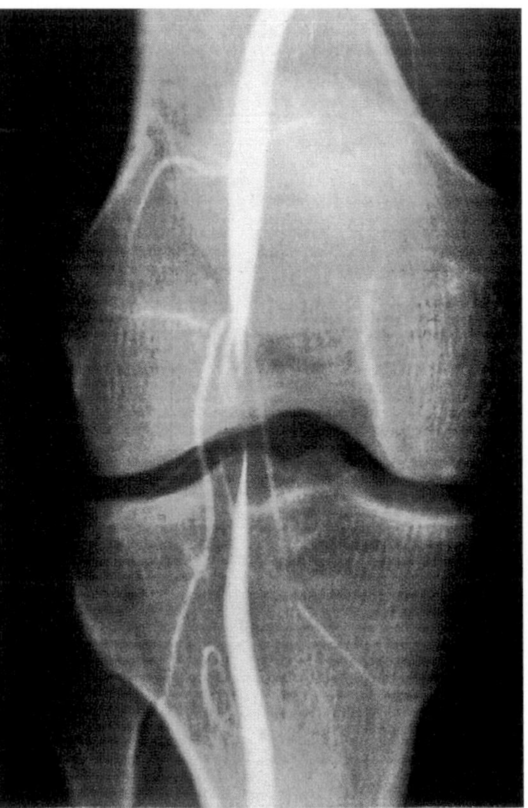

**Figure 2.4** • Smooth 'hourglass' stenosis of popliteal artery due to cystic adventitial disease. A similar appearance may be seen in popliteal entrapment, especially during active plantar flexion.

pulses during active plantar flexion. Duplex scanning or arteriography using this manoeuvre may also demonstrate kinking or compression of the popliteal artery. CT or MR scanning can also demonstrate the anatomical abnormality. Symptomatic patients should be treated by the division of the medial head of gastrocnemius and/or reconstruction of the popliteal artery. Surgery is also indicated for an asymptomatic contralateral limb whenever anatomical entrapment is detected.[12] In the functional variant of the condition, an anatomically normally positioned artery is compressed against a hypertrophied gastrocnemius or the soleal muscle ring. Unlike the anatomical variant, functional entrapment should only be treated when symptomatic.

## Fibromuscular dysplasia (FMD)

Although FMD usually affects the renal and carotid arteries, it can affect the proximal upper and lower limb arteries in young people, causing IC. The external iliac artery appears the commonest site of involvement and arteriography may demonstrate a classic beaded appearance (**Fig. 2.5**). Patients with iliac FMD should be screened for renal involvement. Symptomatic stenoses usually respond well to angioplasty.[13]

## Buerger's disease

Buerger's disease (thromboangiitis obliterans) is a systemic vasculitis that affects medium-sized arteries and veins. It should be considered in any heavy smoking young male claudicant, especially if they are of Middle or Far Eastern origin.[14] Vasospastic symptoms and superficial thrombophlebitis commonly occur and patients may progress rapidly to, or present with, CLI.

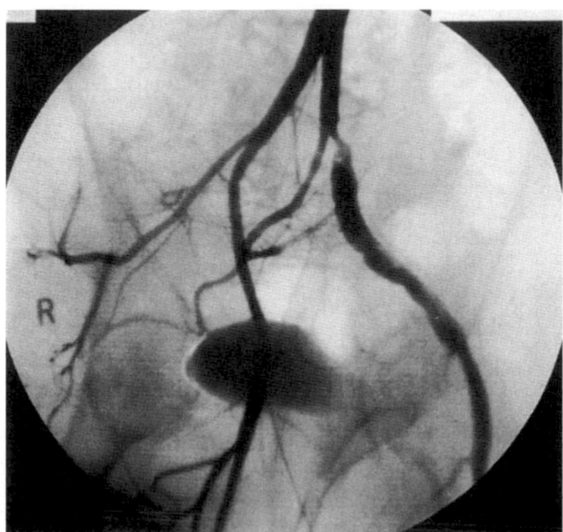


**Figure 2.5** • Fibromuscular dysplasia affecting the left external iliac artery of a 12-year-old boy.

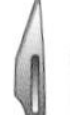

The crural vessels are usually severely affected, with patent arteries to the knee joint and typical 'corkscrew' collaterals in the calf.[15]

The pathophysiology and management of this condition and other causes of vasculitis such as Takayasu's are covered in Chapter 12.

# History and examination

## History

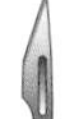

As all patients with PAD are at risk of myocardial infarction or stroke, a full history for other cardiovascular diseases and risk factors is essential (see Chapter 1).

In addition to previous myocardial infarction, stroke, coronary artery bypass grafting and arterial surgery, direct enquiry should include symptoms suggestive of angina or transient cerebral ischaemia. Although approximately 30% of patients with symptoms of limb ischaemia will have a history of myocardial infarction, it is not uncommon that angina or transient ischaemic attacks are diagnosed for the first time. The investigation and treatment of these symptoms usually have a higher priority than PAD (see Chapter 3). The enquiry for cardiovascular risk factors is equally important and obviously covers smoking, diabetes, hypertension, cholesterol or other lipid abnormalities and a detailed drug history.

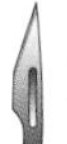

It is surprising how many patients with a history of cardiovascular disease are not taking any antiplatelet agent or a statin when they present with PAD.[16]

Smoking may also cause chronic obstructive pulmonary disease. This will limit exercise capacity, limiting the benefit of any revascularisation, and may render the patient unfit for any open vascular reconstruction.

## Examination

Patients with PAD are usually elderly and often smoke. They are at risk of conditions such as cancer in addition to cardiovascular problems and deserve a full physical examination. Examination, which can be performed also by the general practitioner, should focus on identifying risk factors, on the cardiovascular system generally and then specifically on clinical features to establish the severity and site of PAD. The body mass index (BMI) should be calculated by measuring height and weight.[17] This is a good estimate of obesity, a predictor of life expectancy and anaesthetic risk. The blood pressure, pulse rate and rhythm, and heart sounds should also be recorded. The urine should be tested for sugar and proteins. The abdomen should be palpated for an aortic aneurysm, but an ultrasound investigation is much more sensitive (see Chapter 13). Although carotid bruits may originate from the common, internal or external carotid arteries (as well as the aortic valve), the accurate detection of significant internal carotid artery stenosis requires a duplex ultrasound scan.

Palpation of pulses is subjective and influenced by both the sensitivity of the fingers, the experience of the examiner, the obesity of the patient and the warmth of the room. If there is any doubt, arterial waveforms and ABPIs can be established using a hand-held Doppler, which should be a routine part of the clinical examination. The femoral artery should always be palpable, whether it is pulsatile or occluded, if it is examined properly (**Fig. 2.6**). If it is occluded then it can be palpated as a hard cord due to atherosclerosis. Occasionally, a proximal iliac occlusion in the presence of an undiseased femoral artery, or severe obesity/scarring, can render it impalpable. If the pulse feels weak, auscultation will reveal whether there is a bruit typical of iliac or common femoral stenosis. The popliteal pulse is more difficult to palpate, particularly in a well-muscled or obese subject, but should always be felt to exclude an aneurysm (**Fig. 2.7**). Palpation of the foot pulses may be difficult when the foot is swollen or the room is cold. Describing foot pulses as 'weak' is subjective and only appropriate when clearly different from the contralateral pulse. The absence of a single foot pulse may have little clinical significance and, although it should be recorded, is not an indication for more detailed investigation.

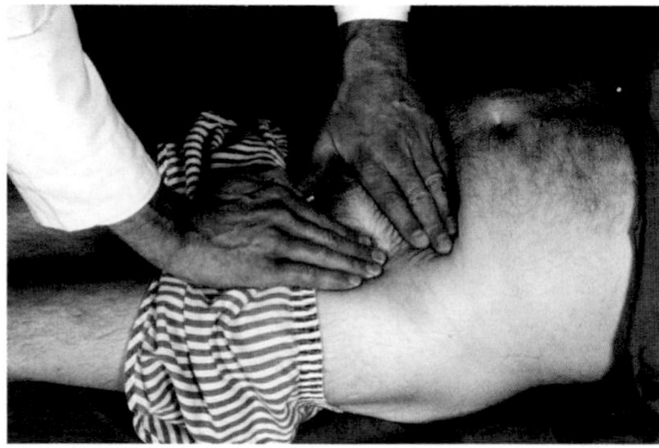

**Figure 2.6** • Palpation of the femoral pulse requires both hands except in the very thin patient. One hand pushes the lower abdomen out of the way and the other palpates the femoral artery/pulse.

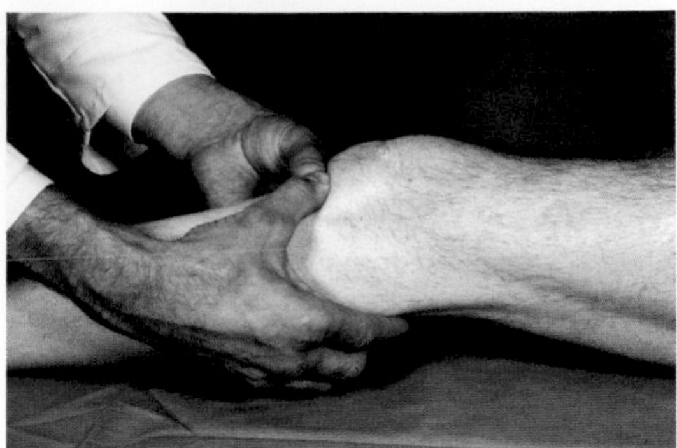

**Figure 2.7** • A popliteal pulse is best felt using both hands with the leg relaxed in slight flexion.

If foot pulses cannot be palpated or are 'weak', then insonation by hand-held Doppler is mandatory. This is particularly useful in patients with reflex sympathetic dystrophy due to immobility of a limb following injury or paralysis. Those with long-standing paralysis, due to polio in childhood or previous stroke, may develop a swollen foot with cyanosis of the toes and absent pulses. On Doppler insonation, there is a healthy biphasic or triphasic Doppler signal and normal arterial pressures will usually be found. Although the foot may appear ischaemic, the cause is merely dystrophy of the microcirculation.

## Exercise challenge

Patients present occasionally with a good history of IC, but with palpable pulses. These patients may have been investigated previously for joint disease or lumbar nerve root irritation, although their patient history may be 'typical' of claudication. Typically, there is proximal aorto-iliac disease with collaterals through the pelvis sufficient to produce adequate or even normal pulses at rest. In patients who complain of symptoms only on exercise, it is rewarding to examine the leg following an exercise challenge. This can be done quite simply in the consulting room. Even elderly patients find it easy to exercise the calf muscle by a repeated 'tiptoe' while leaning on the couch (**Fig. 2.8**). The patient returns to the couch so that the pulses can be examined immediately after exercising for 1 minute. Absent or 'tapping' femoral pulses with a bruit confirms the diagnosis of aorto-iliac disease. A more objective test can be done in the vascular laboratory with a treadmill and formal measurement of pre- and post-exercise ABPIs.

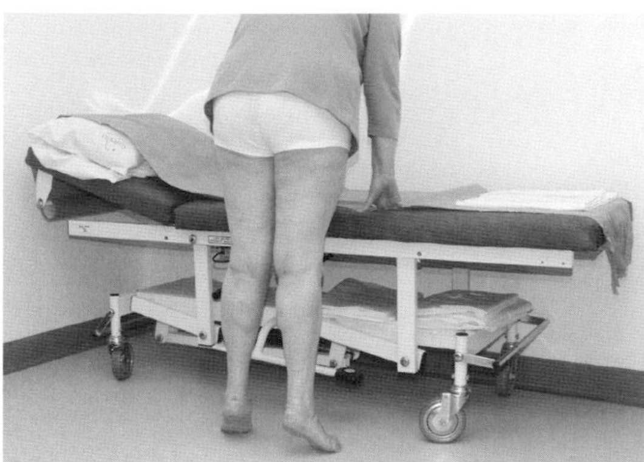

**Figure 2.8** • Simple 'tiptoe' exercise of the calf muscle causes vasodilatation with disappearance of pulses and the emergence of bruits on examination immediately after the exercise.

## Hand-held Doppler examination

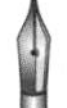

A hand-held Doppler with an 8-MHz continuous-wave Doppler probe should be a routine part of a vascular examination.[6]

The perfusion pressure at the ankle can be measured using a tourniquet and insonating the pedal arteries. The patient should be rested for more than 5 minutes, lying supine, and a standard blood pressure tourniquet applied just above the ankle, with the tourniquet being 50% wider than the limb diameter. The tourniquet cuff is inflated above the systolic pressure, when the pedal Doppler signal should disappear. On gradually lowering the cuff pressure, the Doppler signal reappears at the ankle systolic pressure (**Fig. 2.9**). The probe should be held at a 30° angle to the vessel in order to achieve the optimal signal. The systolic blood pressure is then taken from the brachial artery in the same way and the ABPI calculated as the ratio of the ankle to the brachial systolic pressures.

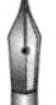

The systolic pressure at the ankle is normally higher, due to superimposed pulse waves down the arterial tree with an ABPI of 1.0–1.2. An ABPI of <0.9 suggests arterial disease, with 0.8 being the lower limit of normal. An ABPI of <0.5 is often associated with critical ischaemia.[6]

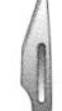

In practice, absolute pressures >60 mmHg are rarely associated with critical ischaemia unless the distal foot arteries are diseased or have been embolised from a proximal source.

As falsely high ankle arterial pressures may be measured if the calf arteries are rigid due to calcification, the pedal signal should also be assessed for normal triphasic or biphasic waveforms. When the Doppler signal in the foot is monophasic due to proximal disease, pressures above the brachial pressure suggest falsely high readings due to vascular calcification. Hand-held Doppler is clearly indicated for all patients with leg ulceration and foot ulcers. The technique is particularly important in diabetic 'neuropathic' ulcers or infection involving the toes or feet where missed proximal arterial disease may lead to amputation due to rapidly progressing infection. Measuring the ABPI is also useful in elderly patients referred with foot symptoms that do not appear to be vascular. Their GP can be reassured by an adequate ABPI and reasonable waveform, even if not completely normal.

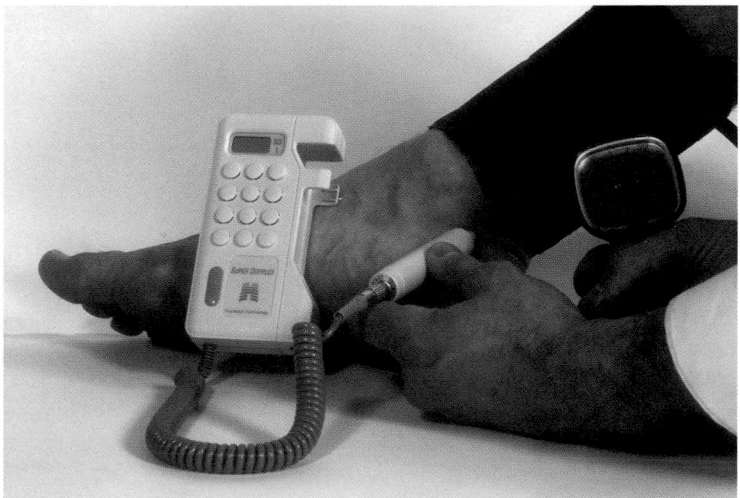

**Figure 2.9** • A hand-held Doppler can be used to detect the presence of an arterial signal at the ankle. Assess the waveform – abnormal (monophasic/damped) or normal (biphasic/triphasic) – and measure the ABPI.

### Toe pressures

Toe pressure measurements may be useful when the calf arteries are incompressible or when severe distal arterial disease in the foot is suspected.

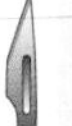

A small 2–3 cm occlusion should be used and the cuff placed around the proximal phalanx of the great, second or third toe with a photoelectric cell on the toe distally.[18]

The toe pressure can be measured using photoplethysmography or laser Doppler to detect the disappearance and reappearance of the pulse as the cuff is inflated and deflated.[19] A warm room is essential to avoid vasospasm. Expressed as a ratio to brachial artery pressure, toe pressures are normally lower than ABPI at 0.8–0.9.

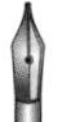

Critical ischaemia is unusual with toe–brachial pressure ratios >0.3 or absolute toe pressures >40 mmHg and two or more serial measurements are of greater value in predicting outcome than an initial single assessment.[20]

### The ischaemic angle

As a refinement to Buerger's test, the level at which a pedal Doppler signal disappears on elevation of the foot may be taken as a crude measure of ankle arterial pressure when the calf arteries are incompressible.[21] This technique has been called the 'pole test' as the foot is raised alongside a calibrated pole marked in mmHg (0.73 mmHg = 1 cmH$_2$O). This technique is only useful in severe ischaemia as it is not possible to raise the foot high enough to measure normal pressures.

## Risk factors

All patients should be investigated for risk factors as modification reduces both the risk of fatal cardiovascular events and the need for arterial reconstruction. The risk factors associated with PAD are essentially the same as those for ischaemic heart disease, and include smoking, hyperlipidaemia, diabetes and hypertension (see Chapter 1). All patients with PAD require a full blood count, erythrocyte sedimentation rate (ESR) or viscosity, urea and electrolytes, plus random blood glucose, and lipids. Anaemia can present with symptoms of leg ischaemia, as can polycythaemia. An elevated ESR or viscosity may indicate raised fibrinogen, which seems an important factor in the development of PAD and vascular thrombosis. Renal impairment is often associated with PAD and requires detection before contemplating arteriography. Arterial thromboembolism is relatively frequent in patients under the age of 50. Young patients with PAD should have a thrombophilia screen as antiphospholipid antibodies or antithrombin III deficiency may lead to repeated rethrombosis following either angioplasty or reconstruction (see Chapter 19). Hyperhomocysteinaemia can cause accelerated atherosclerosis and should be excluded in young patients with PAD. The investigation of cardiovascular risk factors is summarised in Box 2.1. As 25% of patients who claim to have stopped smoking may be 'economical with the truth', measuring a smoking markermay be required, although the effect of such 'proof' on smoking cessation is questionable.[22]

## Vascular laboratory

The majority of patients with IC require no further investigation as precise delineation of the location and extent of arterial disease serves little purpose unless revascularisation is planned. In the past, nearly every patient being considered for revascularisation was investigated by angiography, but minimally invasive investigations in a vascular laboratory have progressively replaced diagnostic angiography.[23]

### Waveform assessment and segmental pressures

Continuous-wave Doppler still has an important role in the investigation of PAD. The elasticity in normal arteries gives a characteristic triphasic waveform. The blood pressure reduces distal to a stenosis

**Box 2.1** • Investigation of cardiovascular risk factors

**All patients**

***Full blood count and ESR (plasma viscosity)***

Anaemia
Polycythaemia
Thrombocythaemia

***Biochemical profile***

Diabetes
Renal impairment
Hypercholesterolaemia
Hypertriglyceridaemia

**Selected patients**

***(Age <50 years or acute unusual thrombosis)***

Thrombophilia screen
Hyperhomocysteinaemia

***'Ex' smokers***

Thiocyanate, carboxyhaemoglobin or urinary cotinine
ESR, erythrocyte sedimentation rate.

and therefore the resistance from the capillary beds is reduced, changing the shape of this waveform. Distal to a 50% stenosis the waveform is biphasic, and with a >70% stenosis the waveform becomes monophasic.[24] Waveform shape can be affected by distal disease, dilatation of arteries, multisegment disease, complete occlusion of an artery and also ambient temperature. Waveform shape can only give an indication of disease and should be used in conjunction with segmental pressures to determine which segments in the leg are diseased.

Clinicians frequently see patients with multisegment disease. Segmental arterial pressures have some additional value in both determining the level of disease and predicting whether proximal arterial reconstruction will be adequate to treat critical ischaemia (**Fig. 2.10**). However, duplex ultrasound or arteriography are more useful in this respect.

## Laser Doppler and transcutaneous oximetry

These are both techniques used to assess the viability of skin perfusion. Laser Doppler measures the Doppler shift in light emitted by a diode and measures overall skin perfusion to a depth of approximately 1.5 mm.

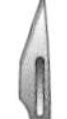

It is most appropriately used as a trend instrument and has failed to gain any useful clinical applications in PAD even though the newer probes, with several measuring points, are more reliable.

Transcutaneous oximetry can be used to measure the partial pressure of oxygen diffusing through the surface of the skin as an indirect measure for oxygen

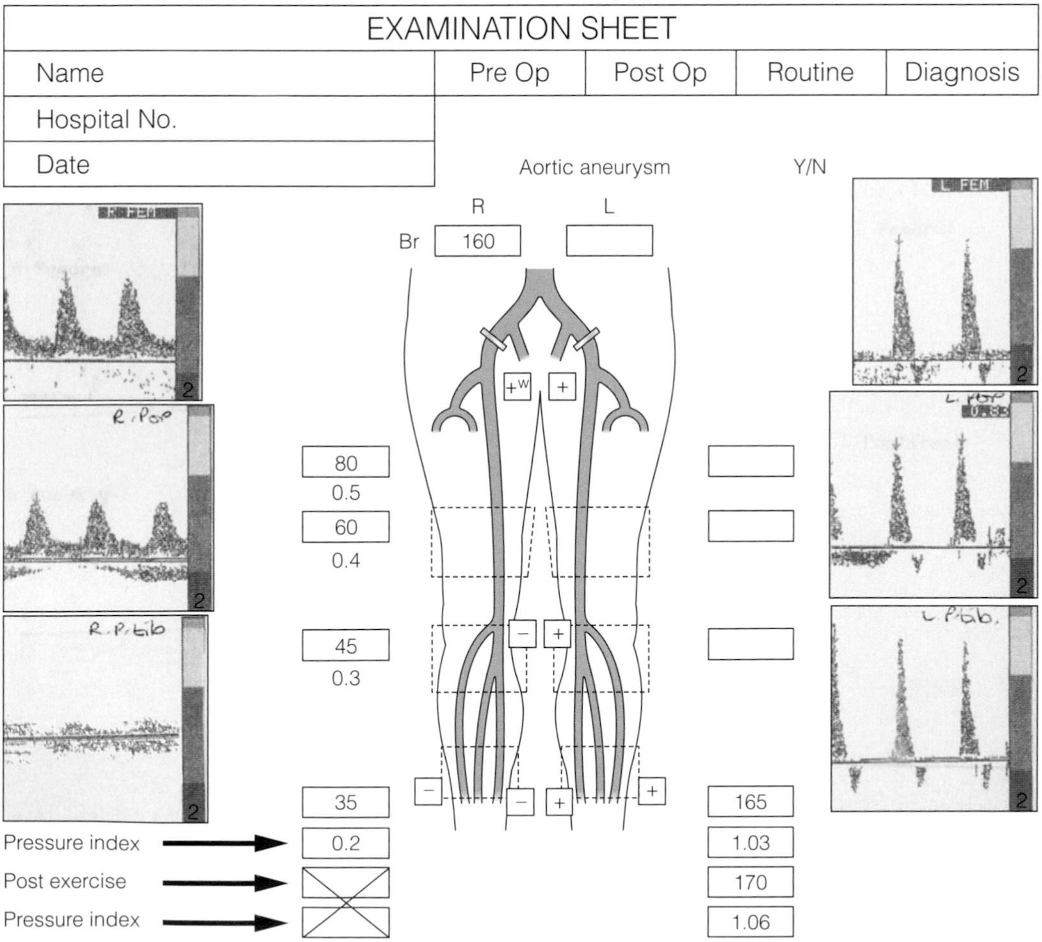

EXAMINATION SHEET

Name | Pre Op | Post Op | Routine | Diagnosis

Hospital No.

Date

Aortic aneurysm Y/N

R L

Br 160

R FEM

R.Pop

R.P.tib

L FEM

L.Pop

L.P.tib.

80 0.5

60 0.4

45 0.3

35

Pressure index 0.2 | 1.03

Post exercise | 170

Pressure index | 1.06

165

**Figure 2.10** • Segmental arterial waveforms may help discriminate the functional significance of multisegment disease, such as the right iliac and superficial femoral occlusions in this patient. Theoretically, normalising the low thigh pressure will approximately double the ankle arterial pressure to a level that should relieve ischaemic rest pain.

tension in the underlying tissue. It was hoped that tc$PO_2$ measurements of calf skin might be used to determine whether healing would occur following below-knee amputation.[25] Unfortunately, neither tc$PO_2$ nor ABPI is reliable for this as the changes in skin perfusion after the distal limb has been removed cannot be predicted. Where there is severe proximal disease, removing the distal limb is unlikely to heal.

## Radiological investigations

The choice of which imaging modality to use, in the investigation of PAD, has been the subject of review by the Scottish Intercollegiate Guidelines Network (SIGN).

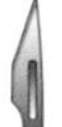

An A-grade recommendation (supported by meta-analyses or systematic reviews of randomised controlled trials (RCTs)) was given for non-invasive imaging modalities that should be employed in the first instance for patients with IC in whom intervention is being considered. They also recommended that digital subtraction angiography should not be used as the primary imaging modality for patients with peripheral arterial disease.[26] In a recent 2007 systematic review of duplex ultrasound (DUS), magnetic resonance angiography (MRA) and computed tomography angiography (CTA) for the diagnosis and assessment of symptomatic lower limb peripheral arterial disease, contrast-enhanced MRA (CE-MRA) showed better overall diagnostic accuracy than CTA or DUS. CE-MRA was also generally preferred by patients over catheter angiography.[27]

Another meta-analysis comparing the accuracy of gadolinium-enhanced MRA versus colour DUS found that the sensitivity for detecting arterial segments with >50% diameter stenosis was better for MRA that for duplex ultrasound (98% vs. 88%), with similar specificities (96% vs. 95%).[28]

Despite the benefits and greater accuracy of CE-MRA, many centres use DUS as the first-line screening imaging modality to investigate PAD. This is mostly due to its greater availability, cost and limited access to MR scanner time. Although some vascular surgeons and interventional radiologists place a high level of faith in DUS, and may intervene on the information it provides alone, most large vascular units perform CE-MRA as the first-line imaging modality for the greater certainty and accuracy it provides in the assessment of challenging vascular territories (for DUS) such as the iliac and crural arteries. CE-MRA also provides an overview 'angiographic' or road-map image of all arterial segments by way of rotated maximal intensity projection (MIP) images of each imaging station. DUS can then be utilised in a complementary role, focused on problem solving to address specific equivocal haemodynamic questions that may remain unanswered. This strategy optimises the sonographer's time and eliminates redundant duplication of imaging normal arterial segments twice.

### Duplex ultrasound (DUS)

DUS allows the visualisation and haemodynamic assessment of arteries using grey-scale also known as B-mode imaging, colour-flow Doppler mapping and pulsed-wave Doppler interrogation of blood flow within the central vessel lumen. It is one of the most operator-dependent radiological examinations; however, in the hands of an experienced sonographer, it can be used to map the length of an artery and identify the severity and location of disease.

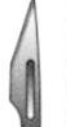

As such, DUS of the extremities has been given a class 1 recommendation (supported by multiple RCTs or meta-analyses) for the diagnosis, the anatomical location and degree of stenosis of PAD, as well as for routine surveillance after femoral–popliteal or femoral–tibial pedal bypass with a venous conduit.[29]

The value of duplex is that the diseased artery may be imaged clearly using grey-scale ultrasound, which visualises echogenic plaques and the anatomy of the artery/disease. Real-time colour-flow Doppler is used to identify blood flow through the colour box positioned in the grey-scale image. Colour filling will only occur where blood is moving and can therefore be used to enhance the grey-scale image by identifying 'soft' echolucent atheroma or thrombus as an area of absent colour filling. Colour flow also allows identification of increased blood velocity by a change in colour within the lumen of the artery. Combining grey-scale and colour-flow mapping, a severe stenosis can be seen as grey echoes reducing the diameter of the colour filling and a 'mosaic' of colours indicating increased velocity and turbulence. Grey-scale and colour flow do not provide a quantitative means of determining the severity of a stenosis other than by direct luminal diameter or area loss measurement (**Fig. 2.11a,b**).

In pulsed-wave Doppler, the ultrasound signal is pinpointed to a specific depth by the sampling box, which is kept small within the central lumen. The change of frequency (Doppler shift) in this reflected signal is determined by the transmitted frequency, angle of insonation and the velocity of blood. Modern DUS machines allow automated calculation of blood velocity but the accuracy of this relies heavily on the correct determination of the position of the pulsed-wave Doppler box and angling of the central cursor to the axis of blood flow. The peak systolic velocity is measured in the normal artery proximal to a stenosis and then in the stenosis identified by colour flow. The shape of the Doppler waveform (triphasic, biphasic or monophasic), degree of spectral broadening (range of velocity profiles within the wave spectra secondary to turbulence) and change in peak systolic velocity relative to the upstream normal artery all help to determine the severity of a given stenosis (Table 2.3).[30] A twofold increase in the peak systolic velocity generally indicates a 50% narrowing of the artery, while a 2.5-fold increase indicates a narrowing of greater than 50%. Distal to a stenosis, the Doppler waveform changes shape due to damping with reduction in peak systolic velocity and a slower acceleration time (time from end diastole to peak systole) (**Fig. 2.11c**).

Certainty of the diagnosis of a complete occlusion as opposed to high-grade stenosis with trickle flow within an artery may be difficult and depends heavily on the experience of the sonographer. The shape of the Doppler wave proximally and distally, colour-flow images and the presence of collaterals all contribute to differentiating these lesions. Difficulties can arise with deep or tortuous arteries, where signal return is reduced and optimum angles of insonation are difficult to obtain. Multiple stenoses along the length of an artery reduce the accuracy of flow velocity measurements in the assessment of more distal stenoses. The sonographer must thus

**Table 2.3** • Diagnostic criteria for peripheral arterial diameter reduction

| | Diameter reduction (%) | Waveform | Spectral broadening | PSV distal/ PSV proximal |
|---|---|---|---|---|
| Normal | 0 | Triphasic | Absent | No change |
| Mild | 1–19 | Triphasic | Present | <2:1 |
| Moderate | 20–49 | Biphasic | Present | <2:1 |
| Severe | 50–99 | Monophasic | Present | >2:1* |

*>4:1 suggests >75% stenosis, >7:1 suggests >90% stenosis.
PSV, peak systolic velocity.

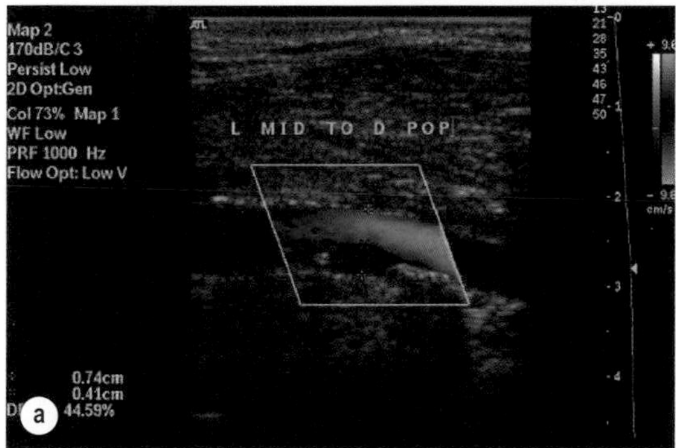


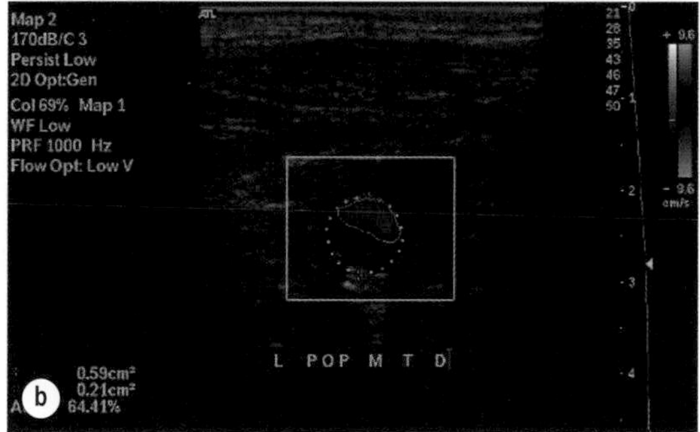


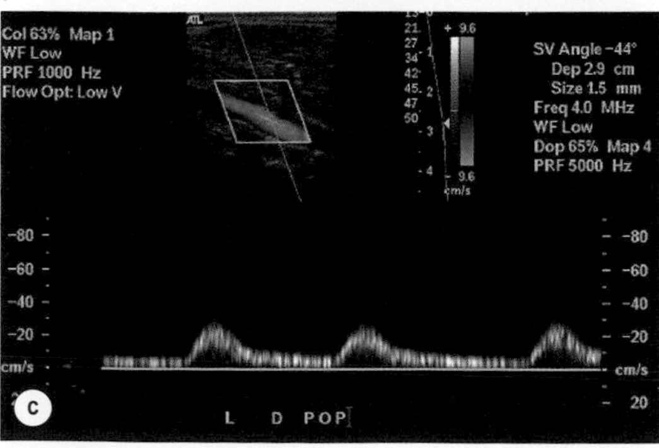


**Figure 2.11** • **(a)** A longitudinal colour Doppler image of a mid to distal left popliteal artery stenosis with a diameter reduction of 45%. **(b)** The area reduction of the same lesion on transaxial imaging is 64%. **(c)** A pulsed-wave Doppler waveform immediately distal to the stenosis. There is dampening of the peak systolic velocity, slowing of the systolic rise time and the waveform is monophasic, indicating a haemodynamically significant stenosis.

use valuable years of experience and knowledge of more subtle changes in blood velocity to determine the severity of a given stenosis when there are tandem or multiple stenosis.

## Assessment of suprainguinal arteries

This can be difficult due to respiratory movements, the depth of arteries, arterial tortuosity, overlying bowel gas and if arterial wall calcification obscures the vessel lumen, particularly in the presence of slow flow. Varying the plane of insonation may occasionally help by 'throwing off' obscuring and distracting anatomy and pathology.

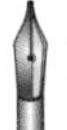

Aorto-iliac DUS arterial assessment has been shown to match catheter angiography, with a sensitivity of 0.89 and specificity of 0.90.[31]

An experienced vascular sonographer will report any study limitations. Changes in the Doppler waveform before and after an inadequately viewed segment give an indication of disease and the need for further investigation.

## Assessment of infrainguinal arteries

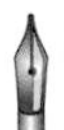

In experienced hands, DUS is accurate at identifying disease from the common femoral to the distal popliteal artery, with a sensitivity of 84–87% and specificity of 92–98% compared to catheter angiography.[31–33]

The crural arteries can be more difficult, especially when there is severe proximal disease.[34,35] In large calves, the depth of insonation attenuates the signal return, making it difficult to visualise the proximal crural arteries.[35] Accuracy can be improved by using a 4.2-MHz curved-array abdominal probe, which allows deeper penetration. Alternatively power Doppler, which is more sensitive to slow flow, can help to detect the optimum tibial artery for revascularisation.[36,37]

## Contrast media

Iodinated intravascular contrast media, whether for use in catheter angiographic procedures or for vascular or tissue enhancement in computed tomography examinations, continue to pose risks for the development of contrast-induced nephrotoxicity (CIN). This is defined as a condition in which an impairment in renal function (an increase in serum creatinine by more than 25% or 44 μmol/L (0.5 mg/dL)) occurs within 3 days following the intravascular administration of a contrast medium in the absence of an alternative aetiology.[38] In a multivariate analysis several risk factors have been identified (Box 2.2).[39] Methods to reduce the incidence of CIN have been highly contentious and have included the choice of contrast, using as little contrast as possible, pharmacological manipulation by stopping nephrotoxic drugs and metformin, and intravenous volume expansion.[40]

A CIN Consensus Working Panel composed of experts in the contrast field undertook an extensive review of the literature and produced ten consensus statements (Box 2.3).[41]

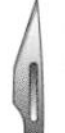

They agreed that for an estimated glomerular filtration rate (eGFR) of 30–59 mL/min, intravenous volume expansion reduces the risk for CIN and that patients should receive adequate intravenous volume expansion with isotonic crystalloid (1.0–1.5 mL/kg per hour) for 3–12 hours before the procedure and for 6–24 hours afterwards. If the eGFR is <30 mL/min a nephrology consultation is recommended with dialysis planning should CIN occur.

Much debate has surrounded which contrast agent might have an advantage in reducing the incidence of CIN with much support for the use of iso-osmolar, non-ionic contrast media over low-osmolar, non-ionic agents.[42]

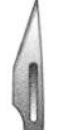

Most recently, new evidence has emerged from the PREDICT study, a randomised double-blind comparison of CIN after low- or iso-osmolar contrast agent exposure; 248 patients with moderate to severe chronic kidney disease and diabetes mellitus were randomised to receive at least 65 mL of iopamidol 370 (low-osmolar) or iodixanol 320 (iso-osmolar) for a CT procedure. There was no significant difference in the incidence of CIN at 48–72 hours after contrast administration.[43]

**Box 2.2** • Risk factors for contrast-induced nephropathy (CIN) identified in multivariate analysis

Chronic kidney disease (stage 3 or greater: eGFR <60 mL/min/1.73 m$^2$)

Diabetes mellitus (type 1 or 2)

Volume depletion

Nephrotoxic drug use (NSAIDs, ciclosporin, aminoglycosides)

Preprocedural haemodynamic instability

Other comorbidities:

- Anaemia
- Congestive heart failure
- Hypoalbuminaemia

eGFR, estimated glomerular filtration rate; NSAIDs, non-steroidal anti-inflammatory drugs.

**Box 2.3** • Consensus statements agreed upon by the CIN Consensus Working Panel

1. CIN is a common and potentially serious complication following the administration of contrast media in patients at risk for acute renal injury.
2. The risk of CIN is elevated and of clinical importance in patients with chronic kidney disease (particularly when diabetes is also present), recognised by an eGFR <60 mL/min/1.73 m$^2$.
3. When serum creatinine or eGFR is unavailable, then a survey may be used to identify patients at higher risk for CIN than the general population.
4. In the setting of emergency procedures, where the benefit of very early imaging outweighs the risk of waiting, the procedure can be performed without knowledge of serum creatinine or eGFR.
5. The presence of multiple CIN risk factors in the same patient or high-risk clinical scenarios can create a very high risk for CIN (50%) and ARF (15%) requiring dialysis after contrast exposure.
6. In patients at increased risk for CIN undergoing intra-arterial administration of contrast, ionic high-osmolality agents pose a greater risk for CIN than low-osmolality agents. Current evidence suggests that for intra-arterial administration in high-risk patients with chronic kidney disease, particularly those with diabetes mellitus, non-ionic, iso-osmolar contrast is associated with the lowest risk of CIN.
7. Higher contrast volumes (100 mL) are associated with higher rates of CIN in patients at risk. However, even small (30 mL) volumes of iodinated contrast in very-high-risk patients can cause CIN and ARF requiring dialysis, suggesting the absence of a threshold effect.
8. Intra-arterial administration of iodinated contrast media appears to pose a greater risk of CIN above that which occurs with intravenous administration.
9. Adequate intravenous volume expansion with isotonic crystalloid (1.0–1.5 mL/kg per hour) for 3–12 hours before the procedure and continued for 6–24 hours afterwards can lessen the probability of CIN in patients at risk. The data on oral fluids as opposed to intravenous volume expansion as a CIN prevention measure are insufficient.
10. No adjunctive medical or mechanical treatment has been proved to be efficacious in reducing the risk of CIN. Prophylactic haemodialysis or haemofiltration have not been validated as effective strategies.

ARF, acute renal failure; CIN, contrast-induced nephropathy; CKD, chronic kidney disease; eGFR, estimated glomerular filtration rate.

Metformin is excreted unchanged in the urine. In the presence of renal failure, either pre-existing or induced by iodinated contrast medium, metformin may accumulate in sufficient amounts to cause lactic acidosis. Metformin does not cause renal failure.[38] Contrast agents should therefore be administered with caution and it is essential that the renal function (serum creatinine) is checked in these patients prior to the examination. If >100 mL of intravenous iodinated contrast is to be administered or intra-arterial contrast, metformin should be withheld for 48 hours after the procedure.

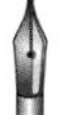

If there is biochemical evidence of renal impairment, i.e. serum creatinine >120 μmol/L, metformin should also be withheld for 2 days before (as well as after) contrast administration and the patient referred for alternative diabetic control. Serum creatinine should be rechecked 48 hours postprocedure and the metformin reinstituted only if the result is <150 μmol/L.

Patients with a baseline serum creatinine of >150 μmol/L should not be on metformin. If patients are referred on metformin despite this level of chronic kidney disease, the metformin should be discontinued indefinitely and the patient referred back for alternative hypoglycaemic therapy prior to the procedure.

Nephrogenic systemic fibrosis (NSF) is a newly described phenomenon of skin, muscle and organ fibrosis that may produce severe disability or even death. Its incidence may vary from negligible up to 2–5% in selected high-risk clinical situations. As of May 2007 the total number of worldwide cases was 215. The cause of NSF is rapidly emerging and has been largely attributed to gadolinium-based contrast agents (GBCAs) used in contrast-enhanced MR imaging and occurs particularly in the setting of moderate to severe renal impairment. Specific subtypes of gadolinium MR contrast agents given to patients with chronic kidney disease (CKD 4 and 5) (Box 2.3) have been implicated in the majority of cases and it is believed that macrocyclic gadolinium chelates are more stable and less likely to release free gadolinium ions,[44] thought to be central to the underlying pathophysiology.

Blood pool contrast agents (BPCAs), which are also GBCAs, have recently emerged and have provided a number of new imaging opportunities in the assessment of vascular disease. Gadofosveset or Vasovist® (Bayer Schering Pharma) is an albumin-bound gadolinium chelate that stays within the vascular compartment allowing vascular imaging up to 30–40 minutes after a single injection. It is 90%

renally excreted and has the highest T1 relaxivity of any gadolinium agent, thus providing good signal strength for first-pass arterial imaging. High-resolution images can subsequently be obtained to interrogate equivocal stenoses or the vessel wall. To date, there have been no cases of NSF attributed to Vasovist®, thought to be due possibly to the lower concentration of gadolinium required.

## Magnetic resonance angiography (MRA)

There are many MR techniques for the assessment of vessels and vessel patency, all of which continue to evolve at a rapid pace. In recent years, phase-contrast and time-of-flight MRA have largely given way to 3D contrast-enhanced MRA (CE-MRA), which employs subtraction, bolus chase and stepping table movements. CE-MRA provides a non-invasive, non-nephrotoxic, three-dimensional luminal assessment of vessels without the use of ionising radiation and has become the preferred first-line imaging technique for the investigation of PAD. This is advocated in international guidelines, as well as by the TASC II document, for the management of PAD.[6,26] Analyses of the accuracy of MRA and comparisons of the merits of differing MR techniques have been performed.

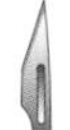

In a meta-analysis of 1090 patients, MRA was shown to be highly accurate for assessment of the entire lower extremity for arterial disease. Three-dimensional gadolinium-enhanced MRA improved the diagnostic performance compared with 2D MRA.[45]

### Technique

There are a wide variety of techniques for performing peripheral lower limb MRA that depend on the MR hardware, software sequences, moving or continuous-table capability, peripheral and surface coils, preferred contrast agent and injection protocols, and of each institution. As crural (tibial) vessel venous contamination has been the Achilles' heel of consistently high-quality peripheral MRA, techniques have been developed to overcome this by obtaining this imaging station either faster using parallel imaging (acceleration techniques) or first, using dynamic time-resolved MRA, followed by the more usual three- or four-station stepping table 'bolus chase' technique (**Fig. 2.12**).

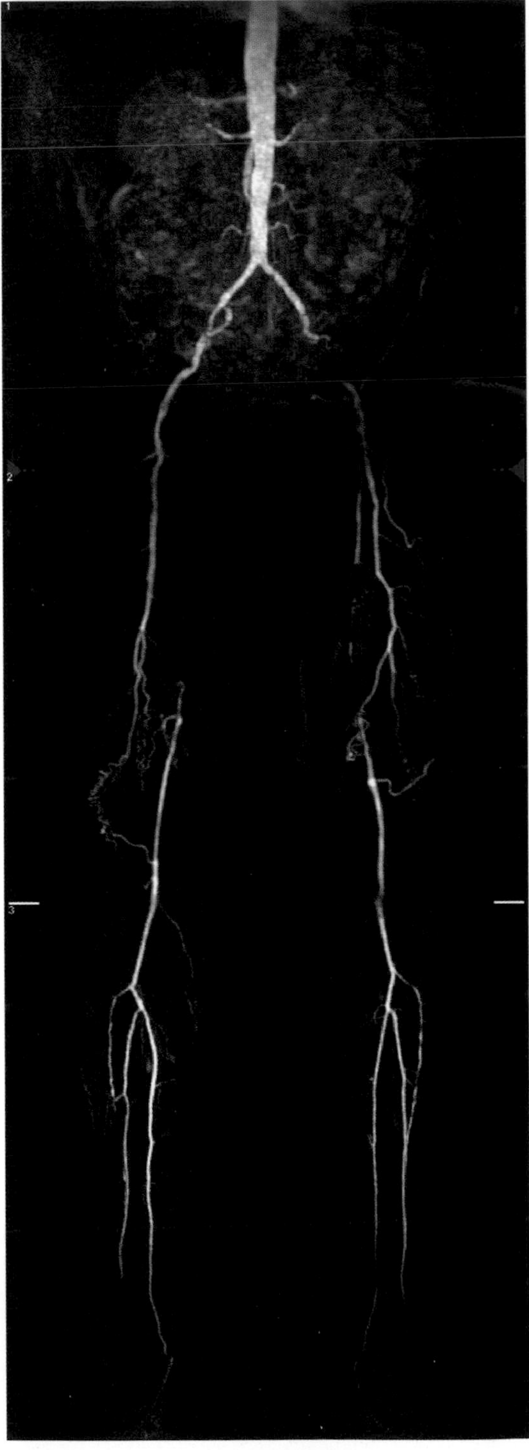

**Figure 2.12** • Bolus chase CE-MRA (using 6 mL of Vasovist® – blood pool contrast agent) coronal MIP showing left external iliac and bilateral superficial femoral artery occlusions. There is also moderate to severe right external iliac disease. Two-vessel run-off to the ankles is seen in the distal station, with severe occlusive anterior tibial artery disease bilaterally.

### Contraindications

Contraindications to MRA include the presence of a pacemaker or certain types of prosthetic cardiac valve implants that contain metal,[45] intracranial aneurysm clips, cochlear implants or metallic intraocular foreign bodies. MRA should be avoided within 6–8 weeks of inserting metal stents to allow endothelialisation to occur and to prevent stent movement. Up to 5% of patients may be claustrophobic in the MR bore, which may be overcome using open bore systems or by using psychotherapy relaxation techniques. Occasionally sedation or rarely a general anaesthetic may be required.[6]

## Computed tomographic angiography (CTA)

Over the last 10 years, CT scanners have developed from single-slice spiral systems to ever increasing numbers of simultaneously acquired multislice systems progressing through 4, 8, 16, 32, 64, dual-energy source systems to 256 slices.

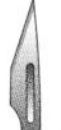

A recent meta-analysis in 2007 of multidetector CTA in lower-extremity arterial disease concluded that CTA was an accurate diagnostic test in the assessment of arterial disease (>50%) of the entire lower extremity.[46]

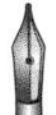

A randomised controlled trial of digital subtraction angiography (DSA) versus multidetector row CTA in PAD randomised 145 patients to either DSA or CTA in the investigation of PAD.[47] Therapeutic confidence was significantly better in the DSA group, but costs were significantly less in the CTA group. There were no patient outcome or quality-of-life differences. It concluded that CTA instead of DSA provided sufficient information for therapeutic decision-making in PAD, was non-invasive and reduced costs.

### Technique

With each of the multislice systems, the tube continuously rotates and acquires information as the patient is fed through the scanner. The volume scanned is then divided into many volume elements (voxels) and the central processor reconstructs slices from this dataset. Because a *volume* of tissue has been scanned, these slices can be reconstructed in any plane (multiplanar and curved planar reconstructions). Complex reconstructions can also be performed, with the subtraction of bone or other detail that may obscure the arteries. As arterial wall calcification is close to the Hounsfield unit of arterially opacified blood, care must be taken to ensure that no normal part of the vessel has been subtracted when using automated subtraction algorithms. This also applies to vessels that lie in close proximity to bone, for example the tibial arteries, that may be subtracted if the bones are automatically removed. The radiologist must therefore review the source data in the plane of greatest spatial resolution (with 0.6-mm slice thickness modern multislice systems, this now includes any plane including oblique planes) as well as the reconstructions.

MIP images can be constructed, selecting the highest density voxel along a given plane or planes (**Fig. 2.13a**). This produces a 2D angiographic-like image that can be rotated to allow multiple viewing angles. A variety of three-dimensional volume rendered reconstructions can also be displayed in colour, with preset colour maps determined to best display the anatomy required (**Fig. 2.13b**). With the exception of complex vascular anatomy, such as arteriovenous malformations or intracranial aneurysms, little additional purely diagnostic information is gained. These images are, however, useful for surgical and endovascular planning, allowing consideration of catheter selection to take place ahead of interventions or to allow planning of optimal angulation of fluoroscopic and digital subtraction angiographic tube positions.

## Catheter angiography

Digital subtraction angiography was for a long time considered the 'gold standard' in the investigation of peripheral vascular disease as well as in most other vascular territories. Although some believe that this remains true (despite the fact that it is a two-dimensional technique), it has been shown that well performed modern non-invasive imaging modalities, including CE-MRA and CTA, have made significant advances in challenging this claim. Although further validation studies are required of many modern imaging techniques, invasive procedures place patients at risk of harm, albeit at low incident levels (Table 2.4). Diagnostic angiography is also expensive, requires informed consent, a day-case bed, ties up numerous members of angiography suite staff and negatively impacts on time available for planned therapeutic interventions.

### Technique

DSA takes the output from an image intensifier and digitises the image. A single image is taken before the injection of contrast (the mask image); following contrast injection, further images are taken that can be subtracted from the mask. This removes bony detail, leaving a clear image of the arterial tree. In CLI, good-quality images of the crural (tibial) arteries and plantar arch are important in planning distal bypass operations. These distal images are prone to movement artefact in the critical limb and adequate analgesia is therefore essential. Occasionally, opiate analgesia is still inadequate, in which case epidural or general anaesthesia may be necessary.

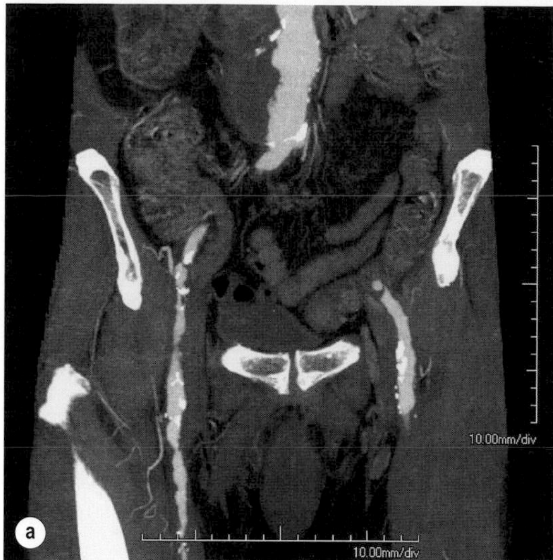


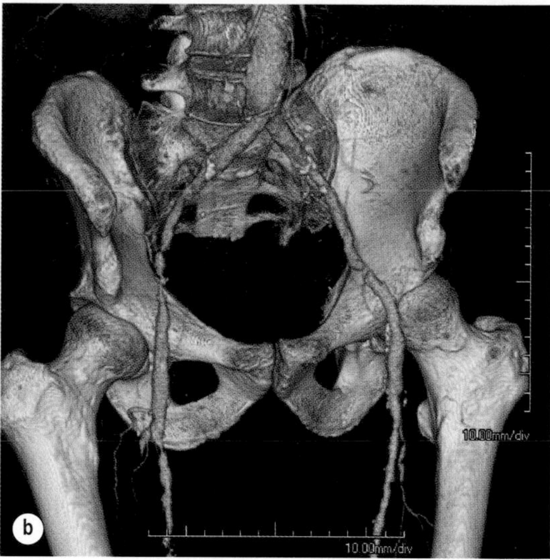


**Figure 2.13 • (a)** An oblique coronal thin MIP reconstruction created for an elderly male patient with chronic bilateral limb ischaemia. **(b)** A volume-rendered CT angiogram of the lower abdominal aorta, iliac and proximal femoral arteries, demonstrating extensive peripheral vascular disease. High-grade stenoses are present in both external iliac arteries and the proximal right superficial femoral artery.

**Table 2.4** • Royal College of Radiologists recommendations for upper limit of complications arising from diagnostic angiography

| | |
|---|---|
| Haematoma (requiring transfusion, surgery or delayed discharge) | 3.0% |
| Occlusion of the artery | 0.5% |
| Pseudo-aneurysm | 0.5% |
| Arteriovenous fistula | 0.1% |
| Distal embolisation | 0.5% |
| Occlusion of distal arteries | 2.0% |

Basic angiographic access is by the modified Seldinger technique[49] using a hollow puncture needle and a floppy guidewire, usually with a J-tip placed down the central lumen of the needle into the artery lumen. A catheter is then passed over the wire once the puncture needle has first been removed. Most angiograms for lower limb ischaemia require the injection of contrast by mechanical pumps using catheters with multiple side holes. This ensures that the contrast is distributed evenly within the circulating blood and that the catheter remains stable in position. Usually, diagnostic angiograms involve placing a pigtail catheter in the abdominal aorta with images from the renal arteries to the foot. More detailed images of the calf and foot arteries may be obtained by selective imaging allowing more definition of the crural vessels, particularly below arterial occlusion. Intra-arterial pressure gradients can also be measured across stenoses of uncertain significance. Anticoagulation should be reversed prior to angiography. With care, diagnostic angiography is safe with 3- or 4-Fr catheters in patients with international normalised ratios of prothrombin time up to 3.0, provided the blood pressure is well controlled.

## Risks and limitations

The risks of conventional catheter angiography may be related to contrast media or technique.

### Contrast related

- Allergic: these are not dose related and probably result from mast cell degranulation. The incidence of severe anaphylactic reactions due to ionic contrast media is 0.01–0.02%, but non-ionic low-osmolar iodinated contrast agents are 5–10 times safer than their predecessors. Patients with severe asthma or hay fever are at increased risk of an allergic reaction, which may be severe. Steroid prophylaxis should be considered. Patients with known contrast allergy should be imaged using alternative techniques.
- Toxic: these are dose related and manifest themselves as a metallic taste in the mouth, feelings of warmth, nausea or vomiting, cardiac arrhythmias and pulmonary oedema. They are more likely to occur in patients with severe vascular disease.
- Renal (CIN – see above).

Technique related

- Pseudo-aneurysm/haematoma: haematoma around the puncture site is common. This can be reduced by using smaller catheters and a good manual haemostasis arterial compression technique for at least 10 minutes. Arterial closure devices are rarely indicated for diagnostic angiography using 3- and 4-Fr catheters, although this may allow faster ambulation of patients and be useful with uncorrected clotting profiles.
- Dissection: a dissection flap is usually caused by poor technique using undue force or hydrophilic guidewires. Although small flaps are rarely a problem, larger or antegrade flaps may significantly slow blood flow or occlude the artery. These will usually then thrombose, which may subsequently embolise down the leg.
- Infection is rare with good aseptic technique.
- Arteriovenous fistula: as the femoral artery and vein are contained within the femoral sheath they may both be punctured during arterial access when a blind puncture is performed. Where ultrasound is available, this should be used to avoid anterior wall plaques and accurately identify the common femoral artery.
- Embolisation: if atheromatous material lining the artery is inadvertently dislodged, it will embolise distally. This may be retrieved using suction aspiration but may need surgical embolectomy or bypass surgery.

## Key points

- The superficial femoral artery in the thigh is commonly affected by atherosclerosis.
- The tibial arteries often become calcified in diabetics and the elderly.
- Rare causes of ischaemia should not be forgotten, especially in younger patients.
- The Fontaine classification for the severity of PAD has the benefit of simplicity and is clinically useful.
- Risk factors must be identified and treated in all patients with PAD.
- A careful history is essential, especially in patients with coexisting spinal problems.
- Patients with a good history of claudication and palpable pulses should be examined after exercise and/or an exercise test performed.
- Documentation of the severity of ischaemia by Doppler pressures/waveforms is mandatory in all patients with absent or weak pulses who are complaining of leg pain, weakness or numbness.
- Further investigation is not warranted unless revascularisation is being considered.
- Critical ischaemia requires urgent investigation and revascularisation in order to avoid limb loss due to progressive tissue necrosis and/or infection.
- Minimally invasive investigation by CE-MRA has largely replaced diagnostic angiography and is supported by international guidelines.
- Contrast-induced nephrotoxiciy remains a serious concern for all procedures requiring iodinated contrast medium. Serum creatinine or eGFRs must be known and provided on all patients at risk for developing this complication and must also be checked at 48 hours post-contrast injection.
- Nephrogenic systemic fibrosis is a rare but potentially serious condition occurring in chronic kidney disease patients receiving gadolinium-based contrast agents. Serum creatinine levels or eGFR must be known and provided on all patients referred for CE-MRA who are at risk of developing this condition (stage 3, 4 and 5 chronic kidney disease).
- CTA provides detailed angiographic imaging in peripheral arterial disease but is limited in severely calcified disease in diabetics and those with known severe PAD. It is particularly useful in the acute assessment of limb ischaemia where potentially embolising sources may be identified.
- Catheter angiography is invasive and is no longer recommended as a first-line imaging modality in the diagnosis of PAD. It should be limited to patients in whom therapeutic intervention is planned at the same time.

## References

1. Porter RW. Spinal stenosis and neurogenic claudication. Spine 1996; 21:2046–52.

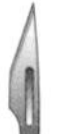

2. Leyk D, Baum K. Cardiac output, leg blood flow and oxygen uptake during foot plantar flexions. Int J Sports Med 1999; 20: 510–15.

   Parallel determinations of cardiac output, leg blood flow (LBF) and pulmonary oxygen uptake were performed in nine healthy male subjects at the onset and cessation of dynamic foot plantar flexions. Within the first 10 seconds of exercise LBF increased from 400 to about 1000 mL/min at all exercise intensities. During the subsequent 5 minutes of exercise, LBF decreased to about 800 mL/min at the lowest intensity. By contrast, it increased to about 1900 mL/min at the highest intensity.

3. Pena CS, McCauley TR. Quantitative blood flow measurements with cine phase-contrast MR imaging of subjects at rest and after exercise to assess peripheral vascular disease. Am J Roentgenol 1996; 167:153–7.

4. Second European Consensus Document on Chronic Critical Leg Ischemia. Eur J Vasc Surg 1992; 6:1–4.

5. Thompson MM, Sayers RD, Varty K et al. Chronic critical leg ischemia must be redefined. Eur J Vasc Surg 1993; 7:420–6.

6. Norgren L, Hiatt WR, Dormandy JA et al. on behalf of the TASC II Working Group. Inter-Society Consensus for the Management of Peripheral Arterial Disease (TASC II). Eur J Vasc Endovasc Surg 2007; 33:S1–75.

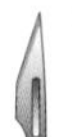

7. Jelnes R, Tonnesen KH. Nocturnal foot blood flow in patients with arterial insufficiency. Clin Sci (Lond) 1984; 67:89–95.

   Twenty-four-hour continuous recording of xenon ($^{133}$Xe) washout from the forefoot was performed on patients with normal circulations ($n$ = 10) and on patients with different degrees of arterial insufficiency ($n$ = 36). During day hours the calculated subcutaneous blood flow in the forefoot was the same in patients with normal circulation and in patients with different degrees of arterial insufficiency (2.0 ± 0.8 mL/min per 100 g). During sleep the blood flow nearly doubled in patients with normal circulation, no systematic change was seen in patients with IC and in patients with severe ischaemia, the blood flow decreased by approximately 50%.

8. Eickhoff JH. Local regulation of subcutaneous blood flow and capillary filtration in limbs with occlusive arterial disease. Studies before and after arterial reconstruction. Dan Med Bull 1986; 33:111–26.

9. Maldini G, Teruya TH. Combined percutaneous endovascular and open surgical approach in the treatment of a persistent sciatic artery aneurysm presenting with acute limb-threatening ischemia – a case report and review of the literature. Vasc Endovasc Surg 2002; 36:403–8.

10. Macfarlane R, Livesey SA. Cystic adventitial arterial disease. Br J Surg 1987; 74:89–90.

11. Levien LJ, Veller MG. Popliteal artery entrapment syndrome: more common than previously recognized. J Vasc Surg 1999; 30:587–98.

12. Turnipseed WD. Popliteal entrapment syndrome. J Vasc Surg 2002; 35:910–15.

13. Hui C, Baker D, Platts A. The role of percutaneous transluminal angioplasty in the treatment of carotid fibromuscular dysplasia. Eur J Vasc Endovasc Surg Extra 2003; 5:102–5.

14. Mills JL. Buerger's disease in the 21st century: diagnosis, clinical features, and therapy. Semin Vasc Surg 2003; 16:179–89.

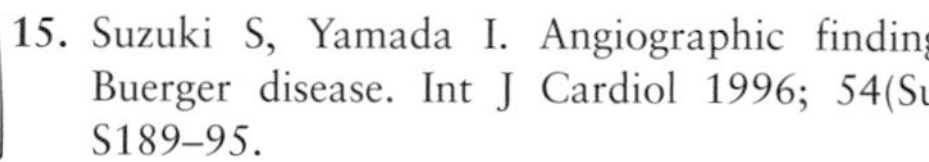

15. Suzuki S, Yamada I. Angiographic findings in Buerger disease. Int J Cardiol 1996; 54(Suppl): S189–95.

    One hundred and forty-four angiographic images of the lower extremities of 119 patients with Buerger's disease were studied. The collateral vessels had a 'corkscrew' appearance in 39 (27%) of 144 limbs affected by Buerger's disease, whereas this appearance was seen in only 2 (3%) of 63 limbs of patients with atherosclerosis ($P < 0.001$). The appearance of corkscrew-shaped vessels is the most characteristic feature of Buerger's disease and represents a dilated vasa vasorum of the occluded main arteries.

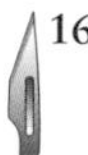

16. Adam AJ, Beard JD, Cleveland T et al. BASIL trial participants. Bypass versus angioplasty in severe ischaemia of the leg (BASIL): multicentre, randomised controlled trial. Lancet 2005; 366:1925–34.

    A prospective RCT of surgery versus angioplasty in patients with severe lower limb ischaemia. At entry into the trial, only one-third were on a statin, over one-third were not on an antiplatelet agent and over one-third were still smoking.

17. NHS Direct. What is the body mass index? 2008; www.nhsdirect.nhs.uk/articles/article.aspx?ArticleId=850

18. Pahlsson HI, Laskar C. The optimal cuff width for measuring toe blood pressure. Angiology 2007; 58:472–6.

    To determine the optimal cuff width for measuring toe blood pressure in patients with lower limb ischaemia, this study examined 20 patients with symptoms of PAD referred for vascular examination or vascular surgery. Toe blood pressure was measured hydrostatically by the pole test using cuffs of different widths. The pole test reflects the true physiological blood pressure value and was the reference method. The 2.5-cm cuff most accurately reflected the pole test.

19. Ubbink DT. Toe blood pressure measurements in patients suspected of leg ischemia: a new laser Doppler device compared with photo-plethysmography. Eur J Vasc Endovasc Surg 2004; 27: 629–34.

20. Varatharajan N, Pillay S. Implications of low great toe pressures in clinical practice. Aust NZ J Surg 2006; 76:218–21.

21. Smith FCT, Shearman CP, Simms MH et al. Falsely elevated ankle pressures in severe leg ischemia. The pole test: an alternative approach. Eur J Vasc Surg 1994; 8:408–12.

22. Silagy C, Mant D, Fowler G et al. Meta analysis on efficacy of nicotine replacement therapies in smoking cessation. Lancet 1994; 343:139–42.

23. Bradbury A, Callum K. ABC of arterial and venous disease: Acute limb ischaemia. BMJ 2000; 320:764–767.

24. Cole SEA, Walker RA, Norris R. Vascular laboratory practice, IPEM Part III. York: Institute of Physics and Engineering in Medicine, 2001.

25. De Graaff JC, Ubbink DT, Legemate DA et al. Evaluation of toe pressure and transcutaneous oxygen measurements in management of chronic critical leg ischemia: a diagnostic randomised clinical trial. J Vasc Surg 2003; 38:528–34.

26. Scottish Intercollegiate Guidelines Network, No. 89, October 2006.

27. Collins R et al. Duplex ultrasonography, magnetic resonance angiography, and computed tomography angiography for diagnosis and assessment of symptomatic, lower limb peripheral arterial disease: systematic review. BMJ 2007; 334(7606):1257.

**A systematic review was performed of high-quality studies, with 58 meeting the inclusion criteria. CE-MRA was more specific that CTA and more sensitive than DUS and was generally preferred by patients over contrast angiography. Where available, CE-MRA might be a viable alternative to contrast angiography.**

28. Visser K, Hunink MG et al. Peripheral arterial disease: gadolinium enhanced MR angiography versus color-guided duplex US – a meta-analysis. Radiology 2000; 216:67–77.

29. ACC/AHA Guidelines for the Management of Patients with Peripheral Arterial Disease (Lower Extremity, Renal, Mesenteric, and Abdominal Aortic): a collaborative report from the American Association for Vascular Surgery/Society for Vascular Surgery, Society for Cardiovascular Angiography and Interventions, Society for Vascular Medicine and Biology, Society of Interventional Radiology, and the ACC/AHA Task Force on Practice Guidelines (Writing Committee to Develop Guidelines for the Management of Patients with Peripheral Arterial Disease). J Am Coll Cardiol 2006; 47(6):1239–312.

30. Gerhard-Hermana M, Gardin JM, Jaff M et al. Guidelines for noninvasive vascular laboratory testing: a report from the American Society of Echocardiography and the Society for Vascular Medicine and Biology. Vasc Med 2006; 11:183–200.

31. Kohler TR, Nance DR, Cramer MM et al. Duplex scanning for the diagnosis of aortoiliac and femoropopliteal disease: a prospective study. Circulation 1987; 76:1074–80.

32. Cossman DV, Ellison JE, Wagner WH et al. Comparison of contrast arteriography to arterial mapping with color-flow duplex imaging in the lower extremities. J Vasc Surg 1989; 10:522–9.

33. Moneta GL, Yeager RA, Antonovic R et al. Accuracy of lower extremity arterial duplex mapping. J Vasc Surg 1992; 15:275–84.

34. Larch E, Minar E, Ahmadi R et al. Value of colour duplex sonography for evaluation of tibioperoneal arteries in patients with femoropopliteal obstruction: a prospective comparison with anterograde intraarterial digital subtraction angiography. J Vasc Surg 1997; 25:629–36.

35. Grassbaugh JA, Nelson PR, Rzucidlo EM et al. Blinded comparison of preoperative duplex ultrasound scanning and contrast arteriography for planning revascularization at the level of the tibia. J Vasc Surg 2003; 37:1186–90.

36. Wain RA, Berdejo GL, Delvalle WN et al. Can duplex scan arterial mapping replace contrast arteriography as the test of choice before infrainguinal revascularization? J Vasc Surg 1999; 29:100–9.

37. Ligush J Jr, Reavis SW, Preisser JS et al. Duplex ultrasound scanning defines operative strategies for patients with limb-threatening ischemia. J Vasc Surg 1998; 28:482–91.

38. European Society of Urogenital Radiology (ESUR) Guidelines on Contrast Media, version 6.0, February 2007.

39. McCullough PA, Adam A, Becker CR et al. Risk prediction of contrast-induced nephropathy. Am J Cardiol 2006; 98(Suppl 6A):27K–36K.

40. Thomsen HS, Morcos SK, Barrett BJ. Contrast-induced nephropathy: the wheel has turned 360 degrees. Acta Radiol 2008; 49(6):646–57.

41. Stacul F, Adam A, Becker CR et al. Strategies to reduce the risk of contrast-induced nephropathy. Am J Cardiol 2006; 98(Suppl 6A):1K–4K.

42. Aspelin P, Aubry P, Fransson S-G et al. Nephrotoxic effects in high-risk patients undergoing angiography. N Engl J Med 2003; 348(6):491–9.

43. Khun MJ et al. The PREDICT study: a randomized double-blind comparison of contrast-induced nephropathy after low- or isoosmolar contrast agent exposure. Am J Roentgenol 2008; 191(1):151–7.

**Two hundred and forty-eight patients with moderate to severe chronic kidney disease and diabetes mellitus were randomised to receive at least 65 mL of iopamidol 370 (low osmolar) or iodixanol 320 (iso-osmolar) for a CT procedure. There was no significant difference in the incidence of CIN at 48–72 hours after contrast administration.**

44. European Society of Urogenital Radiology (ESUR) Guideline. Gadolinium based contrast media and nephrogenic systemic fibrosis (17 July 2007)

opinion of **only** the Academic members of the ESUR Contrast Media Safety Committee.

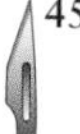

**45.** Koelemay MJ et al. Magnetic resonance angiography for the evaluation of lower extremity arterial disease. JAMA 2001; 285:1338–45.

A total of 34 studies met the inclusion criteria of being of high enough quality and included 1090 patients. 3D gradient echo MRA improved diagnostic performance compared with 2D MRA (relative diagnostic odds ratio 2.8 (95% CI: 1.2–6.4), adjusted for number of subdivisions within arterial tracts).

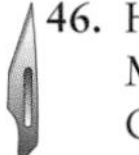

**46.** Heijenbrok-Kal MH, Kock MCJM, Myriam Hunink MG. Lower extremity arterial disease: multidetector CT angiography-meta-analysis. Radiology 2007; 245(2):433–9.

A total of 12 studies met the inclusion criteria. Multidetector CT angiography was used to evalulate 9541 arterial segments in 436 patients. The pooled sensitivity and specificity for detecting a stenosis of at least 50% per segment were 92% (95% CI: 89–95%) and 93% (95% CI: 91–95%) respectively. There was no significant difference in the diagnostic performance in the infrapopliteal segments from that in the aorto-iliac and femoropopliteal segments.

**47.** Kock MR, Adriaensen ME, Pattynama PM et al. DSA versus multi-detector row CT angiography in peripheral arterial disease: randomized controlled trial. Radiology 2005; 237(2):727–37.

**48.** Edwards M-B. 25 years of heart valve replacements in the United Kingdom. A guide to types, models and MRI safety. United Kingdom Heart Valve Registry. London: Hammersmith Hospital, 2000.

**49.** Seldinger S. Catheter replacement of the needle in percutaneous angiography. Acta Radiol 1953; 39:368–76.

# 3

# Medical treatment of chronic lower limb ischaemia

Cliff Shearman

## Introduction

Peripheral arterial disease (PAD) is an extremely common condition.

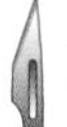

In the Edinburgh Artery Study of men and women aged 55–74 years of age, 4.5% had symptomatic PAD, in other words intermittent claudication. However, a further 8% had evidence of major asymptomatic disease and 16.6% had abnormal haemodynamic parameters suggesting minor PAD.[1] Five years later all new cases of intermittent claudication in the study group were in subjects previously found to have asymptomatic disease.[2]

This is encouraging as it suggests that there may be a window of opportunity in which to identify and try to slow or reverse the progression of PAD. In this study the prevalence of both symptomatic and asymptomatic PAD increased with age and was more common in lower socio-economic groups. Both of these are important issues to consider when comparing the treatment of PAD with other cardiovascular diseases.

Patients with symptomatic PAD have reduced mobility and quality of life which equates to some cancers, but PAD is also a powerful marker of cardiovascular risk, equating to angina.[3] In a survey of 1886 patients with PAD, 58% had coronary artery disease and 34% had suffered a cerebrovascular event.[4]

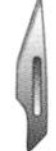

Overall, individuals with PAD are six times more likely to die from cardiovascular disease than those with no PAD.[5] Although the risk of a cardiovascular event increases in symptomatic patients the risk is also present for asymptomatic individuals.

Five years after diagnosis of PAD the mortality risk of the patient is twice that of a patient with breast cancer.

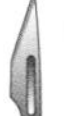

In the Reduction of Atherothrombosis for Continued Health (REACH) registry of patients with either known cardiovascular disease or who are at increased cardiovascular risk, the highest cardiovascular event rate was in the 5986 patients with PAD. At 1-year follow-up 18.2% of PAD patients had suffered a cardiovascular death, myocardial infarction (MI), a stroke or had been hospitalised for a cardiovascular event compared with 13.3% of the coronary artery disease group and 10% of the cerebrovascular disease group.[6] The group that had the highest cardiovascular event rates were those with evidence of polyvascular arterial disease, i.e. disease in three arterial beds (e.g. cerebral, cardiac and peripheral).

In summary PAD is present in over 29% of the adult population and in the majority is asymptomatic. Apart from the impact on the patient in those with symptoms, PAD also identifies patients at extremely high risk of cardiovascular events, particularly

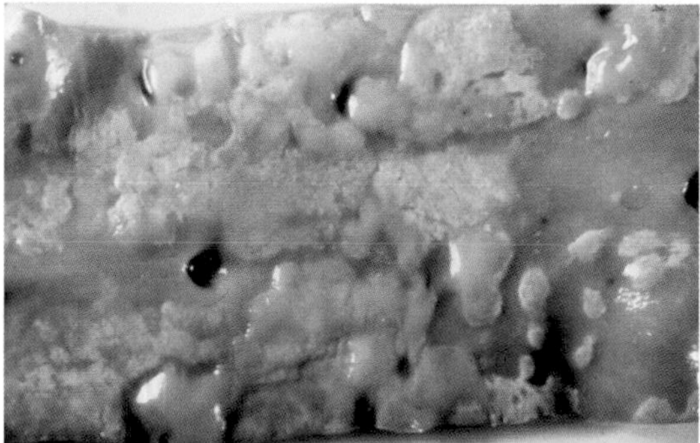

**Figure 3.1** • Early atheromatous changes in aorta of asymptomatic patient. Courtesy of Dr P. Gallagher.

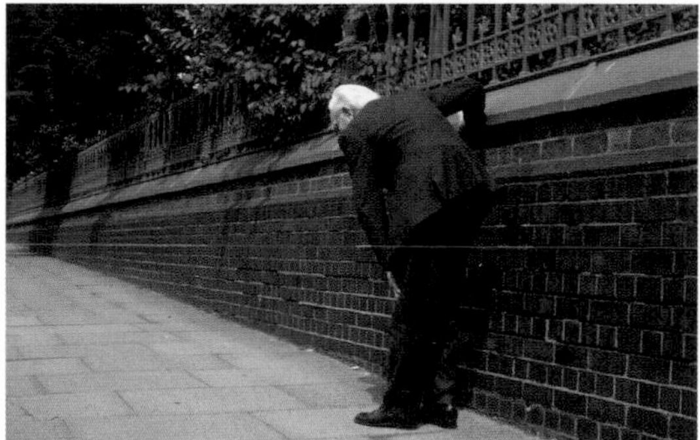

**Figure 3.2** • Patient handicapped by intermittent claudication.

if they have arterial disease elsewhere (**Fig. 3.1**). The key aims of treatment of PAD should be reduction of cardiovascular risk and improvement of the symptoms. Despite these stark figures, evidence suggests that many patients with PAD remain undiagnosed and even those who have been identified get suboptimal treatment especially when compared to patients with coronary artery disease.[7] This chapter will address the diagnosis and detection of PAD, factors affecting cardiovascular risk and medical treatments that may improve the symptoms of PAD.

## PAD diagnosis and screening

Identification of PAD may be relevant to three patient groups. Firstly, in patients who present with primary symptoms affecting the legs who are at increased cardiovascular risk and may also be suitable for treatment of their claudication. Secondly, patients already at increased cardiovascular risk (e.g. after MI or stroke) when the diagnosis of PAD identifies a subgroup (polyvascular disease) who are at extremely high risk of cardiovascular events. The final group is asymptomatic patients in whom the identification of PAD may allow attempts to reduce cardiovascular risk and prevent disease progression. The evidence of identifying arterial disease in each of these groups is examined.

In symptomatic patients the diagnosis of PAD can be made on the history and examination. Typical muscular pain in the calf or thigh and buttocks on walking, combined with absent lower limb pulses, is strongly suggestive of PAD (**Fig. 3.2**). However, many patients have comorbidities, such as arthritis, which can confuse the history and pulse palpation may be difficult. Based on the above clinical criteria PAD will be underdiagnosed, and objective methods of assessment are needed.[8] Measurement of the ankle–brachial pressure index (ABPI) has been shown to be a reproducible method of confirming the diagnosis and is widely applicable in primary and secondary care[9] (**Fig. 3.3**).

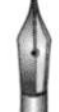

Despite the ease of diagnosis many symptomatic patients go unrecognised and remain at increased cardiovascular risk. Ironically it is often not until the patient with PAD develops coronary heart disease (CHD) or stroke that they begin to receive correct treatment. Even those with identified PAD often go untreated, identifying a lack of awareness amongst physicians and patients.

This lack of awareness of the significance of PAD is also reflected at a national level. In the UK reduction of cardiovascular deaths is a stated aim of the Government. There are financial incentives through the General Medical Services (GMS) contract in primary care to identify and treat risk factors in patients with CHD and stroke. PAD, however, does not appear in this contract and it is estimated that about one-third of patients with PAD will not be picked up by the CHD and stroke registries. This approach contradicts the advice from most expert bodies.

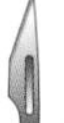

The Inter-Society Consensus for the Management of Peripheral Arterial Disease (TASC II) and a number of international expert bodies have recognised that PAD is a major health issue and should be identified and treated.[10–14]

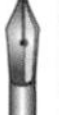

In patients with established CHD or stroke the identification of PAD places them in the highest risk group for further cardiovascular events. At present few patients with stroke or CHD are routinely screened for PAD.

The diagnosis of PAD in these groups would place them in an extremely high-risk group for further cardiovascular events and appropriate attention could be given to modifying their risk factors.

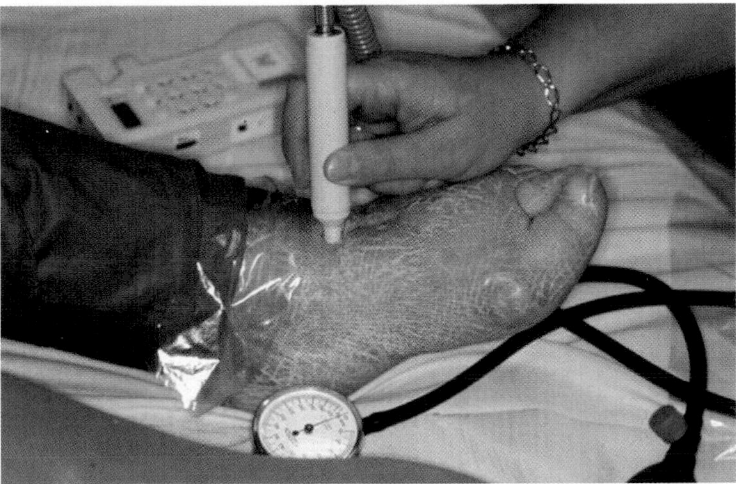

**Figure 3.3** • Measurement of ankle–brachial pressure index in a patient with PAD. The cuff is a standard 15-cm sphygmomanometer cuff just above the malleoli. In this case the anterior tibial artery is being insonated.

The observation that a reduced ABPI, even in asymptomatic patients, correlates with increased cardiovascular risk prompts the concept of screening the adult population.[15]

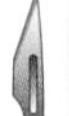

Also, the lower the ABPI the more likely is the patient to have polyvascular disease and hence the greatest cardiovascular risk.[16]

PAD is common in the adult population and identification using ABPI is a simple, inexpensive test. Perhaps one of the most attractive aspects of using ABPI is that it identifies a high-risk individual before they develop clinical problems such as angina, MI or stroke.

Although appealing, at present there is no evidence that screening the adult population in general for PAD using ABPI would be of benefit or cost-effective and further work is needed to clarify this. However, the evidence seems very strong for the measurement of ABPI in all patients with leg pain on walking, or with evidence of coronary or cerbrovascular disease, and patients with risk factors known to increase cardiovascular risk (e.g. diabetes, hypertension and raised cholesterol).

## Modifying cardiovascular risk

There is overwhelming evidence for the benefits of identifying and correcting risk factors such as hypertension, dyslipidaemias, diabetes and obesity in patients with PAD. Active intervention to aid smoking cessation, increased exercise as well as the use of antiplatelet agents will result in a marked reduction in cardiovascular morbidity and mortality (see Chapter 1). Despite such evidence the delivery of this aspect of medical treatment remains poor. In the ongoing REACH registry of patients at increased cardiovascular risk principally being managed in primary care, only a minority of patients with PAD receive adequate medical treatment.[17] Even in patients referred to secondary care only 70% were on antiplatelet therapy and 44% taking a statin.[18] Perhaps most disappointing of all, even after secondary care involvement there still remains a number of patients receiving inadequate treatment. In a retrospective review of 109 patients who had undergone amputation due to PAD at the time of referral for prosthesis fitting only 41% had been prescribed a statin and only 60% were taking an antiplatelet agent; 39% of patients were on both a statin and antiplatelet agent, but 32% had been prescribed neither.[19]

Lay knowledge of PAD too is poor compared to CHD and stroke. In a group of 2501 adult Americans only 26% had ever heard of PAD. Of those with awareness of PAD 56% were aware it was associated with smoking and approximately 25% were aware it was linked to MI, stroke and amputation.[20] Secondary prevention clinics for CHD have been demonstrated to save lives and it seems reasonable to extrapolate this benefit to patients with PAD.[21]

## Medical treatments for symptomatic PAD

### Exercise

Exercise is widely held to be of benefit to patients with PAD and not only improves walking distance but may also help reduce cardiovascular mortality.

Unfortunately only 27% of vascular surgeons have access to such programmes.[22]

There is good evidence for the improvement in muscle function, vascular endothelial cell function and metabolic adaptations with exercise.[23]

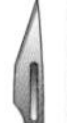

A meta-analysis of 21 studies of the effect of exercise on patients with intermittent claudication suggested an improvement in walking distance of 122%.[24] Supervised programmes in which the patient exercised for 30 minutes at least three times per week for 6 months had the most benefit. Programmes not directly supervised have less, if any benefit.[25]

Numerous mechanisms have been proposed for this apparent benefit including metabolic adaptation of the muscle, transformation of the muscle fibre type, increased muscle capillary blood flow and haemorheological factors such as a reduction in fibrinogen, but the optimum programme or method of exercise remains to be determined.

There are few well-controlled, randomised studies of exercise training compared with other therapies, but from what evidence there is exercise appears as good as, if not better than, other treatment.

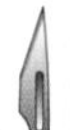

Angioplasty may offer some short-term benefit,[26] but exercise appears more effective at improving walking distance over the longer term. In a randomised controlled study of surgical revascularisation compared to surgery and exercise or exercise alone, the surgery and exercise group had the biggest improvement in walking distance. However, patients undergoing surgery had a 20% excess risk of adverse events.[27]

A sedentary lifestyle is a major risk factor for cardiovascular disease and individuals who undertake exercise on a regular basis have half the cardiovascular mortality risk of those who are inactive.[28] Although intensive exercise such as long distance running reduces cardiovascular risk markedly, moderate increases in activity also confer a significant benefit.[29] The National Institutes of Health conference on physical activity and health concluded that all children and adults should build up to a total of 30 minutes of moderate intense activity such as brisk walking each day.[30] Interestingly there is a direct correlation between levels of activity and ABPI, suggesting that a physically active lifestyle may help prevent PAD.[31] For adults who increase their activity there is evidence of a significant reduction in cardiovascular mortality compared to subjects who maintain a sedentary life style.[32] This benefit is lost if the subject becomes unfit again.

Exercise in patients with claudication is associated with increases in some inflammatory mediators, a type of ischaemia–reperfusion injury. On this basis it has been postulated that exercise may cause endothelial damage and even contribute to the high risk of cardiovascular events suffered by this group. However, regular supervised exercise has been shown not only to improve walking distance, but is associated with a significant reduction in serum markers of the periexercise inflammatory response, suggesting exercise has a positive effect.[33]

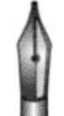

Exercise appears to be of established value in improving walking distance in patients with claudication. Although few patients have access to this therapy and compliance in patient groups remains low, when serious concerted attempts are made to address cardiovascular risk compliance improves.[34]

## Drug treatment

### Vasoactive drugs

A number of drugs have been marketed for the treatment of intermittent claudication and currently appear in the British National Formulary, in particular cilostazol and naftidrofuryl.[35] Currently the evidence base for cilostazol is the probably the strongest. Cilostazol is a phosphodiesterase inhibitor with antiplatelet, metabolic and vasodilatatory effects. In an early study 516 men and women with intermittent claudication were randomised to receive either cilostazol at a dose of 100 mg or 50 mg daily or placebo. After 24 weeks the higher dose treatment group had a 51% mean improvement in walking distance compared to placebo and the lower dose had a similar 38% improvement. The improvement in walking was reflected by an increase in quality-of-life scores.[36]

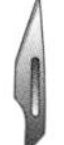

In a review of the evidence available from seven randomised controlled studies of cilostazol compared to placebo, there was again an improvement in walking distance but it tended to be relatively small, with a weighted mean difference between baseline and following treatment of 15.7–41.3 m depending on the dose.[37]

Although side-effects are relatively uncommon it is questionable whether this treatment is cost-effective and also what clinical utility these relatively small improvements have from the patient's perspective.

The results of the use of naftidrofuryl, a 5-hydroxytryptamine type 2 antagonist, have been contradictory, although a large meta-analysis of 888 patients showed a 26% improvement in walking distance above placebo.[38]

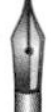

The use of agents such as cilostazol and naftidrofuryl varies across countries and is relatively low in the UK compared to other European countries. The reason for this is not entirely clear, but probably reflects doubt about the clinical value of the small increases in walking distance together with cost.

A range of other drugs and agents have been explored including vitamin E, buflomedil and carnitine without any firm evidence of benefit. Omega-3 fish oils have been found to reduce re-infarct rates after MI and reduce inflammation in atherosclerotic plaques. They have been explored in patients with PAD in uncontrolled studies, but there is no evidence to support their widespread use at present.[39]

Although primarily given for their lipid-lowering properties, plaque regression has been reported in studies when statins are given in high doses. Atovastatin 80 mg/day was shown to improve walking distance in patients with intermittent claudication.[40] Although interesting, it is unclear whether this is likely to be of clinical relevance. In studies of plaque regression in the coronary circulation very high doses of statins have to be administered to see an effect which is likely to be associated with increased side-effects.

### Prostanoids

Prostaglandin $E_1$ ($PGE_1$) and stable prostacyclin ($PGI_2$) have a number of properties which make them theoretically useful in the treatment of PAD. They are powerful vasodilators, have an anti- and disaggregatory effect on platelets and seem to optimise vascular endothelial function. $PGE_1$ is metabolised in the lung on first pass and so is usually administered bound to a carrier. $PGI_2$ has a half-life of 1–2 minutes and itself is of limited value. Iloprost is a stable prostacyclin analogue with a half-life of approximately 30 minutes. Both $PGE_1$ and iloprost are given intravenously and commonly cause side-effects of headaches, nausea, facial flushing and hypotension. Its use, therefore, is effectively confined to patients in a hospital setting and is labour intensive.

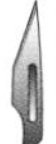

There have been several studies of both these agents in intermittent claudication without any evidence of benefit. In patients with critical limb ischaemia pain reduction, rate of ulcer healing, amputation and survival were advantaged by iloprost.[41] In 133 patients diagnosed with Buerger's disease (thromboangitis obliterans) there were significant improvements in terms of ulcer healing and pain relief compared to aspirin and placebo.[42]

## Angiogenesis

### Gene therapy

The development of new blood vessels in ischaemic tissue, therapeutic angiogenesis, has appeal in patients in whom conventional re-vascularisation procedures are not possible. A number of angiogenic growth factors have been identified and it is thought by raising levels of these at the site of potential collateral formation it may be possible to improve limb blood flow. It is possible to insert a gene coding for a growth factor into a DNA plasmid. These can either be injected as naked plasmids into the muscle of the ischaemic limb or via a viral vector such as human adenovirus. In early human trials using growth factors including vascular endothelial growth factor, fibroblast growth factor and platelet-derived growth factor there has been evidence of increased vascularity and limb blood flow. However, the trials are very small, uncontrolled and there are potential risks of new vessel growth at other sites such as the eye, and malignancy.[43]

### Cell therapy

Endothelial progenitor cells are attracted to sites of endothelial injury and ischaemia. They are involved with endothelial repair and new vessel growth. The origin of these cells is unclear but they can be identified from monocyte or endothelial origins. There is evidence to show that bone marrow-derived mononuclear cells, which include endothelial progenitor cells, are attracted to areas of ischaemia. Early reports suggest some benefit from intramuscular injection of these cells into ischaemic muscle. Studies are in the very early stage at present and it is too early to say whether this approach will have any clinical relevance.[43]

## Spinal cord stimulation

Spinal cord stimulation is a technique that can be used for chronic pain relief. An epidural electrode is inserted and connected to a stimulator box implanted beneath the skin. Based on the gate theory, stimulation of the spinal cord at the level of L3–4 is thought to reduce pain sensation and produces a sensation of warmth and paraesthesia in the limb. Implantation is relatively straightforward, but positioning the electrode to get pain relief can be difficult and getting the correct impulse frequency and strength may be problematic. Spinal cord stimulation is used primarily for intractable pain in patients with unreconstructable PAD. A single, large randomised controlled study of 120 patients failed to identify any benefit in terms of reduction of amputation or survival between the treatment and control groups.[44]

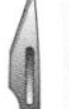

However, in an analysis of six studies involving 450 patients, a significant advantage (0.71 relative risk reduction) was shown in terms of limb salvage for the stimulation group and pain relief was also more marked.[45] However, 17% of patients undergoing spinal cord stimulation suffered complications of the treatment and the average cost of treatment at 2 years was €7900 more than the control group. On this basis the role of spinal cord stimulation seems limited to a few patients in whom reconstruction is not possible and amputation is not imminently threatened. However, the cost of the treatment is high.

## Lumbar sympathectomy

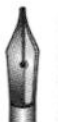

Sympathetic denervation of the lower limbs has been advocated as a treatment for patients unsuitable for reconstruction with critical limb ischaemia for many years. There has been little recent evidence produced for the role of sympathectomy and older studies found variable results in terms of pain relief.

## Intermittent pneumatic compression

Intermittent pneumatic compression of the calf and foot has been shown to increase popliteal artery blood flow. The mechanism for this is unclear but it is thought that the sustained reduction in venous pressure during treatment may be a factor. In one small study sustained benefits in terms of walking ability were found up to 12 months. Since the devices can be used by the patients in their own homes they may prove to be a useful therapy.[46]

## Conclusions

PAD remains underdiagnosed and undertreated. Considering how prevalent it is in the population this seems surprising, but there remains considerable lack of awareness of the significance of the condition amongst both clinicians and the public. The finding of PAD is an indication that the individual is at excess cardiovascular risk and there is overwhelming evidence for the role of risk factor management in this group. Exercise will improve walking distance in patients with claudication, appears as good as any other current therapy, and should certainly be offered to patients prior to other treatments. Other medical therapies may help but generally the benefit is either very modest or unproven. Prostanoids may be of help in some patients such as those with Buerger's disease. The key to improving the treatment of PAD seems to be in raising awareness of the condition and organising risk factor and lifestyle advice clinics.

### Key points

- 29% of the adult population over 55 years have PAD but only 4.5% are symptomatic.
- PAD can be easily identified by a reduced ABPI.
- A low ABPI is a marker of cardiovascular risk.
- Patients with leg pain on walking should have ABPI measured.
- Patients with established cardiovascular disease should have ABPI measured.
- Further evidence is needed to recommend screening of the adult population for reduced ABPI.
- Although all patients with PAD should receive aggressive management of their risk factors, currently less than 50% receive correct medical treatment.
- Exercise should be available and offered to patients with intermittent claudication.
- Drugs such as cilostazol may be of value in a small number of selected patients to improve walking.
- Prostanoids have a limited role but may be of help in patients with Buerger's disease.
- Angiogenesis is an exciting concept but at present needs considerable further evaluation.

## References

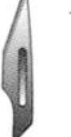

1. Fowkes FGR, Housley E, Cawood EHH et al. Edinburgh Artery Study: prevalence of symptomatic and asymptomatic peripheral arterial disease in the general population. Int J Epidemiol 1991; 20:384–91.

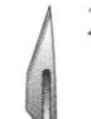

2. Leng GC, Lee AJ, Fowkes FGR et al. Incidence, natural history and cardiovascular events in symptomatic and asymptomatic peripheral arterial disease in the general population. Int J Epidemiol 1996; 25:1172–81.

These two reports from the Edinburgh Artery Study are important as they reveal the true prevalence of PAD in the community. The 5-year follow-up data also reinforce the high risk of cardiovascular events that these patients experience.

3. Belch JJ, Topol EJ, Agneli G et al. Prevention of atherothrombotic disease network. Critical issues in peripheral arterial disease detection and management: a call to action. Arch Intern Med 2003; 163:884–92.
4. Aronow WS, Ahn C. Prevalence of coexistent coronary artery disease, peripheral artery disease and atherothrombotic brain infarction in men and women ≥62 years of age. Am J Cardiol 1994; 74:64–5.
5. Criqui MH, Langer RD, Fronek A et al. Mortality over a period of 10 years in patients with peripheral arterial disease. N Engl J Med 1992; 326:381–6.

This is an important study of 565 men and women over a 10-year period. All subjects with evidence of PAD had a significantly increased risk of cardiovascular death. Those with the most severe disease had a 15-fold increased risk of cardiovascular death.

6. Steg PhG, Bhatt DL, Wilson PWF, et al One-year cardiovascular event rates in outpatients with atherothrombosis. JAMA 2007; 297:1197–206.

The REACH registry is important as it is a contemporaneous registry of the outcome and treatment of over 68000 patients worldwide at increased risk of cardiovascular events. Interestingly the group with PAD appears to have the highest morbidity and mortality compared to coronary heart disease and cerebrovascular disease.

7. Hirsch AT, Criqui MH, Treat-Jacobsen D et al. Peripheral arterial disease detection and awareness and treatment in primary care. JAMA 2001; 286:1317–24.
8. Criqui MH, Fronek A, Klauber MR et al. The sensitivity, specificity, and predictive value of traditional clinical evaluation of peripheral arterial disease: results from noninvasive testing in a defined population. Circulation 1985; 71:516–22.
9. Caruana MF, Bradbury AW, Adam DJ. The validity, reliability, reproducibility and extended utility of ankle to brachial pressure index in current vascular surgical practice. Eur J Vasc Endovasc Surg 2005; 29:443–51.
10. Hirsch AT et al. ACC/AHA 2005 guidelines for the management of patients with peripheral arterial disease (lower extremity, renal mesenteric and abdominal aortic): executive summary. JACC 2006; 47:1239–310.
11. Abrahmson CL et al. Canadian Cardiovascular Society Consensus Conference: peripheral arterial disease – executive summary. Can J Cardio 2005; 21:997–1006.
12. Scottish Intercollegiate Guideline Network (SIGN 89). Diagnosis and management of peripheral arterial disease. A national clinical guideline, 2006.
13. Norgren L, Hiatt WR, Dormandy JA et al. Inter-Society consensus for the management of peripheral arterial disease (TASC II). J Vasc Surg 2007; 45(Suppl S):S5–67.
14. JBS 2. Joint British Societies Guidelines on prevention of cardiovascular disease in clinical practice. Heart 2005; 91:Suppl V.

The guidelines outlined in Refs 10–14 all identify PAD as a major cardiovascular risk which should be treated the same way as other risk factors.

15. Heald CL, Fowkes FG, Murray GD et al. Ankle brachial index collaboration. Atherosclerosis 2006; 189:61–9.
16. Fowkes FGR, Low L-O, Tuta S et al. on behalf of AGATHA Investigators. Ankle brachial index and the extent of atherothrombosis in 8891 patients with or at risk of vascular disease: results of the international AGATHA study. Eur Heart J 2006; 27:1861–7.

This large international study recruited 8891 patients. They found that the ABPI was related to the risk profile of the patient and a low ABPI was associated with arterial disease in more that one bed.

17. Bhatt DL, Steg PG, Ohman E et al. International prevalence, recognition, and treatment of cardiovascular risk factors in outpatients with atherothrombosis. JAMA 2005; 295:180–9.
18. Khan S, Flather M, Mister R et al. Characteristics and treatments of patients with peripheral arterial disease referred to UK vascular clinics: results of a prospective registry. Eur J Vasc Endovasc Surg 2006; 33:442–50.
19. Bradley L, Kirker SGB. Secondary prevention of arteriosclerosis in lower limb vascular amputees: a missed opportunity. Eur J Vasc Endovasc Surg 2006; 32:491–3.
20. Hirsch AT, Murphy TP, Lovell MB et al. Gaps in public knowledge of peripheral arterial disease. The first national PAD public awareness survey. Circulation 2007; 116:2086–94.
21. Murchie P, Campbell NC, Ritchie LD et al. Secondary prevention clinics for coronary heart disease: four year follow up of a randomised controlled trial in primary care. BMJ 2003; 326:84.

Patients with a history of coronary heart disease ($n$ = 1343) were randomised to receive an invitation to attend a secondary prevention clinic or continue usual care. The mean follow-up was 4.7 years. A reduction in deaths and coronary events was found in the intervention group (proportional hazards ratio 0.76 for coronary events).

22. Stewart AHR, Lamont PM. Exercise for intermittent claudication. BMJ 2001; 323:703–4.
23. Stewart K, Hiatt W, Regensteiner J. Exercise training for claudication. N Engl J Med 2002; 347:1941–51.
24. Gardner AW, Peohlman ET. Exercise rehabilitation programs for the treatment of claudication pain. JAMA 1995; 274:975–80.

This meta-analysis still remains the best evidence for advising exercise in patients with claudication. Based on this TASC II (recommendation 14) states: 'supervised exercise should be made available as part of the initial treatment for all patients with peripheral arterial disease'. Attempts at larger studies of the role of exercise failed due to lack of recruitment of patients.

25. Bendermacher BLW, Willigendael EM, Teijink JAW et al. Supervised exercise therapy versus non-supervised exercise therapy for intermittent claudication. Cochrane Database Syst Rev 2006; issue 2, Art. No.:CD005263.DOI:10.1002/14651858.CD005263.pub2.
26. Fowkes FGR, Gillespie IN. Angioplasty (versus non-surgical management) for intermittent claudication. Cochrane Database Syst Rev 1998; issue 2, Art: CD000017.DOI:10.1002/14651858.CD000017.

    There have been two trials involving 98 patients randomised to angioplasty versus exercise or angioplasty compared with medical treatment. At 6 months the angioplasty group had higher ABPIs than the non-angioplasty group. However, despite a long-term follow-up over a year there was no identifiable benefit in terms of walking distance.

27. Lundgren F, Dahllof A-G, Lundholm K et al. Intermittent claudication – surgical reconstruction or physical training? A prospective randomized trial of treatment efficiency. Ann Surg 1989; 209:346–55.

    Seventy-five patients were randomised in this study and follow-up was 1 year. Patients who were operated on generally did better and more were likely to lose their symptoms completely. However, there was morbidity associated with the surgery and a number of patients did not complete exercise training. The added effects of exercise and surgery are interesting, but need further evaluation.

28. Powell KE, Pratt M. Physical activity and health. BMJ 1996; 313:126–7.
29. Winslow E, Bohannon N, Brunton SA et al. Lifestyle modification: weight control, exercise and smoking cessation. Am J Med 1996; 101(Suppl 4A):25S–33S.
30. NIH Consensus Development Panel on Physical Activity and Cardiovascular Health. NIH Consensus Conference: physical activity and health. JAMA 1996; 267:241–6.
31. Gardner AW. Physical activity is related to ankle/brachial index in subjects without peripheral arterial disease. Angiology 1997; 48:883–9.
32. Blair SN, Kohl HW, Barlow CE et al. Changes in physical fitness and all cause mortality: a prospective study of healthy and unhealthy men. JAMA 1995; 273:1093–8.
33. Tisi PV, Husle M, Chulakadabba A et al. Exercise training for intermittent claudication: does it adversely affect biochemical markers of the exercise induced inflammatory response. Eur J Vasc Endovasc Surg 1997; 14:344–50.
34. Noble J, Modest GA. Managing multiple risk factors: a call to action. Am J Med 1996; 101(Suppl 4A):79S–81S.
35. British National Formulary. March 2006; 51:115–16.
36. Beebe HC, Dawson DL, Cutler BS et al. A new pharmacological treatment for intermittent claudication: results of a randomized multicentre trial. Arch Intern Med 1999; 159:2041–50.
37. Robless P, Mikhailidis DP, Stansby GP. Cilostazol for peripheral arterial disease. Cochrane Database Syst Rev 2007; issue 1, Art. No.:CD003748. DOI:10.1002/14651858.CD003748.pub3.

    From all the controlled studies of cilostazol there seems to be a benefit in walking distance above placebo. However, the differences tend to be small and although quality-of-life scores tend to improve the cost-effectiveness of these relatively small increases has not been established.

38. Lehert P, Comte S, Gamand S et al. Naftidrofuryl in intermittent claudication. J Cardiovasc Pharmacol 1994; 23(Suppl 3):S48–52.

    In this meta-analysis of 888 patients the improvement in absolute walking distance remains relatively small.

39. Sommerfield T, Price J, Hiatt WR. Omega-3 fatty acids for intermittent claudication. Cochrane Database Syst Rev 2004; issue 3, Art. No.:CD0038333. DOI:10.1002/14651858.CD003833.pub3.
40. Mohler ER, Hiatt WR, Creager MA. Cholesterol reduction with atorvastatin improves walking distances in patients with peripheral arterial disease. Circulation 2003; 108:1481–6.
41. Loosemore TM, Chalmers TC, Dormandy JA. A meta-analysis of randomized placebo control trials in Fontaine stages III and IV peripheral occlusive disease. Int Angiol 1994; 13:133–42.

    Overall, iloprost seemed to be of benefit in approximately 40% of patients treated. Patients who received iloprost were more likely to survive with their leg (55%) compared to the control group (35%). The response is variable, the treatment time-consuming and side-effects common, possibly explaining the low use of this drug. In the UK it has to be used off-licence on a named patient basis for the treatment of PAD. Based on this data TASC II (recommendation 28) suggests that prostanoids improve healing of ischaemic ulcers and reduce amputations in critical limb ischaemia.

42. Fiessinger JN, Schafer M. Trial of iloprost versus aspirin treatment for critical limb ischaemia of thromboangiitis obliterans. Lancet 1990; 335:555–7.

    In this study 87% of the treated group was thought to respond to treatment. Complete pain relief was obtained in 63% and 35% of the treatment group compared to 28% and 13% of the control group at 6 months.

43. Emmerich J. Current state and perspective on medical treatment of critical limb ischaemia: gene and cell therapy. Int J Lower Extremity Wounds 2005; 4:234–41.

44. Klomp HM, Spincemaille GH, Steyerberg EW et al. Spinal cord stimulation in critical limb ischaemia: a randomised trial. Lancet 1999; 353:1040–4.

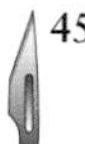
45. Ubbink DT, Vermeulen H. Spinal cord stimulation for non-reconstructable chronic critical leg ischaemia. Cochrane Database Syst Rev 2003; issue 3, Art. No.:CD004001.DOI:10.1002/14651858.CD004001.pub2.

This meta-analysis suggests that spinal cord stimulation may have a role in selected patients in whom the limb is not imminently going to be amputated but pain control is not possible by other means. Although expensive, this technique may be applicable to a small number of selected patients.

46. Ramaswami G, D'Ayala M, Hollier LH et al. Rapid foot and calf compression increases walking distance in patients with intermittent claudication: results of a randomized study. J Vasc Surg 2005; 41: 794–801.

# 4

# Intervention for chronic lower limb ischaemia

Anthony Nicholson
Julian Scott

## Introduction

This chapter will focus upon the role of endovascular and open surgery for chronic lower limb ischaemia. Exercise therapy is considered in Chapter 3. The decision to treat patients with chronic lower limb ischaemia by endovascular or open surgery will depend upon the severity of symptoms, associated comorbidity, technical considerations and evidence-based outcomes. Open surgery is usually reserved for patients in whom conservative or endovascular treatments are not an option or where they have failed to produce significant relief of symptoms. The basic principles of open vascular surgery include the identification of an adequate inflow, a suitable conduit and good run-off. These three elements, along with patient factors (fitness for surgery and lifestyle), should be applied to any decision-making prior to the offer of major reconstructive arterial surgery. In today's healthcare environments the issue of community and hospital acquired infections should be considered and all parties made aware of the implications of such a complication prior to any open vascular procedure.

## Patient selection

The symptoms of patients with chronic lower limb ischaemia can range from mild claudication to limb-threatening ischaemia. The decision to intervene in claudication will depend on walking distance, the patient's current lifestyle and their desire to regain their loss in quality of life. This has to be reviewed against the potential risk of any intervention, the long-term durability of the procedure and the need for further intervention. For instance, a 50-year-old businessman who claudicates at 400 metres might be severely handicapped if he can no longer play golf. Patients in their eighties with a claudication distance of 100 metres might not be handicapped if there is easy access to local amenities and a supportive family. These two scenarios highlight the importance of considering quality of life in the treatment equation. Box 4.1 summarises the factors influencing the decision to intervene in claudication.

Most patients with critical limb ischaemia (CLI) require some form of intervention. There are some situations when this would be inappropriate and these patients should not undergo unnecessary

Box 4.1 • Factors affecting the decision to intervene in claudication

**For**
Short walking distance
Employment affected
No improvement with exercise
Stenosis/short occlusion
Unilateral symptoms

**Against**
Short history
Still smoking
Other limiting conditions
Long occlusion/diffuse disease
Bilateral symptoms

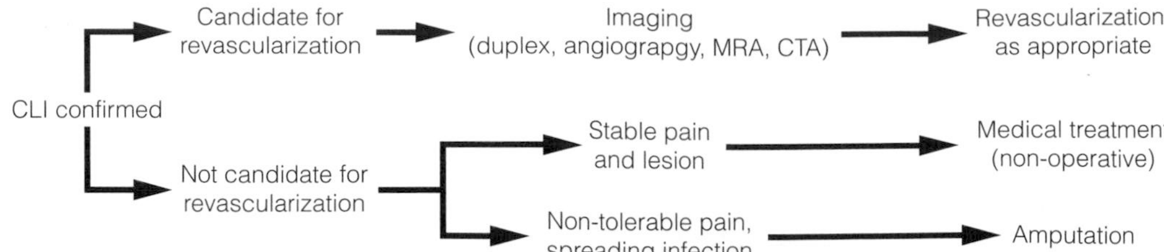


**Figure 4.1** • Algorithm for treatment of patients with critical limb ischaemia. CTA, computed tomography angiography; MRA, magnetic resonance angiography. Adapted from Norgren L, Hiatt WR, Dormandy JA et al. TASC II Working Group. Inter-Society Consensus for the Management of Peripheral Arterial Disease (TASC II). J Vasc Surg 2007; 45(Suppl S): S5–67. With permission from the Society for Vascular Surgery.

investigation. If the general condition of the patient is poor, and the chances of survival limited due to coexistent pathology, it seems reasonable to treat the patient with analgesia alone (**Fig. 4.1**). However, if the patient has a reasonable quality of life and is likely to survive for more than a few months, it is probably better to attempt revascularisation whenever possible. No one wishes to see a patient spend the remaining few months of life struggling with an amputation as well as their primary disease. Some patients present with such advanced ischaemia that there is little viable tissue left on the weight-bearing area of the foot. It is sometimes possible, with revascularisation and a customised forefoot amputation, to achieve a functional foot, but if this is not possible a primary amputation is the better option (see Chapter 5). In a few selected patients the foot can be salvaged with a free tissue transfer combined with revascularisation (**Fig. 4.2**). This is technically demanding and is usually performed in conjunction with the plastic surgeons. The chair- or bed-bound patient can provide a challenge when deciding on whether to intervene. Fixed flexion deformities and extensive tissue loss usually make amputation the best option. However, the rehabilitation team should be involved in this decision, as the patient's ability to transfer from a chair to the bed or toilet may depend on preservation of that limb.

Preoperative independence and mobility have been shown to best predict postoperative independence and mobility after infrainguinal bypass for CLI.[1] Only one of 25 survivors who were not living independently before surgery achieved independent living 6 months postoperatively. Therefore, there seems little point in undertaking extensive revascularisation in the hope of achieving independence for a patient already requiring care in a nursing home.

## Cost-effectiveness

The cost-effectiveness of any intervention requires careful evaluation. A retrospective analysis of CLI in elderly patients found that the hospital cost of reconstruction was nearly twice the cost of primary amputation.[2] However, if the community costs were added, amputation was more than twice as expensive, partly because 66% of reconstructed patients were able to return home compared to only 33% of amputees. A more recent prospective study also found that amputation was more expensive than revascularisation at 1 year.[3] There was little difference between the cost of successful endovascular treatment compared with surgical reconstruction, because the length of inpatient stay was related more to the state of the foot rather than the treatment received.

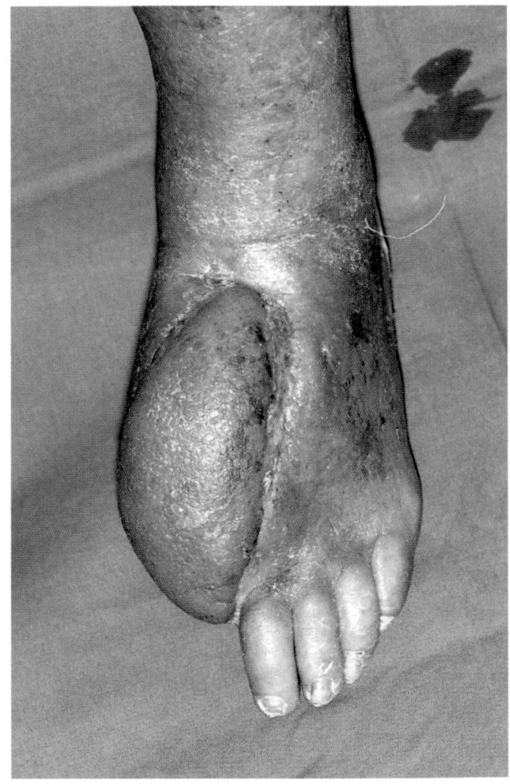

**Figure 4.2** • Lateral arm free flap used to resurface the medial aspect of the foot after femoro-distal bypass and ray amputation.

A prospective study of 150 patients with CLI found that activities of daily living and pain scores improved significantly after successful reconstruction and primary amputation, but mobility was only improved by successful reconstruction.[4] Thus, the improvement in the overall quality of life of those undergoing successful reconstruction seems largely due to better mobility. Patients whose reconstruction fails leading to secondary amputation fare badly, both in terms of quality of life and cost, emphasising the need for a high success rate if undertaking this type of reconstruction. This is especially true for infrainguinal bypass procedures. In one study, the surgical ideal of an uncomplicated infrainguinal bypass operation, with rapid relief of pain, swift wound healing, a rapid return to premorbid function and no further intervention, was only achieved in 16 of 112 patients.[5]

## TASC recommendations

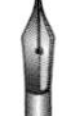

The Trans-Atlantic Inter-Society Consensus (TASC) Working Group and the Society of Interventional Radiology (SIR) have made recommendations for the type of lesion that is suitable or unsuitable for endovascular or open surgical treatment.[6,7]

There are differences between these recommendations but these are not particularly significant; they are summarised in Table 4.1. The recommendations have been updated to account for advances in endovascular techniques. Both classify peripheral arterial disease according to the level of the disease (e.g. aortic, iliac, femoro-popliteal or crural) and by the severity of the disease (e.g. types A–D). As the disease become more severe and/or more diffuse, the recommendations move from endovascular to open intervention:

- type A lesions should usually be treated by endovascular means;
- type B lesions should be preferentially treated by endovascular means;
- type C lesions should be preferentially treated by open revascularisation;
- type D lesions should usually be treated by open surgery.

For types B and C, this depends upon a patient's fitness, fully informed preference and operator's success rates.

## Suprainguinal endovascular intervention

### Abdominal aorta

Haemodynamically significant stenoses of the infrarenal aorta are rare and usually seen in short, obese female smokers with a hypoplastic aorta. Prior to

**Table 4.1** • Endovascular therapy or open surgery: summary of recommendations of the TASC II Working Group

| Segment/ recommendation | Usually PTA (type A) | PTA preferred (type B) | Surgery preferred (type C) | Usually surgery (type D) |
|---|---|---|---|---|
| Infrarenal aorta | | Stenosis ≤3 cm | | Aortic occlusion |
| Iliac (CIA/EIA) | Stenosis ≤3 cm | Stenosis 3–10 cm Unilat. CIA or EIA occlusion | Bilat. CIA occlusions Unilat. CIA + EIA occlusion | Bilat. EIA occlusions Disease extending into aorta and/or CFAs |
| Femoral | SFA stenosis ≤10 cm or | SFA stenosis or occlusion ≤15 cm | SFA stenosis or occlusion >15 cm | Complete SFA or popliteal occlusions |
| Popliteal | Occlusion ≤5 cm | Popliteal stenosis | Recurrent disease | |
| Crural | Crural interventions have severe outcomes if they go wrong. Therefore there is no category A or B | | Stenoses ≤4 cm or occlusions ≤2 cm | Diffuse disease or occlusions >2 cm |
| Outcomes | Excellent results can be expected from an endovascular approach in all segments | | PTA/stent only has modest results and is indicated when surgery is contraindicated for technical or patient reasons | Endovascular approach is not advised unless symptoms are limb-threatening and surgery is not possible |

The presence of calcification or multiple lesions generally moves a recommendation towards open surgery, e.g. type B to type C. CFA, common femoral artery; CIA, common iliac artery; EIA, external iliac artery; PTA, percutaneous transluminal angioplasty; SFA, superficial femoral artery.

the advent of endovascular therapies these patients would have undergone a localised aortic endarterectomy. Over time endovascular techniques have evolved from the 'kissing balloon' angioplasty technique to primary aortic stenting (**Fig. 4.3**). Both balloon angioplasty and primary stenting have acceptable durability, with 5-year patency rates of 50%.[8] Complications are rare and usually relate to embolisation, pseudo-aneurysm formation and recurrent disease.[9] Complete aortic occlusions are best treated by an aorto-bifemoral bypass (see later). In an unfit patient aorto-uni-iliac stenting, combined with a femoro-femoral crossover, may be a better alternative to an axillo-bifemoral bypass. Kissing stents can be used but there is a risk of one stent compressing the other.

## Iliac arteries

To evaluate the evidence base for aorto-iliac intervention the reader requires some knowledge of why interventional radiologists and vascular surgeons turned to percutaneous iliac intervention and why iliac stenting had such an impact from 1990 onwards. Observational and randomised studies have been used to evaluate the role of surgery and radiology; however, there are those who would dismiss observational studies on the basis that randomised controlled trials (RCTs) are seen as more reliable estimators of how well a treatment works. There is, however, evidence that observational studies do not overestimate the size of treatment effect when compared with their randomised counterparts.[10] In many instances concordance is better between RCTs and observational studies than that observed when meta-analysis of small randomised trials is compared to the results of large randomised trials.[11] For interventions that show significant side-effects in observational studies, randomised trials may be justifiably discouraged and never performed. Similarly for interventions that have already shown large beneficial treatment effects in observational trials the ethics of randomisation may be questioned. There are also interventions with such small effects that adequately powered randomised trials would not be possible to perform because of the sample size requirements. Here, only observational evidence may be generated.[12] Where does aorto-iliac evidence fit into this pattern? There would appear to be two aspects to the evidence: endovascular or open surgical reconstruction and percutaneous transluminal angioplasty (PTA) or stent.

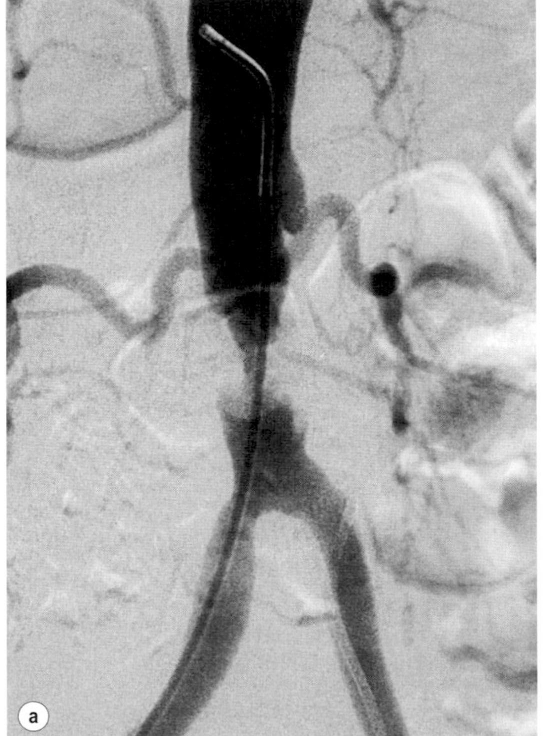


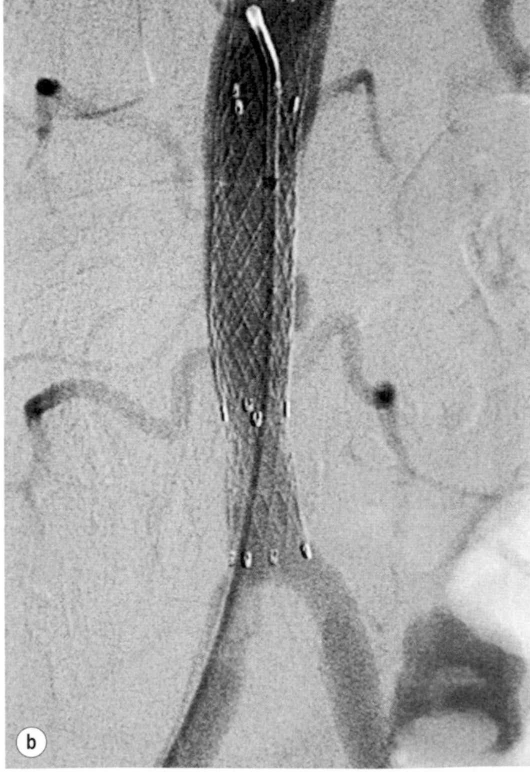


**Figure 4.3** • Localised infrarenal aortic stenosis **(a)** successfully treated with self-expanding nitinol stents **(b)**.

## The evidence for endovascular intervention

There are many observational studies in the literature, which suggest that both surgery and endovascular treatment are safe and efficacious in the aorto-iliac segments. However, the clinical differences shown are not great. Therefore RCTs should be the standard by which we decide which is best.

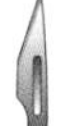

There is only one RCT which compares open surgery to angioplasty in symptomatic iliac disease.[13] In this study 263 men with iliac disease which was a major component to either rest pain or lifestyle-limiting claudication underwent either bypass surgery ($n$ = 123) or angioplasty ($n$ = 129). There were three deaths in the surgery group and none in the angioplasty group. There was no difference in patency and limb salvage rates, at a median follow-up of 4 years. The authors concluded that the lower morbidity and mortality rate in the angioplasty group supported the concept of angioplasty first strategy as outcomes between the two treatments were no different. The study was, however, limited by (i) the absence of women who have smaller arteries and (ii) the relative small numbers which precluded subgroup analysis.

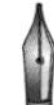

In a second, non-randomised comparative study the complication rate, primary patency and cost of stent deployment were compared with direct surgical reconstruction for the treatment of severe aorto-iliac occlusive disease.[14] Sixty-five patients underwent stent deployment and 54 patients had surgical reconstruction. No significant difference was observed between the groups in terms of clinical presentation, demographics and late complications. The cumulative primary patency rate for bypass grafts was, however, significantly better than for iliac stents at 18 months (93% vs. 73%), 30 months (93% vs. 68%) and 42 months (93% vs. 68%). Multivariate analysis suggested that females, anyone with ipsilateral superficial femoral artery (SFA) occlusion, and patients who had procedure-related vascular complications and hypercholesterolemia were more likely to thrombose their bypass graft or stent. Costs did not differ significantly.

So here we have two studies with very different conclusions. The first is an RCT and the second an observational study. It is difficult to determine which of the many variables in the observational study affected which group, and it is of course possible that patients who were less fit for open surgery were treated by endovascular means. The fact is that the literature regarding surgery or iliac intervention remains controversial.

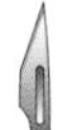

For this reason the TASC Working Group has looked at all the available evidence and concluded that endovascular treatment is the treatment of choice for type A aorto-iliac lesions and open surgical treatment for type D lesions.[7] The TASC considers that the evidence for the efficacy of one treatment instead of another was not sufficient for type B and C lesions.

## When is an iliac lesion significant?

The arteriographic grading of stenoses is hampered by wide intra- and inter-observer variability.[15] Intravascular ultrasound provides better measurements of cross-sectional area but it is expensive and not widely available. In theory, pressure gradient measurements at the time of angiography should be a relatively simple procedure. In practice there are several practical issues which may result in erroneous measurements, including bubbles in the transducer, the diameter of the catheter in comparison to the diameter of the stenosis and whether the catheter has end holes or side holes. As such there remains no consensus in the literature regarding what constitutes a significant pressure gradient[16] and there is little or no information on the role of vasodilators (doses), systolic vs. mean pressures and peripheral resistance in assessing stenotic vessels. Tetteroo et al. reported that they would have stented between 4% and 87% of their patients, emphasising the overall lack of consensus.[17] They suggested that a mean gradient of 10 mmHg at rest or after vasodilation should be used as a marker of significance and this is generally accepted, though there is no evidence at all for this.

## Who should have an angioplasty or a stent?

There are few data on the role of stents in focal aorto-iliac stenotic disease. Early aorto-iliac angioplasty had a high rate of embolic complications, particularly when dealing with occlusive rather than stenotic disease.[18] As a result stenting became the first-line treatment of iliac occlusive disease based on this observation. It could therefore be argued that the RCT is unethical in aorto-iliac occlusive disease. Nevertheless RCTs have been performed, but these have been compounded by flawed design and study methodology. Such a study demonstrated 4-year patency rates of 91.6% for stents and 74.3% for PTA alone, but the results have never been fully published.[19]

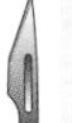

There is only one peer-reviewed, published RCT that compares primary stent placement with PTA followed by stent placement if needed in the iliac arteries. The Dutch Iliac Stent Trial (DIST)[20] randomised patients to either a primary Palmaz stent or PTA alone.

In the latter group stents were reserved for patients with suboptimal PTA results. The authors reported that 43% of patients randomised to PTA received iliac stents and that 2-year cumulative patency rates for the two groups were similar at 71% vs. 70%. They concluded that because angioplasty followed by selective stent placement is less expensive than primary stent placement, the former should be the treatment of choice for lifestyle-limiting intermittent claudication caused by iliac artery occlusive disease. However, only 29 iliac artery occlusions were treated among 279 patients, and by study design, patients with occlusions more than 5 cm in length were ineligible for enrolment. Even with that strict length threshold for eligibility, 10 of the 12 subjects (83%) with occlusions failed PTA alone. Although stents seem to offer special benefits in the treatment of longer segment lesions, little guidance about such patients is therefore provided by this trial. Furthermore, most patients in the DIST study had mild clinical symptoms, and only 22% of patients in each group were classified as having Society for Vascular Surgery/International Society for Cardiovascular Surgery (SVS/ISCVS) grade 3–5 ischaemia. Only 10% of patients had diabetes, and only 10% had simultaneous iliac artery disease and occlusion of the ipsilateral SFA. The mean pretreatment resting ankle brachial index in both groups was 0.77. As a consequence, the milder pattern of atherosclerotic disease observed in the DIST study differed from that encountered in many interventional practices. In addition the study was designed to have a 90% likelihood of detecting a 10% difference in post-treatment arterial patency after 12 months between the two groups (power = 90%). Unfortunately, because of inadequate recruitment and funding, the trial was terminated after less than 80% of the intended sample had been enrolled. Outcome information after as little as 1 year is available in the published report for about 60% of subjects who ultimately enrolled, a fraction that actually represents less than 45% of the intended patient sample. Thus, even though the authors did not observe 'substantial differences' in clinical outcomes between their experimental groups, the DIST study was more likely to miss than to detect the same potential 10% improvement in 12-month patency rates that was used to configure the trial as the actual power was less than 50%. Because of under-recruitment, the authors attempted to amplify their sample by reporting the number of lesions treated, rather than the number of subjects actually involved. For example, a patient with simultaneous common and external iliac stenoses or occlusions was classified as two treated lesions, rather than as a single person. As a result, little information about crucial patient subgroups (e.g. occlusions vs. stenoses, common iliac vs. external iliac lesions) can be gleaned from this report. Despite these problems the authors continued to publish from the original dataset, reporting patency rates and patient survival at 5 years.[21]

There is a recently completed second RCT of stent versus angioplasty in complete iliac occlusions (the STAG Trial). This is not yet published, but a personal communication from the authors suggests that there are significantly fewer major complications, particularly embolisation, following stent compared to PTA, but that stents confer no benefit in terms of patency (P. Gaines, personal communication). If so, we are brought full circle to the original premise that stenting infers benefits in terms of reduced complications in iliac occlusions, rather than improved patency. Though the authors are not in a position to comment until the publication of this study, much will depend on the original design and power of the study in terms of its primary and secondary end-points.

As stated it would be very wrong to ignore observational data when considering the evidence.

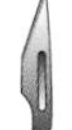

A meta-analysis of such studies has been performed.[22]

This found a better technical success rate for stent (97%) rather than PTA (91%) ($P < 0.05$). It also found a better overall 4-year primary patency for iliac stents in critical limb ischaemia (67% vs. 35%), though this was not the case for claudicants (77% vs. 65%). This emphasises the need for significant subgroup analysis in any study. A cost-effectiveness analysis[23] of aorto-iliac stenotic disease suggested that PTA and selective stent insertion for suboptimal results is the most cost-effective option, but did not deal specifically with technically more difficult and potentially complicated occlusive disease.

## What conclusions can we draw from the evidence?

- We should defer to the TASC recommendations most of the time.
- Consideration should be given to the clinical state of the patient when considering open or endovascular surgery.

- Aorto-iliac stenoses should be angioplastied, reserving stents for residual gradients greater than 10 mmHg after vasodilators.
- Aorto-iliac occlusions are best stented to reduce complications.

## Iliac stenoses

In the case of iliac stenotic disease, PTA alone should be the procedure of choice in stenotic disease. On the basis of the diagnostic angiogram, measurements can be taken from the image to determine the size of the vessel and the length of the lesion. Oversizing should be avoided as this leads to pain and increases the possibility of rupture. Once arterial access has been achieved 3–5000 units of heparin should be administered via the arterial sheath. At the time of balloon inflation the patient should be advised that if they feel any pain then the inflation will be stopped. Pain is indicative of adventitial stretching and may herald arterial rupture (see 'Complications' section).

The end-point for aorto-iliac revascularisation procedures is determined by intra-arterial haemodynamic measurements, which are readily obtained in this arterial segment. Ideally, simultaneous waveforms obtained above and below the treated segment should overlap, with no mean or systolic gradient (**Fig. 4.4**). Generally, most patients have some separation of the waveforms at peak systole, with a slightly more rounded peak observed distally. The systolic gradient usually measures between 1 and 3 mmHg, but the mean gradient may still be zero. Because of the variability in blood pressure over even short intervals of time, repositioning a single catheter across a lesion and measuring pressures at different times is an unreliable way to obtain pressure measurements.

Often, ideal haemodynamic results are not achieved because of recoil or patient intolerance to balloon inflation to a calibre consistent with elimination of the gradient. This situation may demand a stent of suitable diameter and length. Balloon-mounted stents are normally preferred in this situation, though self-expanding stents may be desirable if the problem is intolerance.

It should, however, be understood that in CLI there may be favourable outcomes even when borderline pressure gradients remain after intervention, because almost any haemodynamic improvement tips the scales in favour of wound healing or symptomatic relief. In these patients, such a result is preferred over a prolonged procedure with increased risk of complications. An emergency surgical procedure should clearly be avoided. Conversely, patients who complain of intermittent claudication often have mild residual symptoms if a trans-stenotic gradient of more than a few millimetres of mercury persists. Injection of vasodilators to assess results of an intervention can be informative when the results are borderline in patients with intermittent claudication. A gradient of less than 8–10 mmHg mean after intra-arterial injection of 0.2 mL of nitroglycerine is considered a satisfactory result.

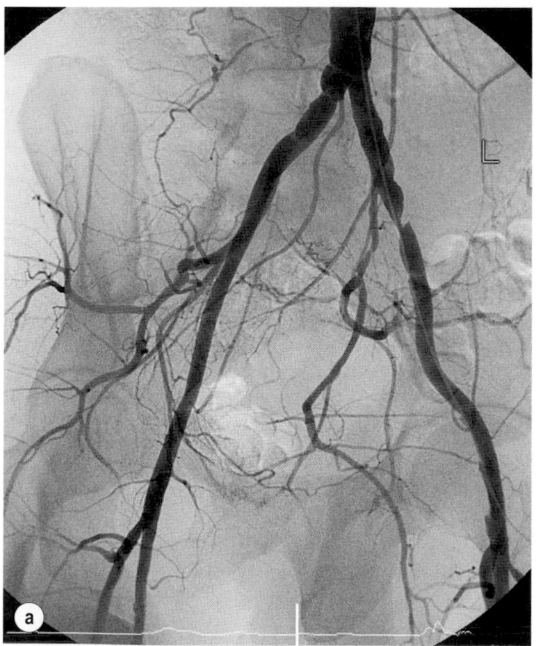


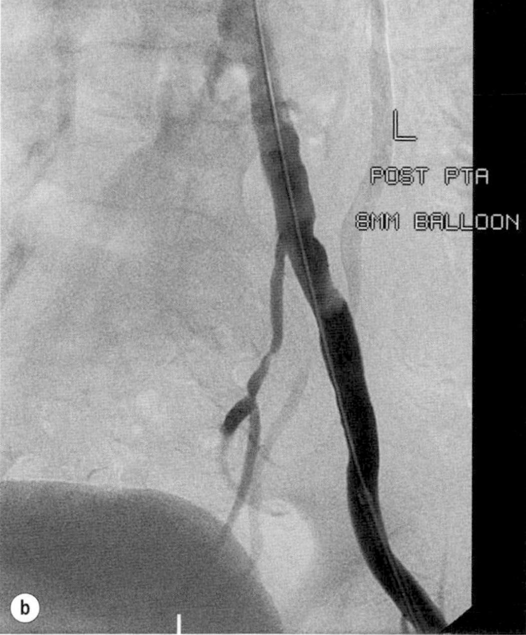


**Figure 4.4 • (a)** There is a severe focal stenosis of the left external iliac artery. **(b)** After balloon dilatation there is minor residual stenosis. However, there is no pressure gradient across the lesion and stenting is not required.

## Iliac occlusions

Chronic iliac occlusions can be crossed from the ipsilateral or contralateral side and stented to reduce the risk of embolic complications. This requires the insertion of a stent prior to PTA (**Fig. 4.5**). Self-expanding stents (e.g. Cook Zilver, Bard Luminexx, Cordis SMART) are indicated and in the authors' experience this will always traverse the chronic occlusion over the wire. Again heparin is mandatory immediately after arterial access. Once a stent of appropriate diameter and length has been deployed it can then be inflated with a suitable sized balloon. If there is a suitable iliac stump of the ostium, a uni-iliac stent will work well. If, however, the occluded iliac artery does not have a stump and the aortic lumen tapers smoothly to the occlusion, then 'kissing' iliac stents may have to be used, even when the contralateral iliac artery does not have a significant stenosis.[24] This should be avoided if at all possible. Early results are good[25] but, in small arteries, the long-term patency is not as good as uni-iliac stenting. The external iliac artery is slightly more prone to rupture than the common iliac, but responds well to stenting.

## Complications

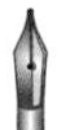

The British Iliac Angioplasty Study (BIAS)[26] followed 1135 patients for 12 months. The complication rate was 20.4%, though no treatment was required in 15.2% of these, of which the majority were small groin haematomas. Only 2.8% required surgery or a transfusion and 2.6% required further endovascular treatment. Importantly, arterial perforation occurred in four patients. Two of these had covered stents inserted and survived. The other two died, giving an overall mortality of 0.17%.

### Bleeding

Bleeding may occur locally at the site of the puncture (haematoma/false aneurysm) or track away (e.g. retroperitoneal space). In the latter, massive blood loss can occur without any obvious immediate clinical signs until they decompensate. Patients who report pain in the groin in the absence of any clinical signs should be carefully observed as this may imply nerve irritation as a result of an expanding haematoma in the retroperitoneal space. A pulsatile mass at the puncture site should be assessed by ultrasound to ascertain (i) the size, (ii) size of the neck and (iii) the presence or absence of an arteriovenous fistula. For small lesions, careful observation may be advocated as many of these lesions will spontaneously close.

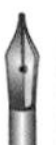

Ultrasound-guided compression can be used; however, success is limited to 60–70% of patients who are anticoagulated.[27]

In addition compression may be limited by a combination of pain and a wide defect in the arterial wall.

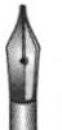

In these situations the management options include (i) thrombin injection, (ii) endovascular stent graft and (iii) open surgery.[28]

### Arterial rupture

One of the most dramatic and (fortunately) infrequent complications of angioplasty and stenting is arterial rupture. Arterial rupture is most often an immediate event with dramatic symptoms of pain and hypotension. However, subacute and chronic presentations are also possible. There are several risk factors for arterial rupture. Steroid therapy is a commonly recognised risk factor. Other conditions that weaken the arterial wall include the presence of fibromuscular dysplasia, adjacent inflammatory arterial changes or infection of the arterial wall. Mechanical factors also contribute. Overdistension of the artery by the use of too large a balloon is a commonly stated concern. However, in most reported cases of rupture, the authors had thought that the balloon was appropriately sized. Rupture of the PTA balloon may also contribute to the arterial rupture. This is caused by sudden delivery of a high-pressure jet at a focal point from the hole in the balloon. In some cases, surgeons operating to repair a rupture have identified large, sharp or densely calcified atherosclerotic plaques that probably sliced though the arterial wall during balloon inflation. Prior mechanical trauma, such as laser recanalisation or balloon thrombectomy, may predispose to arterial rupture either by actual perforation or by weakening of the arterial wall. The most important first step to managing an arterial rupture is recognition of the problem. This allows rapid response and control of the situation before excessive haemorrhaging occurs. Often, when rupture occurs during PTA, the patient experiences severe pain. Interestingly, the pain may relate not to the rupture itself but to the pressure caused by blood leaking out of the artery. Reinflation of the angioplasty balloon to tamponade the leak often leads to immediate relief of the pain. In some cases pain also causes immediate systemic symptoms, such as bradycardia, diaphoresis and decreased level of consciousness. Unfortunately, one cannot rely on such dramatic symptoms to herald a rupture. Cases of rupture have occurred with the patient having no pain or other symptoms. Thus, it is very important to perform an arteriogram immediately after angioplasty. Gross extravasation of contrast is generally seen in cases of frank rupture (**Fig. 4.6**). A secondary fluoroscopic sign is medial displacement and effacement of a contrast-filled bladder secondary to mass effect from the retroperitoneal haemorrhage. Once an arterial rupture is recognised, rapid action is required to prevent death. Maintaining a wire across a PTA site until the result has been assessed is vital.

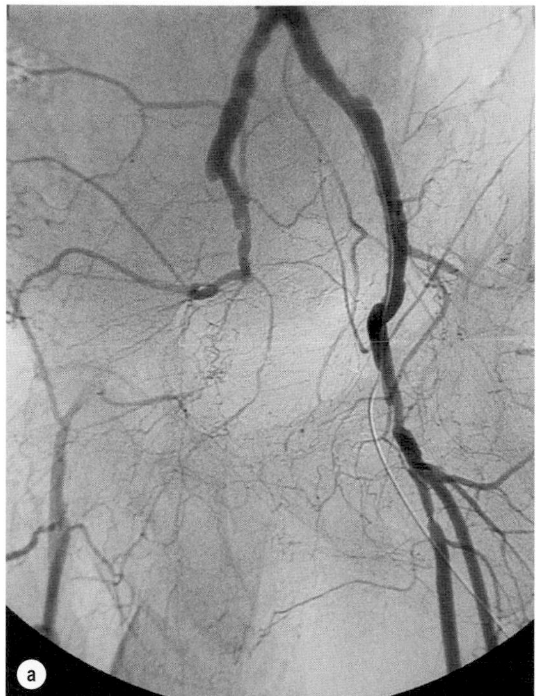


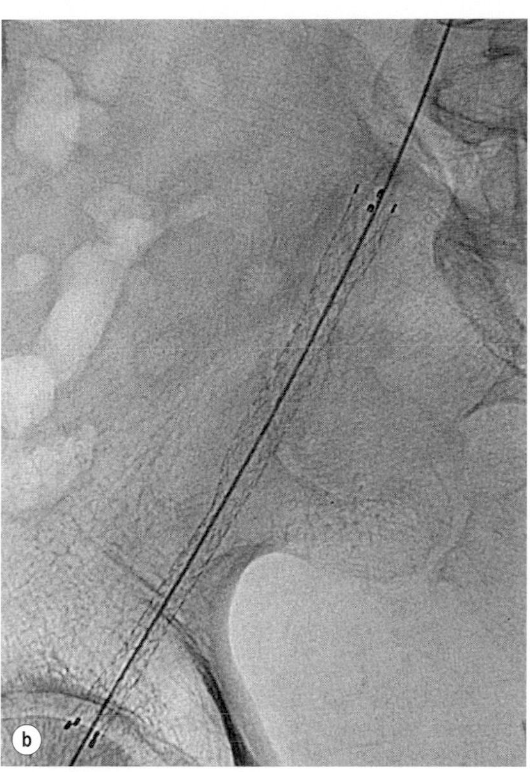


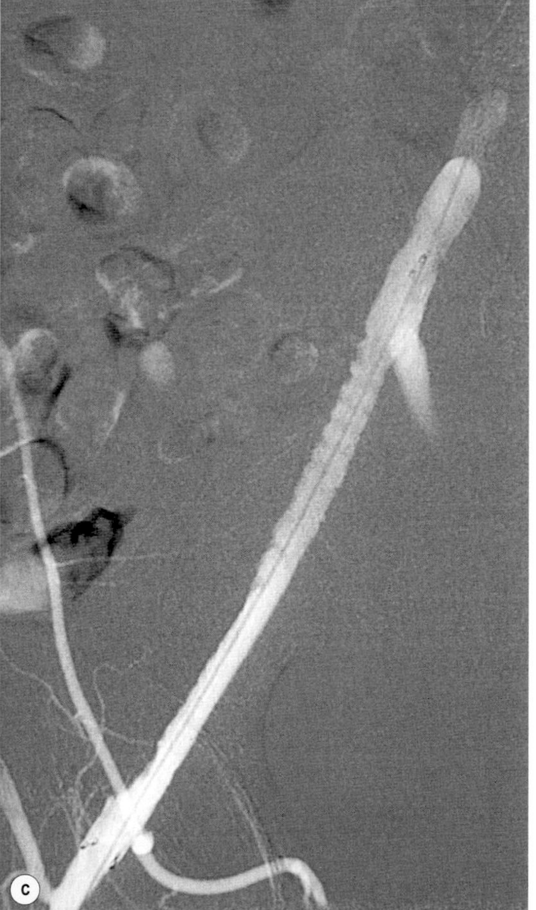


**Figure 4.5** • Long right iliac occlusion **(a)** successfully treated with a self-expanding nitinol stent **(b)**, showing appearance after percutaneous transluminal angioplasty of the stent **(c)**.

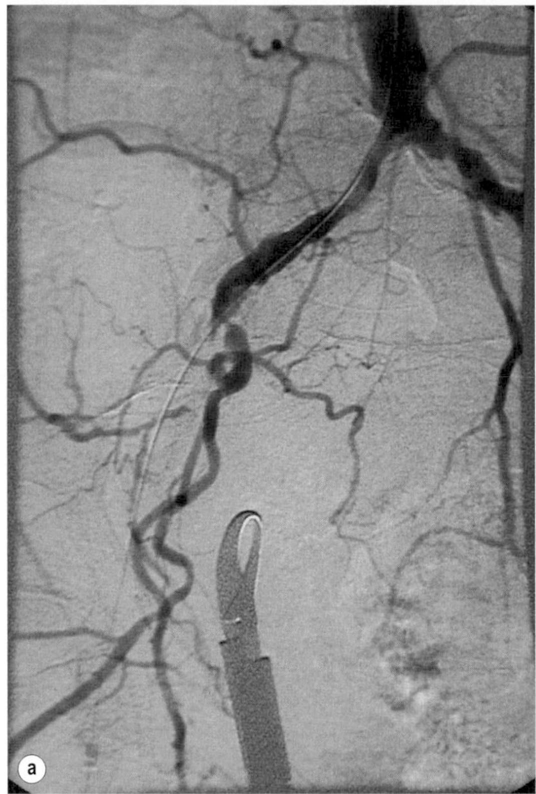


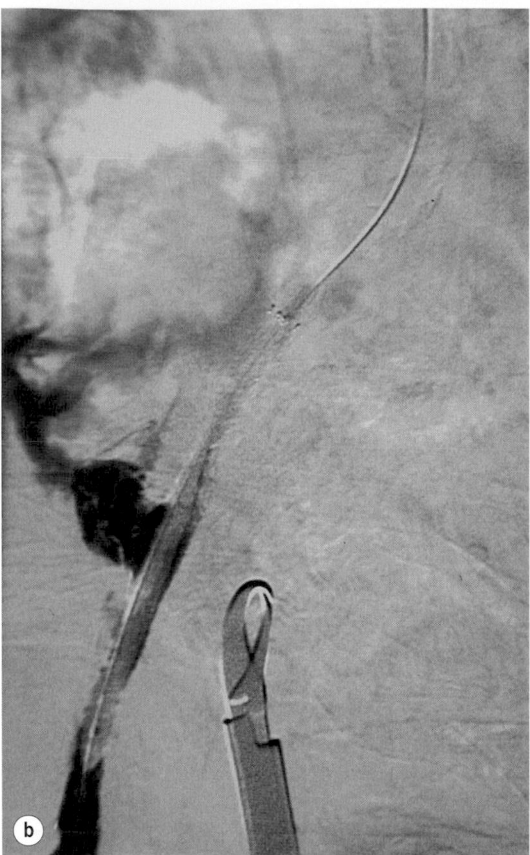


**Figure 4.6** • Angiogram showing an occlusion of the right external iliac artery **(a)** and rupture following balloon dilatation **(b)**. Control was achieved with an occlusion balloon **(c)** and the artery repaired with a covered stent **(d)**.

Having a wire past the disruption will allow one to gain immediate control of the situation. Tamponade of the leak can usually be easily achieved by inflating a balloon across the area of rupture, most often the same balloon that was used for angioplasty. However, one should not assume that this same-size balloon will suffice. Thus, arteriography should be performed both proximally and distally to the rupture to ensure tamponade. Because patients may have hypotension or bradycardia, the operator must also attend to resuscitation with intravenous fluids and/or atropine as needed. Once the haemorrhage is controlled and the patient has been resuscitated, attention can be turned to definitive therapy. In the past ruptures were managed surgically with either patching of the vessel or with ligation and bypass. However, balloon tamponade described above may also provide definitive treatment, though with the risk of thrombus formation and embolisation. In the modern era of endovascular therapy, the most elegant potential solution to arterial rupture is endovascular grafting. Obviously, for this to be a viable option, one must have an endovascular graft readily available. An alternative to stent grafting is the deployment of a bare metallic stent. This probably works by compressing the arterial wall layers against each other, thus sealing the leak. One must remember, however, that several cases of arterial rupture have reportedly occurred during primary stent deployment. Having graft material as an impermeable barrier to cover the arterial rent would certainly seem to be preferable to the use of a bare metal stent. Although arterial rupture would seem to be a catastrophic event, almost all of the reported cases have been successfully managed without loss of life or limb.

## Embolisation

Embolisation occurs in 3–7% of patients,[26] is more common in occlusive disease and may be avoided by preliminary dilatation before deployment of a self-expanding stent. The nature of the emboli (plaque, thrombus, or cholesterol) determines the success of the different therapeutic options. Local thrombolytic infusion works poorly if the embolus is solid material (plaque). Suction thrombectomy is good for either thrombus or plaque. It requires a non-tapered catheter with a large end hole. Occasionally large emboli have to be surgically removed.

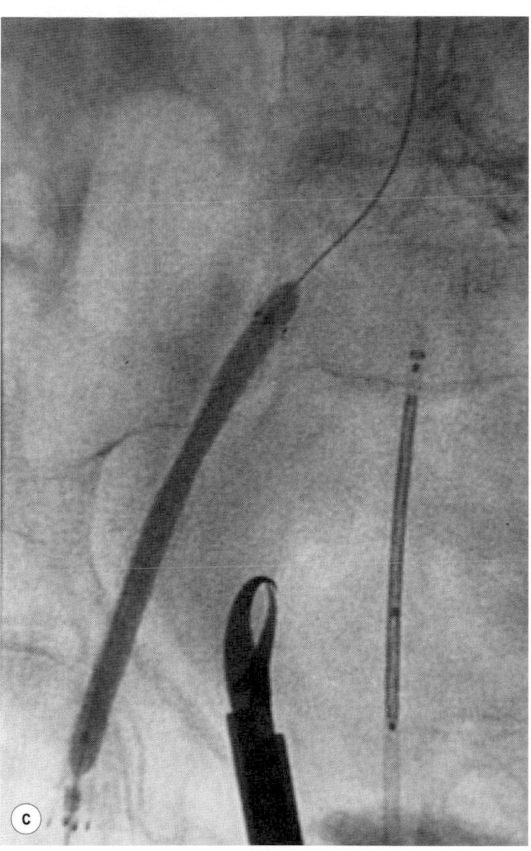


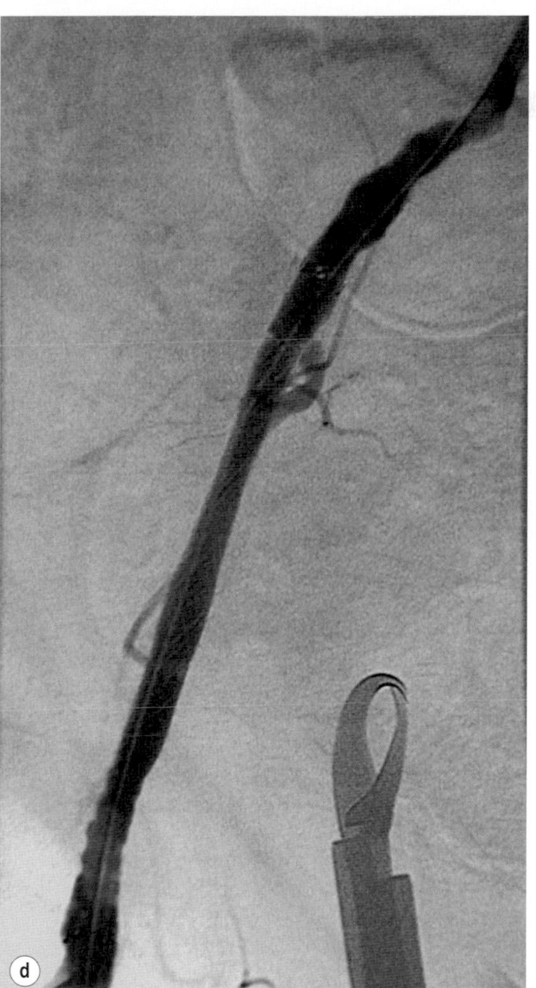


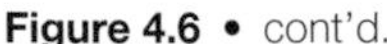

**Figure 4.6** • cont'd.

## Stent-related complications

Device-related problems such as (i) failure to deploy or misplacement and (ii) infection are rare and beyond the scope of this chapter.[29] However, patients with infected stents should be started on intravenous antibiotic therapy and investigated with a view to removal of the stent with revascularisation using autologous vein, preferably via an extra-anatomical route. Fatalities and limb amputations have occurred; however, given the large number of stents that have been placed without infectious sequelae, it is unclear if antibiotics should be used routinely at the time of implantation.

# Suprainguinal open surgery

The surgical approach to patients with significant aorto-iliac disease is determined by the patient's general fitness and whether or not they have had previous abdominal surgery (**Fig. 4.7**). In general terms all patients should undergo cardiorespiratory assessment, e.g. respiratory function tests, left ventricular ejection fraction (echo or Multiple Gated Acquisition Scan MUGA), and preferably a cardiopulmonary exercise test.[30]

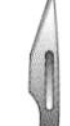

To date there is no evidence for preoperative methicillin-resistant *Staphylococcus aureus* (MRSA) screening, but all patients undergoing prosthetic grafting should either be screened or receive standard MRSA prophylaxis, nasal mupirocin and chlorhexidine bathing. Individual units should consider their admission policy for elective vascular cases.[31]

## Aorto-bifemoral bypass

The infrarenal abdominal aorta can be approached laparoscopically or by conventional open surgery.

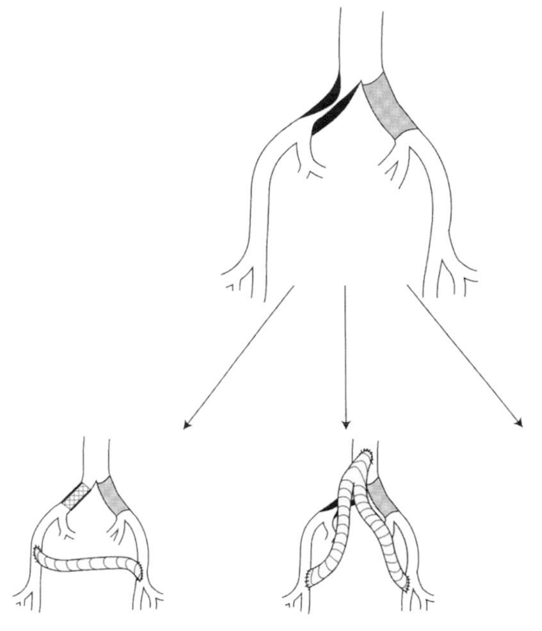


**Figure 4.7** • Possible treatment options in a patient with aorto-iliac disease. Axillo-bifemoral bypass should be reserved for patients with critical ischaemia.

Laparoscopic aortic surgery has been introduced in many European countries and advocates claim lower morbidity and mortality rates and shorter hospital stays.[32,33] There remains no convincing evidence to support these claims as there have been no randomised trials. Laparoscopic aortic surgery requires extensive training and the procedure times are longer than for open surgery. With regard to open surgery, there is little or no evidence to favour either a transperitoneal vs. a retroperitoneal approach or a vertical vs. transverse incision, although transverse incisions are favoured by anaesthetists as the top end of a vertical incision often 'escapes' an epidural. End-to-end anastomoses are used for flush occlusions below the renal arteries (**Fig. 4.8**). If the proximal infrarenal aorta is patent, then an end-to-side anastomosis can preserve flow to a patent inferior mesenteric and/or internal iliac artery, thus reducing the risk of pelvic ischaemia.

The majority of surgeons would favour a Dacron graft over polytetrafluoroethylene (PTFE). There is some theoretical data that PTFE grafts are more resistant to infection than Dacron, but this is outweighed by the superior handling and suturing characteristics of Dacron. Rifampicin soaking and silver impregnation have been shown to improve the infection resistance of Dacron in vitro but there is little or no clinical evidence to support their use.[34] There is some observational evidence

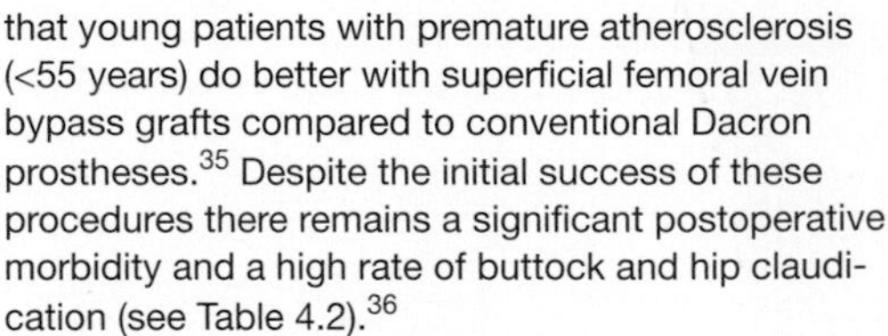
that young patients with premature atherosclerosis (<55 years) do better with superficial femoral vein bypass grafts compared to conventional Dacron prostheses.[35] Despite the initial success of these procedures there remains a significant postoperative morbidity and a high rate of buttock and hip claudication (see Table 4.2).[36]

## Axillo-bifemoral bypass

Often described as the last resort of the destitute, this has its place in the very unfit patient and those with a 'hostile' abdomen.

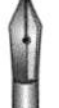

The procedure is associated with a 5% in-hospital mortality, and 5-year limb salvage and patient survival rates of 74% and 34–39% respectively.[37,38]

There appears to be no difference in outcome between axillo-bifemoral or axillo-unifemoral bypass grafts.

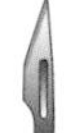

A randomised clinical trial has reported improved 3-year graft patency rates in grafts with a flow-splitter (86%) versus a contralateral limb taken off at 90 degrees (38%).[39]

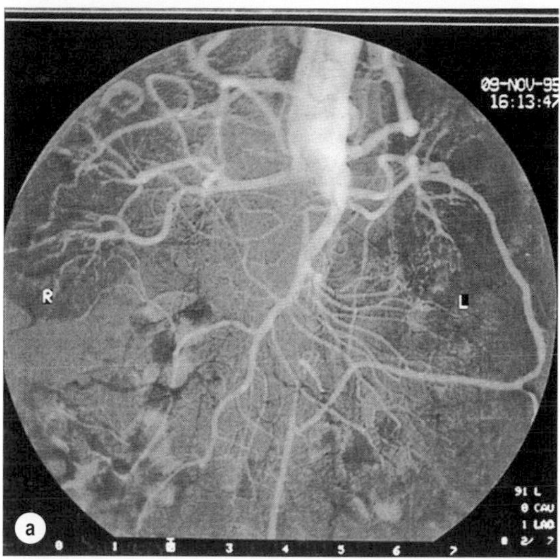


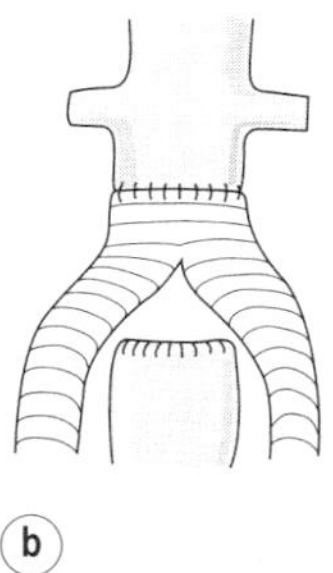


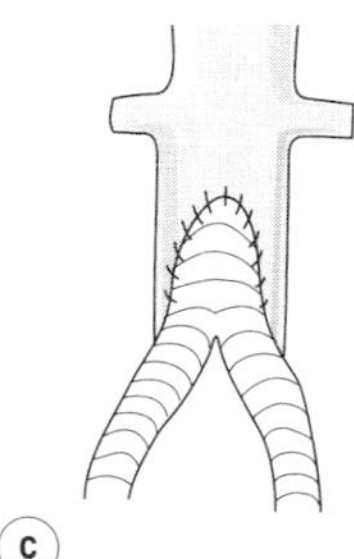


**Figure 4.8 • (a)** Aortogram showing occlusion of the aorta below the level of the renal arteries. In this case the proximal anastomosis of an aorto-bifemoral bypass should be end to end **(b)**. If there is continuity with the inferior mesenteric artery or internal iliac arteries, then an end-to-side anastomosis **(c)** may be preferable.

Table 4.2 • Outcome following aorto-bifemoral grafting[36]

| | |
|---|---|
| Operative mortality | 5% |
| Patient survival | 73–88% at 5 years |
| Primary patency | 85% at 5 years<br>60% at 10 years |
| Re-operation | 33% |
| Graft infection | 1% for 10 years |
| False aneurysm | 1% for 10 years |

## Iliofemoral bypass

### Unilateral iliofemoral bypass

This procedure is indicated where there is extensive disease within the external iliac artery, which has failed to respond to endovascular intervention or where the disease extends into the common femoral artery.

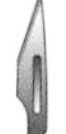

A recent study from France has demonstrated a superior outcome at 4 years in those patients who underwent iliofemoral grafting over femorofemoral crossover grafting.[40]

The key to success is a good inflow in the form of a disease-free common iliac artery and appropriate run-off into the SFA or profunda femoris artery (PFA). In the majority of cases a common femoral artery (CFA) endarterectomy and patch will have to be performed to gain access to the run-off vessels. In the rare cases where the common iliac is poor, the distal aorta can be used as a source of inflow. The common iliac artery is approached through a classical Rutherford–Morrison incision and an Omni-retract is a valuable tool in maintaining exposure of the vessels. Care should be taken to identify and preserve the ureter. Proximal control of the common iliac artery is essential, and some surgeons would avoid dissecting around the back of the vessel, as torrential venous bleeding can ensue, especially if there has been an inflammatory response around the vessels. Some surgeons would therefore advocate not to fully mobilise the vessel, but merely clamp it, without slings. Previous abdominal surgery, e.g. appendicectomy, or inguinal hernia repair may affect access to the retroperitoneal space and should be considered prior to any planned surgery. Externally supported 8-mm Dacron or PTFE are the conduits of choice and are usually sewn end to side to the common iliac. A tunnel is then created from above and below the inguinal ligament and the distal anastomosis completed to the common femoral artery. In those cases where the SFA is occluded it is essential to extend the anastomosis down to at least the first bifurcation of the PFA.

In the rare redo cases where a graft is required from the external iliac artery to the above-knee popliteal artery, usually in the absence of any usable venous conduit, it is recommended that the profunda femoris artery is identified through an incision in the groin.[41] Two separate tunnels can be made, thus avoiding any injury to the femoral vein. The graft can be taken down to the PFA and then extended to the above-knee popliteal artery.

### Iliofemoral crossover

This procedure is indicated where the affected limb has no inflow vessel, i.e. common iliac, but the contralateral limb has a disease-free common or external iliac artery. The approach avoids exposure of both groins. In addition if the donor vessels develop significant atherosclerosis over time, these can be treatment percutaneously via the donor femoral artery, thus avoiding direct puncture of the graft and/or anastomotic site. The donor iliac vessels are approached via a Rutherford–Morrison incision and the graft (Dacron/PTFE externally supported 8 mm) is placed in a lazy S position. It is essential that the patient is catheterised and great care should be taken tunnelling the graft into the contralateral groin as there is the potential to damage the bladder and the iliofemoral veins.

### Femoro-femoral crossover

Femoro-femoral crossover grafting is considered to be a low-risk procedure with an operative mortality between 0% and 5%. However, these figures are influenced by the presence of critical ischaemia, previous surgery and the need for combined iliac interventions.[42] Pursell et al., in a recent review, reported a 22% complication rate including a 6% graft infection rate.[43] Like the iliofemoral graft the procedure can be considered when the affected limb has no inflow and the contralateral iliac and femoral vessels are free of disease. The one contraindication is a large abdominal apron, which can affect the lie of the graft, especially in the seated position. The approach does, however, avoid an abdominal incision, but in theory exposes the patient to a higher rate of wound-related problems in the groin, notably infection. Two types of configuration are described: (1) lazy S and (2) inverted U. There are no convincing data to support either approach and it is often best decided at the time of surgery.

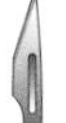

A randomised trial has demonstrated no difference between externally supported 8-mm Dacron or PTFE.[44]

There is some observational evidence that externally supported grafts perform better over time.

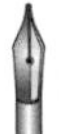

Mingoli et al. reported 5- and 10-year primary patency rates of 80% and 60% respectively for supported grafts versus 69% and 21% for unsupported grafts.[45] Combined or delayed iliac angioplasty at the time of femoro-femoral xover bypass grafting should be avoided in those patients with iliac lesions in excess of 5 cm. Aburahma et al. reported 3-year primary patency rates of 85% and 31% in patients with iliac lesions 3–5 cm and >5 cm respectively.[46]

## Femoral endarterectomy and profundaplasty

The CFA and deep femoral artery (profunda femoris) origin is a common site for exophytic calcific atherosclerotic disease (**Fig. 4.9**). The nature and location of the disease at a bifurcation subject to flexion is not usually amenable to angioplasty or stenting. Femoral endarterectomy and repair using a patch which extends into the profunda is the preferred treatment. The choice of patch includes vein or prosthetic (Dacron or PTFE). If the SFA is occluded, this can be harvested and endarterectomised to form a useful patch, preserving the long saphenous vein and avoiding the risk of infection associated with prosthetic material (**Fig. 4.10**). Femoral endarterectomy can be combined with iliac angioplasty or stenting, if there is proximal disease which would be difficult to access percutaneously. Femoral endarterectomy can also be combined with a femoro-popliteal/distal bypass. In this case, the proximal end of the graft is used as the patch.

It is inadvisable to crossclamp a proximal stent if arterial control is required for distal reconstruction. Clamping may crush the stent or tear the arterial wall. Arterial control can be achieved with an occlusion

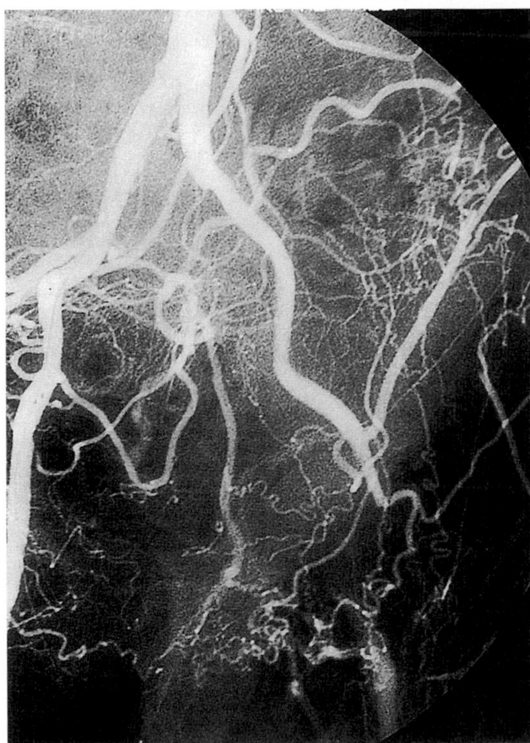

**Figure 4.9** • Arteriogram of a claudicant showing a localised occlusion of the left common femoral artery, suitable for endarterectomy and patch repair.

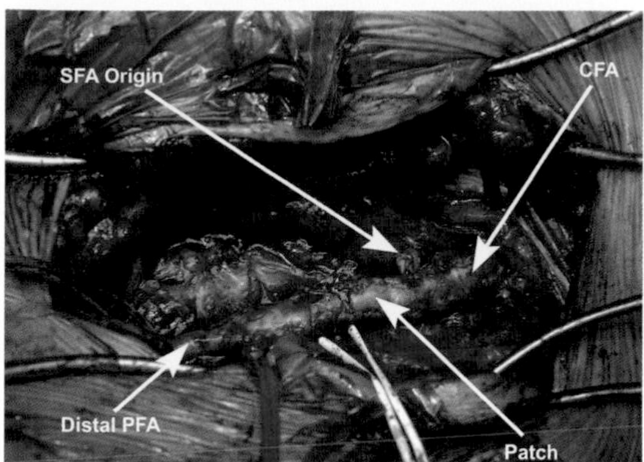


**Figure 4.10** • Femoral and profunda endarterectomy and repair using a patch of endarterectomised SFA. This avoids the infection risk associated with prosthetic material and preserves the long saphenous vein.

balloon, passed up the artery over a J-tip guidewire. This trick is also useful whenever the proximal inflow is heavily calcified.

### Infrainguinal reconstruction

There are several treatment options for patients with isolated disease of the SFA (**Fig. 4.11**). Multilevel infrainguinal disease often requires more extensive revascularisation, and would normally only be justified in a patient with critical ischaemia (**Fig. 4.12**). Over the last decade there has been a significant reduction in the number of infrainguinal bypass grafts. The reasons for this are unclear, but may well relate to improvements in general medical care and risk factor modification, earlier referral, better access to interventional vascular radiology and improved endovascular techniques (see later).

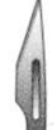

Smoking cessation is vital as continued smoking results in a threefold increased risk of graft failure.[47] Preoperative screening for hypercoagulability is also important as this adversely affects graft patency, limb salvage and survival.[48]

Successful infrainguinal bypass is dependent upon a good inflow, a reasonable size conduit and adequate run-off. It is important to have access to a contemporary set of images (usually within 6 months) and all inflow issues resolved either before or at the time of surgery. The CFA is the usual site for the proximal anastomosis, but if the vein will not reach, then either the profunda femoris or SFA can be used. If the SFA is diseased, it can be endarterectomised.

In terms of the outflow, grafts to the above-knee popliteal should only be undertaken if there is limited vein available or if there is no evidence of disease in that segment. As such, the below-knee popliteal is the preferred site of the distal anastomosis. By contrast, the tibioperoneal trunk is often diseased and represents a poor alternative to a crural vessel. Restoration of foot pulses is usually required to heal necrosis, especially in the presence of diabetes. If there are concerns about the run-off vessels, antegrade angiography or dedicated calf and foot magnetic resonance angiography may provide additional information. The posterior tibial artery is the easiest crural artery to access as it lies deep to the long saphenous vein (LSV). The mid-peroneal artery is also accessible from the medial side between the posterior tibial and soleus muscles. Access to the lower peroneal artery requires resection of a short length of fibula (**Fig. 4.13**). The anterior tibial artery is reached via an incision 4 cm lateral to the anterior edge of the fibula.

## Choice of graft material

### Saphenous vein

The LSV is the conduit of choice in femoro-popliteal grafting. Preoperative ultrasound mapping is essential. In general a single non-varicose LSV is usable as long as it is not too small.

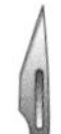

Small LSV <3 mm is associated with a twofold risk of early failure and should be discarded or used as a venous patch or cuff.[49]

By contrast, large veins (>6 mm) are often associated with focal varicosities which may require excision and splicing or alternatively plication of a local blowout. The use of complex LSV systems (two or more) is associated with increased dissection, local haematoma formation and skin necrosis. If the LSV has been removed or is of poor quality one should consider removing the contralateral LSV. If this is not an option the short saphenous veins (SSVs) can be scanned; however, for most femoro-popliteal grafts, both will be needed. Bilateral SSV harvesting is best approached with the patient in the prone position (**Fig. 4.14**).

### Arm vein

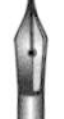

In general these veins should only be used for rest pain, ulceration and/or gangrene; however, there are odd exceptions but patients need to be aware of the lower patency rates and the increased technical difficulties in harvesting and anastomosing these veins.[50]

It is important to remind junior doctors and phlebotomists not to use the anticubital vein for blood

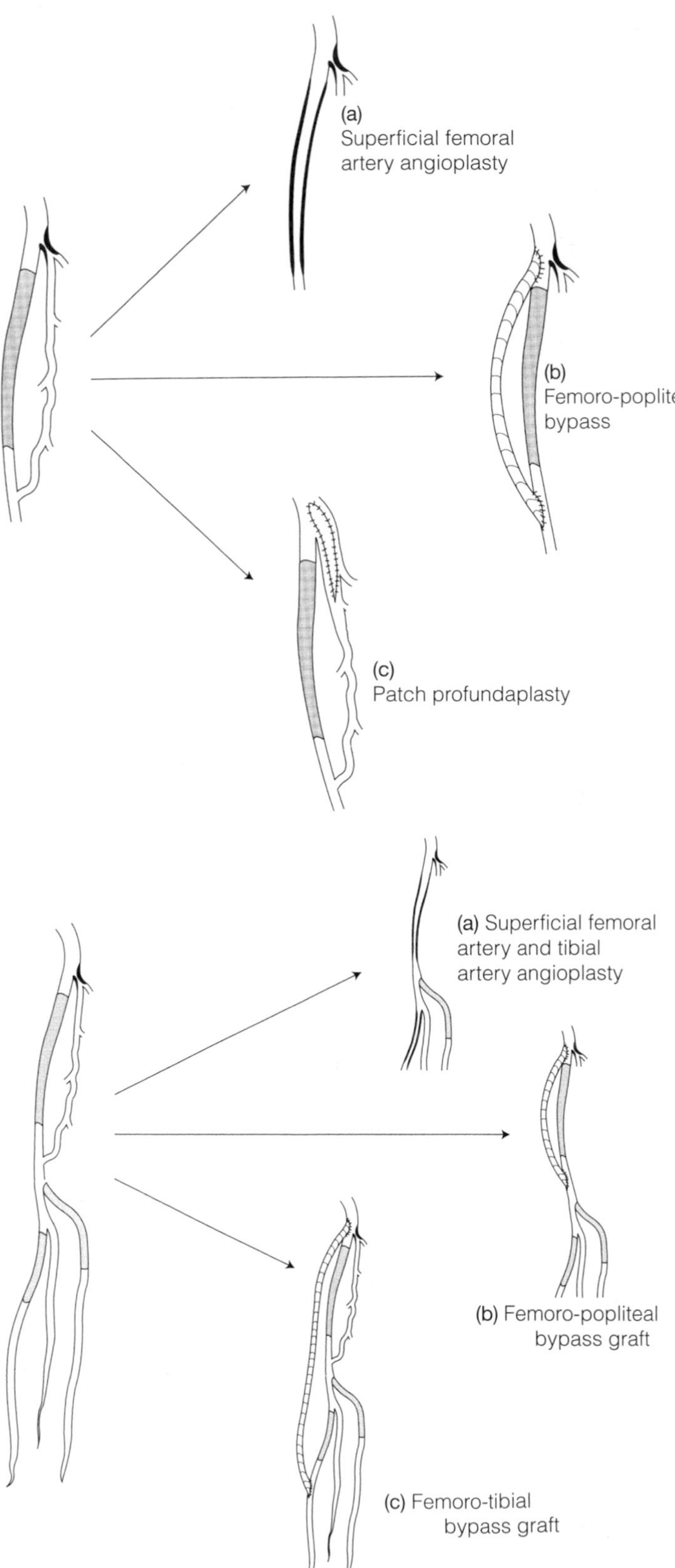


**Figure 4.11** • Possible treatment options for a patient with localised SFA disease. Angioplasty **(a)** should be the first line of treatment for stenoses and occlusions less than 15 cm in length. Longer lesions will require a femoro-popliteal bypass graft **(b)**. Profundaplasty **(c)** may be sufficient to improve claudication or rest pain, but will not usually heal ulceration or necrosis.

**Figure 4.12** • Possible infrainguinal revascularisation options in a patient with critical limb ischaemia due to multilevel disease. Angioplasty **(a)** should be attempted if possible but may need to be extensive, with the risk of early re-occlusion. Femoro-popliteal bypass **(b)** may fail to reperfuse the foot unless at least one calf artery is patent into the foot. Extensive tissue loss or sepsis usually requires a femoro-tibial bypass graft **(c)**, especially in a diabetic.

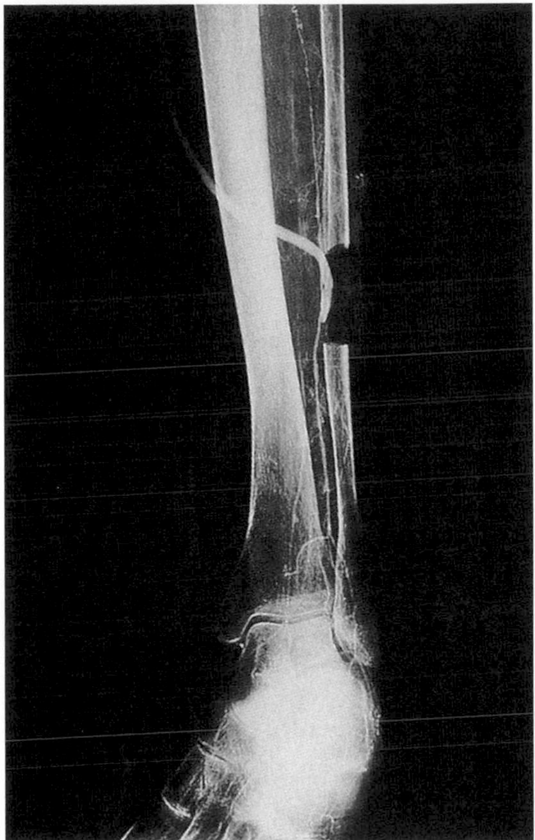

**Figure 4.13 •** Completion arteriogram of a femoro-peroneal vein bypass graft showing the fibulectomy required to access the peroneal artery from the lateral side of the leg.

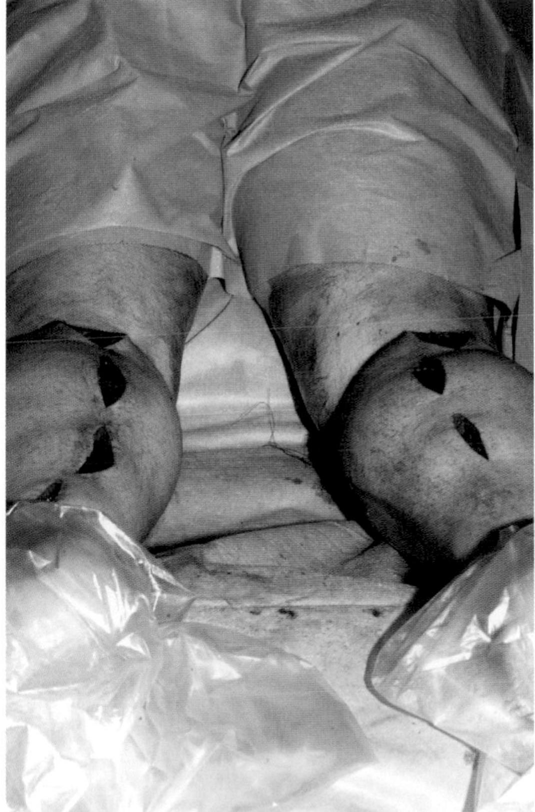

**Figure 4.14 •** Bilateral short saphenous vein harvesting for a redo left femoro-anterior tibial vein graft.

sampling; as a result the arm should be marked with a waterproof pen: 'Do not touch'.

In general, the cephalic vein harvested from the wrist to the deltopectoral grove is sufficient for a below-knee femoro-popliteal graft. If the forearm cephalic vein is of poor quality the basilic vein can be harvested along with the median cubital vein and upper arm cephalic vein and used as an intact conduit. This will require removal of the valves in one segment. Alternatively the vein can be divided at the level of median cubital vein and one length of vein reversed and re-anastomosed in a spatulated fashion. In the case of femoro-tibial grafting, a single arm vein is usually too short for mid to distal calf anastomoses and so both arms should be prepared. After removal of the arm veins the wounds should be closed and bandaged with velband and crepe prior to the administration of i.v. heparin.

## In situ versus reversed vein

There is no good clinical evidence to suggest that either technique is better than the other. However, the in situ technique is less forgiving than the conventional reverse graft, especially with uniform good-quality veins. The in situ technique lends itself to femoro-tibial bypass grafts to the posterior tibial, peroneal and dorsalis pedis arteries. By contrast, grafts to the anterior tibial artery are best tunnelled in the lateral position. Grafts tunnelled via the medial to lateral aspect via the interosseous membrane can be difficult to access if they develop a stenosis within this segment. The key step to success is the correct use of the valvulotome and one should be familiar will all types, including the disposable versions (LeMaitre). If the reversed technique is preferred it is essential to follow a strict tunnelling protocol to avoid twisting or kinking, especially if simultaneous anastomoses are undertaken. The use of a tourniquet is particularly useful in femoro-distal bypass surgery as it reduces the need for extensive dissection and facilitates the anastomosis, as no clamps are required because of the bloodless field (**Fig. 4.15**). Alternatively, fine silastic slings or intraluminal occluders are preferable to clamps, and magnifying loupes are essential.

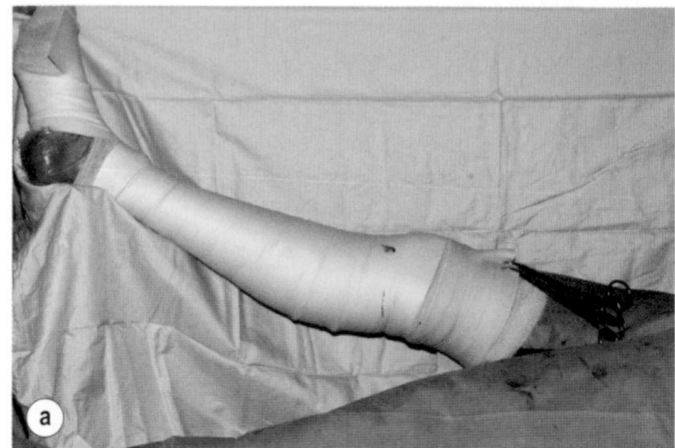

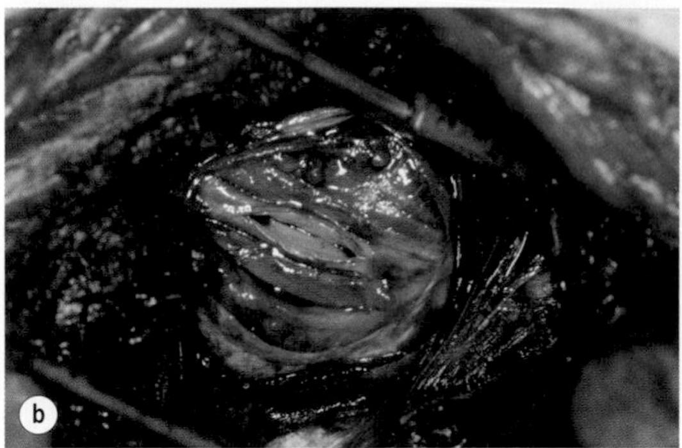

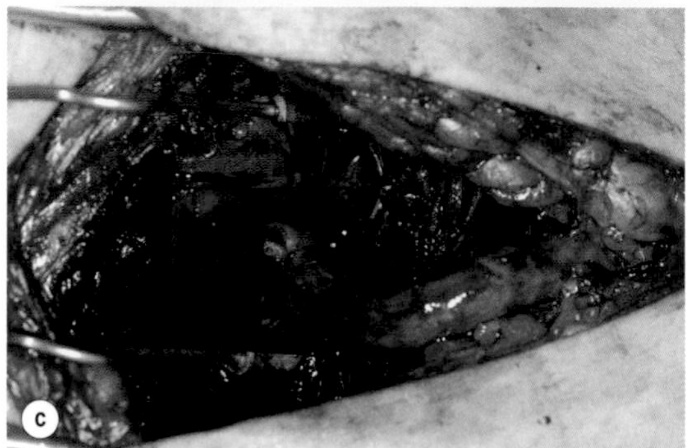

**Figure 4.15 • (a)** Esmarch tourniquet applied over a crepe bandage. **(b)** Exposed posterior tibial artery and venae commitantes after the application of the tourniquet. Note no clamps and no bleeding which facilitates the anastomosis. **(c)** Completed distal anastomosis to the posterior tibial artery. A Boazul cuff can be used in the same way (see Chapter 17).

## Prosthetic grafts

The use of prosthetic material for both intermittent claudication and critical ischaemia has fallen dramatically because of poor patency rates and concerns about graft infection.[51]

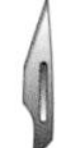

The patency rates for femoro-popliteal bypass for CLI from a meta-analysis by Hunink et al. gave primary patencies of 66% for vein (any level), 47% for above-knee PTFE and 33% for below-knee PTFE at 5 years.[52] The pooled weighted data for primary patency rates for femoro-distal (tibial or pedal) bypass are reported in TASC as 85%, 80% and 70% for femoro-distal bypass with vein and 70%, 35% and 25% for femoro-distal bypass with prosthetic at 1, 3 and 5 years respectively.[7]

A Cochrane review reported no differences between PTFE and Dacron.[53] However, a subsequent multicentre randomised study of PTFE or Dacron for above-knee femoro-popliteal bypass has reported a significant difference in the 2-year secondary patency rates for Dacron over PTFE.[54]

When no vein is available, most surgeons favour a vein cuff at the distal anastomosis.

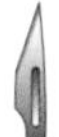

The Joint Vascular Research Group RCT of Miller vein cuff vs. non-cuff for femoro-popliteal PTFE grafts demonstrated significantly higher patency rates for prosthetic grafts with a vein cuff at the below-knee level at 3 years.[55]

# Graft surveillance

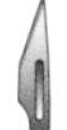

This remains a controversial subject. Three randomised clinical trials demonstrated no benefit from a graft surveillance programme.[56–58]

These studies were, however, criticised on the basis of the duplex criteria for an 'at-risk' graft and the timing of the initial scan (see Table 4.3).[59]

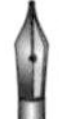

On the basis of these observations, Mofidi et al., in an observational study using rigid duplex criteria, reported that a duplex scan at 6 weeks could predict those patients who require continued graft surveillance.[60] In addition patients undergoing grafting using arm veins should be targeted as they are prone to develop stenoses and aneurysms.[61]

Further work is required to define this population in more detail, but for the present time a 6-week scan should identify those grafts which require continued surveillance.

**Table 4.3** • Ultrasound criteria for 'at-risk' femoro-distal vein grafts

| Authors | Year | Machine | PSV (cm/s) | V2/V1 |
|---|---|---|---|---|
| Lundell et al.[56] | 1995 | Diasonics CV 400 | >200 | – |
| | | Acuson XP10 | < 45 | – |
| Ihlberg et al.[57] | 1998 | ATL ultramark 9 | <45 | >2 |
| Davies et al.[58] | 2005 | – | <45 | >2 |

PSV, peak systolic velocity.

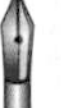

In the case of PTFE grafts the data are limited, but there is observational evidence to support the practice of an early duplex to identify those with low graft flow. These patients can then be considered for long-term anticoagulation.[62]

# Endovascular intervention

## Femoro-popliteal angioplasty

The angioplasty literature would claim a 1-year patency rate for femoro-popliteal stenosis of 70% and for occlusions of 50%. The literature is, however, generally poor and rarely defines the type of lesion that is being treated. The TASC document[7] is probably more realistic about the type of lesion that should be treated. In order to improve outcomes, many different alternatives to angioplasty have been proposed, including stents, cutting balloons,[63] cryoplasty[64] and drug-eluting stents. Analysis of the literature on cryoplasty would suggest it is no better than angioplasty alone.[65]

## Subintimal angioplasty

Although often described as a novel technique, subintimal angioplasty has been around for more than 20 years. It is perhaps considered novel because it has only been described in detail in the last 10 years. Using an antegrade catheter and a hydrophilic guidewire the subintimal space above a femoro-popliteal occlusion is accessed and the wire pushed down like a surgical ring stripper (**Fig. 4.16**). If the artery is not too calcified the wire will invariably re-enter the true lumen below the obstruction and dilatation with a 5- or 6-mm angioplasty balloon will produce a patent though dissected channel offering a clean surface to blood flow. As a limb salvage procedure this technique works extremely well, with salvage rates of >75% being reported.[66,67]

## Femoro-popliteal stents

The results of femoro-popliteal stents are variable and depend on an adequate inflow, the size of the artery treated and good run-off.

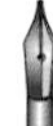

Patency rates of nearly 90% at 1 year and 78% at 3 years have been reported.[68–70] These good results are mainly in claudicants. Stent fractures also occur more commonly in the femoro-popliteal segment due to flexion and overlapping of multiple stents. Stent fractures are associated with a higher risk of re-stenosis and occlusion.[71]

The incidence of stent fractures may be reduced by the use of long stents that are designed to withstand flexional forces.

Early results from placement of stents did not demonstrate advantage over simple angioplasty, in part probably due to a poor understanding of the biomechanics of the SFA. However, improved stent graft design and better use of adjuvant pharmaceuticals may have changed the way we now approach femoro-popliteal disease. Two randomised trials have now been undertaken. One published study[72,73] compared the patients with severe claudication or chronic CLI and SFA disease of >3 cm long to either angioplasty or Guidant Dynalink or Absolute self-expanding nitinol stent. All patients were placed on dual antiplatelet therapy. At 6 and 12 months the walking distance and re-stenosis rates were better in the stent group. There were no amputations in either group. A similar, as yet unpublished, study (the RESILIENT Trial) has been undertaken using the Edwards (now Bard) Lifestent, which again demonstrated improved clinical and re-stenosis outcomes in the stent group at 6 months. There are some caveats to be considered. Both trials had a dominance of claudicants and patients with very good tibial artery run-off, and both treated limited length disease (average 13 and 6 cm respectively). There is also doubt as to whether these data can be transferred to all stents since there are data to indicate that design does matter.[74]

## Drug-eluting stents/balloons

Sirolimus-eluting stents have been tested and results from animal models demonstrated marked effects on smooth muscle proliferation and cell migration, with reduction in intimal hyperplasia following stent placement.

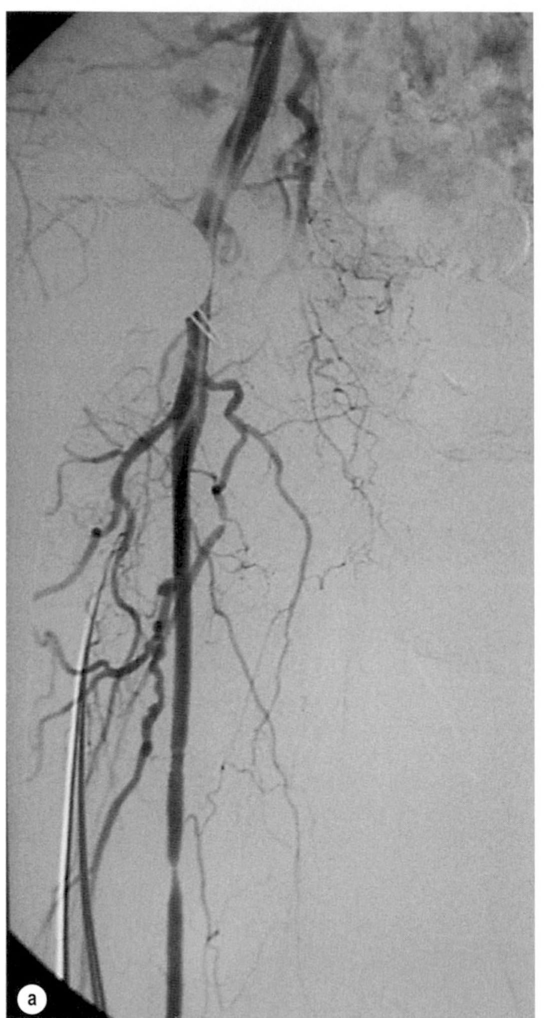

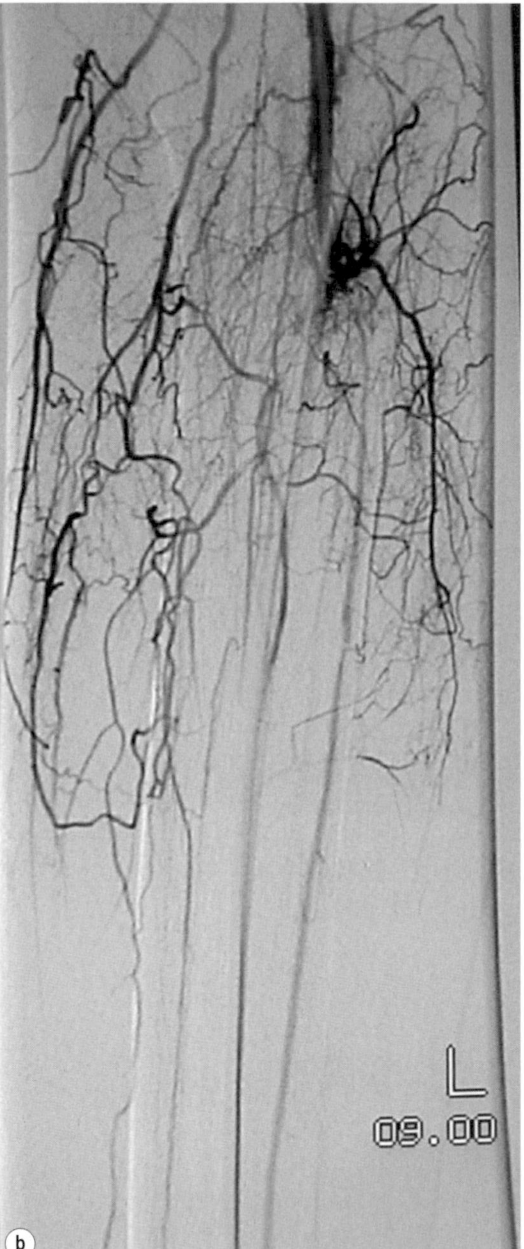


**Figure 4.16 • (a,b)** Angiograms of a patient with right-sided tissue loss demonstrating an occluded SFA with a stenosed left profunda femoris, an isolated popliteal segment, and patent peroneal and anterior tibial arteries. **(c)** This captured image demonstrates the classic loop of hydrophilic wire used to strip a passage through the subintimal space. **(d,e)** Following 6-mm PTA the femoro-popliteal segment is patent with good flow. The irregularities are caused by the deliberately dissected intimal flap. These are rarely (but occasionally) flow limiting.

In the SCIROCCO trial of sirolimus-eluting stents versus bare SMART nitinol stents for TASC C lesions, the re-stenosis rate at 24 months was 22.9% and 21.1% respectively.[75,76] In a recent multicentre study from Germany, angioplasty balloons coated in paclitaxel produced significantly better results at 6 and 24 months in terms of late lumen loss and target lesion revascularisation.[77]

## Covered stent grafts

A small single-centre randomised trial of Viabahn expanded PTFE/nitinol stent grafts vs. femoral to above-knee popliteal expanded PTFE or Dacron bypass grafts showed no difference in primary and secondary patency rates at 12 months (73.5% and 83.9% vs. 74.2% and 83.7% respectively).[78]

This trial has been criticised for the large proportion of patients with claudication and the preferential use of prosthetic bypass material, rather than autologous vein. Nevertheless, if a patient does not have a suitable vein, then a stentgraft seems a reasonable, but expensive, option. The superiority of stentgrafts over open stents has not been demonstrated and there are no trials of stents versus bypass grafts to the below-knee popliteal level, which is more commonly required in patients with CLI.

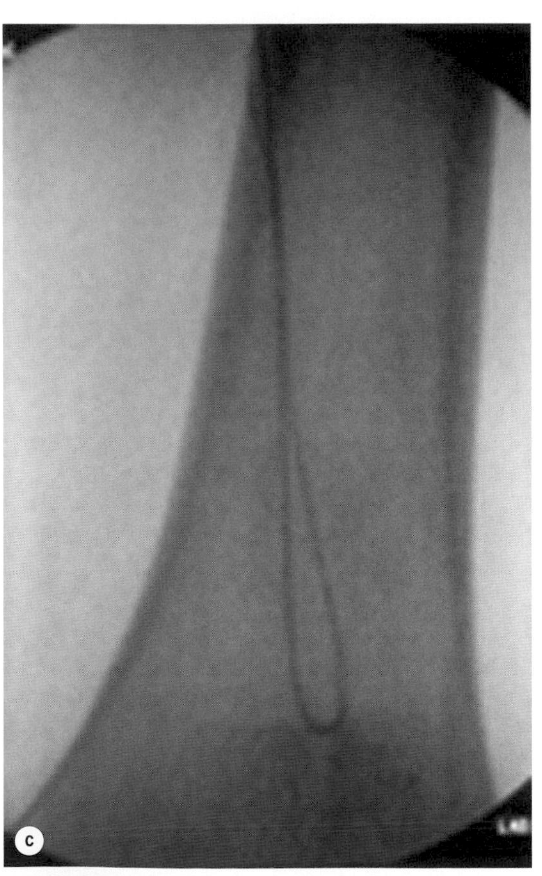


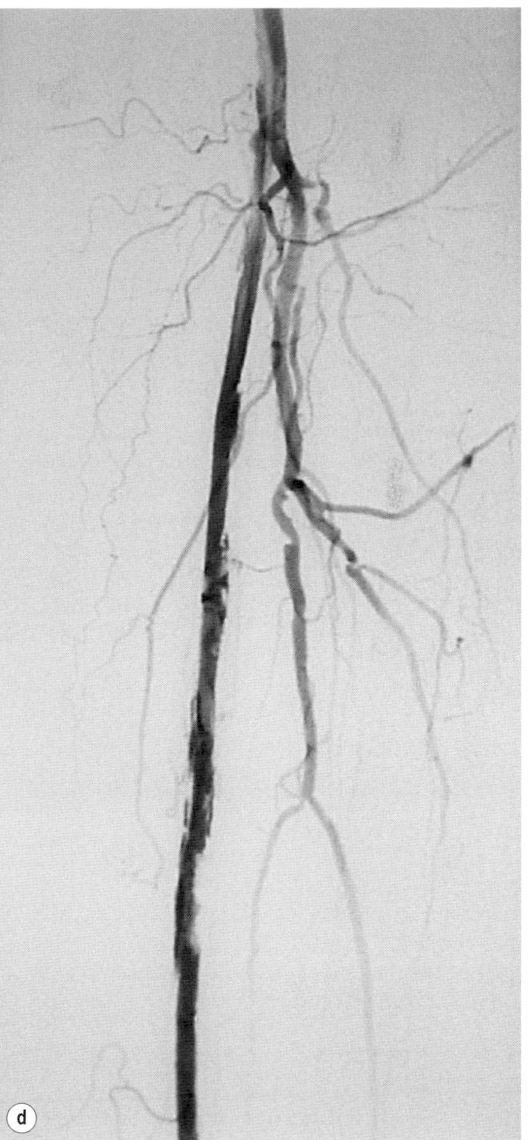


**Figure 4.16** • cont'd.

*(Continued)*

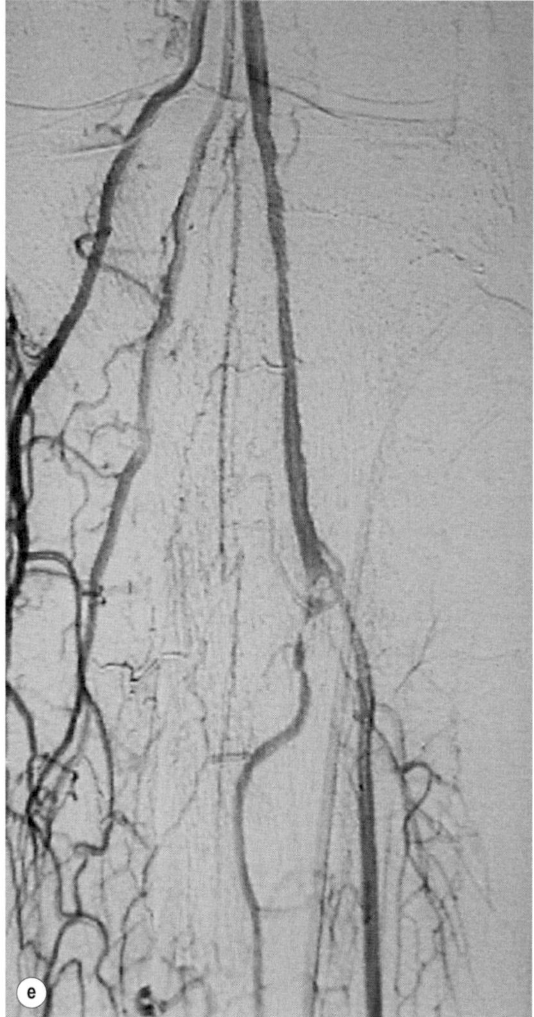

Figure 4.16 • cont'd.

## Crural artery interventions

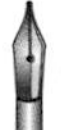

Interventions in the crural arteries are confined to those patients who have rest pain or tissue loss and in whom surgical options are limited because of anatomical considerations or comorbidities.[79]

The success of the procedure is dependent upon a good inflow, stenotic rather than occlusive disease and focal rather than widespread atherosclerosis.

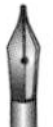

Limb salvage rates of 81% have been reported at 12 months;[80] the use of self-expandable stents have shown additional benefit at 1 year.[81]

## The evidence for endovascular intervention

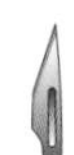

In the BASIL trial (Bypass versus Angioplasty in Severe Ischaemia of the Leg) angioplasty was compared against infrainguinal bypass.[82] The primary outcome measure was amputation-free survival. Secondary outcome measures included all-cause mortality, morbidity and reintervention, quality of life and hospital costs. A total of 452 patients were randomised; 30-day mortality was low in both groups (5% for surgery and 3% for angioplasty). Surgery was associated with a significantly higher morbidity (57% vs. 41%), mainly due to myocardial infarction and wound infection. Those having surgery also stayed in hospital longer and this contributed to the cost of surgery being one-third higher than angioplasty at 1 year. However, by 3 years there was no significant difference in costs because those having angioplasty had a significantly higher failure rate (20% vs. 3% within 12 months), resulting in a higher reintervention rate (28% vs. 17%). There was no difference in quality of life, amputation-free survival or all-cause mortality at any time interval out to 2 years, and by 5 years 36% of patients had died. Subgroup analysis suggests that surgery is the best option for fit patients with a usable vein.

The trial has been criticised for the combined end-point, the high mortality which accounted for 75% of the end-points, the failure to address the secondary risk factors and the absence of data on diabetic control.

# Non-interventional treatment

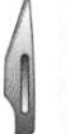

A meta-analysis of six randomised controlled studies of Iloprost, involving more than 700 patients with CLI, suggests a significant reduction in death and amputation at 6 months (35% vs. 55%) for those patients receiving the drug.[83]

However, the long-term benefit remains unclear for this expensive drug and its use in the UK has declined over the last few years.

## Gene therapy

Gene therapy uses recombinant formulations of angiogenic growth factors to produce therapeutic angiogenesis.

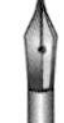

However, a recent large-scale phase II double-blind, placebo-controlled study using AdVEGF21, in a group of 105 subjects with unilateral claudication, demonstrated no difference between the two groups at 26 weeks.[84] A recent phase I trial has used a standard adenoviral delivery system with a constitutively active form of the transcription factor hypoxia-inducible factor-1$\alpha$ (HIF-1$\alpha$).

At 1 year, 14 of the 32 patients treated with HIF-1α had resolution of their rest pain and 5 of 18 patients had complete healing of their ulcers.[85]

Stem therapy using either bone marrow mononuclear cells or autologous peripheral blood CD133+ purified stem cells is an alternative method of promoting neorevascularisation, but the results are confusing.[86–88] An alternative approach combines basic fibroblast growth factor with a biodegradable gelatin hydrogel microsphere, which is injected into the gastrocnemius muscle. A phase I–IIa study in seven patients with critical limb ischaemia has demonstrated improvements in walking distance, rest pain scores and transcutaneous oxygen levels. Moderate improvements in ulcer healing were seen in three of the five patients.[89] These studies confirm the general principle, but there is a long way to go before these technologies are widely available.

## Spinal cord stimulation

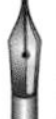

Two controlled studies of spinal cord stimulation have demonstrated no improvement in ulcer healing, limb salvage and mortalilty rates.[90,91] More recently a further study has confirmed the role of spinal cord stimulation in non-reconstructable vascular disease. The authors reported that preoperative transcutaneous $PO_2$ measurements and preoperative sceening improved the probability of limb salvage.[92]

## Sympathectomy

Lumbar sympathectomy is an option in patients with unreconstructable occlusive disease and rest pain. The duration of the benefit remains, however, in question. In those patients with rest pain and tissue loss, sympathectomy is of limited use. Published results are old and variable: some report long-term pain relief in 78% of cases, with 11% requiring amputation;[93] others report pain relief in only 6%, with 70% requiring early amputation.[94]

## Calf and foot compression

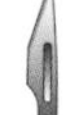

In a small-scale community-based observation study, Kavros et al. reported their experience of intermittent pneumatic compression (IPC) of the foot, calf or both in patients with chronic lower limb ischaemia. IPC was delivered at an inflation pressure of 85–95 mmHg, applied for 2 seconds with rapid rise (0.2 seconds), three cycles per minute; three 2-hourly sessions per day were requested. Significant improvements in wound healing and limb salvage rates were noted over a control group.[95]

## Key points

- The TASC offers sensible guidelines for the treatment of both supra- and infrainguinal disease.
- Unilateral iliac occlusions should be treated by primary stenting. Complication rates are low.
- Suprainguinal surgery remains a useful treatment option for bilateral/diffuse disease, but great care should be taken in the new era of MRSA.
- Infrainguinal surgery is in decline but autologous vein remains the conduit of choice.
- In the absence of leg vein, arm vein should be considered.
- Prosthetic grafts should only be used as a last resort and only with a venous cuff.
- Graft surveillance remains contentious and requires further research.
- Infrainguinal endovascular intervention requires further study.
- The long-term results of the BASIL trial favour surgery if there is a good vein and the patient is fit.
- There is no role for vasodilators in critical limb ischaemia.
- Gene therapy to stimulate angiogenesis remains an elusive treatment option.
- Sympathectomy continues to be used despite little or no evidence.
- Some patients are best treated by primary amputation.

# References


1. Abou-Zamzam AM Jr, Lee RW, Moneta GL et al. Functional outcome after infrainguinal bypass for limb salvage. J Vasc Surg 1997; 25(2):287–95; discussion 295–7.
2. Humphreys WV, Evans F, Watkin G et al. Critical limb ischaemia in patients over 80 years of age: options in a district general hospital. Br J Surg 1995; 82(10):1361–3.


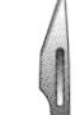


3. Singh S, Evans L, Datta D et al. The costs of managing lower limb-threatening ischaemia. Eur J Vasc Endovasc Surg 1996; 12(3):359–62.
4. Johnson BF, Singh S, Evans L et al. A prospective study of the effect of limb-threatening ischaemia and its surgical treatment on the quality of life. Eur J Vasc Endovasc Surg 1997; 13(3):306–14.

5. Nicoloff AD, Taylor LM Jr, McLafferty RB et al. Patient recovery after infrainguinal bypass grafting for limb salvage. J Vasc Surg 1998; 27(2):256–63; discussion 264–6.
6. Society of Interventional Radiology Standards of Practice Committee: Guidelines for percutaneous transluminal angioplasty. J Vasc Interv Radiol 2003; 14:S209.
7. Norgren L, Hiatt WR, Dormandy JA et al. TASC II Working Group. Inter-Society Consensus for the Management of Peripheral Arterial Disease (TASC II). J Vasc Surg 2007; 45(Suppl S):S5–67.

   Comprehensive guidelines on the treatment of PAD.
8. Stoeckelhuber BM, Meissner O, Stoeckelhubr M et al. Primary endovascular stent placements of focal infrarenal aortic stenosis. Initial and mid term results. J Vasc Interv Radiol 2003; 14:1443–7.
9. Simons PC, Nawijn AA, Bruijninckx CM et al. Long-term results of primary stent placement to treat infrarenal aortic stenosis. Eur J Vasc Endovasc Surg 2006; 32:627–33.
10. Benson K, Hartz AJ. A comparison of observational studies and randomised control trials. New Engl J Med 2000; 342:1878–86.
11. Concato J, Shah N, Howitz RI. Randomised control trials, observational studies in the hierarchy of research design. New Engl J Med 2000; 342:1887–92.
12. Ioannidis JPA, Haidich AB, Lau J. Any casualties in the clash of randomised and observational evidence? Br Med J 2001; 322:879–90.
13. Wolf GL, Cross AP et al. Surgery or balloon angioplasty for peripheral vascular disease; a randomised clinical trial. J Vasc Interv Radiol 1993; 4:639–48.

   A multicentre prospective trial comparing PTA versus surgery for both supra- and infrainguinal disease. Both treatment arms were successful in terms of improving quality of life and haemodynamics; however, no difference was observed in outcomes at 4 years.
14. Ballard JL, Burgen JJ, Singh P et al. Aorto iliac stent deployment vs surgical reconstruction; analysis of outcome and cost. J Vasc Surg 1998; 28:94–101.
15. Kaufmann SL, Barth KH, Kadir S et al. Haemodynamic measurements in the evaluation and follow up of transluminal angioplasty of the iliac and femoral arteries. Radiology 1982; 142:329–36.
16. Kamphius AG, van Engelen AD, Tetteroo E et al. Impact of different haemodynamic criteria for stent placement after suboptimal iliac angioplasty. Dutch Iliac Stent Trial Study Group. J Vasc Interv Radiol 1999; 10:741–6.
17. Tetteroo E, Haaring C, van der Graaf Y. Randomised comparison of primary stent placement versus primary angioplasty followed by selective stent placement in patients with iliac-artery occlusive disease. Lancet 1998; 341:1153–9.
18. Ring EJ. Percutaneous recanalisation of common iliac occlusions; an unacceptable complication rate. Am J Roentgenol 1982; 139:587–9.
19. Richter GM. RCT comparing iliac stenting and PTA in stents; state of the art 1989. Pub Plyscience, pp. 30–35.
20. Tetteroo E, van der Graaf Y, Bosch JL et al. Randomised comparison of primary stent placement versus primary angioplasty followed by selective stent placement in patients with iliac-artery occlusive disease. Dutch Iliac Stent Trial Study Group. Lancet 1998; 351:1153–9.

   A multicentre randomised clinical trial (1993–7) comparing direct stent placement versus primary angioplasty with or without subsequent stent placement in patients with intermittent claudication. No difference was observed in the quality of life, patency and reintervention rates.
21. Klein WM, van der Graaf Y, Seegers J et al. Dutch Iliac Stent Trial: long-term results in patients randomized for primary or selective stent placement. Radiology 2006; 238:734–44.
22. Bosch JL Hunink MG. Stent or PTA in iliac "occlusive" disease meta-analysis of the results of PTA and stent placement in aortoiliac occlusive disease. Radiology 1997; 204:87–96.

   A meta-analysis of data from 1990 onwards, which included six PTA studies (1300 patients) and eight stent placement studies (816 patients). No differences were observed between the two groups in terms of mortality and complications, but technical success was higher in the stented group.
23. Bosch JL. Iliac arterial disease: cost effectiveness analysis of stent placement vs PTA. Radiology 1998; 208:641–81.
24. Dyet JF, Cook AM, Nicholson AA. Self expanding stents in iliac arteries.Clin Radiol 1993; 48:117–19.
25. Dyet JF, Gaines PA, Nicholson AA. Treatment of chronic iliac occlusions by means of percutaneous endovascular stent placement. J Vasc Interv Radiol 1997; 8:349–53.
26. British Society of Interventional Radiology. Iliac Angioplasty Study (BIAS) 2001. Oxfordshire: Dendrite Clinical Systems. ISBN 1–903968–01–1; http://www.bsir.org
27. Lewis DR, Davies AH, Irvine CD et al. Compression ultrasonography for false femoral artery aneurysms: hypocoagulability is a cause of failure. Eur J Vasc Endovasc Surg 1998; 16:427–8.
28. Tisi PV, Callam MJ. Surgery versus non-surgical treatment for femoral pseudoaneurysms. Cochrane Database Syst Rev 2006; 1:CD004981.
29. Hogg ME, Peterson BG, Pearce WH et al. Bare metal stent infections: case report and review of the literature. J Vasc Surg 2007; 46:813–20.
30. Carlisle J, Swart M. Mid-term survival after abdominal aortic aneurysm surgery predicted by

cardiopulmonary exercise testing. Br J Surg 2007; 94:966–9.

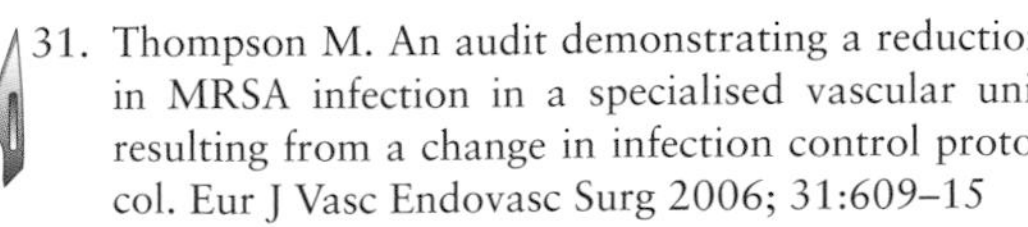

31. Thompson M. An audit demonstrating a reduction in MRSA infection in a specialised vascular unit resulting from a change in infection control protocol. Eur J Vasc Endovasc Surg 2006; 31:609–15

    **A prospective audit which demonstrated the effectiveness of an isolation policy on MRSA infection rates.**

32. Coggia M, Javerliat I, Di Centa I et al. Total laparoscopic bypass for aortoiliac occlusive lesions: 93-case experience. J Vasc Surg 2004; 40:899–906.
33. Štádler P, Šebesta P, Vitásek P et al. A modified technique of transperitoneal direct approach for totally laparoscopic aortoiliac surgery. Eur J Vasc Endovasc Surg 2006; 32:266–9.
34. Schmacht D, Armstrong P, Johnson B et al. Graft infectivity of rifampin and silver-bonded polyester grafts to MRSA contamination. Vasc Endovasc Surg 2005; 39:411–20.
35. Jackson MR, Ali AT, Bell C et al. Aortofemoral bypass in young patients with premature atherosclerosis: is superficial femoral vein superior to Dacron? J Vasc Surg 2004; 40:17–23.
36. Jaquinandi V, Picquet J, Bouyá P et al. High prevalence of proximal claudication among patients with patent aortobifemoral bypasses. J Vasc Surg 2007; 45:312–18.
37. Hertzer NR, Bena JF, Karafa MT. A personal experience with direct reconstruction and extra-anatomic bypass for aortoiliofemoral occlusive disease. J Vasc Surg 2007; 45:527–35.
38. Harrington ME, Harrington EB, Haimov M et al. Axillofemoral bypass: compromised bypass for compromised patients. J Vasc Surg 1994; 20:195–201.
39. Wittens CH, van Houtte HJ, van Urk H. European Prospective Randomised Multi-centre Axillo-bifemoral Trial. Eur J Vasc Surg 1992; 6:115–23.

    **A prospective multicentre RCT comparing two designs: (i) contralateral branch at an angle of 90 degrees and (ii) a flowsplitter. At a median follow-up of 12 months the flowsplitter group had a significantly better patency rate at 2 years. No differences were observed in terms of mortality and graft infection.**

40. Ricco JB, Probst H. Long-term results of a multicenter randomized study on direct versus crossover bypass for unilateral iliac artery occlusive disease. J Vasc Surg 2008; 47:45–53.

    **A prospective multicentre RCT (France and Switzerland) between 1986 and 1991, which demonstrated superior assisted primary and secondary patency rates for iliofemoral grafting over femoro-femoral bypass. The latter should be reserved for high-risk cases not amenable to interventional radiology.**

41. Ascer E, Kirwin J, Mohan C et al. The preferential use of the external iliac artery as an inflow source for redo femoropopliteal and infrapopliteal bypass. J Vasc Surg 1993; 18:234–9.
42. Kim YW, Lee JH, Kim HG et al. Factors affecting the long-term patency of crossover femorofemoral bypass graft. Eur J Vasc Endovasc Surg 2005; 30:376–80.
43. Pursell R, Sideso E, Magee TR et al. Critical appraisal of femorofemoral crossover grafts. Br J Surg 2005; 92:565–9.
44. Eiberg JP, Røder O, Stahl-Madsen M et al. Fluoropolymer-coated Dacron versus PTFE grafts for femorofemoral crossover bypass: randomised trial. Eur J Vasc Endovasc Surg 2006; 32:431–8.

    **A randomised multicentre clinical trial comparing Dacron versus PTFE in femoro-femoral reconstruction demonstrated no differences in outcome.**

45. Mingoli A, Sapienza P, Feldhaus RJ et al. Femorofemoral bypass grafts: factors influencing long-term patency rate and outcome. Surgery 2001; 129:451–8.
46. Aburahma AF, Robinson PA, Cook CC et al. Selecting patients for combined femorofemoral bypass grafting and iliac balloon angioplasty and stenting for bilateral iliac disease. J Vasc Surg 2001; 33(2, Suppl):S93–9.
47. Willigendael EM, Teijink JAW, Bartelink M-L et al. Smoking and the patency of lower extremity bypass grafts: a meta-analysis. J Vasc Surg 2008; 42:67–74.

    **A meta-analysis of 29 studies that evaluated the influence of smoking on the patency rates of lower limb arterial reconstruction.**

48. Curi MA, Skelly CL, Baldwin ZK et al. Long term outcome of infrainguinal bypass grafting in patients with serologically proven hypercoagulability. J Vasc Surg 2003; 37:301–6.

    **A retrospective analysis of consecutive patients from January 1994 to January 2001which demonstrated that patients with evidence of hypercoagulability have a worse outcome in terms of long-term patency, limb salvage and survival rates.**

49. Shanser A, Hevelone N, Owens CD et al. Technical factors affecting autogenous vein graft failure: observations from a large multicentre trial. J Vasc Surg 2007; 46:1180–90.

    **Analysis of the PREVENT III trial database of 1404 North American patients who underwent lower limb arterial reconstruction with autogolous vein.**

50. Faries PL, Arora S, Pomposelli FBJr et al. The use of arm vein in lower-extremity revascularization: results of 520 procedures performed in eight years. J Vasc Surg 2000; 31:50–9.
51. Veith FJ, Gupta SK, Ascer E et al. Six-year prospective multicenter randomized comparison of autologous saphenous vein and expanded polytetrafluoroethylene grafts in infrainguinal arterial reconstructions. J Vasc Surg 1986; 3(1):104–14.
52. Hunink MG, Wong JB, Donaldson MC et al. Patency results of percutaneous and surgical

revascularization for femoropopliteal arterial disease. Med Decis Making 1994; 14(1):71–81.

The authors used a method based on the proportional hazards model and the actuarial life-table approach; the results were adjusted for differences in case mix of the study populations. Adjusted 5-year primary patencies after surgery varied from 33% to 80%, the best results being for saphenous vein bypass performed for claudication.

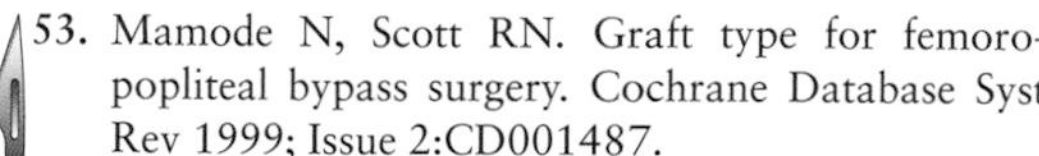

53. Mamode N, Scott RN. Graft type for femoropopliteal bypass surgery. Cochrane Database Syst Rev 1999; Issue 2:CD001487.

A Cochrane review of nine trials which included 1334 patients. No clear evidence was identified as to which type of graft is best. No difference was observed between in situ and reversed. Vein cuffs offer better primary patency rates for below-knee femoro-popliteal PTFE grafts.

54. Jensen LP, Lepäntalo M, Fossdal JE et al. Dacron or PTFE for above knee femoropopliteal bypass. A multicenter randomised study. Eur J Vasc Endovasc Surg 2007; 34:44–9.

A prospective multicentre RCT (1993–8) comparing Dacron versus PTFE. No difference was observed in terms of limb salvage, mortality and major complications. Secondary patency rates were better in the Dacron group.

55. Griffiths GD, Nagy J, Black D et al. Randomized clinical trial of distal anastomotic interposition vein cuff in infrainguinal polytetrafluoroethylene bypass grafting. Br J Surg 2004; 91:560–2.

A prospective RCT of cuff versus no cuff for femoropopliteal PTFE reconstructions. Three-year patency rates were significantly better in the cuff group in the below-knee setting; however, no differences were observed in limb salvage rates (above and below knee).

56. Lundell A, Lindblad B, Bergqvist D et al. Femoropopliteal–crural graft patency is improved by an intensive surveillance program: a prospective randomised study. J Vasc Surg 1995; 21:26–34.

A prospective RCT of intensive versus routine surveillance. Primary and secondary patency rates were better in the intensive group, but no difference was observed in the PTFE grafts.

57. Ihlberg L, Luther M, Tierala E et al. The utility of duplex scanning in infrainguinal vein graft surveillance: results from a randomised controlled study. Eur J Vasc Endovasc Surg 1998; 16:19–27.

Entry into this trial was based upon a patent graft at 1 month. Patients were prospective randomised to clinical observation versus duplex. No beneficial effect was noted in the duplex group.

58. Davies AH, Hawdon AJ, Sydes MR et al. on behalf of the VGST participants. Is duplex surveillance of value after leg vein bypass grafting. Circulation 2005; 112:1985–91.

A multicentre prospective RCT where patients with a patent graft at 1 month were randomised to clinical versus duplex assessment. No differences were observed between the two groups in mortality, primary and secondary patency rates and limb salvage rates.

59. Bandyk D. Surveillance after lower extremity arterial bypass. Perspect Vasc Surg Endovasc Ther 2007; 19:376–83.

60. Mofidi R, Kleman J, Berry O et al. Significance of early postoperative duplex results in infrainguinal vein bypass surveillance. Eur J Vasc Endovasc Surg 2007; 34:327–32.

61. Armstrong PA, Bandyk D, Wilson JS et al. Optimizing infrainguinal arm vein bypass patency with duplex ultrasound surveillance and endovascular therapy. J Vasc Surg 2004; 40:724–31.

62. Brumberg RS, Back MR, Armstrong PA et al. The relative importance of graft surveillance and warfarin therapy in infrainguinal prosthetic bypass failure. J Vasc Surg 2007; 46:1160–6.

63. Raby JF, Kiran RP, Gersten G et al. Early results with infra-inguinal cutting balloon angioplasty limits distal dissection. Ann Vasc Surg 2004; 18:640.

64. Laird J, Jaff MR, Biamino G et al. Cryoplasty for the treatment of femoro-popliteal arterial disease; results of a prospective multi-centre registry. J Vasc Interv Radiol 2005; 16:1067–73.

65. Karthik S, Tuite DJ, Nicholson AA et al. Cryoplasty for arterial restenosis. Eur J Vasc Endovasc Surg 2007; 33:40–3.

66. Spinosa DJ, Leung DA, Matsumoto AH et al. Percutaneous intentional extraluminal recanalization in patients with chronic critical limb ischemia. Radiology 2004; 232:499–507.

67. Lazaris AM, Salas C, Tsiamis AC et al. Factors affecting patency of subintimal infrainguinal angioplasty in patients with critical lower limb ischemia. Eur J Vasc Endovasc Surg 2006; 32:668–74.

68. Sabeti S, Schillinger M, Amighi J et al. Primary patency of femoro-popliteal arteries treated with Nitinol stainless steel self expanding stents: propensity score adjusted analysis. Radiology 2004; 232:516–21.

69. Vogel TR, Shindelman LE, Nackman JB et al. Efficacious use of Nitinol stents in the femoral and popliteal arteries. J Vasc Surg 2003; 38:1178–84.

70. Jahnke T, Voshage G, Müller-Hülsbeck S et al. Endovascular placement of self expanding Nitinol coiled stents for the treatment of femoro-popliteal obstructive disease. J Vasc Interv Radiol 2002; 13:257–66.

71. Rits J, van Herwaarden JA, Jahrome AK et al. The incidence of arterial stent fractures with exclusion of coronary, aortic and non-arterial settings. Eur J Vasc Endovasc Surg 2008; 36:339–45.

72. Schillinger M et al. Balloon angioplasty versus implantation of nitinol stents in the superficial femoral artery. N Engl J Med 2006; 354(18):1879–88.

73. Schillinger M et al. Sustained benefit at 2 years of primary femoropopliteal stenting compared with balloon angioplasty with optional stenting. Circulation 2007; 115(21):2745–9.

74. Sabeti S et al. Primary patency of femoropopliteal arteries treated with nitinol versus stainless steel self-expanding stents: propensity score-adjusted analysis. Radiology 2004; 232(2):516–21.

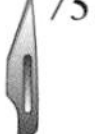

75. Duda SH, Bosier SM, Lammer J et al. Sirolimus eluting vs bare Nitinol stents for obstructive superficial femoral artery disease. The SIROCCO II trial. J Vasc Interv Radiol 2005; 16:331–8.

**A randomised double-blind trial comparing bare stents against sirolimus-eluting stents. No difference was observed between the groups in terms of the primary end-point of in-stent lumen diameter at 6 months.**

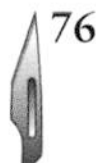

76. Duda SH, Bosiers M, Lammer J et al. Drug-eluting and bare nitinol stents for the treatment of atherosclerotic lesions in the superficial femoral artery: long-term results from the SIROCCO trial. J Endovasc Ther 2006; 13:701–10.

**A randomised double-blind trial comparing bare stents against sirolimus-eluting stents. At 24 months no difference was observed between the two groups in terms of mortality, ankle brachial index and re-stenosis rates.**

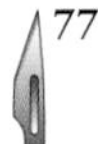

77. Tepe G, Zeller T, Albrecht T et al. Local delivery of paclitaxel to inhibit restenosis during angioplasty of the leg. N Engl J Med 2008; 14:689–99.

**A randomised multicentre trial which compared paclitaxel-coated angioplasty balloons and paclitaxel dissolved in the angiographic contrast medium during angioplasty of the leg. At 6 months there was a significant reduction in late lumen loss and requirement for target lesion revascularisation.**

78. Kedora J, Hohmann S, Garrett W et al. Randomised comparison of percutaneous Viabahn stent grafts vs prosthetic femoro-popliteal bypass in the treatment of superficial femoral arterial occlusive disease. J Vasc Surg 2007; 45:10–16.

79. Soder HK, Manninen HI, Jaakkola P et al. Prospective trial of infrapopliteal artery balloon angioplasty for critical limb ischemia: angiographic and clinical results. J Vasc Interv Radiol 2000; 11:1021–31.

80. Vraux H, Hammer F, Verhelst R et al. Subintimal angioplasty of tibial vessel occlusions in the treatment of critical ischaemia: mid-term results. Eur J Vasc Endovasc Surg 2000; 20:441–6.

81. Peregrin JH, Smirová S, Koznar B et al. Self-expandable stent placement in infrapopliteal arteries after unsuccessful angioplasty failure: one year follow up. Cardiovasc Interv Radiol 2008 (Epub ahead of print).

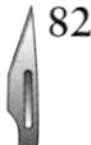

82. Adam AJ, Beard JD, Cleveland T et al. BASIL trial participants. Bypass versus angioplasty in severe ischaemia of the leg (BASIL): multicentre, randomised controlled trial. Lancet 2005; 366:1925–34.

**A prospective RCT of surgery versus angioplasty in patients with severe lower limb ischaemia. The primary end-point of the study was amputation. At the end of 6 months there was no difference between the two groups in terms of amputation-free survival rates and quality of life.**

83. Loosemore TM, Chalmers TC, Dormandy JA. A meta-analysis of randomized placebo control trials in Fontaine stages III and IV peripheral occlusive arterial disease. Int Angiol 1994; 13:133–42.

**A meta-analysis of six RCTs of Iloprost in the treatment of patients with Fontaine stage III and IV peripheral arterial occlusive disease unsuitable for arterial reconstruction. Significant ($P$ < 0.05) beneficial effects with regards to the probability of being alive with both legs at 6 months follow-up were reported.**

84. Rajagopalan S, Mohler ER 3rd, Lederman RJ et al. Regional angiogenesis with vascular endothelial growth factor in peripheral arterial disease: a phase II randomized, double-blind, controlled study of adenoviral delivery of vascular endothelial growth factor 121 in patients with disabling intermittent claudication. Circulation 2003; 108:1933–8.

85. Rajagopalan S, Olin J, Deitcher S et al. Use of a constitutively active hypoxia-inducible factor-1alpha transgene as a therapeutic strategy in no-option critical limb ischemia patients: phase I dose-escalation experience. Circulation 2007; 115:1234–43.

86. Tateishi-Yuyama E, Matsubara H, Murohara T et al. Therapeutic Angiogenesis using Cell Transplantation (TACT) Study Investigators. Therapeutic angiogenesis for patients with limb ischaemia by autologous transplantation of bone-marrow cells: a pilot study and a randomised controlled trial. Lancet 2002; 360:427–35.

87. Cañizo MC, Lozano F, González-Porras JR et al. Peripheral endothelial progenitor cells (CD133+) for therapeutic vasculogenesis in a patient with critical limb ischemia. One year follow-up. Cytotherapy 2007; 9:99–102.

88. Kajiguchi M, Kondo T, Izawa H et al. Safety and efficacy of autologous progenitor cell transplantation for therapeutic angiogenesis in patients with critical limb ischemia. Circ J 2007; 71:196–201.

89. Marui A, Tabata Y, Kojima S et al. A novel approach to therapeutic angiogenesis for patients with critical limb ischemia by sustained release of basic fibroblast growth factor using biodegradable gelatin hydrogel: an initial report of the phase I–IIa study. Circ J 2007; 71:1181–6.

90. Jivegard LE, Augustinsson LE, Holm J et al. Effects of spinal cord stimulation (SCS) in patients with inoperable severe lower limb ischaemia: a prospective randomised controlled study. Eur J Vasc Endovasc Surg 1995; 9:421–5.

91. Klomp HM, Spincemaille GH, Steyerberg EW et al. Spinal-cord stimulation in critical limb ischaemia: a randomised trial. ESES Study Group. Lancet 1999; 353:1040–4.

92. Amann W, Berg P, Gersbach P et al. European Peripheral Vascular Disease Outcome Study SCS-EPOS. Spinal cord stimulation in the treatment of non-reconstructable stable critical leg ischaemia: results of the European Peripheral Vascular Disease

Outcome Study (SCS-EPOS). Eur J Vasc Endovasc Surg 2003; 26:280–6.

**93.** Persson AV, Anderson LA, Padberg FTJr. Selection of patients for lumbar sympathectomy. Surg Clin North Am 1985; 65:393–403.

**94.** Fulton RL, Blakeley WR. Lumbar sympathectomy: a procedure of questionable value in the treatment of arteriosclerosis obliterans of the legs. Am J Surg 1968; 116:735–44.

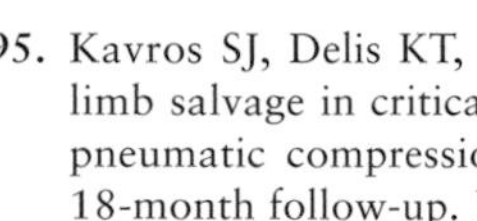

**95.** Kavros SJ, Delis KT, Turner NS et al. Improving limb salvage in critical ischemia with intermittent pneumatic compression: a controlled study with 18-month follow-up. J Vasc Surg 2008; 47:543–9.

A retrospective observational study looking at the efficacy of intermittent pneumatic compression (IPC) in the community in patients with chronic limb ischaemia. Wound healing and limb salvage were significantly better in the IPC group.

# 5

# The diabetic foot

Edward B. Jude
Andrew J.M. Boulton

## Introduction

The diabetic foot is one of the most common complications of diabetes, resulting in increased morbidity and mortality.[1–4] With increasing prevalence of diabetes mellitus, in particular type 2 diabetes, it is a major burden on healthcare systems due to microvasulcar and macrovascular complications as a result of end-organ damage caused by long-term hyperglycaemia.[1] Diabetic peripheral neuropathy and peripheral vascular disease are the main aetiological factors in foot ulceration and may act alone, together or in combination with other factors such as microvascular disease, biomechanical abnormalities, limited joint mobility and increased susceptibility to infection. Foot problems in diabetic patients account for more hospital admissions than any other long-term complication of diabetes.[2–4] The 'diabetic foot syndrome' encompasses a number of pathologies, including diabetic neuropathy, peripheral vascular disease, Charcot neuroarthropathy, foot ulceration, osteomyelitis and the potentially preventable end-point, amputation.[5] Patients with the diabetic foot can also have multiple diabetic complications, including retinopathy, nephropathy and cardiovascular disease. Caring for such patients is complicated and involves specialities across boundaries; a multidisciplinary approach is required and involvement of physicians, surgeons and other healthcare professionals should be sought.

## Epidemiology

The burden of diabetic foot disease will increase due to the increasing prevalence of diabetes.[6] Prevalence and incidence studies of foot ulceration have looked at a number of different community-based populations. Kumar et al.[7] found a history of current or previous ulceration in 5.3% of patients with type 2 diabetes, a study from Oxford found foot ulceration in 7% of diabetic patients over the age of 60 years,[8] and Borssen et al.[9] reported a history of ulceration in 3% of type 1 diabetic patients aged 15–50 years. In a recent study in the north-west of England, the annual incidence of foot ulceration was reported to be 2.2% among 10000 community-based diabetic individuals with type 2 diabetes,[10] and in the Wisconsin study the 4-year incidence of ulcers in diabetic patients with type 1 and type 2 diabetes was 9.5% and 10.5% respectively.[11] In another study from the USA, 5.8% of 8905 patients followed up over a 3-year period developed a foot ulcer, or in other words nearly 2% per year.[12]

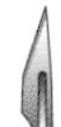

With regard to the aetiology of foot ulceration, 45–60% are purely neuropathic, about 10% purely ischaemic and 25–45% of mixed neuroischaemic origin. In a more recent study we found a slight increase in the incidence of neuroischaemic (52.3%) and ischaemic (11.7%) foot ulcers, with a reduction in neuropathic ulcers (36%).[13] This changing pattern in the presentation of diabetic foot ulcers may be an indication of the greater awareness created by the initiation of multidisciplinary foot clinics as well as the importance placed on the education of patients who are 'at risk' of foot ulceration.

Lower limb amputation is performed 15 times more frequently in diabetic than non-diabetic patients;[14] after unilateral amputation, rates for both mortality and contralateral amputation are depressingly high.

Like neuropathy and peripheral vascular disease, both amputation and ulceration are more common in males. Racial differences exist, with the amputation rate in Asian subjects being only one-quarter that in Caucasians.[15]

# Aetiology of foot ulceration

## Diabetic neuropathy

The numerous manifestations of diabetic neuropathy affect up to 50% of patients, but despite much intensive research the pathophysiology remains unclear and opinion is divided between microvascular disease leading to nerve hypoxia, and the direct effects of hyperglycaemia on neuronal metabolism. Recently, attempts to unite these two hypotheses have demonstrated abnormalities in nitric oxide metabolism, resulting in perineural vasoconstriction and nerve damage.

There are a number of manifestations of diabetic neuropathy, including mononeuropathies and polyneuropathies. In the lower limbs, distal sensory polyneuropathy is the commonest presentation of neuropathy. However, the motor and autonomic fibres may also be involved. The development of neuropathy is linked to poor glycaemic control over many years and thus increases in frequency with both age and duration of diabetes. Estimates of the prevalence of neuropathy vary because of different diagnostic criteria and populations. A number of studies have indicated a prevalence of neuropathy of approximately 30% among diabetic patients attending hospital,[16] with lower rates closer to 20% seen in population-based samples.[10,17] Among the elderly, the prevalence may be as high as 50%. Regular foot examination is essential to identify the presence of neuropathy so that treatment and education can be instituted to prevent complications resulting from loss of protective sensation.[18] Unless proper foot examination is carried out the diagnosis can be missed in a significant number of patients.[19]

Symptoms of neuropathy do not occur in every patient and a significant number of patients are completely unaware of their marked sensory loss, which can therefore only be detected by regular and annual screening of the asymptomatic diabetic patient. Over time, as the neuropathy evolves, patients will experience symptoms, although these may simply be 'negative' and might comprise 'numbness' or 'deadness' in the lower limbs. Positive symptoms most commonly include burning pain, altered and uncomfortable temperature perception, paraesthesiae, shooting, stabbing and lancinating pain, hyperaesthesiae and allodynia. Many patients find the symptoms difficult to describe, but most report them to be extremely uncomfortable, distressing and prone to nocturnal exacerbation. The feet and lower legs are most commonly affected, although some patients with long-standing neuropathy may experience similar though less severe symptoms in the upper limbs. About an equal number of patients report no symptoms and distal symmetrical polyneuropathy cannot be excluded without a careful neurological examination. These can be differentiated from intermittent claudication most easily by the nocturnal exacerbations, the lack of relationship to exercise and the location of symptoms mainly in the foot rather than the calf (Table 5.1).

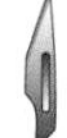

Although no drugs have been demonstrated to improve the underlying neuropathy, painful symptoms are often well controlled by tricyclic antidepressants (e.g. amitryptylline), anticonvulsants (e.g. gabapentin, pregabalin and carbamazepine) or the serotonergic noradrenaline reuptake inhibitors (e.g. duloxetine).[20–22] Topical creams containing capsaicin may also provide relief, especially at night.[23]

Autonomic neuropathy reduces sweating in the skin and opens arteriovenous shunts, leading to increased blood flow to the leg.[24] Thus, the neuropathic foot is typically warm with bounding pulses and has dry, sometimes cracked, skin. Motor neuropathy mainly affects the intrinsic muscles of the foot (as they are the most distal) and can lead to wasting (guttering between the metatarsals) and an altered foot shape, with clawed toes and prominent metatarsal heads. It can be seen therefore that the insensitive neuropathic foot is at risk from unperceived

**Table 5.1** • Comparison of signs and symptoms of neuropathic and ischaemic pain

| | Neuropathic pain | Intermittent claudication | Ischaemic rest pain |
|---|---|---|---|
| Site | Foot/shin | Calf/thigh | Foot/calf |
| Nature | Tingling/burning/shooting | Cramping | Aching |
| Exacerbating factors | Night time | Exercise | Elevation |
| Relieving factors | Exercise | Rest | Dependency of foot |
| Clinical signs in the foot | Warm, bounding pulses | Weak/absent pulses | Cold/pulseless |

external trauma (e.g. ill-fitting shoes), repetitive painless injury to high-pressure areas under the metatarsal heads during walking, and easy access to infection through dry cracked skin. Although vascular disease and infection were once thought to be the main causes of foot ulceration, prospective studies have now clearly demonstrated the important role of neuropathy.[25,26] Neuropathy is responsible for a high proportion of foot ulcers,[27,28] and leads to a seven- to tenfold increase in the risk of ulceration.

The diagnosis of neuropathy is usually simple and can be made by clinical examination, which reveals a 'stocking' distribution of sensory loss to one or more of pain, temperature and vibration modalities with absent ankle reflexes. If present, neuropathic symptoms and the typical appearance (described above) are useful. Quantitative sensory testing (of vibration, pressure and temperature perception thresholds) may provide a useful adjunct, and of the different tests available, measurement of the pressure perception threshold is the simplest. Using a nylon monofilament pressed against the skin until it buckles, a load of 10 g can be accurately applied. Patients unable to feel this on the sole of the foot are at high risk of ulceration. Simple bedside tests are all that is required to identify the foot at risk of neuropathic ulceration, and nerve conduction studies are rarely needed in clinical practice.[29]

## Peripheral vascular disease

Atherosclerotic vascular disease is probably present (at least in subclinical form) in all patients with long-duration diabetes.[30]

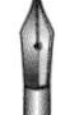

Vascular disease is responsible for up to 70% of deaths in type 2 diabetes, the premenopausal protection from vascular disease is lost in female diabetic patients, and peripheral vascular disease may be 20 times more common in diabetes.[31]

The basic pathophysiology of atherosclerosis is probably no different in diabetes and is characterised by endothelial damage followed by platelet aggregation, lipid deposition and smooth muscle proliferation with plaque formation. The same risk factors also operate and include smoking, hypertension, dyslipidaemia, abnormal fibrinolysis and altered platelet function. Although some of these risk factors are much more prevalent in the diabetic population, a full explanation of the excess of vascular disease in diabetes remains elusive.

The distribution of vascular disease in the lower limb is thought to be different in diabetes, with more frequent involvement of vessels below the knee (**Fig. 5.1**a). Surprisingly, however, there are few good studies available to support this widely held belief, although Strandness et al.[32] reported that two-thirds of diabetic patients with peripheral vascular disease had infrapopliteal disease, and King et al.[33] found that involvement of the profunda femoris was increased in diabetes (Fig. 5.1b).

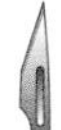

In our random study of patients referred for angiography, no difference was seen in proximal disease (iliac, femoropopliteal vessels) but distal disease (calf vessel) was twice as high in diabetic compared with non-diabetic patients.[34]

The difficulties posed by the distribution may be further complicated by a reduced ability to develop a contralateral supply, but despite these problems revascularisation procedures are frequently successful, although a more distal anastomosis may be required. Indeed, comparative studies have shown similar long-term outcomes of revascularisation for patients with and without diabetes,[35] and a number of centres have reported reduced amputation rates due to an increase in the number of bypass procedures.

Diabetic patients with peripheral vascular disease may develop intermittent claudication, but often this is absent and the first clinical presentation may be ischaemic foot ulceration.[30] Typically, this is at the ends of the toes, and in the absence of neuropathy is painful. The foot is usually cool with absent pulses, but presence of warmth in a neuroischaemic foot with swelling may suggest deep infection. The most helpful non-invasive investigation is measurement of the ankle–brachial pressure index (ABPI).[36] When below 0.9 this is clearly indicative of ischaemia, but often it may be falsely elevated due to medial calcification of vessel walls, a phenomenon frequently seen in diabetic neuropathy (**Fig. 5.2**). In this situation, the Doppler waveform seems useful, as loss of the normal triphasic waveform indicates vascular disease. Measurement of toe pressures provides additional information, as the digital arteries are less frequently affected by calcification (see Chapter 2). Finally, transcutaneous oxygen tension (measured by an electrode placed on the foot) accurately reflects skin oxygenation and can be used to determine the severity of ischaemia, the likelihood that an ulcer will heal, and an appropriate level for amputation.[37] Despite advances in non-invasive investigations, arteriography (which must include pedal arteries) remains the gold standard for both diagnosis and planning of treatment. However, care is needed with contrast media in patients with renal impairment, since they can precipitate an acute deterioration in renal function. If the serum creatinine is >200 μmol/L, a nephrologist should be consulted prior to contrast arteriography (see Chapter 2).

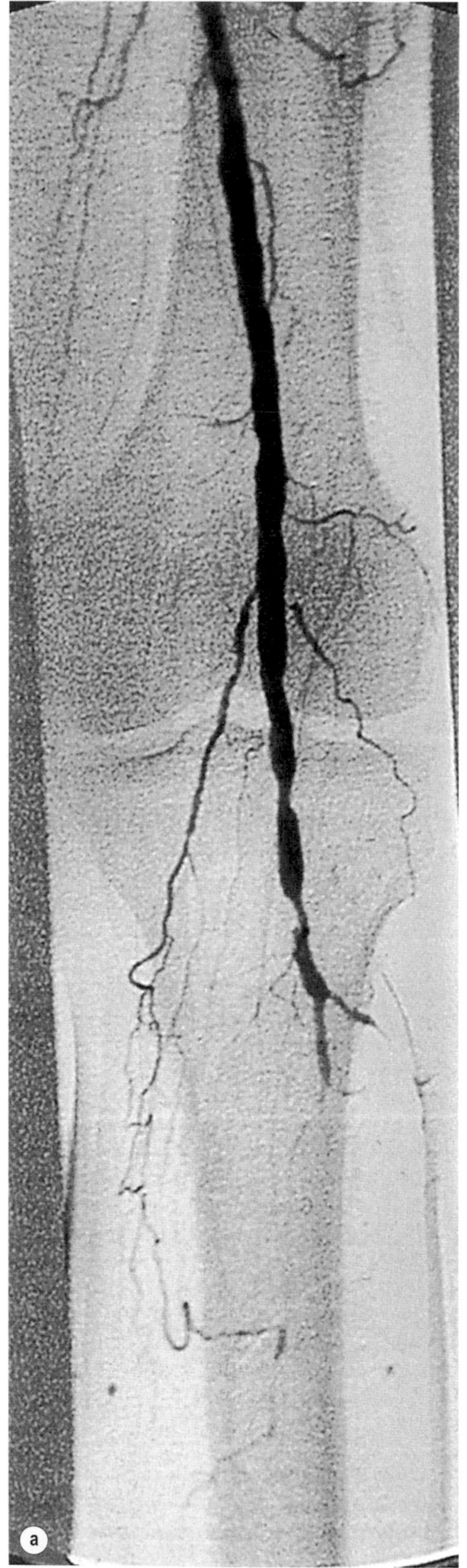


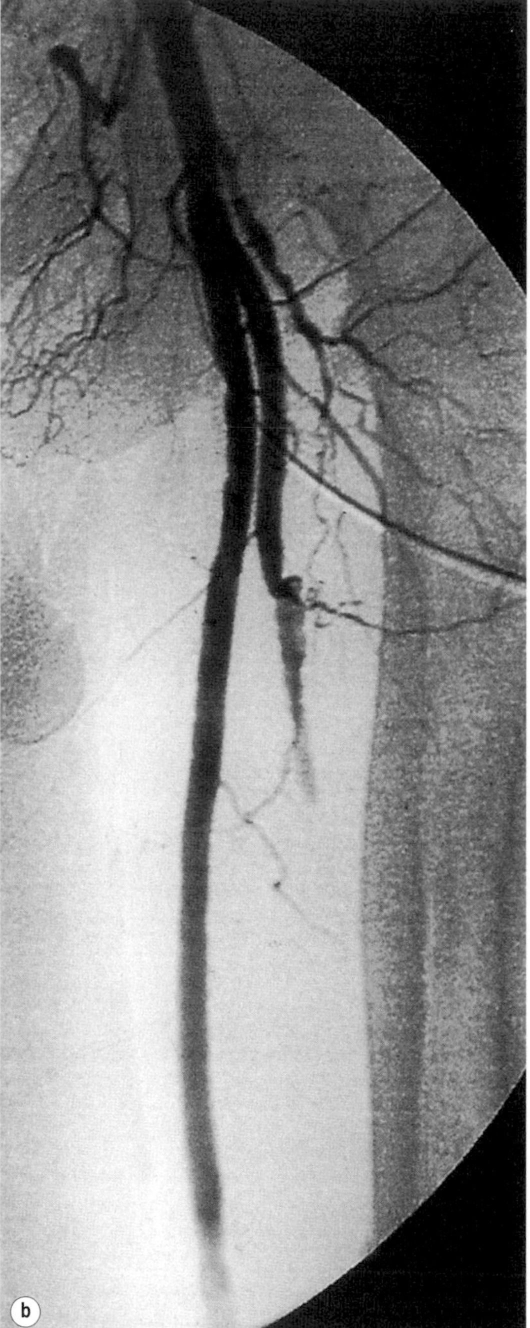


**Figure 5.1** • Typical distribution of atherosclerosis affecting the popliteal trifurcation and tibial arteries **(a)**. The distal profunda is also often affected **(b)**, which reduces the ability for collaterals to develop around a superficial femoral occlusion.

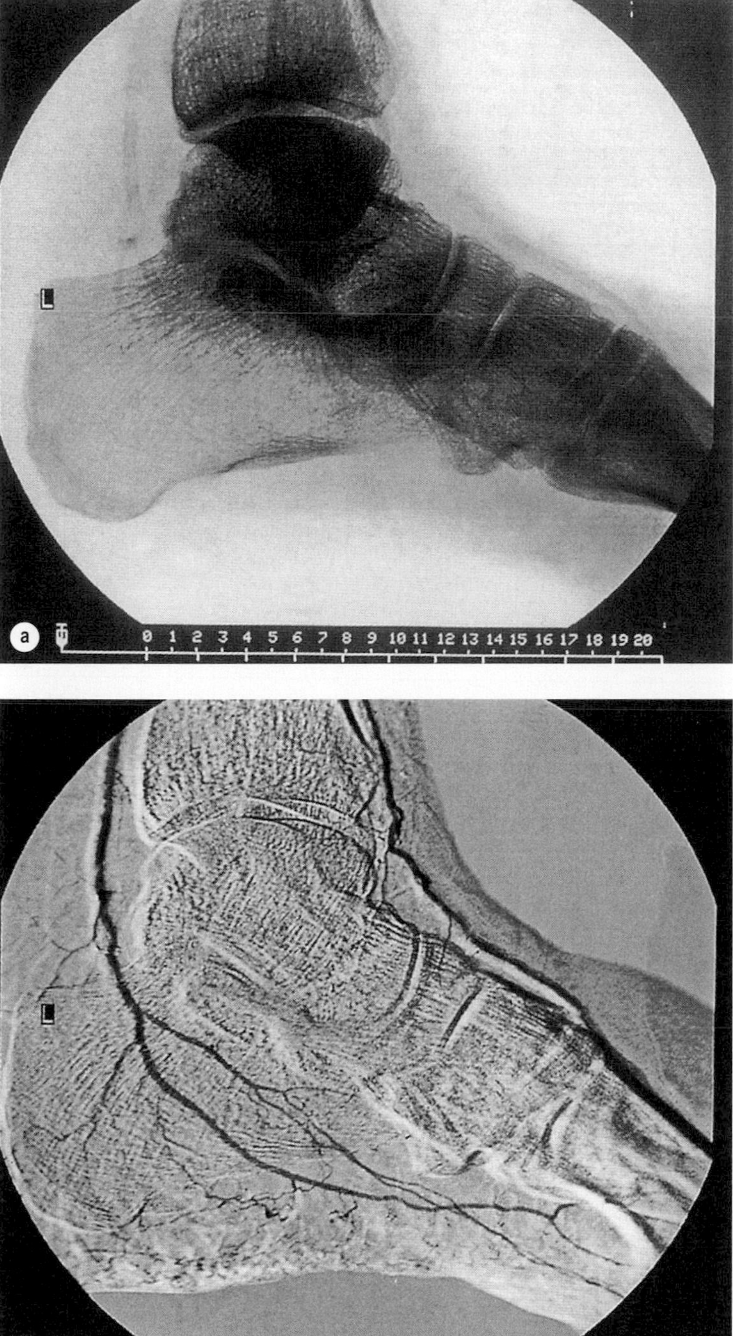


**Figure 5.2** • Calcification of the posterior tibial, anterior tibial and dorsalis pedis arteries in diabetes **(a)**. The calcification is in the media and may falsely elevate Doppler pressures and make pulses difficult to palpate. However, good arterial flow may still be present **(b)**.

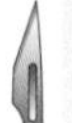

An antiplatelet agent such as aspirin, dipyridamole or clopidogrel will lower the risk of thrombotic vascular events, and has been shown to reduce vascular death in patients with intermittent claudication by about 25%.[38] Hypertension should be treated to target (130/80 mmHg for patients with diabetes),[39] with an angiotensin-converting enzyme (ACE) inhibitor probably being the treatment of choice. The HOPE study showed that the ACE inhibitor ramipril reduces cardiovascular morbidity and mortality in patients with peripheral arterial disease by around 25%.[40] Patients with hyperlipidaemia should have their cholesterol levels lowered to target. The Heart Protection Study showed that lowering total and low-density lipoprotein (LDL) cholesterol by 25% with a statin reduces cardiovascular mortality and morbidity in patients with peripheral arterial disease by around one-quarter.[41]

Three indicated therapies are available to improve walking distance. Two of these (naftidrofuryl, pentoxifylline) are considered to be less suitable for prescribing.[42] Cilostazol has been shown to significantly improve maximal and pain-free walking distance in patients with intermittent claudication, both in patients with diabetes and in those without diabetes.[30]

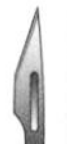

Regular exercise has been shown to be beneficial in diabetic patients with intermittent claudication, where it more than doubled the symptom-free walking distance.[43] Based on current evidence, the most effective exercise regimen consists of walking sessions approximately 1 hour long three times a week during which the patient walks to near maximal pain (preferably on a treadmill during supervised therapy), stops until the pain is relieved and then resumes walking to near maximal pain again.[44] Exercise training in patients with intermittent claudication can produce a significant improvement in walking distance in those patients who adhere to the programme. Unfortunately, compliance in such patients is often poor and only a minority are able to attend supervised exercise classes.

Cilostazol, a selective phosphodiesterase III inhibitor, has vasodilating, antithrombotic and antiplatelet properties but its exact mechanism of action in patients with intermittent claudication is unknown.[45]

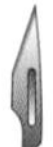

A pooled analysis of the results of eight phase III controlled clinical trials of 436 patients with intermittent claudication who also had diabetes showed that the 216 patients who received cilostazol (100 mg b.d.) increased their maximal walking distances, initial claudication distance and absolute claudication distance significantly more than the 220 patients who received placebo.[46,47]

Patients with diabetes showed no significant differences from those without diabetes who had taken cilostazol with respect to improvements in walking distances and response rates. Mean percentage change in maximal walking distance from baseline was 53% for patients with diabetes versus 60% for patients without diabetes. However, increases in maximal walking distance were slightly lower in patients with diabetes, as these patients had a lower baseline walking distance and a higher incidence of concomitant cardiovascular disease. Safety data in the patients with diabetes were in line with those seen in patients without diabetes. Cilostazol is contraindicated in several subpopulations of patients, particularly those with congestive heart failure and severe hepatic or renal impairment. However, current data would appear to support the use of cilostazol as a promising therapy for patients with intermittent claudication and diabetes, among the limited options available for these patients.

The indications for invasive treatment of peripheral vascular disease are progressive claudication and ischaemic or neuroischaemic ulceration. Suitability of an individual for vascular reconstruction needs to be considered and depends on appropriate anatomy and the presence of other medical conditions. Thus, a decision to amputate rather than revascularise in a patient with renal failure and ischaemic heart disease may be based on their substantial perioperative risk from a prolonged distal bypass, rather than the availability of a vessel to graft onto. However, an aggressive approach to revascularisation is known to save limbs, and other conditions may need treating or controlling before vascular surgery. Finally, when severe foot infection is present, this needs treating promptly with incision, drainage and debridement. Only when the infection has been controlled can revascularisation be performed.

## Biomechanical aspects

The most important cause of foot ulceration is loss of protective pain sensation, permitting 'painless' repetitive trauma and tissue injury. However, vertical pressure applied to the plantar surface of the feet during walking and standing predisposes to ulceration. Plantar pressures can be measured by various methods, dynamic and static. Dynamic measurements are made using optical pedobarograph, Podotrack,[48] in-shoe or in-sole pressure transducers and static measurements using a Harris mat or a polytechnic-modified force plate. Patients with peripheral neuropathy and particularly ulcer patients have high plantar pressures,[49] although high pressures alone in the absence of insensitivity do not lead to ulceration.[50] Using an optical pedobarograph, Van Schie et al.[48] showed that plantar ulcers developed in one-third of patients with foot pressures >12.3 kg/cm$^2$, whereas no ulcers developed in patients with pressures <12.3 kg/cm$^2$. However, Frykberg et al.,[51] using an F-scan mat system, identified patients at risk of ulceration with foot pressures >6 kg/cm$^2$. Using the Pedar in-shoe pressure analysis system, Stacpoole-Shea et al.[52] demonstrated its ability to predict sites of potential foot ulceration, with a sensitivity of 83% and a specificity of 69%. Additionally, neuropathy with altered proprioception and small muscle wasting leads to alteration in foot shape, clawing of the toes, prominent metatarsal heads and a high arch, all of which result in changes in foot pressures.[53] Patients with previous amputations have higher foot pressures and greater risk of foot ulceration.[54] The more severe deformity of the Charcot foot, with joint dislocation and bony deformities, can also result in increased foot pressures and foot ulceration.

Limited joint mobility is a further contributing factor to elevated plantar pressures. Chronic hyperglycaemia results in glycosylation of proteins and when collagen is involved the collagen bundles become thickened and cross-linked. This results in thick, tight, waxy skin and restriction of joint movement. Limited joint mobility of the subtalar joint alters the mechanics of walking and is strongly associated with high plantar pressure.[55]

Neuropathy alone does not lead to spontaneous ulceration. It is only the combination of trauma and insensitivity that results in tissue damage. The trauma sometimes takes the form of a single event, such as standing on a nail, but more frequently occurs as repeated minor trauma, such as unperceived shoe rubbing to the toes or increased pressure beneath the metatarsal heads during walking. It is now possible to measure dynamic vertical plantar pressure accurately, and a number of studies have clearly demonstrated that this is elevated in diabetic neuropathy and especially in patients with a history of plantar ulceration.[56,57] More importantly, a prospective study has shown that elevated plantar pressures are predictive of plantar ulceration, with 28% of neuropathic feet with high foot pressures ulcerating during a 30-month follow-up period.[49] Plantar ulcers only occurred in those who had both neuropathy and high foot pressures. The presence of callus (produced in response to pressure) may exacerbate the problem both by acting as a foreign body and by increasing plantar pressures.[58] Thus, removal of callus significantly reduces foot pressures.[59] Increased plantar tissue thickness has also been demonstrated in the neuropathic foot, thus making these patients at higher risk of foot ulceration.[60]

The main cause of increased pressure is thought to be the alteration in foot shape (described earlier), resulting in prominent metatarsal heads. Neuropathy causes atrophy of the intrinsic muscles of the foot (predominantly plantar flexors of the toes), altering the flexor/extensor balance at the metatarsophalangeal joints. This results in clawing of the toes and may be associated with subluxation at the metatarsophalangeal joints. There is also anterior displacement of the submetatarsal fat pads and indeed reduced subcutaneous tissue thickness at the metatarsal heads has been confirmed in diabetic neuropathy.[61]

The accurate measurement of foot pressures requires sophisticated and expensive systems, which are currently available only in specialised centres. However, clinical examination that both inspects foot shape and identifies the presence of callus provides very valuable information, which can be used to select patients in need of pressure relief (see below). Indeed, the presence of callus may in some ways be superior to pressure measurement, as it results not only from vertical pressure but also from shear forces, which cannot currently be measured. Furthermore, the presence of haemorrhage into callus should be seen as a pre-ulcerative phenomenon and requires urgent attention.

## Other risk factors

A number of inherent immunological abnormalities have been documented in diabetes. Neutrophil function is impaired, with abnormalities of adherence, chemotaxis, phagocytosis and killing ability,[62] and these may be partly due to ascorbic acid transport defects.[63] Several studies have shown an increased infection rate in postoperative wounds.[64] Thus, although no study has specifically examined reduced immunity in the context of diabetic foot ulceration, it seems likely that this forms part of the explanation of the common clinical problem of infection in the diabetic foot.

Advancing age is frequently accompanied by impaired vision and immobility, both of which make foot inspection more difficult and delay the time when help is sought for an ulcer. The prevalence of neuropathy and peripheral vascular disease is also high among the elderly. Thus, lower limb amputation is more common among older diabetic patients.[14]

Diabetic nephropathy and renal failure are usually associated with numerous other problems, including diabetic retinopathy, neuropathy, macrovascular disease, reduced resistance to infection and peripheral oedema, all of which place such patients at very high risk of ulceration.

## The pathway to ulceration

As evidenced by the number of different risk factors (Box 5.1), the pathway to ulceration and amputation is often complex, and two or more elements are nearly always required. Ulceration of the insensitive foot only occurs when it is subjected to trauma, and the addition of peripheral vascular disease reduces the external pressure required to cause local ischaemia and tissue breakdown. Conversely, in patients with elevated plantar pressures due to rheumatoid arthritis, ulceration does not occur because sensation is intact and pain protects the feet from repeated injury.

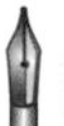

A two-centre prospective study confirmed that the commonest factors leading to foot ulceration were neuropathy, deformity (e.g. claw toes, prominent metatarsal heads) and trauma (e.g. ill-fitting shoes).[28]

The corollary of this multifactorial aetiology is that the pathways can be interrupted at any point. Tight glycaemic control in the first 10–20 years of diabetes will prevent the development of neuropathy and other complications, but the provision of good education about foot care to patients with high-risk feet may be equally successful at preventing ulceration.

## Management

The management of diabetic foot problems requires input from a number of different healthcare professionals, and the evidence strongly suggests that specialised diabetic foot clinics can significantly reduce ulceration and amputation rates.[65] Such a clinic requires a doctor with an interest in diabetes, a nurse, a podiatrist and orthotist, as well as rapid access to the services of vascular and orthopaedic surgeons. Before considering the details of the management of foot ulcers it is essential to recognise the crucial role of prevention, which initially involves identification of the 'at-risk' foot.

**Box 5.1** • Risk factors for diabetic foot ulceration

- Previous ulceration
- Neuropathy
- Peripheral vascular disease
- Altered foot shape
- High foot pressures
- Increasing age
- Visual impairment
- Living alone

## The 'at-risk' foot

The identification of patients at risk of foot ulceration is most easily done on an annual basis and must be performed on all patients with diabetes. Screening does not involve expensive equipment or testing and can be done in an ordinary clinic setting. However, foot examination is frequently overlooked,[19,66] perhaps because doctors are reassured by the patient not reporting any symptoms. However, as discussed earlier, neuropathy, vascular disease and even ulceration are frequently asymptomatic but can be easily diagnosed by simple clinical examination.[67] Peripheral neuropathy can be recognised with standard clinical tools by finding reduced or absent vibration, pin-prick or thermal (cold tuning fork) sensation in the foot, usually accompanied by the loss of the ankle reflex. As described earlier, quantitative sensory testing is a useful adjunct. Dry and cracked skin on the feet usually signifies autonomic neuropathy, and neuropathic symptoms (burning, paraesthesiae, etc.) should be sought. The peripheral vascular status is usually indicated by palpation of peripheral pulses and it should be remembered that absent foot pulses may be due to arterial wall calcification not absent flow. The ABPI should be measured whenever there is any doubt, but further investigations will be dictated by individual clinical requirements. If a patient is at risk by virtue of having either neuropathy or peripheral vascular disease, then a more detailed assessment of additional risk factors is required. Foot inspection may reveal deformities of foot shape and areas of callus that indicate sites exposed to high pressure or friction. Immobility and social circumstances may influence a patient's ability to understand and carry out appropriate foot care. Finally, a history of previous ulceration should be sought, as this is probably the strongest single predictor of ulceration.

As most of the risk factors (apart from vascular disease) are not directly modifiable by treatment, the most important element of the management of at-risk patients is the provision of good education on foot care.

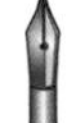

Even a simple approach can have considerable success, as demonstrated by Malone et al.,[68] who reported a two-thirds reduction in amputation and ulceration as a result of a 1-hour educational session.

A number of different educational approaches have been used and options include group sessions, printed material, videos and opportunistic education. Areas covered by education need to include both the correction of patient misconceptions[69] and advice on foot care. With regard to the latter, it is important to concentrate on positive recommendations rather than prohibitions. The basic elements of foot-care advice are shown in Box 5.2. Patients also need to know how to gain rapid access to advice and treatment from the foot-care team.

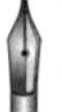

Areas of high pressure need to be accommodated in appropriate footwear and the evidence suggests that when high-risk patients wear the footwear provided, ulceration rates are reduced.[70] A small randomised study showed that injecting liquid silicone under areas of callus and high pressure resulted in reduced ulceration at these sites.[71]

Extra-depth shoes provide enough room for clawed toes, and cushioned insoles reduce plantar pressures. It is not clear whether flat insoles provide greater pressure relief than custom-moulded insoles. Padded hosiery may further reduce pressure and also protect the dorsum of the toes.[72] Most patients can be fitted with 'off-the-shelf' extra-depth shoes, with custom-made shoes being reserved for patients with major foot deformity. Further shoe modifications are possible, for example a rigid rocker bottom sole can be added. With the rocker axis posterior to the metatarsal heads, metatarsal head pressure can be reduced by up to 40%.[73] Regular podiatry is required for most at-risk patients. Callus needs to be debrided regularly because although it develops in response to pressure and friction, its removal reduces pressure.[59] Furthermore, callus can sometimes hide ulceration, which will only be revealed when the callus is removed. Without its removal, infection and abscess formation are encouraged, but it is important to explain to the patient that the podiatrist has not caused the ulcer. The presence of callus should always prompt a search for its cause, and shoe modification may be necessary.

The surgical correction of specific foot deformities is sometimes necessary to prevent ulceration. However, this should only be done after confirming that there is a good peripheral circulation and it is important to bear in mind that the correction of a hallux valgus may leave a rigid hallux with high plantar pressures. Metatarsal head resection (through a dorsal incision) is sometimes used to reduce pressures; the only study that has examined the results of this procedure showed a 40–70% fall in pressure, with no evidence of transfer of pressure to other metatarsal heads.[74] However, the follow-up period was short and our own observations suggest that, after a few months, pressures may start to increase again. Correction of deformity is usually only performed in patients with a history of ulceration, rather than for primary prevention.

**Box 5.2** • Principles of foot-care education

1. Target the level of information to the needs of the patient. Those not at risk require only general advice about foot hygiene and footwear
2. Make positive rather than negative recommendations

   DO inspect the feet daily

   DO report any problems, even if painless

   DO buy shoes with a square toe box and laces

   DO inspect the inside of shoes for foreign objects every day before putting them on

   DO attend a fully trained podiatrist regularly

   DO cut your nails straight across and not rounded

   DO keep your feet away from heat (fires, radiators, hot-water bottles) and check the bath water with your hand or elbow

   DO always wear something on your feet to protect them and never walk barefoot
3. Repeat the advice at regular intervals and check for compliance
4. Disseminate the advice to other family members and other healthcare professionals involved in the care of the patient

## Ulcer management

All diabetic patients presenting with foot ulcers need at the very least a clinical examination of peripheral sensation and circulation (supplemented with measurement of ABPI if there is any doubt at all about the circulation) in order to classify the ulcer.

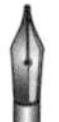

The Wagner classification[75] is probably the most widely used in the literature and grades ulcers on the depth of penetration and extent of tissue necrosis. However, it makes no reference to aetiology and, for clinical practice, a more helpful classification is to divide ulcers into neuropathic, neuroischaemic and purely ischaemic, combined with an assessment of the presence and severity of infection. Radiography of the foot should also be carried out if the ulcer is deep or resistant to therapy to exclude underlying osteomyelitis (**Fig. 5.3**). Any type of ulcer can be infected and the management of infection will be considered separately.

A second commonly used classification is the University of Texas Wound Classification system. This assesses ulcer depth, the presence of wound infection and the presence of clinical signs of lower-extremity ischaemia.[76] The system uses a matrix of grade on the horizontal axis and stage on the vertical axis. Grade 0 is a pre- or post-ulcerative site that has healed; Grade 1 a superficial wound not involving tendon, capsule or bone; Grade 2 a wound penetrating to tendon or capsule; and Grade 3 a wound penetrating bone or joint. Within each wound grade there are four stages: clean wounds (A), non-ischaemic infected wounds (B), ischaemic non-infected wounds (C) and ischaemic infected wounds (D). This classification system has recently been shown to be a better predictor of outcome in terms of healing and amputations compared with the Wagner system.[77]

## Neuropathic ulcers

Typically, the foot is warm and well perfused with bounding pulses and distended veins. The ulcer is usually at the site of repetitive trauma and most commonly due to a shoe rub on the dorsum of the toes or a high-pressure area under the metatarsal heads. The ulcer may be hidden under callus and only revealed when this is removed by a podiatrist. Occasionally, a foreign body causes ulceration: either a nail penetrates the sole of the shoe and the skin, or a stone or other object gets into the shoe. Neuropathic patients may walk on a foreign body for hours or even days without being aware of it.

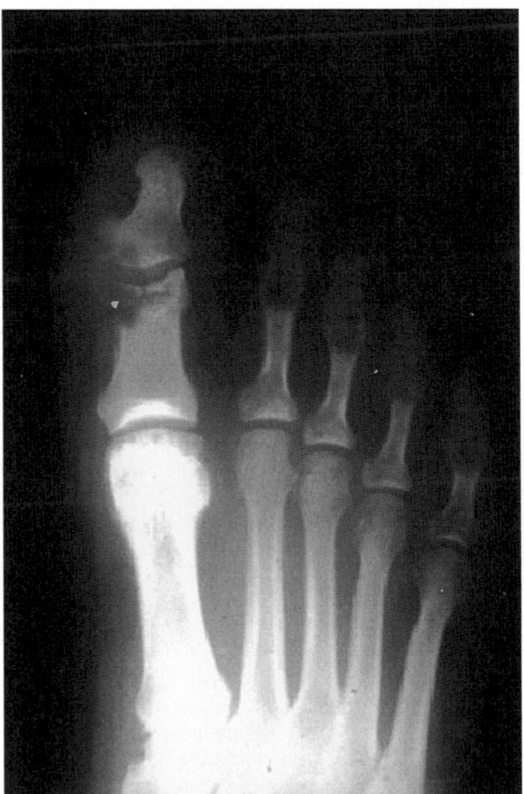

**Figure 5.3** • Osteomyelitis of the first toe causing bony destruction.

The key to management is pressure relief. With shoe-induced ulcers, appropriate footwear must be provided, irrespective of patients' protestations that their own shoes (which caused the ulcer) are comfortable. However, merely providing shoes may not be enough, as many patients do not wear prescribed shoes on a regular basis. Failure to wear the provided shoes may be because of their appearance or the belief (common in the elderly) that they are only for outdoors and that slippers are suitable footwear in the home.

In order to relieve pressure from a plantar ulcer, a more aggressive approach is required. Bed rest is simple and attractive, but is expensive in hospital and difficult to enforce in a patient who feels well and is free of pain. Therefore, several ambulatory methods have been designed.

The total contact cast was originally used for patients with neuropathic ulcers due to leprosy and was modified by Paul Brand for use in diabetic neuropathy. The cast extends from below the knee and encases the whole foot. Only minimal padding is used, except in the forefoot.

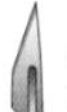

Excellent healing rates have been reported and in a randomised controlled trial total contact cast was associated with faster healing compared with other removable devices.[78]

The cast works by transferring load from the forefoot to the heel and directly to the leg via the cast walls,[79] as well as by reducing oedema and shear forces. Its main disadvantages are that it is labour intensive, as it may need frequent changes, and signs of wound infection or ulceration secondary to the cast may not be seen. An alternative is the Scotch cast boot.[80] This is a removable fibreglass boot that is moulded to the contours of the plantar surface of the foot (**Fig. 5.4**). A number of commercially produced pressure-relieving boots are now available and although their capacity to reduce pressure has been demonstrated, only the total contact cast has been tested in trials of ulcer healing. However, since these are removable patients may remove the cast when at home and when they might do a lot of walking, thus impeding healing. These can be made non-removable by wrapping the removable cast walker with fiberglass casting material. Studies have shown that the healing with this form of offloading was almost on a par with total contact casting.[81,82]

The second important element of management of neuropathic ulcers is debridement of callus. Wounds heal from the margins and callus prevents the migration of epidermal cells from the wound margin, and encourages wound infection. Debridement of callus and necrotic tissue is usually required on a weekly basis and the continued presence of callus should prompt a review of the pressure relief being employed.

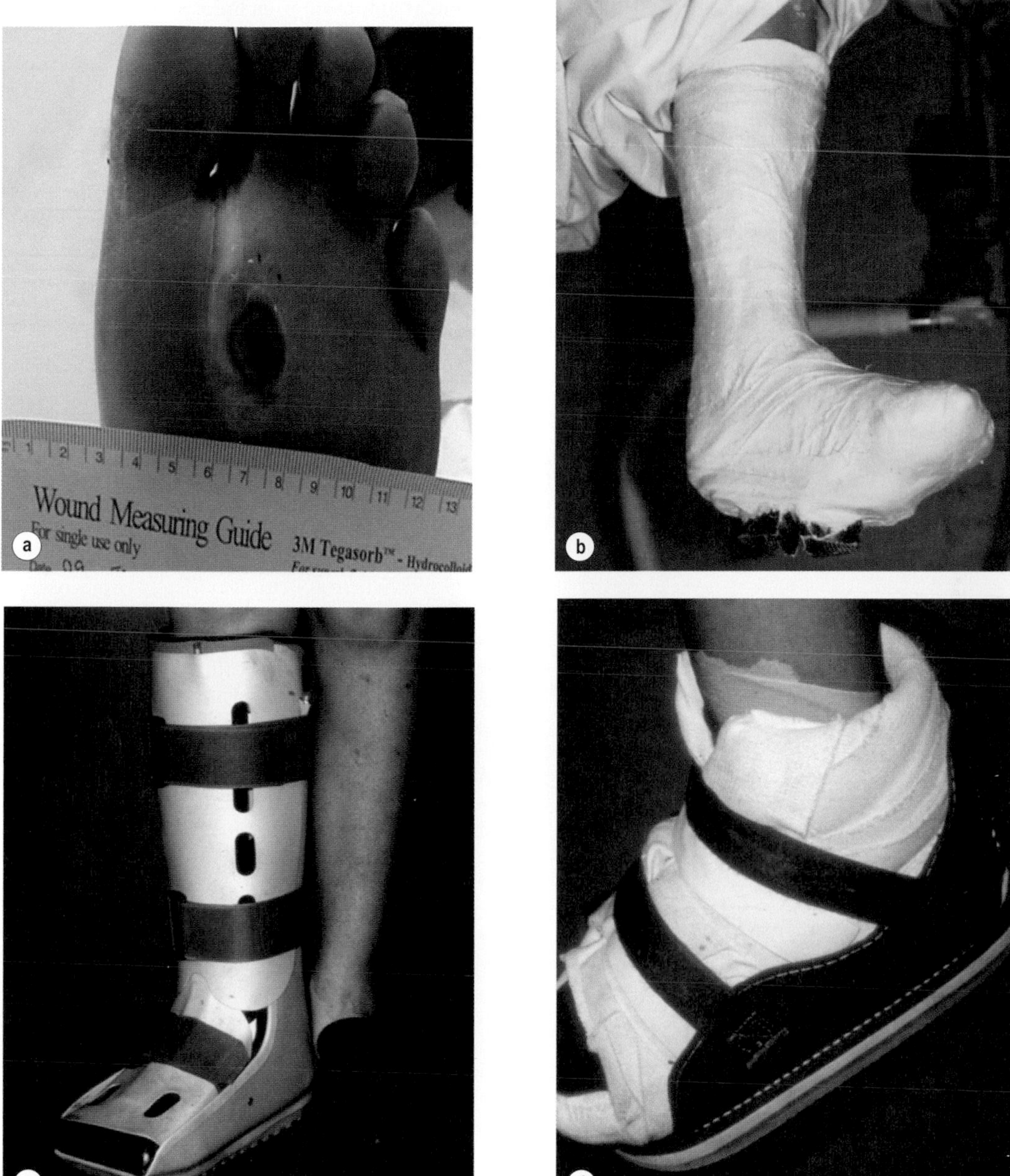


**Figure 5.4** • Plantar ulcer due to neuropathy **(a)** treated with total contact cast **(b)** Aircast **(c)** scotch cast boot **(d)**.

## Ischaemic and neuroischaemic ulcers

The purely ischaemic ulcer is relatively rare and most are in fact neuroischaemic. Typical sites include the toes, heel and medial aspect of the first metatarsal head. Callus is usually absent and the ulcer is often surrounded by a rim of erythema and may have a necrotic centre. The presence of pain depends on the degree of neuropathy. Ulceration is often precipitated by minor trauma and the most common culprit is ill-fitting shoes. Prompt vascular assessment is crucial and angiography is often required. Revascularisation should be performed whenever possible, both for ulcer healing (ischaemic and neuroischaemic ulcers only rarely heal without improvements in blood flow) and to prevent future ulceration. As described earlier, this may involve a distal bypass, although the outcome of vascular surgery is just as good in patients with and without diabetes.[35]

Gangrene and amputation are among the most feared complications of diabetes. Although gangrene may complicate neuropathic ulceration (micro-organisms in infected digital ulcers may produce necrotising toxins, which lead to thrombotic occlusion of digital arteries and subsequent gangrene), it usually only occurs when significant vascular disease is present. Gangrenous tissue must be removed, and when it involves a dry digit with a clear demarcation line this will usually occur spontaneously, leaving a healed stump (**Fig. 5.5**). However, when these conditions are not met, local amputation is mandatory. Local amputation includes simple removal of a toe, ray amputation (of a toe and metatarsal), or a transmetatarsal amputation. The general rule is to remove all necrotic tissue, ensuring that no bone is left exposed, while leaving part of the wound open to allow drainage. If arterial reconstruction is possible, then this can be combined with amputation to enable the healing of the amputation site. This is not possible when major sepsis is present, and in such circumstances revascularisation should be done at a second procedure when infection has been controlled by debridement and antibiotics. The amputation site is determined by both the extent of tissue involvement and the level at which the circulation will support wound healing. With regard to the latter, the transcutaneous oxygen tension provides useful information; in a large study, values under 40 mmHg were strongly associated with failure of healing at the amputation site.[37]

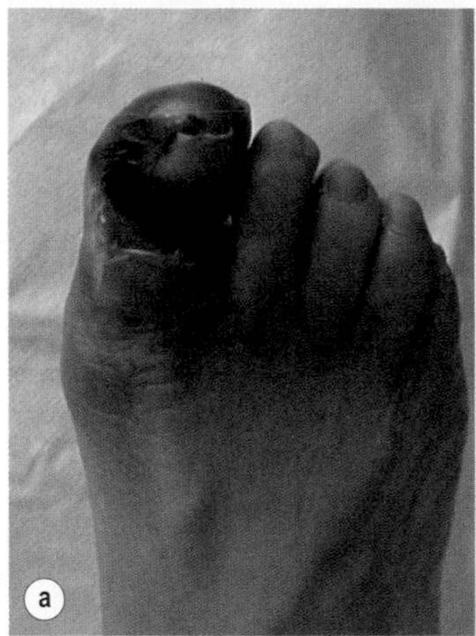

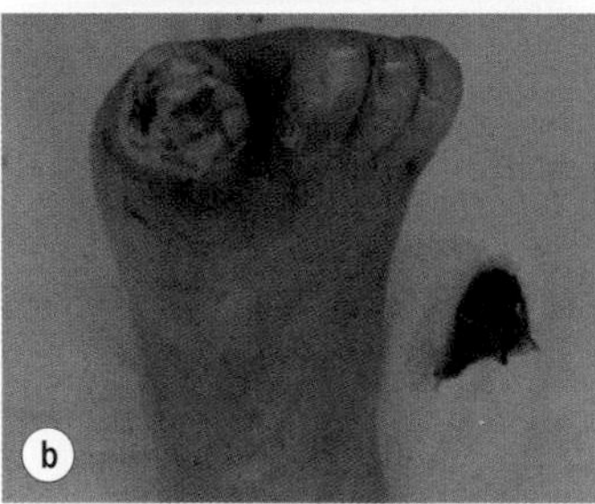

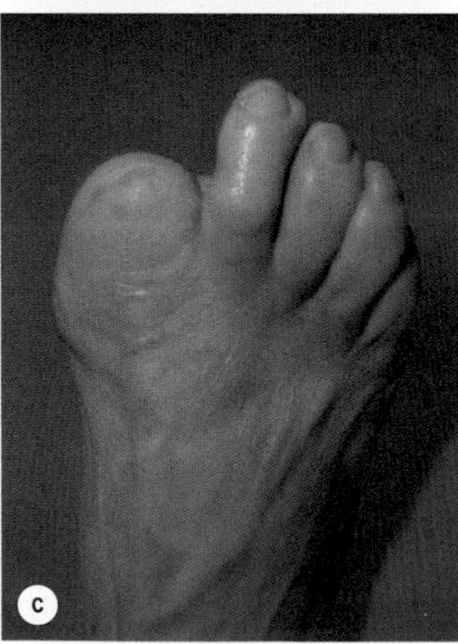

**Figure 5.5** • Patient with digital gangrene **(a)** resulting in autoamputation **(b)** and healing of the wound **(c)**.

## Infection

An infected diabetic foot ulcer can lead to limb loss in a matter of days, but by no means are all ulcers infected, although bacterial colonisation seems universal. The distinction between colonisation and infection can be difficult and is not aided by microbiological investigations. Clinical signs are the most reliable indicators of infection. Evidence of systemic upset (e.g. fever, leucocytosis) is frequently absent, and signs of local inflammation, swelling and the presence of pus are usually used to dictate the need for antibiotics. With severe infection, there may be crepitus due to gas formation and fluctuance indicating the presence of an abscess. Infections are usually polymicrobial, with typically three to six organisms isolated per ulcer.[83,84] The most commonly found organisms include staphylococci, streptococci, Gram-negative species such as *Proteus* and *Pseudomonas* and anaerobes such as *Bacteroides*, and synergy between organisms may increase pathogenicity. Recently, methicillin-resistant *Staphylococcus aureus* (MRSA) has posed an increasing problem, and was found to be present in over 20% of ulcers in a specialised diabetic foot clinic and increasing in prevalence.[85,86] In non-limb-threatening infections, microbiological investigation is not essential, but when swabs are taken the method is important. Superficial swabs are likely to isolate colonising rather than pathogenic bacteria[83] and the deeper the sample, the more reliable the results. Ideally, curettings from the ulcer base should be transported and cultured aerobically and anaerobically.

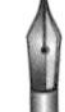

Osteomyelitis should be suspected in any deep ulcer if a sinus tract is present or if an ulcer fails to heal despite adequate pressure relief.

Osteomyelitis is an important predisposing factor for amputation. Though sometimes obvious from plain radiographs, the sensitivity and specificity of radiography in diagnosing osteomyelitis are only about 70%.[87,88] This may be improved with serial radiographs taken at 2-weekly intervals or by using isotope scans. Three-phase bone scans and indium-labelled white cell scans improve the sensitivity but not necessarily the specificity.[87,88] However, by combining bone and white cell scan images, sensitivity is over 90% and specificity greater than 80%.[89] Magnetic resonance imaging is now also proving useful by showing marrow oedema before cortical bone loss occurs, and is particularly valuable in differentiating infection from Charcot neuroarthropathy. Interestingly, a simple clinical test (the ability to probe to bone with a blunt instrument at the base of an ulcer) has proved to be a useful test for osteomyelitis,[90] with a sensitivity of 66% and positive predictive value of 89% (i.e. bone can be probed in 66% of all cases of osteomyelitis, and in all ulcers where bone can be probed 89% have osteomyelitis). Simple laboratory markers, such as erythrocyte sedimentation rate and C-reactive protein, may assist in the diagnosis.

The threshold for initiating antibiotic treatment should be low, and the agents used should have a broad spectrum of activity to include the known common pathogenic organisms.[91,92] There is limited evidence on which to base the choice of antibiotic regimen, although it has been demonstrated that antibiotic treatment is not required in neuropathic ulcers that are not clinically infected.[93]

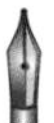

In limb-threatening diabetic foot infections, amoxicillin or ampicillin combined with a β-lactamase inhibitor (clavulanic acid or sulbactam) are effective and give very similar results to those achieved with either ofloxacin used alone[94] or imipenem combined with cilastatin.[95]

Clindamycin or the combination of amoxicillin with flucloxacillin are also suitable outpatient treatments and cover most of the required spectrum, although they do not have trial data to support their use. Preferably the antibiotic of choice should be against common organisms causing infection in the diabetic foot and the most frequent organism found is *S. aureus*. Caution should be exercised in patients with pencillin hypersensitivity and clindamycin can be the first choice in these patients.

Organisms that are commonly isolated are shown in Table 5.2. MRSA is also being seen increasingly, causing a major problem in antibiotic choices. A new class of antimicrobial agents has been identified, represented by linezolid, an oxazolidinone, which acts against bacteria by inhibiting the initiation of protein synthesis at the ribosomal subunit.[95] Linezolid has excellent activity against staphylococci, including MRSA, streptococci and other Gram-positive organisms.[96] It can also be used in patients with penicillin allergy. It has recently been approved for use in skin and soft-tissue infection but is not currently licensed for the treatment of osteomyelitis. However, pharmacological data, supported by case reports, suggest that linezolid may be a useful option in the treatment of bone infection due to resistant Gram-positive bacteria.[97] Furthermore, linezolid has excellent oral absorption, giving the potential for oral therapy of deep-seated infections. However, it can be used intravenously in the initial period and then converted to oral dosage when the patient is less toxic or able to take medications by mouth. Regular monitoring of blood counts is required for patients on this antibiotic.

However, antibiotics should be used with care. Aminoglycosides are potentially nephrotoxic, and clindamycin (as well as other agents) can cause *Clostridium difficile* diarrhoea. Quinolones (such as ofloxacin) sometimes have limited potency against Gram-positive cocci. Serious limb-threatening infections often demand multiple drug regimens, which should be administered carefully with monitoring for adverse effects, and in consultation with a microbiology department. Infected and necrotic tissue must be aggressively debrided, and when osteomyelitis is

**Table 5.2** • Organisms isolated from diabetic foot ulcers in a specialised diabetic foot clinic

| | |
|---|---|
| Gram-positive aerobes | 59 (56.7%) |
| *Staphylococcus aureus* | 30 (28.8%) |
| Coagulase-negative *Staphylococcus* | 5 (4.8%) |
| *Streptococcus* spp. | 11 (10.6%) |
| Gram-negative aerobic bacilli | 31 (29.8%) |
| *Enterobacter* spp. | 22 (21.1%) |
| *Pseudomonas* spp. | 4 (3.8%) |
| Anaerobic species | 14 (13.5%) |
| Cases with mixed skin flora | 12 (17.9%) |
| **Results by category** | |
| Aerobes only | 53 (79.1%) |
| Anaerobes only | 3 (4.5%) |
| Aerobes and anaerobes | 11 (16.4%) |
| Monomicrobial infection | 35 (52.2%) |
| Methicillin-resistant *Staphylococcus aureus* | 12 (15.2%) |

Reproduced from Tentolouris N, Jude EB, Smirnof I et al. Methicillin-resistant *Staphylococcus aureus:* an increasing problem in a diabetic foot clinic. Diabetic Med 1999; 16:767–71. With permission from Blackwell Publishing.

present infected bone nearly always needs resecting, although prolonged antibiotic courses may successfully eradicate the bone infection. Limb-threatening infections require urgent hospitalisation, bed rest, surgical debridement and broad-spectrum antibiotics.

The choice of dressings remains controversial due to the lack of large well-controlled comparative studies. When slough is present, desloughing agents are often effective (although more expensive than a scalpel) and hydrocolloid dressings are useful in cleaner ulcers. Interest has recently focused on actively influencing the complex environment that exists within chronic wounds. Growth factors are central to this process, and are responsible for triggering and controlling the events that finally result in healing and skin closure. Silver-containing dressings have also been found to have antibacterial activity and may be used in certain foot ulcers where antibiotics may not be necessary or in conjunction with antibiotics.

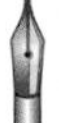

Various newer topical therapies have been researched recently and have been shown to be of some benefit in the healing of chronic diabetic foot ulcers. These include platelet-derived growth factor (becaplermin), living dermal equivalent (Dermagraft) and living human skin equivalents (Graftskin). However, they are not appropriate for all patients and should be used judiciously, with good wound care being paramount.

Becaplermin, a formulation of platelet-derived growth factor that is applied directly to the ulcer, has recently been shown to improve healing times for neuropathic diabetic foot ulcers,[98] and studies of other growth factors are currently under way. Living dermal replacements can now be manufactured from neonatal fibroblasts, which are cultured in vitro onto a bioabsorbable mesh. The product is applied as a dressing to the wound, and the fibroblasts within it are metabolically active, producing a full array of growth factors. Evidence is now available that this skin substitute may also improve healing,[99] although some uncertainty remains about the validity of the data. Hyperbaric oxygen therapy has been used for a variety of conditions including wound healing. It improves tissue oxygenation, enhances the killing capacity of neutrophils and directly inhibits the growth of anaerobic organisms. A controlled trial of this treatment modality in limb-threatening diabetic foot ulcers indicated its efficacy, especially when ischaemia was a major problem.[100]

The recent development of living human skin equivalents, produced by tissue engineering techniques, offers new opportunities for wound healing in chronic ulcers caused by venous disease and diabetic neuropathy. Graftskin is a bilayered cultured skin equivalent, consisting of human epidermis and a collagenous dermal layer containing human fibroblasts. A prospective, randomised, controlled trial has demonstrated the efficacy of Graftskin in the management of chronic neuropathic diabetic foot ulcers.[101] Graftskin or a standard treatment (saline-moisturised gauze) was applied to more than 200 patients who also received standardised foot care for their foot ulcers, which comprised sharp debridement and offloading. After 12 weeks of treatment, 56% of Graftskin-treated patients achieved complete healing compared with 38% of the controls.

It appears therefore that treatments such as Graftskin and possibly Dermagraft might be useful adjuncts in the treatment of diabetic neuropathic foot ulcers. These new treatments offer a variety of exciting options, but are expensive and are limited in their indications (e.g. growth factors and skin substitutes should only be used in non-infected ulcers). Their availability should not obscure the fact that most ulcers respond to simple care, comprising pressure relief, debridement and control of infection, and must not be seen as a replacement but as an addition to good wound care.

### Granulocyte colony-stimulating factor (G-CSF)

Neutrophil superoxide generation, a crucial part of neutrophil bactericidal activity, is impaired in diabetes. G-CSF increases the release of neutrophils from the bone marrow and improves neutrophil function. In a placebo-controlled trial, G-CSF (filgrastim) treatment was associated with improved clinical outcome of foot infection in diabetic patients. This improvement may be related to an increase in neutrophil superoxide production.[102]

### Larva debridement therapy

Larva debridement therapy (the use of maggots to cleanse wounds) is hardly new. Indeed, an early reference to larval therapy was made during the Napoleonic wars, when it was observed that those wounds accidentally infected by maggots did not become infected and appeared to heal better.

In recent years the use of sterile larvae (of the greenbottle fly, *Lucilia sericata*) has been investigated with encouraging results, and is becoming increasingly popular as therapy for infected and necrotic wounds.[103,104] It is thought that maggots remove necrotic tissue by secreting powerful enzymes that break down dead tissue into a liquid form, which is then ingested.[105] The mechanisms by which larvae prevent or combat infection are also complex but there is anecdotal evidence that they may also help in combating antibiotic-resistant strains of bacteria. There is a growing body of clinical experience with the use of larval therapy that suggests that it is useful in the management of patients with necrotic, sloughing and often neuroischaemic ulcers. The use of this therapy is now quite widespread in foot care for infected diabetic ulcers, with some recent evidence that it may be effective in eradicating MRSA.[106]

## Medical problems on the surgical ward

By the time that a diabetic patient reaches the vascular surgeon, numerous complications will often have developed. Apart from somatic neuropathy and peripheral vascular disease, coronary artery disease, diabetic nephropathy (with or without renal failure) and cardiac autonomic neuropathy are frequently present in this population and may play a major role in determining the overall outcome. Thus patients need careful screening to identify potential problems. All patients with a significant degree of renal impairment should ideally be reviewed by a renal physician prior to any procedures.

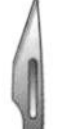

Angiography with contrast media carries a risk of worsening renal function (see Chapter 2).

Metformin must also be stopped for 48 hours before elective angiography because of the risk of lactic acidosis, which carries a high mortality. Coronary artery disease and cardiac autonomic neuropathy increase the risk of perioperative cardiac events. Invasive monitoring (e.g. Swan–Ganz catheterisation) and regional anaesthetic techniques help to reduce this risk. The hormonal and metabolic changes associated with surgery present a particular problem in diabetes. Intravenous insulin (plus dextrose and potassium) is usually needed for the perioperative period, unless the duration of anaesthesia is short (<45 minutes) and the patient is not on insulin. It is mostly simply administered as part of a 'GKI' regimen,[107] in which 15 units of soluble insulin and 10 mmol of potassium chloride are added to 500 mL of 10% dextrose, the solution being infused at 100 mL/hour. Despite its simplicity, this regimen provides remarkably stable glycaemic control, although many centres prefer the insulin to be administered separately, allowing adjustment of the rate according to capillary glucose measurements, using a sliding scale.

Patients with neuropathy are at great risk of developing posterior heel ulcers when lying in bed immobile for several days. These can be very difficult to heal, are entirely preventable and medicolegally indefensible. The simple provision of foam leg troughs is all that is needed to relieve the pressure on the heels while the patient is in bed. This should be done routinely in patients at risk. Pressure-relieving boots (**Fig. 5.6**) seem useful for wheelchair-bound patients.

## Charcot neuroarthropathy

Charcot neuroarthropathy is characterised by bone and joint destruction, fragmentation and remodelling. It can be one of the most devastating foot complications of diabetes, and was first described as a complication of tabes dorsalis. It can develop in any joint and has been reported in most sensory neuropathies, but diabetes is now the commonest cause of the Charcot foot. Although once thought to be very rare, it is now known to affect nearly 10% of patients with neuropathy and over 16% of those with a history of neuropathic ulceration.[108] The exact mechanism remains unclear. Unperceived trauma, followed by weight-bearing on an injured limb, is thought by some to account for the fractures and joint destruction; however, there is evidence that increased blood flow to bone, resulting from autonomic

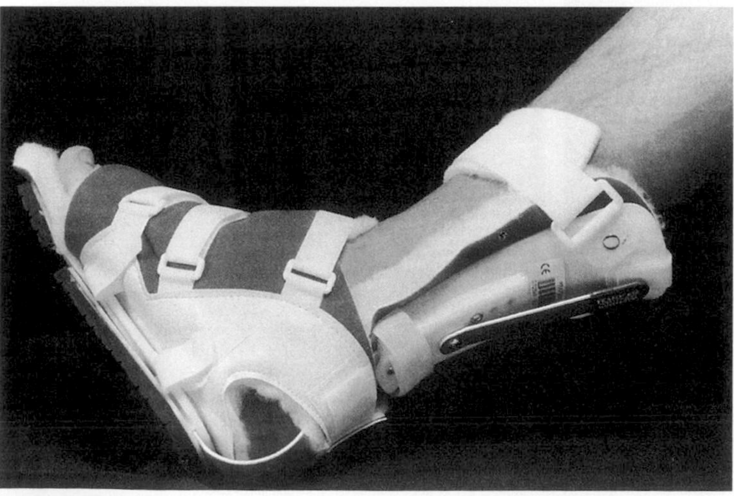

**Figure 5.6** • Routine use of pressure-relieving boots reduces the risk of pressure ulcers in bed- or chair-bound patients.

neuropathy, activates osteoclasts and leads to localised osteoporosis,[109,110] perhaps allowing fractures to occur with minimal trauma. The matter is further complicated by the observation that fractures may not develop until several weeks after the foot becomes swollen. We have noted that periarticular erosions are common around affected joints and sometimes precede fractures and fragmentation, suggesting that an inflammatory arthropathy (possibly secondary to trauma) is the first stage of the process and that continued weight-bearing prolongs this phase, allowing periarticular bone resorption and fractures. Typically, patients present with a warm swollen foot. Although most textbooks describe it as a painless condition, there is frequently discomfort but not enough to prevent walking. The presentation is often several weeks after the onset of symptoms and, because of the lack of significant pain, simple radiographs may unfortunately not be performed. However, plain radiography is usually adequate to make the diagnosis, but isotope scans and magnetic resonance imaging are sometimes necessary to exclude osteomyelitis. The natural history is such that after a matter of months, during which bone resorption continues, the swelling and warmth begin to resolve. Treatment is aimed at shortening this time in order to minimise bone and joint destruction. The midfoot is a common site of Charcot neuroarthropathy and when affected can result in midfoot collapse, with a plantar bony prominence and 'rocker' foot, which has a very high risk of ulceration (**Fig. 5.7**). The mainstay of treatment is rest and immobilisation, usually in a total contact cast, which may need to be continued for many months until disease activity has subsided. Disease activity is usually judged by measuring the temperature of the overlying skin with an infrared thermometer; when this is 2°C warmer than the other foot, an inflammatory response is still present. The only treatment directed at the excessive osteoclastic activity is with the intravenous bisphosphonate pamidronate. In an open study, pamidronate led to a rapid clinical improvement, together with a decrease in foot temperature and alkaline phosphatase.[111]

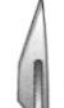

In a randomised trial a single infusion of pamidronate resulted in a significant reduction in symptoms and an additional improvement in disease activity, as well as a reduction in bone turnover markers compared with standard care.[112] The oral bisphosphonate, alendronate (70 mg weekly), has also been shown to reduce bone markers and symptoms but no difference in disease activity was demonstrated.[113]

Surgery to the foot is contraindicated in the early stages, due to the gross hyperaemia of involved bone and the risk that it (like trauma) will trigger bone resorption. However, corrective surgery may be useful at a later stage in order to remove bony prominences. At this stage, appropriate (usually custom-made) footwear is required, and great care should be taken of the other foot as there is a high risk of contralateral Charcot changes. Therefore, medical treatment must be instituted immediately a diagnosis of Charcot foot is made. The cornerstone of treatment of acute Charcot neuroarthropathy is immediate effective offloading,

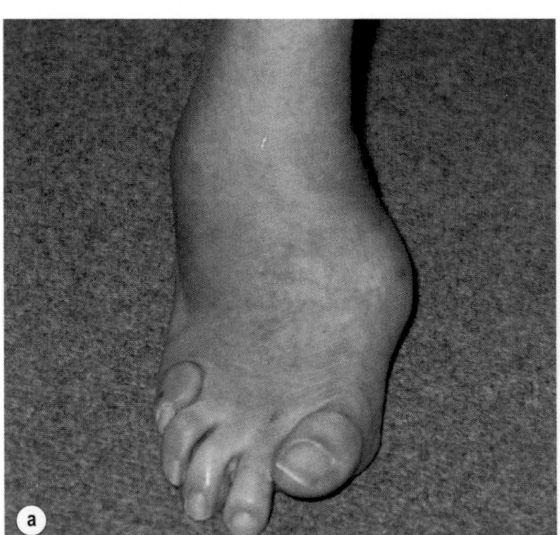

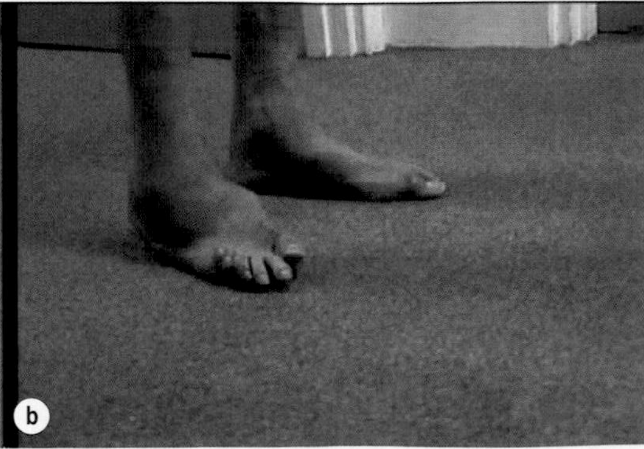

**Figure 5.7** • Charcot neuroarthropathy resulting in midfoot collapse with plantar bony prominence.

typically with total contact casting, and reduction in weight-bearing. The main current targets of pharmacological intervention are the inhibition of excess osteoclast activation and suppression of an excess proinflammatory cytokine response. Antiresorptive therapy, especially with bisphosphonates, has been used in randomised trials and may be tried early in the disease phase. Long-term follow-up is necessary as recurrence is common as well as complications such as foot ulceration, with high mortality.[114,115]

## Key points

- The management of the diabetic foot is challenging and requires a multidisciplinary approach, ideally coordinated by a specialised clinic.
- Identification of high-risk patients requires screening that must be both comprehensive and regular, and patient education should be part of this process.
- Once ulceration has developed, aggressive management can achieve excellent results with a significant reduction of both amputation and re-ulceration rates.
- Future research may ultimately enable the prevention of foot ulcers and the predisposing factors that lead to ulceration and may demonstrate superior ways of healing ulcers. However, the dissemination of current 'best practice' is already starting to have a major impact on the outlook for this condition.

## References


1. Wild S, Roglie G, Green A et al. Global prevalence of diabetes: estimates for 2000 and projections for 2030. Diabetes Care 2004; 27:1047–53.
2. Boyko EJ, Ahroni JH, Smith DG et al. Increased mortality associated with diabetic foot ulcer. Diabetic Med 1996; 13:967–72.
3. Krentz AJ, Acheson P, Basu A et al. Morbidity and mortality associated with diabetic foot disease: a 12-month prospective survey of hospital admissions in a single UK centre. Foot 1997; 7:144–7.
4. Tentolouris N, Al-Sabbagh S, Walker MG et al. Mortality in diabetic and non-diabetic patients after amputations performed from 1990 to 1995: a 5-year follow-up study. Diabetes Care 2004; 27:1598–604.
5. Jude EB, Boulton AJM. End stage complications of diabetic neuropathy. Diabetes Rev 1999; 7:395–410.
6. Boulton AJ, Vileikyte L, Ragnarson-Tennvall G et al. The global burden of diabetic foot disease. Lancet 2005; 366:1719–24.
7. Kumar S, Ashe HA, Parnell LN et al. The prevalence of foot ulceration and its correlates in type 2 diabetic patients: a population-based study. Diabetic Med 1994; 11:480–4.
8. Neil HA, Thompson AV, Thorogood M et al. Diabetes in the elderly: the Oxford Community Diabetes Study. Diabetic Med 1989; 6:608–13.
9. Borssen B, Bergenheim T, Lithner F. The epidemiology of foot lesions in diabetic patients aged 15–50 years. Diabetic Med 1990; 7:438–44.
10. Abbott CA, Carrington AL, Ashe H et al. The North West Diabetic Foot Care Study: incidence of, and risk factors for, new diabetic foot ulceration in a community-based patient cohort. Diabetic Med 2002; 19:377–84.
11. Moss SE, Klein R, Klein B. The prevalence and incidence of lower extremity amputation in a diabetic population. Arch Intern Med 1992; 152:610–13.
12. Ramsey SD, Newton K, Blough DK et al. Incidence, outcomes, and cost of foot ulcers in patients with diabetes. Diabetes Care 1999; 22:382–7.
13. Oyibo SO, Jude EB, Voyatzoglou D et al. Clinical characteristics of patients with diabetic foot problems: changing patterns of foot ulcer presentation. Pract Diabetes Int 2002; 19:10–12.

    **This study showed the increase in ischaemic and neuroischaemic ulcers in patients presenting to the foot clinic.**
14. Most RS, Sinnock P. The epidemiology of lower extremity amputations in diabetic individuals. Diabetes Care 1983; 6:87–91.
15. Gujral JS, McNally PG, O'Malley BP et al. Ethnic differences in the incidence of lower extremity amputation secondary to diabetes mellitus. Diabetic Med 1993; 10:271–4.
16. Young MJ, Boulton AJ, MacLeod AF et al. A multicentre study of the prevalence of diabetic peripheral neuropathy in the United Kingdom hospital clinic population. Diabetologia 1993; 36:150–4.
17. Walters DP, Gatling W, Mullee MA et al. The prevalence of diabetic distal sensory neuropathy in an English community. Diabetic Med 1992; 9:349–53.
18. Boulton AJ, Vinik A, Arezzo J et al. For the American Diabetes Association. Position Statement: diabetic neuropathies. Diabetes Care 2005; 28:956–62.

19. Herman WH, Kennedy L. Underdiagnosis of peripheral neuropathy in type 2 diabetes. Diabetes Care 2005; 28:1480–1.

20. Backonja M, Beydoun A, Edwards KR et al. Gabapentin for the symptomatic treatment of painful neuropathy in patients with diabetes mellitus: a randomised controlled trial. JAMA 1998; 280:1831–6.

**Gabapentin is effective in reducing painful symptoms in patients with painful neuropathy and improves quality of life.**

21. Rull JA, Quibrera R, Gonzalez-Millan H et al. Sympathetic treatment of peripheral diabetic neuropathy with carbamazepine (Tegretol). Diabetologia 1969; 5:215–18.

22. Wernicke JF, Pritchett YL, D'Souza DN et al. A randomized controlled trial of duloxetine in diabetic peripheral neuropathic pain. Neurology 2006; 67:1411–20.

**Duloxetine treatment was shown to reduce painful symptoms in diabetic patients with painful neuropathy.**

23. Capsaicin Study Group. The effect of treatment with capsaicin on the daily activities of patients with painful diabetic neuropathy. Diabetes Care 1992; 15:159–65.

**Capsaicin treatment was associated with reduced pain in patients with painful neuropathy.**

24. Boulton AJM, Scarpello JH, Ward JD. Venous oxygenation in the neuropathic diabetic foot: evidence of arteriovenous shunting. Diabetologia 1982; 22:6–8.

25. Young MJ, Breddy JL, Veves A et al. The prediction of diabetic neuropathic foot ulceration using vibration perception thresholds. A prospective study. Diabetes Care 1994; 17:557–60.

26. Rith-Najarian SJ, Stolusky T, Gohdes DM. Identifying diabetic patients at high risk for lower-extremity amputation in a primary health care setting. A prospective evaluation of simple screening criteria. Diabetes Care 1992; 15:1386–9.

27. Pecoraro RE, Reiber GE, Burgess EM. Pathways to diabetic limb amputation: basis for prevention. Diabetes Care 1990; 13:513–21.

28. Reiber GE, Vileikyte L, Boyko EJ et al. Causal pathways for incident lower-extremity ulcers in patients with diabetes from two settings. Diabetes Care 1999; 22:157–62.

29. Boulton AJM, Malik RA, Arezzo JC et al. Diabetic somatic neuropathy: a technical review. Diabetes Care 2004; 27:1458–86.

30. Jude EB. Intermittent claudication in the patient with diabetes. Br J Diabetes Vasc Dis 2004; 4:238–42.

31. National Diabetes Advisory Board. The prevention and treatment of five complications of diabetes: a guide for primary care practitioners. HHS publ. no. 83–8392. Atlanta, GA: Centers for Disease Control, 1983.

32. Strandness DE, Priest RE, Gibbons RE et al. Combined clinical and pathological study of diabetic and non diabetic peripheral artery disease. Diabetes 1961; 13:366–72.

33. King TA, DePalma RG, Rhodes RS. Diabetes mellitus and atherosclerotic involvement of the profunda femoris artery. Surg Gynecol Obstet 1984; 159:553–6.

34. Jude EB, Oyibo SO, Chalmers N et al. Peripheral arterial disease in diabetic and non-diabetic patients: a comparison of severity and outcome. Diabetes Care 2001; 24:1433–7.

**Diabetic patients have greater involvement of the infrapopliteal vessels when compared to non-diabetic patients, with poorer outcome and increased amputations and mortality.**

35. Karacagil S, Almgren B, Bowald S et al. Comparative analysis of patency, limb salvage and survival in diabetic and non-diabetic patients undergoing infrainguinal bypass surgery. Diabetic Med 1995; 12:537–41.

36. Weitz JL, Byrne J, Clagett GP et al. Diagnosis and treatment of chronic arterial insufficiency of the lower extremities: a critical review. Circulation 1996; 94:3026–49.

37. Jacobs MJ, Ubbink DT, Kitslaar PJ et al. Assessment of the microcirculation provides additional information in critical limb ischaemia. Eur J Vasc Surg 1992; 6:135–41.

38. Robless P, Mikhailidis DP, Stansby G. Systematic review of antiplatelet therapy for the prevention of myocardial infarction, stroke or vascular death in patients with peripheral vascular disease. Br J Surg 2001; 88:787–800.

**Antiplatelet agents can reduce vascular deaths by up to 25% in patients with intermittent claudication.**

39. Chobanian AV, Bakris GL, Black HR et al. Seventh report of the Joint National Committee on Prevention, Detection, Evaluation and Treatment of high blood pressure. Hypertension 2003; 42:1206–52.

40. Heart Outcomes Prevention Evaluation Study Investigators. Effects of an angiotensin-converting enzyme inhibitor, ramipril, on cardiovascular events in high-risk patients. N Engl J Med 2000; 342:145–53.

**The HOPE study showed that the ACE inhibitor ramipril reduces cardiovascular morbidity and mortality in patients with peripheral arterial disease by around 25%.**

41. Heart Protection Study Collaborative Group. MRC/BHF Heart Protection Study of cholesterol lowering with simvastatin in 20,536 high-risk individuals: a randomised placebo-controlled trial. Lancet 2002; 360:7–22.

**The Heart Protection Study showed that lowering total and LDL cholesterol by 25% with a statin reduces cardiovascular mortality and morbidity in patients with peripheral arterial disease by around one-quarter.**

42. British Medical Association and Royal Pharmaceutical Society of Great Britain. British National Formulary 43, March. London: BMA and RPSGB, 2002.

43. Ubels FL, Links TP, Sluiter WJ et al. Walking training for intermittent claudication in diabetes. Diabetes Care 1999; 22:198–201.

Regular exercise is beneficial in diabetic patients and can double walking distance in patients with intermittent claudication.

44. TASC Working Group. Management of peripheral arterial disease: TransAtlantic Inter-Society Consensus (TASC). J Vasc Surg 2000; 31(Suppl):S1–296.
45. Chapman TM, Goa KL. Cilostazol. A review of its use in intermittent claudication. Am J Cardiovasc Drugs 2003; 3:117–38.
46. Hittel N, Donnelly R. Treating peripheral arterial disease in patients with diabetes. Diabetes Obes Metab 2002; 4(Suppl 2):S26–31.
47. Rendell M, Cariski AT, Hittel N et al. Cilostazol treatment of claudication in diabetic patients. Curr Med Res Opin 2002; 18:479–87.

Cilostazol increases walking distance in diabetic patients by 53%.

48. Van Schie CHM, Abbott CA, Vileikyte L et al. A comparative study of the Podotrack, a simple semi-quantitative device, and the optical pedobarograph in the assessment of pressures under the diabetic foot. Diabetic Med 1999; 16:154–9.
49. Veves A, Murray HJ, Young MJ et al. The risk of foot ulceration in diabetic patients with high foot pressures: a prospective study. Diabetologia 1992; 35:660–3.
50. Masson EA, Hay EM, Stockley I et al. Abnormal foot pressure alone does not cause ulceration. Diabetic Med 1989; 6:426–8.
51. Frykberg RG, Lavery LA, Pham H et al. Role of neuropathy and high foot pressures in diabetic foot ulceration. Diabetes Care 1998; 21:1714–19.
52. Stacpoole-Shea S, Shea G, Lavery L. An examination of plantar pressure measurements to identify the location of diabetic forefoot ulceration. J Foot Ankle Surg 1999; 38:109–15.
53. Boulton AJM. The pathogenesis of diabetic foot problems: an overview. Diabetic Med 1996; 13(Suppl 1):S12–16.
54. Armstrong DG, Lavery LA. Plantar pressures are higher in diabetic patients following partial foot amputation. Ostomy Wound Manage 1998; 44:30–2.
55. Fernando DJ, Masson EA, Veves A et al. Relationship of limited joint mobility to abnormal foot pressures and diabetic foot ulceration. Diabetes Care 1991; 14:8–11.
56. Ctercteko GC, Dhanendran M, Hutton WC et al. Vertical forces acting on the feet of diabetic patients with neuropathic ulceration. Br J Surg 1981; 68:608–14.
57. Boulton AJM, Hardisty CA, Betts RP et al. Dynamic foot pressure and other studies as diagnostic and management aids in diabetic neuropathy. Diabetes Care 1983; 6:26–33.
58. Murray HJ, Young MJ, Hollis S et al. The association between callus formation, high pressures and neuropathy in diabetic foot ulceration. Diabetic Med 1996; 13:979–82.
59. Young MJ, Cavanagh PR, Thomas G et al. The effect of callus removal on dynamic plantar foot pressures in diabetic patients. Diabetic Med 1992; 9:55–7.
60. Abouaesha F, van Schie CH, Griffiths GD et al. Plantar tissue thickness is related to peak plantar pressure in the high-risk diabetic foot. Diabetes Care 2001; 24:1270–4.
61. Young MJ, Coffey J, Taylor PM et al. Weight bearing ultrasound in diabetic and rheumatoid arthritis patients. Foot 1995; 5:76–9.
62. Sapico FL, Bessman AN. Diabetic foot infections. In: Frykberg RG (ed.) The high risk foot in diabetes mellitus. New York: Churchill Livingstone, 1991; p. 173.
63. Pecoraro RE, Chen MS. Ascorbic acid metabolism in diabetes mellitus. Ann NY Acad Sci 1987; 498:248–58.
64. Grossi EA, Esposito R, Harris LJ et al. Sternal wound infections and use of internal mammary artery grafts. J Thorac Cardiovasc Surg 1991; 102:342–6.
65. Edmonds ME, Blundell MP, Morris ME et al. Improved survival of the diabetic foot: the role of a specialized foot clinic. Q J Med 1986; 60:763–71.
66. Bailey TS, Yu HM, Rayfield EJ. Patterns of foot examination in a diabetes clinic. Am J Med 1985; 78:371–4.
67. Apelqvist J, Bakker K, van Houtum WH et al. Practical guidelines on the management and prevention of the diabetic foot: based upon the International Consensus on the Diabetic Foot (2007). Prepared by the International Working Group on the Diabetic Foot. Diabetes Metab Res Rev 2008; 24(Suppl 1):S181–7.
68. Malone JM, Snyder M, Anderson G et al. Prevention of amputation by diabetic education. Am J Surg 1989; 158:520–3.
69. Vileikyte L. Psychological aspects of diabetic neuropathic foot complications. An overview. Diabetes Metab Res Rev 2004; 20(Suppl 1):513–18.
70. Uccioli L, Faglia E, Monticone G et al. Manufactured shoes in the prevention of diabetic foot ulcers. Diabetes Care 1995; 18:1376–8.
71. Van Schie CHM, Whalley A, Vileikyte L et al. Efficacy of injected liquid silicone in the diabetic foot to reduce risk factors for foot ulceration. Diabetes Care 2000; 23:634–8.
72. Veves A, Masson EA, Fernando DJ et al. Use of experimental padded hosiery to reduce abnormal foot pressures in diabetic neuropathy. Diabetes Care 1989; 12:653–5.
73. Schaff PS, Cavanagh PR. Shoes for the insensitive foot: the effect of a 'rocker bottom' shoe modification on plantar pressure distribution. Foot Ankle 1990; 11:129–40.
74. Patel VG, Wieman TJ. Effect of metatarsal head resection for diabetic foot ulcers on the dynamic plantar pressure distribution. Am J Surg 1994; 167:297–301.

75. Wagner FW Jr. The dysvascular foot: a system for diagnosis and treatment. Foot Ankle 1981; 2:64–122.

76. Lavery LA, Armstrong DG, Harkless LB. Classification of diabetic foot wounds. J Foot Ankle Surg 1996; 35:528–31.

77. Oyibo S, Jude EB, Tarawaneh I et al. Comparison of two diabetic foot ulcer classification systems: the Wagner and University of Texas systems. Diabetes Care 2001; 24:84–8.

78. Armstrong DG, Nguyen HC, Lavery LA et al. Offloading the diabetic foot: a randomised clinical trial. Diabetes Care 2001; 24:1019–21.

Proper offloading of the diabetic foot ulcer was shown to enhance wound healing.

79. Shaw JE, Hsi WL, Ulbrecht JS et al. The mechanism of plantar unloading in total contact casts: implications for design and clinical use. Foot Ankle Int 1997; 18:809–17.

80. Knowles EA, Armstrong DG, Hayat SA et al. Offloading diabetic foot wounds using the scotchcast boot: a retrospective study. Ostomy Wound Manage 2002; 48:50–3.

81. Armstrong DG, Lavery LA, Wu S et al. Evaluation of removal and irremovable cast walkers in the healing of diabetic foot wounds: a randomized controlled trial. Diabetes Care 2005; 28:551–4.

82. Katz IA, Harlan A, Miranda-Palma B et al. A randomized trial of two irremovable off-loading devices in the management of plantar neuropathic diabetic foot ulcers. Diabetes Care 2005; 28:555–9.

83. Lipsky BA, Pecoraro RE, Wheat LJ. The diabetic foot. Soft tissue and bone infection. Infect Dis Clin North Am 1990; 4:409–32.

84. Wheat LJ, Allen SD, Henry M et al. Diabetic foot infections. Bacteriologic analysis. Arch Intern Med 1986; 146:1935–40.

85. Tentolouris N, Jude EB, Smirnof I et al. Methicil lin-resistant *Staphylococcus aureus*: an increasing problem in a diabetic foot clinic. Diabetic Med 1999; 16:767–71.

86. Dang CN, Prasad YDM, Boulton AJM et al. Methicillin-resistant *Staphylococcus aureus* in the diabetic foot clinic: a worsening problem. Diabetic Med 2003; 20:159–61.

87. Park HM, Wheat LJ, Siddiqui AR et al. Scintigraphic evaluation of diabetic osteomyelitis: concise communication. J Nucl Med 1982; 23:569–73.

88. Keenan AM, Tindel NL, Alavi A. Diagnosis of pedal osteomyelitis in diabetic patients using current scintigraphic techniques. Arch Intern Med 1989; 149:2262–6.

89. Crerand S, Dolan M, Laing P et al. Diagnosis of osteomyelitis in neuropathic foot ulcers. J Bone Joint Surg Br 1996; 78:51–5.

90. Grayson ML, Gibbons GW, Balogh K et al. Probing to bone in infected pedal ulcers. A clinical sign of underlying osteomyelitis in diabetic patients. JAMA 1995; 273:721–3.

91. Jude EB, Unsworth PF. Optimal treatment of infected diabetic foot ulcers. Drugs Aging 2004; 21:833–50.

92. Lipsky BA, Berendt AR, Deery HG et al. Diagnosis and treatment of diabetic foot infections. Clin Infect Dis 2004; 39:885–910.

93. Chantelau E, Tanudjaja T, Altenhofer F et al. Antibiotic treatment for uncomplicated neuropathic forefoot ulcers in diabetes: a controlled trial. Diabetic Med 1996; 13:156–9.

94. Grayson ML, Gibbons GW, Habershaw GM et al. Use of ampicillin/sulbactam versus imipenem-cilastatin in the treatment of limb-threatening foot infections in diabetic patients. Clin Infect Dis 1994; 18:683–93.

95. Lipsky BA, Itani K, Norden C. Linezolid Diabetic Foot Infections Study Group. Treating foot infections in diabetic patients: a randomized, multicentre, open-label trial of linezolid versus ampicillin–sulbactam/amoxicillin–clavulanate. Clin Infect Dis 2004; 38:17–24.

96. Perry CM, Jarvis B. Linezolid: a review of its use in the management of serious Gram-positive infections. Drugs 2001; 61:525–51.

97. Melzer M, Goldsmith D, Gransden W. Successful treatment of vertebral osteomyelitis with linezolid in a patient receiving hemodialysis and with persistent methicillin-resistant *Staphylococcus aureus* and vancomycin-resistant *Enterococcus* bacteremias. Clin Infect Dis 2000; 31:208–9.

98. Wieman TJ, Smiell JM, Su Y. Efficacy and safety of a topical gel formulation of recombinant human platelet-derived growth factor-BB (becaplermin) in patients with chronic neuropathic diabetic ulcers. A phase III randomized placebo-controlled double-blind study. Diabetes Care 1998; 21:822–7.

99. Gentzkow GD, Iwasaki SD, Hershon KS et al. Use of dermagraft, a cultured human dermis, to treat diabetic foot ulcers. Diabetes Care 1996; 19:350–4.

100. Faglia E, Favales F, Aldeghi A et al. Adjunctive systemic hyperbaric oxygen therapy in treatment of severe prevalently ischemic diabetic foot ulcer. A randomized study. Diabetes Care 1996; 19:1338–43.

101. Veves A, Falanga V, Armstrong DG et al. Graftskin, a human skin equivalent, is effective in the management of noninfected neuropathic diabetic foot ulcers: a prospective randomised multicentre clinical trial. Diabetes Care 2001; 24:290–5.

102. Gough A, Clapperton M, Rolando N et al. Randomised placebo-controlled trial of granulocyte-colony stimulating factor in diabetic foot infection. Lancet 1997; 350:855–9.

103. Thomas S, Jones M, Shutler S et al. Using larvae in modern wound management. J Wound Care 1996; 5:60–9.

104. Thomas S. New drugs for diabetic foot ulcers: larval therapy. In: Boulton AJM, Connor H, Cavanagh

PR (eds) The foot in diabetes, 3rd edn. Chichester: John Wiley & Sons, 2000; pp. 185–91.

105. Casu RE, Eisemann CH, Vuoclo T et al. The major excretory/secretory protease from *Lucilia cuprina* larvae is also a gut digestive protease. Int J Parasitol 1996; 26:623–8.

106. Bowling FL, Salgami EV, Boulton AJ. Larval therapy: a novel treatment in eliminating methicillin-resistant *Staphylococcus aureus* in diabetic foot ulcers. Diabetes Care 2007; 30:370–1.

107. Husband DJ, Thai AC, Alberti KG. Management of diabetes during surgery with glucose–insulin–potassium infusion. Diabetic Med 1986; 3:69–74.

108. Cavanagh PR, Young MJ, Adams JE et al. Radiographic abnormalities in the feet of patients with diabetic neuropathy. Diabetes Care 1994; 17:201–9.

109. Edmonds ME, Clarke MB, Newton S et al. Increased uptake of bone radio-pharmaceutical in diabetic neuropathy. Q J Med 1985; 57:843–55.

110. Young MJ, Marshall A, Adams JE et al. Osteopenia, neurological dysfunction, and the development of Charcot neuroarthropathy. Diabetes Care 1995; 18:34–8.

111. Selby PL, Young MJ, Boulton AJ. Bisphosphonates: a new treatment for diabetic Charcot neuroarthropathy? Diabetic Med 1994; 11:28–31.

112. Jude EB, Selby PL, Mawer B et al. Pamidronate in diabetic Charcot neuroarthropathy: a randomised placebo controlled trial. Diabetologia 2001; 44:2032–7.

**This trial showed the efficacy of bisphosphonates in treating acute Charcot neuroarthropathy.**

113. Pitocco D, Ruotolo V, Caputo S et al. Six-month treatment with alendronate in acute Charcot neuroarthropathy: a randomized controlled trial. Diabetes Care 2005; 28(5):1214–15.

**This trial showed the reduction in symptoms, bone turnover markers and improvement in bone density in the bones of the feet of Charcot patients treated with the bisphosphonate, alendronate.**

114. Gazis A, Pound A, Macfarlane R et al. Mortality in patients with diabetic neuropathic osteoarthropathy (Charcot foot). Diabetes Med 2004; 21:1243–6.

115. Fabrin J, Larsen K, Holstein PE. Long-term follow-up in diabetic Charcot feet with spontaneous onset. Diabetes Care 2000; 23:796–800.

# 6

# Amputation, rehabilitation and prosthetic developments

Dipak Datta
Gillian Atkinson

## Introduction

In some patients with lower limb ischaemia, amputation seems the best option. This may be because revascularisation appears impracticable or unjustified, or because it has not succeeded. Amputation should not be regarded as 'failure' of treatment but should be seen by patients as well as clinicians as a positive procedure. Amputation should achieve relief of symptoms, removal of dead, severely ischaemic or infected tissue, as well as restoring function and quality of life. This is true even for the patients who may not be able to return to walking with a prosthesis.

The planning and process of rehabilitation of amputees should start prior to amputation and continue into the community. Expert and holistic assessment of the patient leading to careful selection of the level of amputation, good surgical technique and optimal postoperative management are all vital in the initial stage of amputee rehabilitation. The process then dovetails into postamputation early rehabilitation, e.g. use of early walking aids, wheelchair and home assessments, prosthetic rehabilitation where appropriate, and continuing follow-up and support to patients and their families in the community.

This chapter concentrates on the rehabilitation of patients undergoing amputation because of lower limb ischaemia, although the principles involved are similar for amputations due to other causes.

## Epidemiology

Peripheral arterial occlusive disease accounts for the vast majority of lower limb amputations in westernised societies. More than 80% of all amputations carried out in the UK are said to be due to vascular causes, of which 20–30% are due to diabetes mellitus.[1] The overall risk of amputation is six times higher in insulin-dependent diabetics compared with non-insulin-dependent diabetics. A global study group also reported a marked difference in the incidence of amputation between 10 centres in six different countries. Rates were highest in the North American and northern European centres and lowest in Spain, Taiwan and Japan. In the Navajo population, a very high prevalence of diabetes was thought to be the explanation for their high amputation rates.[2]

The National Amputee Statistical Database for the UK reported that dysvascularity is the most common reason for referral to prosthetic services centres following a lower limb amputation, accounting for 72% of all lower limb referrals in 2005–6.[3] In this group referred to the prosthetic centres in the UK, 52% were transtibial and 38% were transfemoral amputees. In this 1-year period a total of 15 391 of lower limb amputations were carried out in the UK, of which amputation of toe(s) was recorded in 7417 (48.19%) and amputation of foot (total or partial) in 1209 (6.6%).[3] The annual incidence of critical limb ischaemia is 500–1000 per million population and up to one-quarter of these patients undergo major amputations.[4]

There is some evidence that the impact of modern vascular surgery may reduce the incidence of amputation.[5] The Danish National Amputation Register has demonstrated a 27% fall in the number of major amputations due to peripheral vascular disease in the decade 1980–90. This decline was attributed to the increased use of infrainguinal bypass operations.[6] A paper from Finland also reported that it was possible to reduce amputation rates with an aggressive reconstruction policy in critical limb ischaemia.[7] However, the West Coast Vascular Surgeons Study Group in Sweden failed to demonstrate a negative correlation between amputation and revascularisation rates.[8]

It has been quoted that 30% of vascular amputees may be expected to lose the opposite leg within 2 years and 50% to die within 5 years.[9,10] In a more recent study in Scotland, the overall survival of patients who had an amputation as a result of peripheral vascular disease was found to be 4 years. Median survival was significantly lower in patients with diabetes mellitus (3 years 8 months) than in those without diabetes (4 years 2 months). In this study, analysis of two 10-year cohorts of amputees indicates that overall survival is improving.[11]

## Indications for amputation

The decision to perform amputation seems straightforward where there is extensive tissue loss or no reasonable prospect of revascularisation. However, the precise role of amputation in the management of critical limb ischaemia remains controversial. If it is predicted that vascular reconstruction is likely to be unsuccessful, then primary amputation perhaps offers the best outcome in terms of quality of life and cost benefit.[12] (Chapter 3 discusses the treatment of chronic lower limb ischaemia and covers these issues of economics and quality of life in more detail.) Where patients with critical limb ischaemia also have coexisting disabilities or other medical conditions that would render them unable to make use of a salvageable limb, then primary amputation and appropriate rehabilitation offers the best option. Examples of such patients include those with severe dementia, dense hemiplegia or spinal paralysis, severe arthritis and severe cardiorespiratory disease.

## Level selection

Selection of the ideal level of amputation depends on the healing potential, rehabilitation potential and prosthetic considerations. The potential for rehabilitation and likely goals can only be set by a holistic assessment of the patient by the specialist amputee rehabilitation team. This assessment should include other illnesses and disabilities, cognitive state and motivation, likely discharge destination, lifestyle, as well as the patient's own aspirations and wishes.

In general terms, the more proximal the level of amputation, the more difficult it will be for the patient to achieve independent walking. Therefore the more distal the amputation site, the better the rehabilitation potential for walking, as this provides longer stump length and preserves more joints and hence more control of the prosthesis. **Figure 6.1** is an algorithm dealing with level selection.

Except in diabetics with good foot pulses (see Chapter 7), amputation of single or multiple toes generally does not heal unless the foot can be revascularised. Transmetatarsal or ray amputation, if technically feasible, produces excellent functional results. Chopart's mid-tarsal amputation and Symes' through-ankle amputation are rare in chronic limb ischaemia and are not recommended because of the risks of developing equinus deformity (in Chopart's), movement of the distal flap (in Symes'), poor long-term flap viability and considerable technical difficulties in prosthetic fitting. Thus, the commonest major levels of amputation in limb ischaemia are transtibial, knee disarticulation, Gritti–Stokes and transfemoral. Hip disarticulation and hindquarter amputation are rare and in 2001–2 accounted for just over 1% of all cases of lower limb amputations referred to the prosthetic centres in the UK. Dysvascularity was given as the cause for this level of amputation in only 18% of cases.[3]

Preservation of the knee joint has enormous advantages in terms of mobility. In one study, 80% of transtibial amputees achieved unlimited household mobility or better compared with 40% of above-knee amputees.[13] In a Sheffield study, only 26% of transfemoral vascular amputees achieved community ambulation compared with 50% of transtibial vascular amputees at 1-year follow-up of a group of amputees who underwent prosthetic rehabilitation. In this study group, the figures for household mobility were 48% and 63% respectively for transfemoral and transtibial vascular amputees at 1-year follow-up.[14]

Transcutaneous oximetry (tc$P_{O_2}$),[15] photoplethysmography,[16] laser Doppler velocimetry,[17] thermography[18] and isotope clearance rates[19] have all been shown to correlate with subsequent stump healing. However, while all these methods seem superior to Doppler ankle pressures,[20] a review concluded that sensitivities and specificities were inadequate to recommend their clinical use.[21]

The energy cost of walking with prostheses for vascular amputees is increased by 63% and 117% respectively in unilateral transtibial and transfemoral amputees compared with non-amputees.

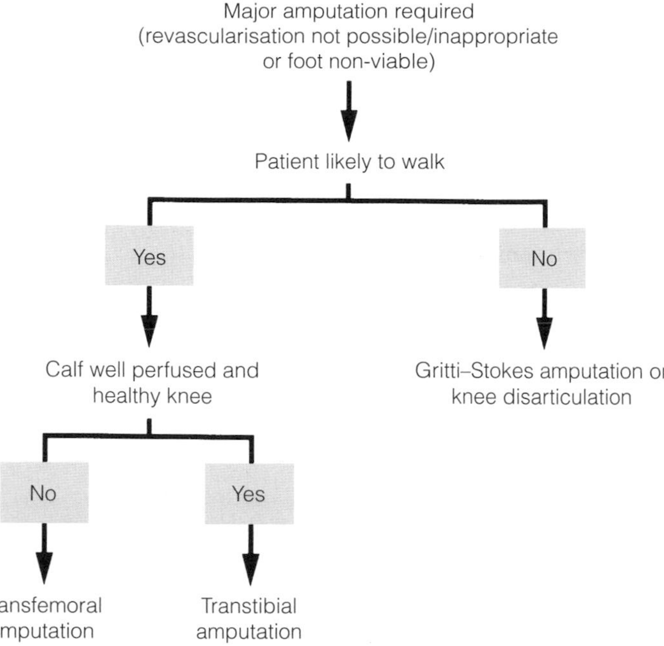


**Figure 6.1** • Algorithm for the selection of amputation level.

In bilateral transfemoral amputees, it is calculated that energy cost is 280% higher.[22] Therefore, it should not seem surprising that even in a selected group of bilateral transfemoral amputees who were successfully trained to walk with prostheses in an inpatient rehabilitation facility, the majority of them abandoned walking when they returned home and preferred to be wheelchair-dependent.[23]

Thus, for patients in whom major lower limb amputations are necessary, the following points should be remembered:

- Preserve the knee joint whenever possible if it is anticipated that the patient has the potential to achieve prosthetic walking or has the potential to use a prosthetic limb for assisting transfers from chair, bed, etc.
- In patients likely to remain chair- or bed-bound following amputation, a transtibial amputation risks non-healing and may become a hindrance to transfers if flexion contractures of the knee and hip joints develop. In such patients, knee disarticulation or Gritti–Stokes amputation seems a better option.
- Where there is a fixed knee flexion deformity of 35° or more, satisfactory fitting of a prosthesis is not possible. In such cases, a more proximal amputation should be undertaken.
- For patients likely to remain wheelchair- or bed-bound, including bilateral amputees, knee disarticulation or Gritti–Stokes amputation is preferable to transfemoral or transtibial as longer lever lengths and larger surface area are more conducive to transferring and provide a much better seating balance.
- In patients where a transtibial amputation is not possible but the patient has the potential to walk, most amputee rehabilitation units prefer a transfemoral rather than knee disarticulation or Gritti–Stokes amputation. This is because of problems of prosthetic fitting compromising cosmetic appearance and function.

## Surgical considerations

All amputations should be carried out by surgeons experienced in the procedure and should not be delegated to unsupervised and inexperienced junior staff. The following important general principles should be followed:

- tissues must be handled with care;
- flaps should be oversized initially and then shaped and trimmed as required;

- good-quality sensate skin coverage of stump without tension;
- bone edges should be smoothed off and bevelled;
- skin and muscle flaps should be trimmed and shaped to prevent dog ears, redundant tissue or a bulbous stump;
- creating the correct shape of the stump is the responsibility of the surgeon at the time of surgery;
- the use of a thigh tourniquet can reduce blood loss significantly during fashioning of muscle flaps.

## Transfemoral amputation

Ensure adequate muscle (myoplastic) cover over the cut end of femur to prevent pain and discomfort and allow balanced action of flexors and extensors.[24] The technique of myodesis, where drill holes are made in the bone to fix muscles, may not be applicable in ischaemic limbs due to poor tissue quality. However, this minimises the risk of the muscles slipping off the end of the femur. The myoplasty and myodesis need to be performed with the hip joint in the neutral and naturally adducted position.

Allow at least 12 cm of clearance from the distal end of stump to knee-joint level in order to allow space for incorporating a prosthetic knee joint. The exact level of bone section will depend on thickness of the myoplasty and subcutaneous tissue. This will prevent the unacceptable cosmetic and functional disability of a lowered knee centre in the prosthetic limb.

## Gritti–Stokes and through-knee amputation

These seem useful options for patients in whom transtibial amputation will not heal and who are deemed incapable of walking.[25] The longer stump assists transfers and sitting balance and maintains muscle attachment and proprioception. Limitations in prosthetic fitting due to a lowered knee centre, and limited availability of stance and swing phase control mechanism in the prosthetic knee joint at this level, make these procedures unpopular with prosthetists, although good ambulation can be achieved.[26]

In the Gritti–Stokes amputation, the femoral condyles are removed to avoid a bulbous stump. Adequate fixation of patella is vital as a mobile and non-united patella prevents end bearing. In the modified Gritti–Stokes amputation there is a long anterior semicircular flap, which transects the patellar tendon to enter the knee joint. The patella is then retracted and the femur divided just above the condyles at a 30° backward angle. This allows the patella to lock over the end of the femur once the articular surface has been removed (**Fig. 6.2**).

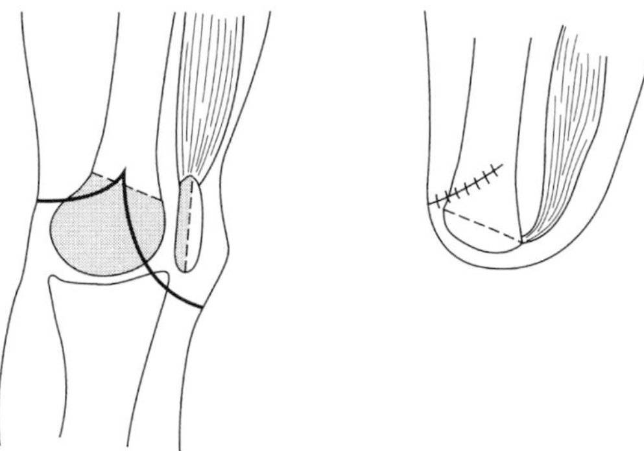

**Figure 6.2** • Transection of the femur with a backward angle results in a more stable attachment of the patella in the modified Gritti–Stokes amputation.

In the through-knee amputation, mediolateral flaps should be devised to allow the scar to retract into the condylar notch away from the end-bearing area. The bulbous end of the stump may make fitting and cosmesis of a prosthesis unacceptable.

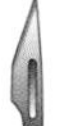

A randomised study of through-knee versus Gritti–Stokes amputation has reported poorer healing rates with the former as a result of synovial fluid leakage.[27]

## Transtibial amputation

Many surgeons now favour the skew flap technique[28] rather than the traditional Burgess long posterior flap.[29] In the skew flap technique, the flaps are based on the arteries that run with the long and short saphenous veins, which provide the main blood supply to the skin. In a small study of posterior flap and skew flap techniques, evaluation of flap hypoxia demonstrated that the posterior flap was associated with greater and more persistent reduction in tc$P_{O2}$.[30]

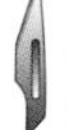

Randomised trials have shown no difference in healing between the skew flap and traditional Burgess long posterior flap.[31] However, the time to limb-fitting and early mobility was shorter in the skew flap group due to a less bulbous stump (**Fig. 6.3**).

The Burgess amputation still seems useful when skew flaps might be compromised by the medial skin incision of a failed femoro-distal bypass graft or following fasciotomies (**Fig. 6.4**).

A tibial section at about 15 cm is considered ideal. The fibula should be divided around 1.5 cm proximal

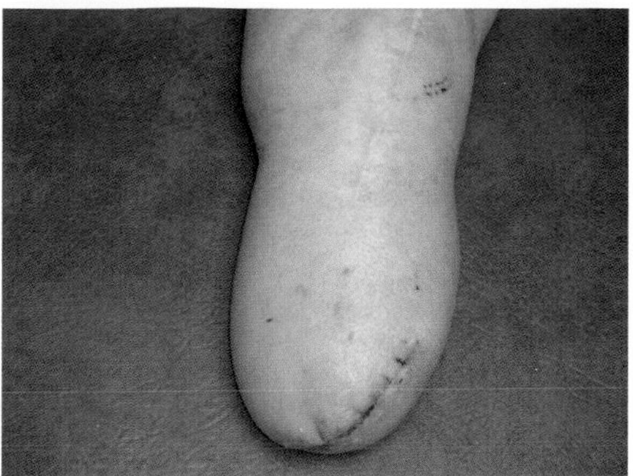

**Figure 6.3 •** Skew flap transtibial amputation at two and a half weeks showing a nicely shaped stump suitable for early limb fitting.

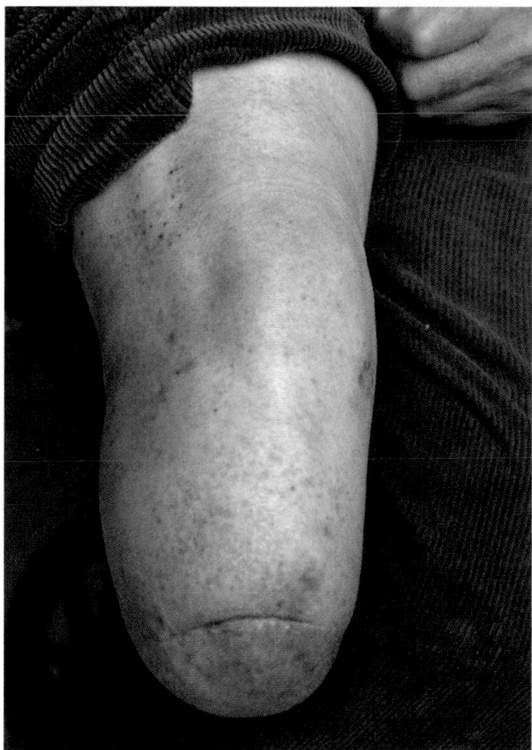

**Figure 6.4 •** An excellent transtibial amputation stump with a long posterior flap myoplasty.

to the level of the tibial section. A short bevel and rounding off the sharp corners of the tibia must be undertaken. Much shorter transtibial stumps (up to 8 cm), though not ideal, can be fitted with supracondylar or ICEROSS sockets. Avoidance of a bulbous distal end of stump is vital for this level of amputation.

## Foot amputation

Digital amputation is most commonly performed in diabetics because of their susceptibility to infection. In general, a digital amputation will only heal if foot pulses are present or can be restored. Therefore it is better to leave toes with partial dry gangrene alone. Amputation is best performed through the base of the proximal phalanx, leaving the wound open to heal by secondary intention. When infection extends beyond the proximal phalanx, a 'ray amputation' is indicated, especially in diabetics. After excision of the relevant toes, the line of excision is carried back through the infected tissue until healthy tissue is reached. The underlying metatarsal head is excised and the wound left open like a 'fish mouth'.

Infection of the first or fifth metatarsophalangeal joint requires a 'tennis-racquet' incision; the handle of the racquet can usually be closed after excision of the metatarsal head. A transmetatarsal amputation can be useful when all the toes are gangrenous but when the plantar skin is still viable. A dorsal skin incision is made at mid-metatarsal level with a long plantar flap and bone transection through the metatarsal bases. As much soft tissue as possible should be preserved and the flaps left open with delayed closure, as infection and gangrene of the flaps may occur if primary closure is attempted. Vacuum-assisted closure systems may facilitate the healing of such open-foot amputations.

## Rehabilitation

The process of rehabilitation for vascular amputees, who are usually elderly and often have a number of other concurrent disabilities and illnesses, can pose a considerable challenge. A 'team approach' in amputee rehabilitation is gaining popularity and has been shown to be cost-effective.[32] The core members of the team should include a vascular surgeon, a specialist in rehabilitation medicine, specialist physiotherapist and occupational therapist, and a prosthetist. Ready availability of a social worker, a community nurse, a clinical psychologist and a chiropodist is invaluable. Other multidisciplinary team members include wheelchair personnel, housing and adaptation officers, social services and orthotists. Close liaison and cooperation between all members of the team are vital. Counsellors and amputee volunteers, if available, can be extremely valuable.

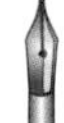

The British Society of Rehabilitation Medicine has recently updated and published standards and guidelines in amputee and prosthetic rehabilitation based on national consensus.[33]

In smaller district general hospitals where fewer amputations are carried out, it is not practical to develop such a multidisciplinary team. In such situations an experienced senior physiotherapist specialising in amputee rehabilitation should be given the coordinating role with the surgical team, liaising closely with the nearest regional or subregional amputee rehabilitation centre.

## Planning

A preamputation consultation by specialists in rehabilitation medicine and their team is ideal but impractical for every patient for whom an amputation is planned. However, a member of the amputee rehabilitation team (usually a therapist) should see all patients prior to amputation in order to make an initial assessment and prepare the patient for the likely programme to be implemented, instil realistic expectations and resolve any specific questions or anxieties. Other members of the multidisciplinary team may be involved at this stage if specially required. In our unit, specialist physiotherapists cover the boundary between the vascular and rehabilitation units and we find that this works extremely effectively. In cases where amputation is a treatment option rather than a necessity, and in situations where there is some uncertainty regarding level selection, we recommend that the surgical team obtain advice from an appropriate consultant in rehabilitation medicine.

## Stump management

Tight or elasticated stump bandaging should not be used in vascular amputees as it can generate unacceptable pressures and cause tissue breakdown.[34] Rigid dressings of plaster of Paris are not generally used for vascular amputees in the UK, although some studies have suggested that they reduce the knee contracture rate following transtibial amputation. Adhesive clear-plastic film dressing applied postoperatively can be very useful as this allows easier and regular wound inspection. This type of dressing makes life easier for the physiotherapist when inspecting wounds before and after application of early walking aids. Where a more conventional dressing for the wound is required, an elasticated tubular bandage (e.g. Tubifast) is usually placed on the stump to hold these dressings in place. If the wound is healed or healing satisfactorily, then elasticated and graduated pressure stump shrinker socks (e.g. Juzo) are applied to the stump (**Fig. 6.5**). A survey of amputee physiotherapists in the UK (unpublished) revealed that the current practice is moving forward using the stump shrinker socks earlier than previously. In Sheffield, if the vascular surgeons are satisfied with the stump wound and the patient is able to tolerate, the Juzo sock is applied on the fourth postoperative day. On the first day it is applied for 1 hour and then the wearing time is gradually increased over the next few days until the patient is wearing it all day and night. This process is carefully monitored by experienced staff. Appropriate stump supports are fitted to the wheelchair so that the patients can keep their below-knee stumps elevated. Sometimes appropriate stump supports may also be necessary for long transfemoral or knee disarticulation stumps. Appropriate and specialist footwear to protect the other leg from damage by the wheelchair may be an important consideration. In our centre we find pressure-relieving ankle foot orthoses effective for this purpose and also relieve pressure on the heel whilst lying down.

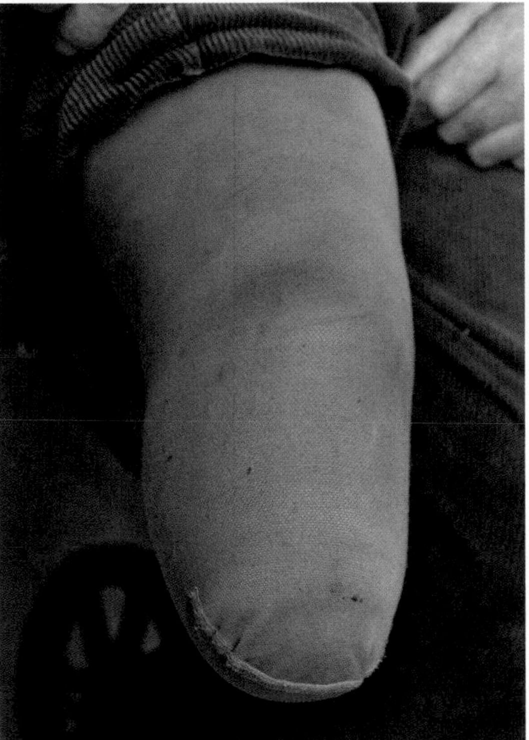

**Figure 6.5** • A stump shrinker sock applied over a transtibial amputation stump.

## Pain management

Controlling stump and phantom pains is vital for the patient to participate successfully in a rehabilitation programme. Houghton et al.[35] found a significant relationship between preamputation pain and phantom pain in the first 2 years after amputation in vascular amputees. Nikolajsen et al.,[36] in a study of mostly vascular amputees, found a relationship between preoperative pain and incidents of phantom pain at 1 week and 3 months after amputation, but not after 6 months. Early involvement of the 'pain team' in appropriate cases is most beneficial. Numerous medical interventions have been proposed over the years but tricyclic antidepressants and sodium channel blockers are currently considered to be the drugs of choice for neuropathic pain.[37] The anticonvulsant carbamazepine, a non-specific sodium channel blocker, has been reported to be effective in phantom pain.[38,39]

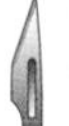

In a randomised, double-blind, placebo-controlled, crossover study of 19 patients, gabapentin monotherapy was better than placebo in relieving postamputation phantom limb pain.[40] In a randomised study of 25 patients undergoing amputation, Bach et al. established that incidents of phantom pain were reduced 6 months after amputation but not after 1 week or after 12 months in the group receiving epidural analgesia for 72 hours prior to amputation compared with a controlled group.[41] In a blinded and placebo-controlled trial of 60 patients who received epidural analgesia for 1 day before amputation, it was concluded that it is not possible to prevent phantom pain by an epidural block of short duration.[42]

In addition to the medical treatment of stump and phantom pains, various non-invasive treatments such as transcutaneous electrical nerve stimulation, vibration therapy, acupuncture, hypnosis and biofeedback can prove useful, although evidence of efficacy is limited.

## Early rehabilitation

The occupational therapist and physiotherapist should work closely together to ensure an effective and timely rehabilitation programme. Following amputation the physiotherapist usually sees the amputee on the first postoperative day and will begin a programme of bed mobility, joint movements, transferring and wheelchair mobility, depending on the patient's general condition and pain control. Stump exercises, exercises for the remaining limb and upper limbs, muscle strengthening, maintaining range of movements of the proximal joints, sitting balance and improvement of general cardiovascular fitness will all be incorporated into the programme. Each amputee will be assessed for an appropriate wheelchair and cushion as early as possible to facilitate discharge. The amputee will be taught the skills necessary for independent use of the wheelchair. By around the 1-week assessment, the therapist is usually reasonably sure of a patient's potential ability to use a prosthesis or not; however, some amputees are too unwell at the early postoperative stage but later may recover sufficiently to benefit from prosthetic rehabilitation. Therefore appropriate follow-up assessment may need to be arranged for this group of amputees.

Extreme frailty, severe dementia, severe cardiorespiratory disease, gross fixed flexion contractures and severe arthritis are contraindications to prosthetic rehabilitation. It is generally the practice in our unit to guide elderly bilateral vascular transfemoral amputees away from prosthetic rehabilitation.

Assessing the home environment and adaptations, advice regarding driving, hobbies and employment also need addressing as an integral part of the rehabilitation.

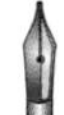

Evidence-based guidelines on the early rehabilitation phase have been published by the British Association of Chartered Physiotherapists in Amputee Rehabilitation.[43]

## Primary prosthetic rehabilitation

All amputees who receive a prosthesis should undergo prosthetic rehabilitation to achieve the best prosthetic outcome. The physiotherapist will play a key role in this. Prosthetic rehabilitation should aim to establish an energy-efficient gait based on normal physiological walking patterns. The physiotherapist should teach efficient control of the prosthesis through postural control, weight transference, use of proprioception, and specific muscle strengthening and stretching exercises to prevent and correct gait deviations. Prosthetic rehabilitation will work towards the individual's own realistic goals, and should include functional activities relevant to that person and his or her lifestyle. All encouragement should be given to enable the individual to resume hobbies, sports, social activities, driving and return to work.

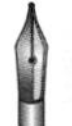

The British Association of Chartered Physiotherapists in Amputee Rehabilitation have published useful evidence-based clinical guidelines for the physiotherapy of adults with lower limb prostheses.[44]

## Sport activities for amputees

Amputation does not prevent an individual actively participating in sport. We often think of running, cycling, swimming and football, but there are others which may be more appropriate for the older, vascular amputee including darts, snooker, bowls, fishing and golf.

Specialised componentry/prostheses are available for amputees who may want to run or swim. They may enable amputees to participate in more comfort and at a higher level than previously. However, most sports will not require special prostheses and can be played alongside the able-bodied.

Previous and current fitness, concurrent disabilities (e.g. diabetic complications) and determination will all be important factors in the individual returning to or engaging in a new sport. Amputees may seek advice from professionals at their amputee rehabilitation centre, from peers, from groups such as British Amputee Les Autre Sports Association (BALASA) and, ever increasingly, the internet. Many local areas have groups who specialise in disabled sport and leisure which the amputee could access. The English Federation of Disability Sports (EFDS) keep a list of all the disabled clubs nationally who deal with sports and leisure.

## Prostheses

There are two main types of early walking aids used in the UK (**Figs 6.6** and **6.7**). The best known is the pneumatic postamputation mobility aid (PPAM Aid). The PPAM Aid is widely used and can be used for transtibial, through-knee and transfemoral levels of amputation. Until recently another type of early walking aid known as amputee mobility aid (AMA), designed for transtibial amputation only, has been in use which allows amputees to flex and extend their knee during the gait cycle. It has a foot rather than a rocker end, allowing a more natural gait. Unfortunately the production for AMA has now ceased and no new ones are now available commercially. The Femurette is an excellent early walking aid for transfemoral amputees; it mimics a definitive transfemoral prosthesis in terms of ischial tuberosity-bearing socket configuration and knee joint and it also has a foot.[45] The early walking aids are excellent morale boosters and are also used as assessment tools to estimate an amputee's potential for walking. They allow stump desensitisation, assist in reduction of stump oedema and may promote wound healing, and allow re-education of postural reflexes, balance and gait. The early walking aids should be considered around 1 week after amputation, under the judicious supervision of experienced therapists. However, in some cases where wound healing is very poor, introduction of early walking aids needs to be delayed.

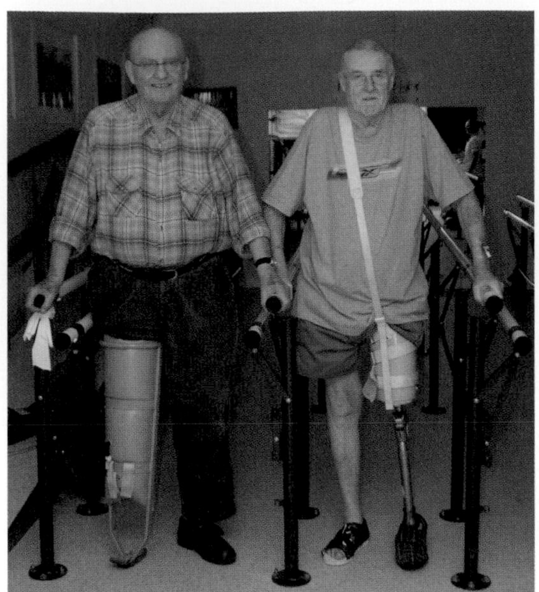

**Figure 6.7** • A patient wearing Femurette (right) and a patient wearing PPAM Aid (left).

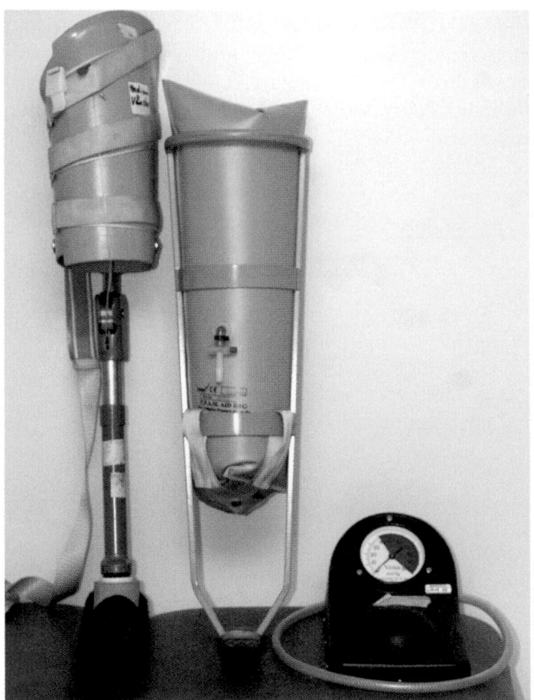

**Figure 6.6** • A selection of early walking aids: Femurette (left) and pneumatic postamputation mobility aid (PPAM Aid; centre). A foot pump to inflate the PPAM Aid is shown on the right.

### Prosthetic developments

The lower limb prostheses used in the UK are mainly of endoskeletal modular construction (**Fig. 6.8**). This system allows much speedier manufacture, socket change, adjustments and repairs compared with old conventional exoskeletal and labour-intensive prostheses. A complete new limb, from measurement to delivery, is now usually available within five working days for primary patients, or even quicker if needed. The modern prostheses usually incorporate thermoplastic materials like polypropylene or laminated

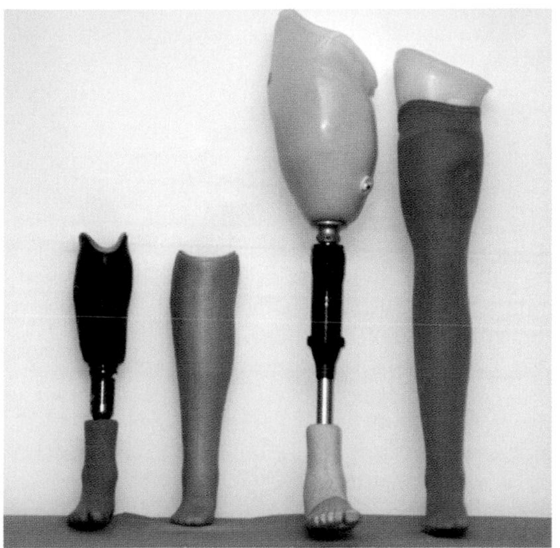

**Figure 6.8** • Modular endoskeletal prostheses for transfemoral and transtibial amputation, with and without cosmetic covers.

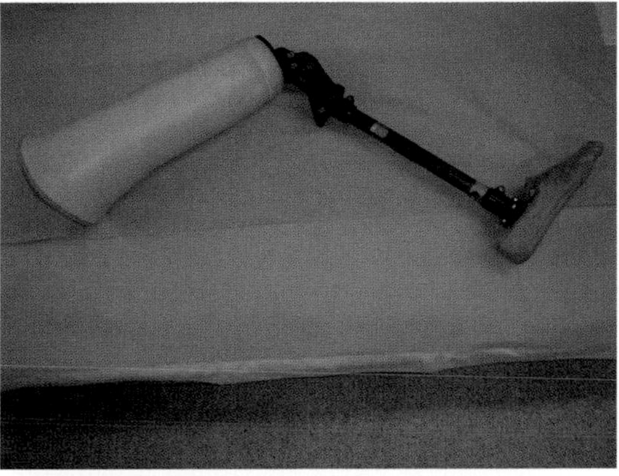

**Figure 6.9** • A knee disarticulation prosthesis (without cosmetic cover) incorporating a four-bar linkage polycentric knee joint.

plastics as socket materials and carbon fibre or lightweight alloy for fabrication of the weight-bearing structures.

Usually, vascular amputees are measured for their first prosthesis at about 6–8 weeks from amputation, although earlier fitting can take place subject to wound-healing status and the general condition of the stump. It is not imperative that the stump be completely healed before a prosthesis can be provided.

Younger dysvascular transfemoral amputees may have good musculature of the stump and adequate hand function and agility to benefit from prostheses with suction socket fitting and sophisticated 'free knee' mechanisms like pneumatic or hydraulic swing phase controls. Microchip-controlled 'intelligent' knee joints providing improved swing and stance phase control are used to some benefit for transfemoral amputees, but experience so far has been generally limited to younger and more active amputees.[46] In the UK, most elderly and dysvascular transfemoral amputees, if they are accepted for a prosthetic rehabilitation programme, are provided with non-suction prostheses with some form of waist-belt suspension and a 'locked' knee (bends only to sit down). More active dysvascular transfemoral amputees may also benefit from modern microchip-controlled knee mechanisms and self-suspending sockets.

For knee disarticulation, Gritti–Stokes or long transfemoral amputees, prosthetic options are limited. Use of polycentric knee joints like four-bar linkage knee mechanisms has eased some of the difficulties, though prostheses at these levels still create cosmetic as well as functional difficulties (**Fig. 6.9**).

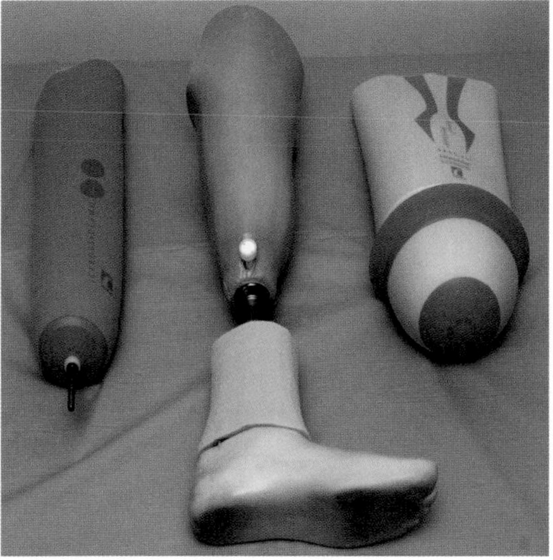

**Figure 6.10** • From left to right: an ICEROSS liner with a distal locking pin which is applied by rolling onto the stump; a transtibial prothesis on which the stump with the liner is inserted and locked in; and a Seal-in silicone liner which provides excellent suspension by suction without the necessity of a locking pin.

For transtibial amputees the introduction of the ICEROSS prosthesis has found favour with some patients as it provides much improved suspension as well as reducing friction and shear forces at the stump–socket interface[47] (**Fig. 6.10**). This type of prosthesis uses a silicone sleeve directly on the stump, which is then locked into the prosthetic socket. Currently several other types of gel liners are also available using locking pin or suction suspension system. Much shorter transtibial amputation stumps can now be fitted successfully, which was not possible previously with the traditional patellar tendon-bearing prosthesis.

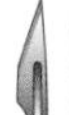

Direct casting of socket on the amputation stump using the pressure-casting method of ICECAST has been available more recently. This type of socket and prostheses for transtibial amputation can be made much more speedily but it is considerably more expensive and has been shown not to improve gait and to give only minor comfort preference in a randomised controlled study.[48]

Computer-aided socket design and manufacture are also being used more frequently in the UK, eliminating the need for plaster models.

Energy-saving prosthetic feet, e.g. Dynamic Response Foot (Blatchford), Flex Foot, Seattle Foot, are generally provided to younger active amputees – Flex Foot prostheses have been known to be less energy consuming to walk for transtibial amputees.

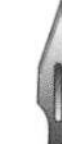

More recently these high-energy return feet have also been found to offer significant help to transfemoral amputees.[49,50]

They are more expensive than the usual uniaxial or multiaxial ankle joints and moulded foot provided for the vast majority of lower limb amputees. A patient-adjustable heel height device is available when shoes with different heel height are to be worn. Special components are also available and may be of benefit in appropriate cases, such as a torsion device and vertical shock absorber in the shin of a prosthesis that absorbs vertical forces and rotational torque, turntables that allow sitting cross-legged on the floor, or individually created, highly life-like silicone cosmetic cover, swimming or shower legs. Selection of the prostheses and components will be determined by the amputee's wishes, realistic goals, progress in rehabilitation and ability to benefit from a prescribed device.

## Key points

- In the UK, 80% of all amputations carried out are due to vascular disease, of which 20–30% are due to diabetes.
- Vascular reconstruction may reduce the incidence of amputation.
- Selection of the ideal level of amputation depends on healing potential, rehabilitation potential and prosthetic considerations.
- Transtibial amputees have a much higher potential to achieve prosthetic mobilisation compared with those undergoing transfemoral amputation.
- For patients who are not likely to achieve prosthetic walking, a Gritti–Stokes amputation is preferable to the transfemoral level.
- A comprehensive and holistic assessment of amputees or prospective amputees, followed by multidisciplinary rehabilitation, is likely to provide the optimal outcome.
- Amputation surgery should be considered as a constructive procedure to create the best possible amputation stump and should therefore be carried out by surgeons who have had proper training in these procedures.
- Stump bandaging with elasticated bandages is not recommended.
- Appropriate use of early walking aids during the early postamputation period is an essential part of rehabilitation.
- Modern prostheses are modular and can be made quickly using modern materials technology.
- Increasingly more sophisticated components are becoming available, although they tend to be applicable only for the more active amputee.
- The types of prostheses and their components will be determined by the amputee's realistic goals, progress in rehabilitation and ability to benefit.

## References


1. Fyfe NCM. Amputation and rehabilitation. In: Davies AH, Beard JD, Wyatt MG (eds) Essential vascular surgery. London: WB Saunders, 1999; pp. 243–51.
2. The Global Lower Extremity Amputation Study Group. Epidemiology of lower extremity amputation in centres in Europe, North America and East Asia. Br J Surg 2000; 87:328–37.
3. Amputee Statistical Database for the United Kingdom 2005–06: Information Services Division. Edinburgh: National Health Service Scotland, Edinburgh, 2007.
4. Price JF, Fowkes FGR. Epidemiology of peripheral vascular disease. In: Davies AH, Beard JD, Wyatt MG (eds) Essential vascular surgery. London: WB Saunders, 1999; pp. 18–30.
5. Gutteridge W, Torrie P, Galland R. Trends in arterial reconstruction, angioplasty and amputation. Health Trends 1994; 26:88–91.
6. Ebskov LB, Scroeder TV, Holstein PE. Epidemiology of leg amputation: the influence of vascular surgery. Br J Surg 1994; 81:1600–3.
7. Luther M. The influence of arterial reconstruction surgery on the outcome of critical leg ischaemia. Eur J Vasc Surg 1994; 8:682–9.
8. The West Coast Vascular Surgeons Study Group. Variations of rates of vascular surgical procedures for chronic critical limb ischaemia and lower limb amputation rates in Western Swedish counties. Eur J Vasc Endovasc Surg 1997; 14:310–14.
9. English AWG, Dean AAG. The Artificial Limb Service. Health Trends 1980; 12:77–82.
10. Couch NP, David JK, Tilney NL et al. Natural history of the leg amputee. Am J Surg 1977; 133:469–73.
11. Stewart CPU, Jain AS, Ogden SA. Lower limb amputee survival. Prosthet Orthot Int 1992; 16:11–18.
12. Johnson B, Evans L, Datta D et al. Surgery for limb threatening ischaemia. A reappraisal of costs and benefits. Eur J Vasc Endovasc Surg 1995; 9:181–8.
13. Houghton AD, Taylor PR, Thurlow S et al. Success rates for rehabilitation of vascular amputees: implications for preoperative assessment and amputation level. Br J Surg 1992; 79:753–5.
14. Davies B, Datta D. Mobility outcome following unilateral lower limb amputation. Prosthet Orthot Int 2003; 27:186–90.
15. Ratcliffe DA, Clyne CAC, Chant ADB et al. Prediction of amputation wound healing: the role of transcutaneous pO2 assessment. Br J Surg 1984; 71:219–22.
16. Van Den Broek TAA, Dwars BJ, Rauwerda JA et al. Photoplethysmographic selection of amputation level in peripheral vascular disease. J Vasc Surg 1988; 8:10–13.
17. Karanfilian RG, Lynch TG, Zinsl VT et al. The value of laser Doppler velocimetry and transcutaneous oxygen tension determination in predicting healing of ischaemic forefoot ulcerations and amputations in diabetic and non-diabetic patients. J Vasc Surg 1986; 4:511–16.
18. Stoner HB, Taylor L, Marcuson RW. The value of skin temperature measurements in forecasting the healing of below-knee amputation for end-stage ischaemia of the leg in peripheral vascular disease. Eur J Vasc Surg 1989; 3:355–61.
19. Moore WS, Henry RE, Malone JM et al. Prospective use of xenon Xe-133 clearance for amputation level selection. Arch Surg 1981; 166:86–8.
20. Welch GH, Leiberman DP, Pollock JG et al. Failure of Doppler ankle pressure to predict healing of conservative forefoot amputations. Br J Surg 1985; 72:888–91.
21. Savin S, Sharni S, Shields DA et al. Selection of amputation level: a review. Eur J Vasc Surg 1991; 5:611–20.

    **The authors reviewed the evidence for many tests (Doppler indices, segmental pressures, skin blood flow, skin perfusion pressure, tc$P_{O2}$, thermography) to predict the likelihood of successful healing of an amputation stump. They concluded that the foremost requirement to raise the below-knee/above-knee ratio is to promote awareness among surgeons of the value of medical management and encourage the use of routinely available tests such as ankle–brachial pressure index and Doppler segmental pressures. The value of more specialised tests remains to be established.**
22. Huang CT, Jackson JR, Moore NB et al. Amputation: energy cost of ambulation. Arch Phys Med Rehab 1979; 60:18–24.
23. Datta D, Nair PN, Payne J. Outcome of prosthetic management of bilateral lower limb amputees. Disabil Rehab 1992; 14:98–102.
24. Chadwick SJD, Lewis JD. Above-knee amputation. Ann R Coll Surg Engl 1991; 73:152–4.
25. Dovan J, Hopkinson BE, Makin GS. The Gritti–Stokes amputation in ischaemia: a review of 134 cases. Br J Surg 1978; 65:135–6.
26. Houghton A, Allen A, Luff R et al. Rehabilitation after lower limb amputation: a comparative study of above-knee and Gritti–Stokes amputations. Br J Surg 1989; 76:622–4.
27. Campbell WB, Morris PJ. A prospective, randomised comparison of healing in Gritti–Stokes and through-knee amputations. Ann R Coll Surg Engl 1986; 69:1–4.

    **In this study, 22 patients with a median age of 79 years had 24 amputations about knee-joint level. The patients were randomised to undergo either Gritti–Stokes or through-knee amputation; 12 (75%) Gritti–Stokes amputations underwent uncomplicated primary**

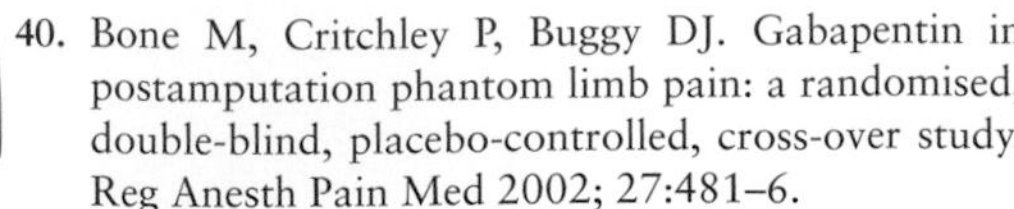


healing compared with only 2 of 12 (17%) through-knee procedures ($P$ = 0.04). Two through-knee amputations required revision to above the knee (17%), whereas all Gritti–Stokes amputations healed.

28. Robinson KP, Hoile R, Coddington T. Skew flap myoplastic below knee amputation: a preliminary report. Br J Surg 1992; 69:554–7.
29. Burgess EM. The below knee amputation. Bull Prosth Res 1968; 10:19–25.
30. Johnson WC, Watkins MT, Hamilton J et al. Transcutaneous partial oxygen pressure changes following skew flap and Burgess-type below knee amputations. Arch Surg 1997; 132:261–3.
31. Ruckley CV, Stonebridge PA, Prescott RJ. Skewflap versus long posterior flap in below-knee amputations: multicenter trial. J Vasc Surg 1991; 13:423–7.

    A multicentre trial – 191 patients with end-stage occlusive vascular disease needing transtibial amputation were randomised to skew flap technique in 98 and long posterior flap technique in 93 patients. The two groups were well matched: 30-day mortality rate, date of wound at 1 week and need for surgical revision at the same or higher level were not statistically significant between the groups. Follow-up information at 6 months showed 64 (84%) of the skew flaps and 50 (77%) of the long posterior flaps were fitted with prostheses. Walking, alone or with support, was achieved in 59 (78%) and 46 (71%) respectively. None of these differences reached statistical significance.

32. Ham RO, Thornberry DJ, Regan JF et al. Rehabilitation of the vascular amputee: one method evaluated. Physiother Pract 1985; 1:6–13.
33. British Society of Rehabilitation Medicine. Amputee and prosthetic rehabilitation standards and guidelines, 2nd edn. Report of the Working Party (chair Hanspal RS). London: British Society of Rehabilitation Medicine, 2003.
34. Isherwood PA, Robertson JC, Rossi A. Pressure measurements beneath below-knee stump bandages. Elastic bandaging, the Puddifoot dressing and a pneumatic bandaging technique compared. Br J Surg 1975; 62:982–6.
35. Houghton AD, Nicholls G, Houghton AL et al. Phantom pain: natural history and association with rehabilitation. Ann R Coll Surg Engl 1994; 76:22–5.
36. Nikolajsen L, Ilkjaer S, Kroner K et al. The influence of preamputation pain on postamputation stump and phantom pain. Pain 1997; 72:393–405.
37. Nikolajsen L, Jensen TS. Phantom limb pain. Br J Anaesth 2001; 87:107–16.
38. Elliott F, Little A, Milbrandt W. Carbamazepine for phantom limb phenomena. N Engl J Med 1976; 295:678.
39. Patterson JF. Carbamazepine in the treatment of phantom limb pain. South Med J 1988; 81:1101–2.
40. Bone M, Critchley P, Buggy DJ. Gabapentin in postamputation phantom limb pain: a randomised, double-blind, placebo-controlled, cross-over study. Reg Anesth Pain Med 2002; 27:481–6.

    In this study, 17 patients attending a multidisciplinary pain clinic with phantom limb pain were randomised to a double-blind, placebo-controlled, crossover study. A daily dose of gabapentin was administered in increments of 300–2400 mg or the maximum tolerated dose. Fifteen patients completed both arms of the study. It was concluded that, after 6 weeks, gabapentin monotherapy was better than placebo in relieving postamputation phantom pain. There were no significant differences in mood, sleep interference and activities of daily living.

41. Bach S, Norenz MF, Tjellden NU. Phantom limb pain in amputees during the first twelve months following limb amputation after pre-operative lumbar epidural seventy-two hours pre-operation. Pain 1988; 33:297–301.

    The aim of this study was to investigate if it was possible to reduce postoperative phantom limb pain by lumbar epidural blockade (LEB) with bupivacaine and morphine for 72 hours prior to the operation. Twenty-five patients were interviewed about their limb pain before limb amputation and about their phantom limb pains 7 days, 6 months and 1 year after limb loss. Seven patients received LEB, so that they were pain-free 3 days prior to operation. The control group of 14 patients all had preoperative limb pain. After 6 months, all patients in the LEB group were pain-free, whereas five patients in the control group had pain ($P < 0.05$).

42. Nikolajsen L, Ilkjaer S, Kroner K et al. Randomized trial of epidural bupivacaine and morphine in prevention of neuropathic pain following amputation. Lancet 1997; 350:1353–7.

    In a randomised double-blind trial, 60 patients scheduled for lower limb amputation were randomly assigned to epidural (bupivacaine and morphine) 18 hours before and during the operation (29 patients) or epidural saline and oral or intramuscular morphine (31 patients). All patients had general anaesthesia for the amputation and were asked about stump and phantom pain after 1 week and then at 3, 6 and 12 months. The authors concluded that perioperative epidural blockade did not prevent phantom or stump pain.

43. Broomhead P, Davies D, Hancock A et al. Clinical guidelines for the pre and post operative physiotherapy management of adults with lower limb amputation. London: British Association of Chartered Physiotherapists in Amputee Rehabilitation, 2006.
44. Broomhead P, Dawes D, Hale C et al. Evidence based clinical guidelines for physiotherapy management of adults with lower limb prostheses. London: British Association of Chartered Physiotherapists in Amputee Rehabilitation, 2003.
45. Ramsay EM. A clinical evaluation of the LIC Femurette as an early training device for the primary above knee amputee. Physiotherapy 1988; 74:598–601.

46. Datta D, Howitt J. Conventional versus microchip controlled pneumatic swing-phase control for transfemoralamputees. Prosthet Orthot Int 1998; 22:129–35.

47. Datta D, Vaidya S, Howitt J et al. Outcome of fitting of ICEROSS prosthesis: views of transtibial amputees. Prosthet Orthot Int 1996; 20:111–15.

48. Datta D, Harris I, Heller B et al. Gait cost and time implications for changing from PTB to ICEX® sockets. Prosthet Orthot Int 2004; 28:115–20.

In this study, 27 established transtibial amputees were randomised to be fitted with either a conventional patella tendon-bearing socket by conventional plaster-casting methods (control) or were fitted with a new ICEX socket created directly on the patients' amputation stump by using air pressure (experimental). Twenty-one subjects completed the trial. No significant difference was found in the gait parameters in the two groups. ICEX prostheses were considerably more expensive, although they could be manufactured more quickly. Patients showed only minor comfort preference for ICEX prostheses.

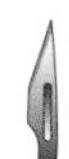

49. Graham LE, Datta D, Heller B et al. A comparative study – Oxygen consumption and energy storing prosthesis in transfemoral amputees. Clin Rehab 2008 ; 22(10–11):896–901.

This experimental crossover trial established transfemoral amputees wearing Multiflex foot initially and then Variflex foot and concluded that a high functioning transfemoral amputee who wears an energy-storing prosthetic foot may have significantly reduced oxygen consumption at normal walking speed.

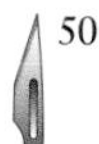

50. Graham LE, Datta D, Heller B et al. A comparative study of conventional and energy storing prosthetic feet in high functioning transfemoral amputees. Arch Phys Med Rehab 2007; 88(6):801–6.

In this study of the same subjects as in Ref. 49 it was shown that a transfemoral amputee who wears an energy-storing foot can have a more symmetrical gait in regard to some measures of spatial symmetry, kinetics and kinematics than one who wears a conventional prosthetic foot.

# 7

# Revision vascular surgery

Andre Nevelsteen

## Introduction

Revision of vascular reconstructions is frequently required beyond the first 6 weeks because of progressive atherosclerosis, graft occlusion, aneurysm formation or infection. Up to 40% of infrainguinal bypass surgery grafts require reintervention within 5 years.[1] The same is true for endovascular intervention, where it has been shown that up to 20% of the patients need a reintervention within 2 years after endovascular aortic aneurysm reconstruction (EVAR).[2] Revision surgery requires experience and judgement; it is technically more difficult because of fibrosis and the loss of easily definable tissue planes, which necessitates careful sharp dissection to gain arterial control. Operating times, blood loss, infection rates and operative risk are increased.

## Graft occlusion

Graft thrombosis usually presents acutely but is occasionally heralded by increasing ischaemic symptoms, ranging from mild claudication through to critical ischaemia. Asymptomatic graft occlusion can also occur. Occasionally, simultaneous distal embolisation causes digital ischaemia (blue toe syndrome or gangrene). Graft thrombosis with loss of run-off due to distal embolisation is associated with a high risk of limb loss. Whereas graft thrombosis in the first 6 weeks is generally due to technical error or poor run-off, most late occlusions result from intimal hyperplasia within the bypass or progressive inflow or run-off disease (see Chapter 4). Graft stenoses are usually asymptomatic and occur in 20–30% of infrainguinal vein grafts, mostly in the first year. Stenoses of greater than 70% (velocity >3 m/s or velocity ratio >3.0) compromise flow and often occlude if left untreated.[3]

## Factors influencing graft occlusion

### Local factors

- These are essentially the quality of the inflow, the run-off and the conduit itself (see Chapter 4).

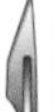

Patency is better for suprainguinal than infrainguinal grafts and graft occlusion is more frequent in femorotibial than femoropopliteal bypasses.[4] Infrainguinal bypass patency of autologous vein is better than Dacron, polytetrafluoroethylene (PTFE) or human umbilical vein. The role of heparin-bonded prostheses remains under discussion.[4,5] The results of reversed and in situ vein grafts are equivalent.[6,7]

- Arm veins are similar to the long saphenous vein provided that angioscopically detected defects are corrected.[8]

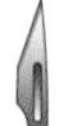

Vein cuffs and patches[9,10] or an expanded hood[11] at the lower anastomosis improve PTFE graft patency.

- The risk of ischaemic complications and the need for emergency limb revascularisation are greater with occlusion of prosthetic grafts compared to venous grafts. This is because the thrombus in the prosthetic graft extends into the outflow artery. Vein cuffs at the distal anastomosis reduce the risk of outflow impairment after thrombosis of PTFE grafts (**Fig. 7.1**).[12]

- The quality and number of run-off vessels strongly predicts outcome.[13] Bypasses for gangrene occlude more frequently than for ulceration, rest pain or claudication.[14] This is probably related to the poorer run-off associated with worsening ischaemia.

## General factors

- Continued smoking increases graft thrombosis three- to fivefold.[15]

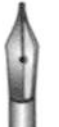

Diabetes and renal failure compromise patient survival but not graft patency.[16,17]

- Raised fibrinogen, hyperlipidaemia, thrombophilias (e.g. protein C, protein S or antithrombin III deficiency, antiphospholipid antibodies, factor V Leiden mutation) and increased platelet aggregation favour graft thrombosis.[15]
- Graft occlusion and recurrent stenoses are commoner in women and hormone replacement therapy potentiates this.[18,19]

# Prevention of graft thrombosis

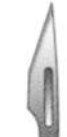

Antiplatelet agents should promote graft patency but good evidence exists only for aspirin.[20] Aspirin is more effective for infrainguinal prosthetic grafts, whereas warfarin is better for vein grafts.[21]

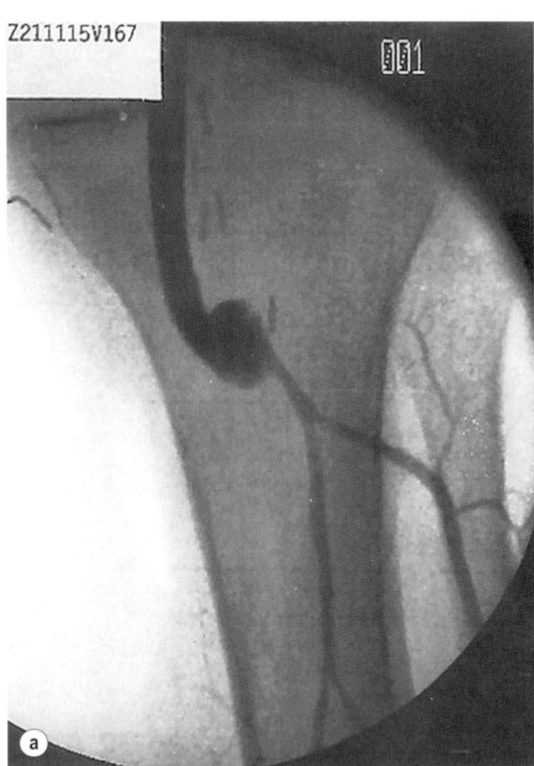


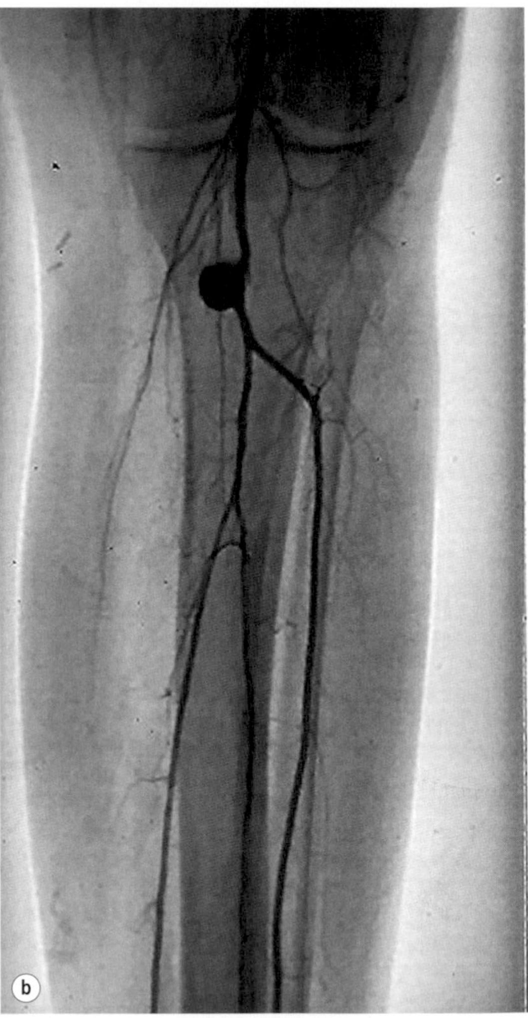


**Figure 7.1 • (a)** Femoropopliteal bypass with venous cuff (Miller cuff) at the distal anastomosis: perioperative angiography. **(b)** Preservation of outflow vessels after thrombosis at 3 years.

Surveillance for suprainguinal bypass grafts is not cost-effective. Occlusion is far more frequent after infrainguinal bypass grafting and, since most of the occlusions occur within 2 years after the implantation, patients should be carefully followed during this time period. This includes medical history, clinical examination and Doppler pressure measurements. Additional duplex scanning is not effective after prosthetic bypass.

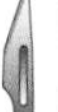

Although some smaller trials report duplex scanning to be advantageous after venous bypass surgery, this has been challenged by a recent large randomised trial where intensive surveillance with duplex scanning did not show any additional benefit in terms of limb salvage rates for patients undergoing venous bypass operations.[22]

## Management of graft stenosis (the failing graft)

Although there is some discussion about asymptomatic stenosis, it is clear that symptomatic graft stenosis should be treated by either angioplasty or surgical revision. Surgical revision is probably more durable in the long term, but an endovascular approach is actually preferred because of the acceptable short-term patency and a low rate of complications, particularly for short (<2 cm) stenoses.[23,24] In addition, angioplasty as first treatment rarely compromises subsequent surgery.

Short graft stenosis, whether midgraft or anastomotic, usually responds well to angioplasty with high inflation pressures (up to 2020 kPa; **Fig. 7.2**). Cutting balloons have been advocated, but seem to offer only small benefit at the expense of an elevated complication rate.[25,26] Stents (preferably self-expandable bare nitinol) should be used only

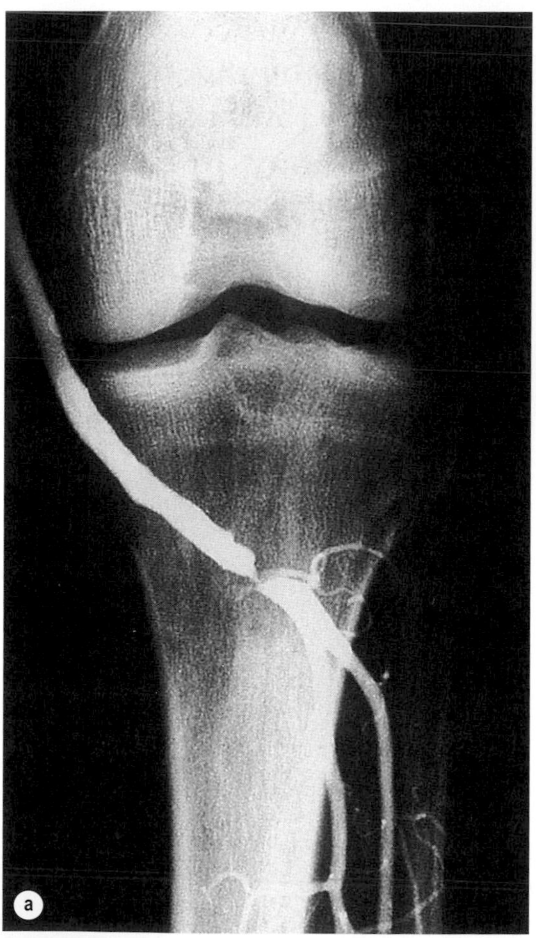



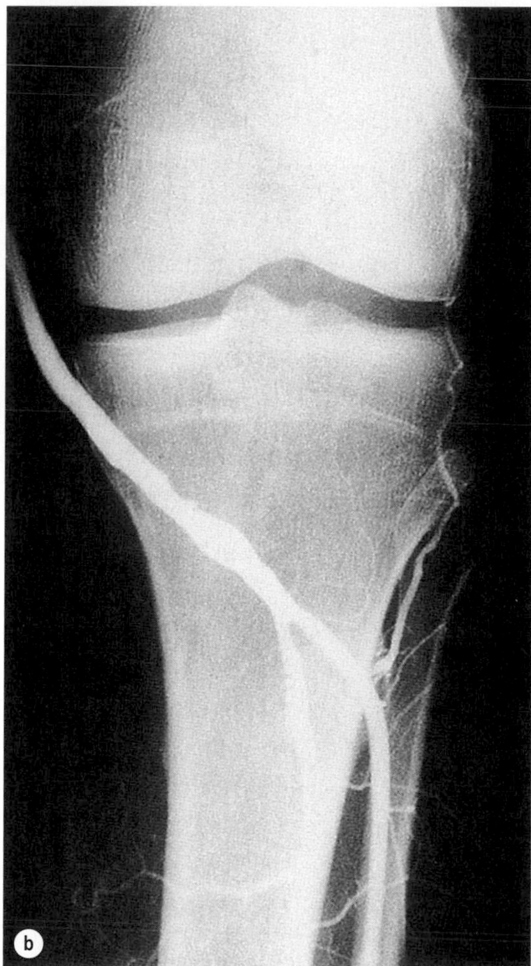



**Figure 7.2** • Vein graft stenosis near the below-knee popliteal anastomosis **(a)**, successfully treated by balloon angioplasty **(b)**.

selectively and there is no evidence for drug-eluting stents.[27]

Longer graft stenoses are best treated by open surgery and may be bypassed using the contralateral long saphenous or superficial femoral vein.[8] Tibial or distal popliteal anastomotic stenoses resistant to angioplasty are best treated by a jump graft to a fresh run-off vessel to avoid scar tissue or adherent tibial veins (**Fig. 7.3**).

## Management of the failed graft

If graft occlusion causes non-disabling claudication, a conservative approach might be preferred. Acute subcritical ischaemia allows time for thrombolysis or elective surgery but an anaesthetic paralysed limb demands emergency revascularisation within a few hours (see Chapter 8).

### Role of thrombolysis

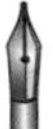

Local catheter-directed thrombolysis might be a valuable tool for a viable limb within 14 days of graft occlusion provided that the patient has undergone surgery within 3 months.[28]

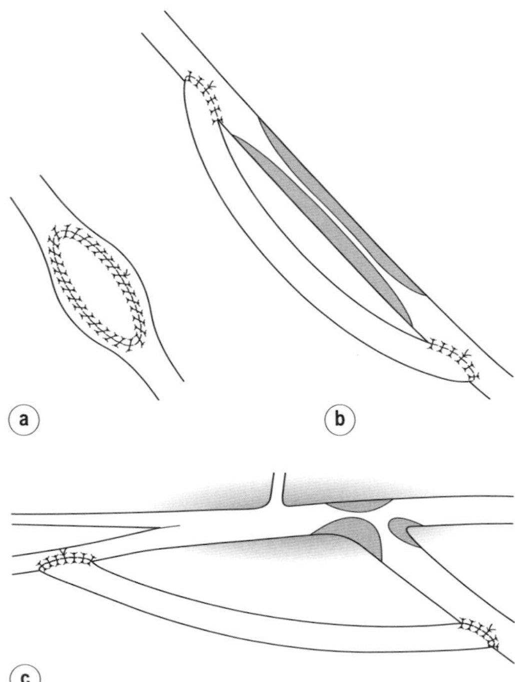


**Figure 7.3** • Vein patch angioplasty **(a)**, bypass of long vein graft stenosis **(b)** and jump graft around stenosed distal anastomosis of a femoropopliteal bypass graft to the popliteal artery **(c)**.

Although not applicable for suprainguinal grafts, thrombolysis is still frequently used for infrainguinal graft occlusion. The advantages are that redo surgery may be avoided and the graft will be cleared, unmasking the underlying cause of thrombosis, which can often be treated endovascularly during the same session. The outflow vessels might also be cleared more effectively than with open surgery. If thrombolysis is unsuccessful or reveals a problem that is not amenable to endovascular treatment, then open surgery can be performed with a clear knowledge of the cause of the problem and the state of the run-off. Mechanical thrombectomy or the use of high bolus therapy can reduce the duration of the procedure.[29] Although thrombolysis has a high initial success rate, it is also characterised by contraindications, haemorrhagic complications, poor long-term patency and persistent ischaemia.[30,31] This explains the reduced popularity of thrombolysis. A pragmatic solution is to reserve thrombolysis for patients with associated extensive thrombosis of the outflow vessels.[32]

### Suprainguinal graft thrombosis

A unilateral limb thrombosis of an aorto-bifemoral graft can be thrombectomised through the groin even months after the occlusion. Thrombectomy is performed with Fogarty embolectomy catheters, an adherent clot catheter or a ring stripper. During these manoeuvres, the contralateral groin is compressed to avoid contralateral embolisation. The underlying cause is most frequently stenosis at the distal anastomosis, which should be repaired by extension of the graft into the profunda femoris artery (**Fig. 7.4**). Graft thrombectomy by a femoral approach is usually not possible in bilateral graft occlusion. Here the graft should be replaced in situ or by an extra-anatomical bypass.

The underlying cause of occlusion in case of axillofemoral or femorofemoral grafting is most frequently anastomotic stenosis or stenosis of the inflow vessel.[33] Thrombectomy can also be performed by the groin. The underlying cause needs to be taken care of. The inflow vessels (subclavian artery for axillofemoral graft, iliac artery for femorofemoral graft) are checked pre- or perioperatively and inflow stenosis is treated if necessary. A new graft in clean tissues offers the best solution in the case of long-standing thrombosis or when thrombectomy is insufficient.

### Infrainguinal graft thrombosis

In the case of chronic occlusion, the decision regarding revascularisation should be taken in the light of the clinical examination and results of investigations (Doppler, duplex scan, angiography).

In patients with acute ischaemia, an immediate decision should be taken regarding thrombolysis or open surgery. Prosthetic grafts can usually be

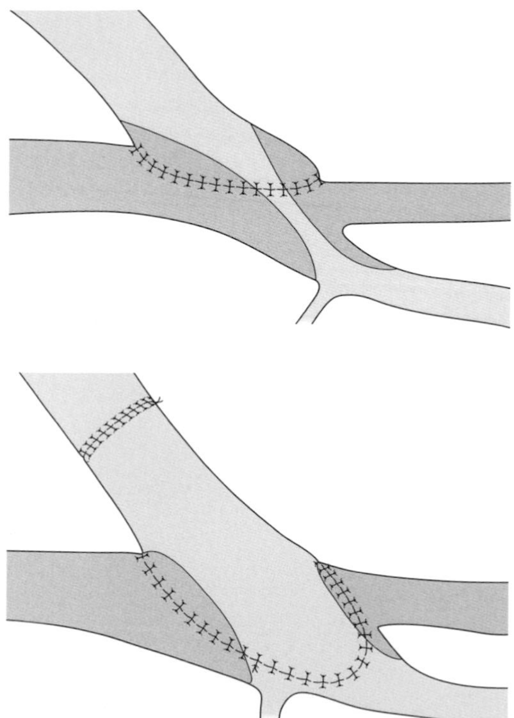

**Figure 7.4 •** Extension graft to one limb of an aortobifemoral graft to treat a stenosis at the profunda femoris origin. In this case the superficial femoral artery is occluded.

thrombectomised by a groin approach if the occlusion is less than 1 week old. Anastomotic stenosis must be corrected. Inflow and outflow vessels need to be checked by perioperative angiography. If necessary, outflow vessels can be selectively approached by an infragenicular approach. Intraoperative thrombolysis might be an alternative in selected cases (see Chapter 8).[34] Venous grafts are usually more difficult to thrombectomise. Here it might be wise to place a new graft, as is the case in prosthetic grafts where thrombectomy is insufficient. If at all possible, a venous graft should be used. Following thrombectomy for acute ischaemia, four-compartment fasciotomy should be considered to relieve pressure and improve distal perfusion, especially if there is any calf swelling or tenderness preoperatively.[35]

## Graft infection

Graft infection is relatively uncommon (1–5%) but has a high amputation and mortality risk.[36] In a recent multicentre audit of 55 graft infections, 31% died, 33% underwent amputation and only 45% left the hospital alive without amputation.[37]

Treatment has therefore to focus on patient's survival, eradication of infection and revascularisation by a method which is durable and does not become infected itself.

### Causes

Most graft infections originate at surgery due to a breakdown of sterility or from pre-existing bacteria (e.g. skin commensals), but some occur by extension from superficial wound infections or from haematogenous spread.

Patients with gangrene, those who are elderly obese and those undergoing re-operation during the same hospital admission have a higher risk. Preoperative shaving, open surgical drainage for more than 3 days, operations lasting over 2 hours, emergency surgery, diabetes, steroids, renal failure, recent angiography and wound haematoma are all risk factors. Blood-borne bacteria from intravenous lines or systemic infections may also cause graft sepsis.

Venous grafts are more resistant to infection than prostheses but direct bacterial erosion can occur, especially when exposed in an open wound.

### Prevention

Patients should be admitted as near to surgery as possible and isolated from patients with known infections, especially methicillin-resistant *Staphylococcus aureus* (MRSA). Many hospitals are adopting a policy of screening elective surgical patients for MRSA colonisation before admission and eradicating any infection before proceeding with the surgery.

Strict aseptic technique and laminar flow theatres minimise infection rates. Iodine-impregnated adhesive drapes help isolate the operative field.

Prophylactic antibiotics (cephalosporin or coamoxyclav) reduce wound and graft infection. There is no evidence for using more than three doses (one intraop and two postop). Some surgeons add a single dose of gentamicin as this is active against many strains of MRSA. Vancomycin should be used if the patient is MRSA positive.

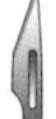

Antibiotic-bonded grafts (rifampicin) are attractive on theoretical and experimental grounds, but randomised clinical trials have failed to demonstrate any prophylactic effect.[38,39] The same is true for the more recently developed silver-coated grafts.

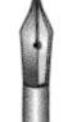

Randomised trials failed to show any advantage of closed suction drains in the incidence of inguinal wound infection.[40,41] Neither do they prevent wound haematomas, so there is no point in using them.

There is also little evidence regarding the need for prophylactic antibiotics before other surgical or dental procedures in the presence of prosthetic grafts.

## Presentation

Wound infections after vascular surgery are classified according to the depth of tissue involvement: type 1 involves the skin only, type 2 the subcutaneous tissue and type 3 the graft itself. Prosthetic graft infection can present at any time from days to years after surgery with pyrexia, systemic sepsis, local abscesses and sinuses, graft exposure, thrombosis or anastomotic haemorrhage. On rare occasions septic emboli can be the first sign (**Fig. 7.5**). Septic erosion of exposed vein grafts can occur at any point.

Infrarenal aortic grafts can erode the third or fourth parts of the duodenum causing aortoduodenal fistula, which may present with one or two sentinel gastrointestinal bleeds before the inevitable catastrophic haemorrhage. Occasionally, an aortic graft can also erode any other part of the bowel, including the appendix, and also the ureter. Such aortoenteric erosion will lead to localised peritonitis with retroperitoneal or groin abscesses and ultimately catastrophic bleeding. The mortality rate of aortoenteric complications is high (>50%) with recurrent infection or aortic stump blowout in over 25%.[42]

## Bacteriology

Most graft infections are due to skin organisms.[43] *Staphylococcus epidermidis* is the least virulent, producing a biofilm or an infected seroma after months or years. It is difficult to culture, requiring homogenisation of explanted graft material to dislodge adherent bacteria. *Staphylococcus aureus* is more virulent and usually presents earlier. MRSA infections have a particularly high morbidity and mortality. The incidence is increasing. Apart from staphylococci, there is a wide variety of organisms which can cause graft infection. Gram-negative species include *Escherichia coli* and *Pseudomonas aeruginosa*, which is recognised by a high tendency of anastomotic disruption and bleeding. It may be difficult or even impossible to culture the causative organism, particularly after prolonged periods of antibiotic therapy.

## Diagnosis

In most cases there is a perigraft collection or sinus. Aspiration of frank pus or turbid fluid from around the graft and the subsequent culture of a causative organism are diagnostic. Computed tomography (CT), magnetic resonance imaging (MRI) or ultrasound usually demonstrates perigraft fluid and inflammation but can underestimate the extent of infection, especially if a sinus is present, when sinography may be useful. For wholly intra-abdominal prostheses there may be few signs, but the leucocyte count, erythrocyte sedimentation rate and C-reactive protein are often raised. Perigraft fluid after 3–6 months or gas beyond 7–10 days on ultrasound, CT or MRI suggests infection. One in four anastomotic aneurysms result from graft infection, but this is not always evident from CT. Where doubt exists, indium-labelled leucocyte or positron emission tomography scanning is occasionally helpful. In aortoenteric fistulas, the graft may be seen eroding the duodenum at endoscopy (**Fig. 7.6**).

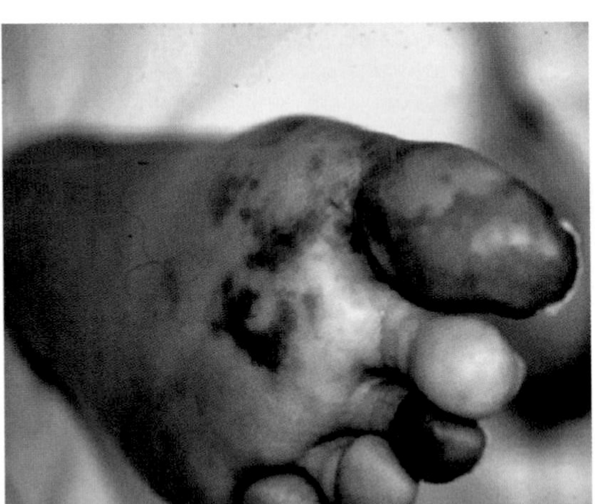

**Figure 7.5** • Septic emboli at the foot as the presenting sign of aortofemoral graft infection.

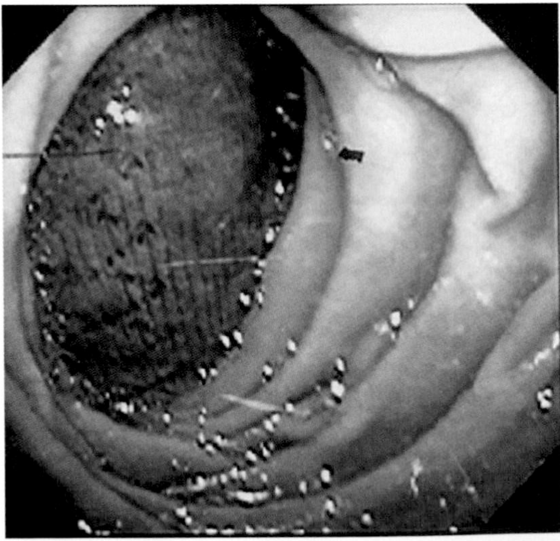

**Figure 7.6** • Aortic graft, eroding the duodenum as seen during endoscopy.

Definitive confirmation is sometimes only made at operation by the presence of pus around the graft and the absence of tissue incorporation.

## Management

### General principles

Once infection is confirmed, semi-urgent treatment is required to pre-empt catastrophic haemorrhage, graft thrombosis or systemic sepsis. An infected prosthesis acts as a foreign body, rendering bacteria inaccessible to antibiotics. Conservative measures (including prolonged antibiotic therapy, drainage and irrigation of abscesses, muscle flaps) may be helpful and can buy time, but they are rarely curative.

The mainstay of treatment is complete graft excision and adequate debridement of all infected tissues. Partial graft resection usually requires later replacement.[44] Simple graft excision without revascularisation can heal infection but usually results in major amputation, even in patients operated on initially for claudication.

Revascularisation is traditionally preformed by extra-anatomical bypass (axillofemoral graft for infrarenal aortic graft infection, obturator bypass for infection at the groin, lateral bypass for infection of a femoropopliteal graft).[36]

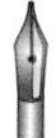

There is growing evidence that in situ reconstruction produces equal or better results with regard to reinfection rate and particularly late patency and amputation rates.[45,46] An autologous conduit is preferable for in situ reconstruction.[47]

Arterial homografts are an alternative but they are prone to late complications such as stenosis, occlusion or aneurysmal degeneration.[45,48] There are a few encouraging reports on the use of rifampicin-bonded grafts or silver-impregnated grafts, but they should be reserved for patients with low-grade infections (e.g. *Staphylococcus epidermidis*).[49,50]

The duration of postoperative antibiotic therapy is still under discussion. Most authors will accept a period of 2–6 weeks depending on the causative organism.

### Infrarenal aortic graft infection

Infection remains the most catastrophic complication after infrarenal aortic graft reconstruction. In the beginning of the 1990s we started a programme of total graft excision and in situ reconstruction with the superficial femoral veins. Our results have been published in 1995 and 2003.[51,52] The basic steps in this operation are as follows.

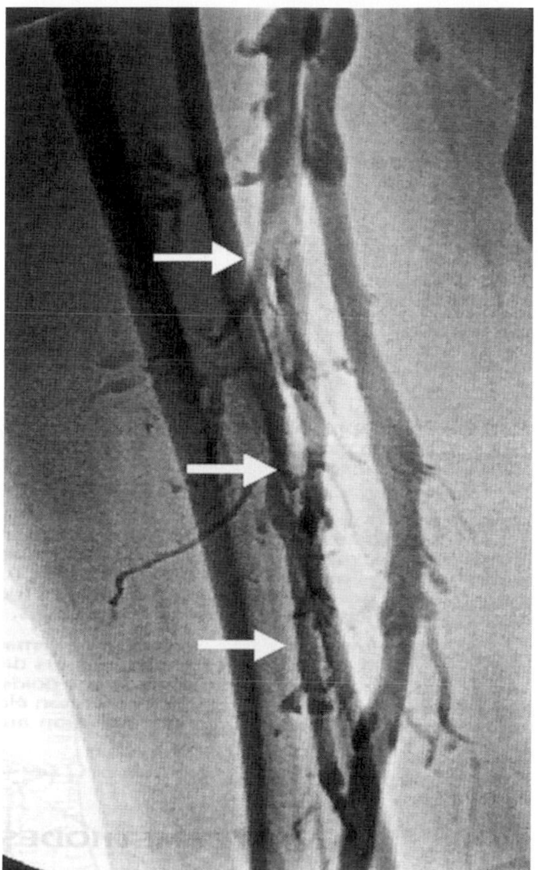

**Figure 7.7** • Phlebography showing the femoral vein. Important collaterals by the profunda femoris vein (white arrows) protect from venous hypertension after harvest.

1. Harvesting of the superficial femoral vein (**Fig. 7.7**)

The patency of the femoral veins is checked preoperatively by duplex scanning. The superficial femoral vein itself is approached by an incision anteromedially on the thigh, commonly used for harvesting of the greater saphenous vein. After incision of the fascia the vein is identified just next to the superficial femoral artery. The bifurcation with the profunda femoris vein is situated in the groin a couple of centimetres below the arterial bifurcation. When working in a medial direction, this means that the venous bifurcation can be approached without entering the original and mostly infected groin incision. Distally the adductor canal is opened and the dissection is continued to the level of the mid-popliteal artery. The vein is transected at the level of the knee joint and then freed upwards with ligation of different side branches. At the level of the adductor canal there are usually dense adhesions with the artery and multiple fragile side branches. Proximally the excision extends to the level of the venous bifurcation and the profunda femoris vein is carefully preserved since it provides important collateral circulation to the popliteal vein.

Excision of one superficial femoral vein will usually be sufficient for aorto(bi)iliac reconstruction. In the event of an aorto(bi)femoral reconstruction the veins need to be harvested from both lower limbs. After excision, the veins are preserved in cold (4 °C) heparinised blood with papaverine (40 mg). The wounds are closed primarily with suction drains.

2. Excision of the infected graft

The preferred approach is median xyphopubic laparotomy. The retroperitoneal approach might be an alternative in selected cases but the disadvantage is that it hampers a complete debridement and coverage of the new reconstruction with healthy tissue (omentoplasty). In addition, it renders the approach to the femoral vessels and reconstruction in this area more difficult. The infrarenal aorta is approached in the traditional way, but in the case of dense adhesions, the right retrocolic approach can be a good option. It is frequently necessary to obtain aortic control at the suprarenal or supracoeliac level. Once the aorta has been freed, the distal anastomoses at the iliac or femoral level are exposed. The aorta is clamped after systemic heparinisation and the infected graft is excised completely. The periaortic tissues and any other sites of infection are generously debrided in order to achieve a healthy bed for the new graft. Existing retroperitoneal tunnels are irrigated with polyvidone–iodide solution and mechanically debrided by pulling open-gauze sponges through them. Finally the aorta itself and the femoral vessels are debrided to achieve a clean anastomotic site.

3. In situ reconstruction with the deep vein (**Fig. 7.8**)

The veins can be used in reversed or non-reversed position, after fracture of the valves with a valvulotome. Our preferred configuration for the proximal aortic anastomosis is that we simply suture one vein end to end to the aorta. Taking into account the discrepancy in diameter between the aorta and

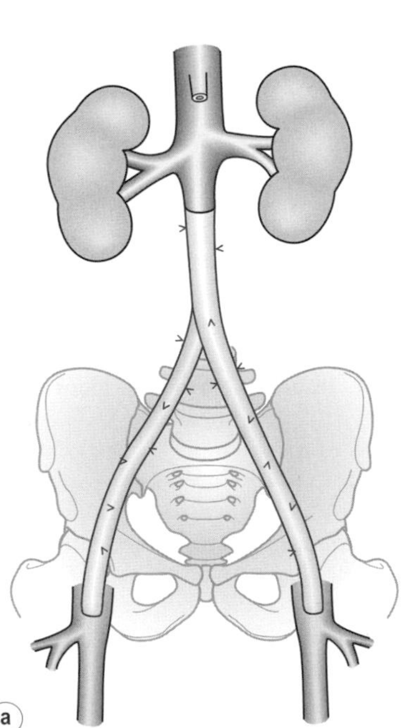


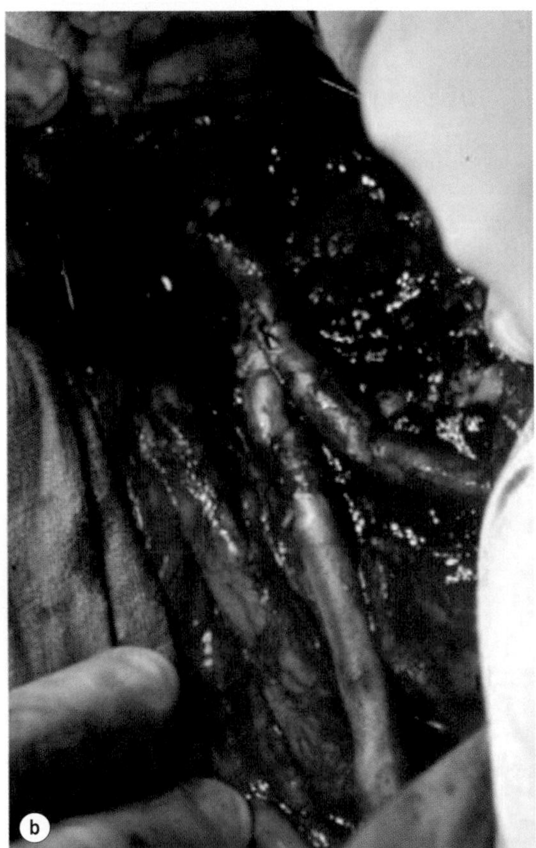


**Figure 7.8** • The reversed Y technique for in situ reconstruction of an infected aortobifemoral graft. **(a)** Schematic drawing. **(b)** Perioperative view.

*(Continued)*

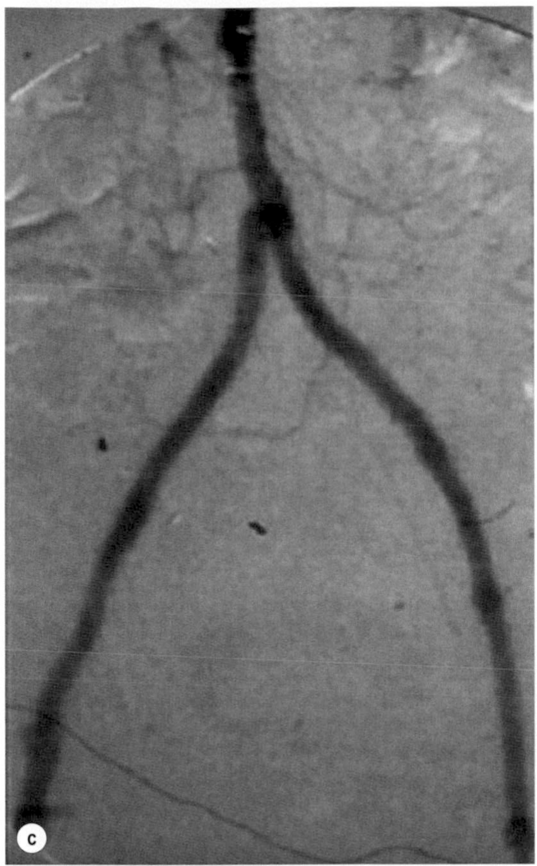

**Figure 7.8** • Cont'd **(c)** Postoperative angiography.

the veins, it is frequently necessary to downsize the aortic cuff with two or three separate through-and-through stitches. The second vein graft is subsequently anastomosed to the first one some 5 cm below this proximal anastomosis. When replacing an infected aortobifemoral bypass, the vein grafts are brought to the groin through the old tunnels and anastomosed to the femoral vessels in the usual way. Afterwards, the vein grafts are covered both in the abdomen and at the femoral level with viable tissues, leaving no residual cavities. Omentoplasty is generally used at the proximal anastomosis and muscle flaps are provided in the groin in cases of extensive infection.

It is agreed that in situ reconstruction with the superficial femoral veins represents a technically demanding and time-consuming operation. The operation has also been criticised because of the risk of venous hypertension in the lower limbs and an increased need for fasciotomy.[53] In our series, 4.5% of the patients required a fasciotomy within 30 days of the operation.[54]

The role of endovascular reconstruction in graft infection, and particularly infrarenal aortic graft infection, seems limited. An endoprosthesis can, however, be an excellent tool to buy time in an unstable patient with catastrophic bleeding due to aortoduodenal fistula (**Fig. 7.9**). However, this is usually only a temporary solution and reinfection will occur in about 60% of the patients.[56]

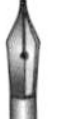

The important point, however, is that despite mortality and limb loss of about 10% after femoral vein replacement, infection is eliminated in the survivors, which makes it the procedure of choice for most patients.[47,51,52,55]

There are few data on infection after endovascular aneurysm reconstruction. A recent review reported an incidence of 0.43%.[57] Two-thirds of the infections were classified high grade and 31% were associated with aortoenteric fistulas (**Fig. 7.10**). Mortality after conservative treatment was 36.4%. The surgical mortality was 14%, ranging from 5.8% with in situ reconstruction to 16% after resection and extra-anatomical bypass.

# Graft aneurysms

## True aneurysms

Following repair of a true aneurysm, the adjacent artery may also become aneurysmal. Aneurysms were frequent within some early PTFE grafts but manufacturing improvements have almost eliminated this. Biological grafts such as the human umbilical vein graft frequently became aneurysmal before the addition of a Dacron wrap.[58] Xenografts such as bovine mesenteric vein and cryopreserved venous or arterial allografts are particularly subject to aneurysmal degeneration.[45,48] Dacron undergoes late degradation and dilatation, which becomes clinically significant in 2–3%. After 5–10 years, disruption can occur at points of stress (e.g. under the inguinal ligament) causing false aneurysms,[59] which may present with haemorrhage or thrombosis. Distraction during shoulder abduction may cause spontaneous rupture or axillary anastomotic disruption of PTFE axillofemoral grafts.[60] Vein graft aneurysms are rare but more frequent in bypasses for popliteal aneurysms than for occlusive disease.[61] Information on the natural history of untreated graft aneurysms is lacking but repair is generally recommended and is essential for rupture, thrombosis or embolism. Treatment is either with a covered endovascular stent or by graft replacement.

## False aneurysms

False aneurysms are essentially pulsating haematomas, which may occur at the arterial puncture

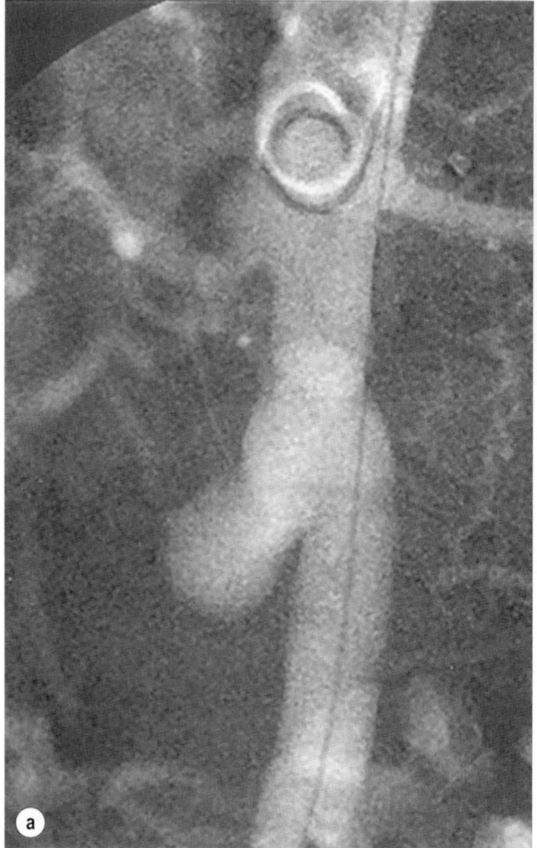

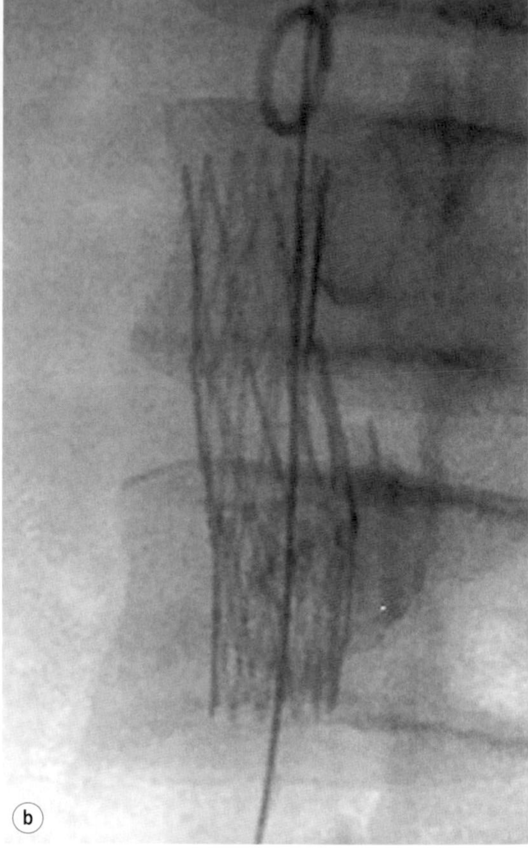

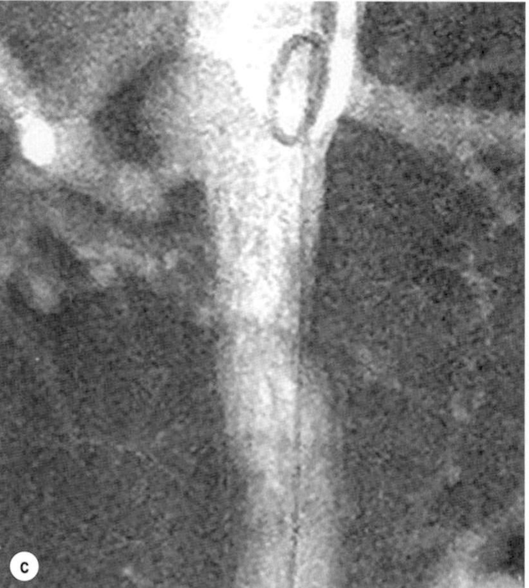

**Figure 7.9** • Anastomotic aortic aneurysm resulting in bleeding aortoduodenal fistula after infrarenal aortic graft treated by endoprosthetic insertion. **(a)** Perioperative angiography showing false aneurysm. **(b)** Deployed endoprosthesis (AneurX). **(c)** Completion angiography: false aneurysm completely excluded.

site after angiography (or intervention), following intra-arterial injection by intravenous drug users, after trauma (usually penetrating), due to primary arterial infection (e.g. salmonella and HIV) and at disrupted arterial anastomoses. Puncture-site aneurysms often thrombose spontaneously. Ultrasound-guided compression occludes over 80% and most others will thrombose following

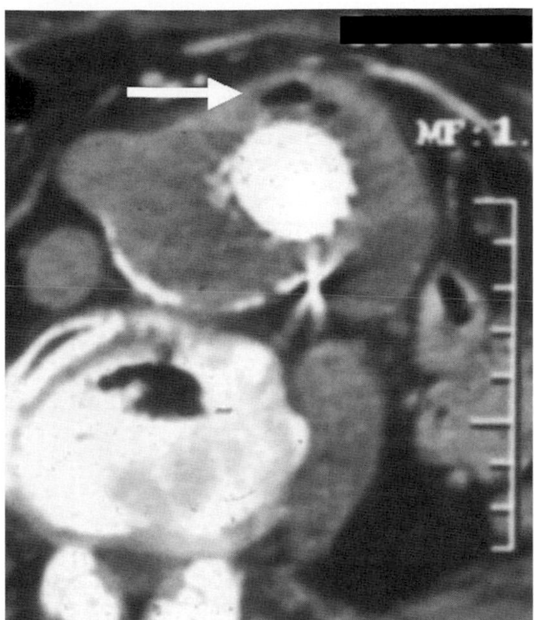


**Figure 7.10** • CT scan demonstrating aortoduodenal fistula 5 years after EVAR. Note air bubbles in the neighbourhood of the graft (arrow).

thrombin injection.[62] Direct surgical repair or a covered stent are rarely necessary. The management of infected (mycotic) aneurysms is dealt with in Chapter 13.

Anastomotic aneurysms result from mechanical distraction or graft infection. They occur most frequently at femoral anastomoses and they predispose to rupture, thrombosis and embolisation. Anastomotic aneurysms appear typically late during follow-up, and the incidence at the femoral anastomosis after aortofemoral grafting is around 3%.[63] Aortic anastomotic aneurysms are not easily discovered by clinical examination, but the incidence with CT follow-up may be as high as 4%.[64] Some feel this justifies the need for lifelong follow-up after aortic reconstruction, but many patients who develop an aneurysm above a previous aortic graft never come to revision because they are too old or the repair is too complex (involving the renal/visceral arteries).

Anastomotic aneurysms at the femoral level are best handled by open surgery and graft interposition, although there are anecdotal reports of endovascular reconstruction.[65] The treatment of choice for iliac anastomotic aneurysms is now stentgraft placement by the groin. The procedure can be done under local anaesthesia and mortality and morbidity is minimal. Late complications include endoleak and occlusion in a minority of cases.[66,67] Preoperative embolisation of the internal iliac artery is frequently required, which may lead to gluteal claudication and other pelvic complications (see Chapter 13).

Graft interposition for aortic anastomotic aneurysms is done by laparotomy or a preferentially retroperitoneal approach. It is, however, associated with a higher surgical risk than a primary vascular operation: perioperative mortality in the elective setting ranges from 0% to 17% and is definitely higher than 50% in cases of rupture.[68,69]

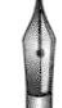

Endovascular reconstruction is actually preferred if the patient is a morphological candidate (**Fig. 7.11**).[70,71] A recent comparative study also confirmed reduced blood loss, reduced procedural time and shorter hospital stay in the endovascular group. The operative mortality was 19% in the surgical group versus 10% in the endovascular series.[72] Although a tubular stentgraft from a technical point of view can handle most aneurysms, there are indications that a bifurcated graft might be more effective at midterm follow-up.[73]

## Revision surgery after EVAR

EVAR is associated with a significant risk of late complications, which occur at a rate of 5–10% per annum. Endoleaks are the most frequent complication and are described in more detail in Chapter 13. Most complications can be treated by endovascular reintervention, if required.[74] Surgical techniques such as laparoscopic clipping of the side branches and remodelling of the aneurysm have not generated much enthusiasm (**Fig. 7.12**).[75,76] Open surgery, on the other hand, is well accepted for graft limb thrombosis, e.g. graft thrombectomy or femorofemoral crossover grafting.[74]

The need for early conversion was around 5% in the starting years of EVAR, but this has decreased to well below 1%.[77] Late conversions might be necessary because of persistent endoleaks, disintegration of the stentgraft, endotension with growing aneurysms, aneurysm rupture or infection. The need is around 1% per year.[78,79] Although the operation is more challenging, the procedure is essentially performed according to the guidelines of primary aneurysm surgery. Dissection of the proximal infrarenal aortic neck might be more difficult because of periaortic inflammation caused by the stentgraft. Suprarenal and preferably supracoeliac clamping are frequently required, particularly in stentgrafts with suprarenal fixation. Endografts with infrarenal fixation are easily removed once the aneu-

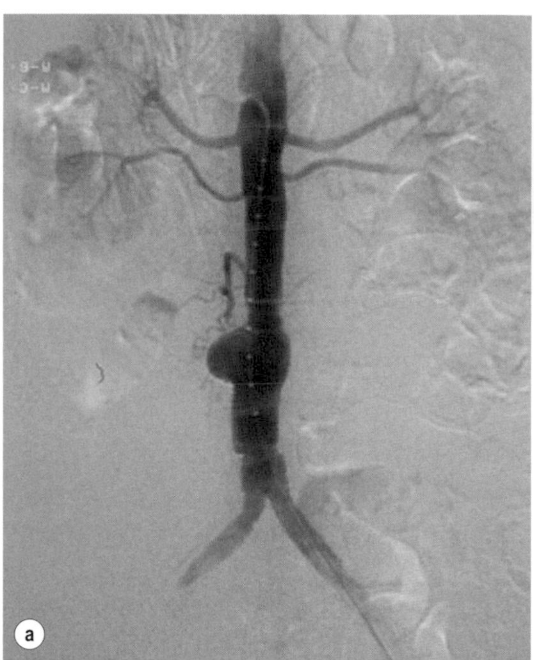
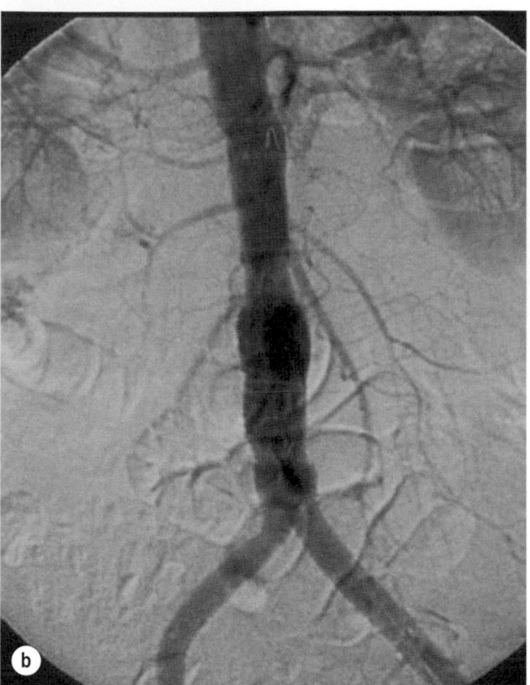

**Figure 7.11** • Aortic false aneurysm after previous aortofemoral Dacron graft. **(a)** Preoperative calibrated angiography. **(b)** Angiography after placement of tubular endoprosthesis.

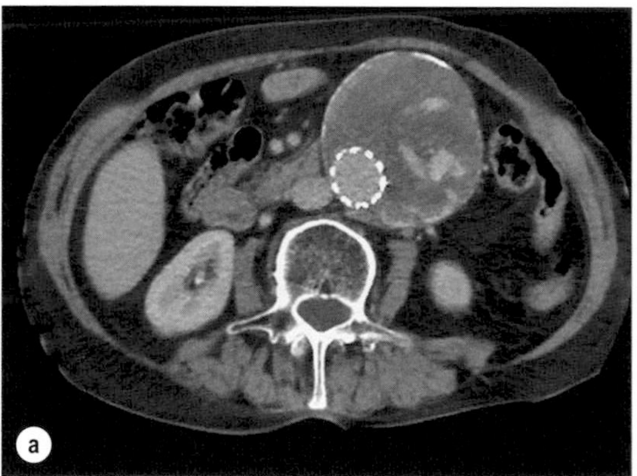
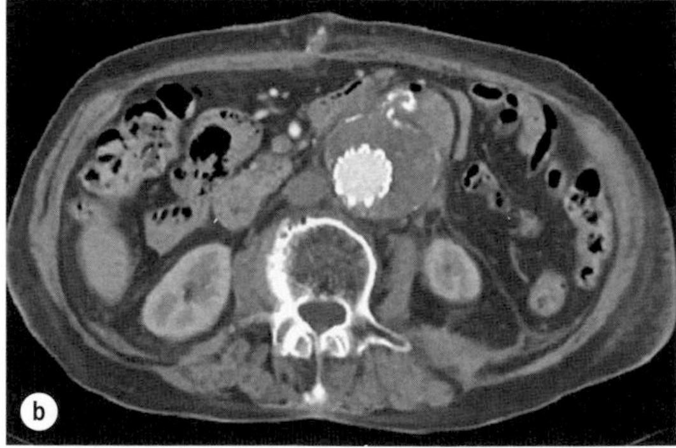

**Figure 7.12** • An 82-year-old female presenting with endoleak type II and growing aneurysm, 4 years after endoprosthesis. **(a)** Preoperative CT scan. **(b)** CT scan 6 months after laparoscopic remodelling and ligature of lumbar arteries. Note the difference in aneurysm diameter and absence of endoleak.

rysm sac has been opened and the aorta is clamped below the renal arteries (**Fig. 7.13**). In grafts with suprarenal fixation, particularly in those with barbs and hooks, it might be wise to leave the suprarenal portion in place and to amputate the infrarenal portion of the endoprosthesis by cutting the metal frame of the suprarenal attachment system.[80] The suprarenal fixation system is then incorporated into the proximal anastomosis, which is performed under supracoeliac aortic clamping. Preferably the graft should be removed completely. In the usual case of a bifurcation graft this means that the iliac arteries have to be dissected and that the external and internal iliac arteries have to be clamped selectively in order to perform a reconstruction to the iliac bifurcation.

Although it is understood that conversion is associated with increased risk of mortality and morbidity, different teams have reported a 0% mortality rate for elective late conversion. Mortality rates for early conversion range from 7% to 25%, rising to 40% in cases of rupture.[78,79,81]

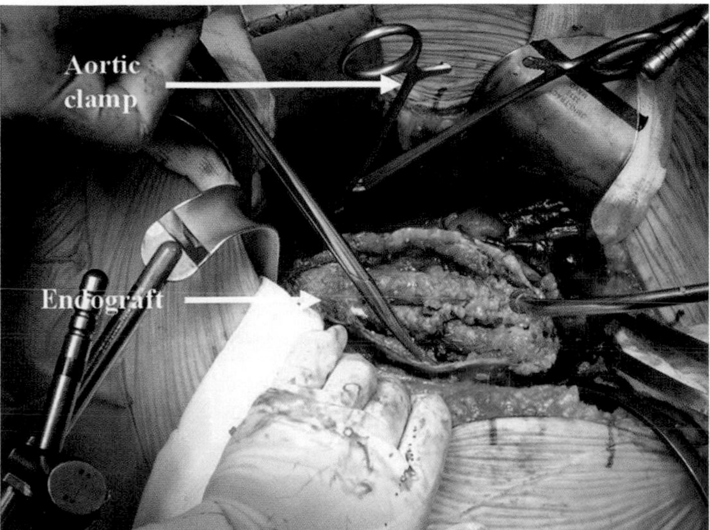


**Figure 7.13** • Explantation of Gore Excluder graft because of endotension. The aortic clamp is placed (but not closed) just below the renal arteries. The aneurysm is opened; the body of the graft is mobilised and extracted, during which the aorta will be cross-clamped.

## Key points

- Late graft occlusion is caused by intimal hyperplasia or progression of atherosclerosis of the inflow or outflow.
- Graft stenoses occur in 20–30% of infrainguinal vein grafts. Symptomatic stenoses require treatment. Angioplasty offers excellent early results. In the long term, open surgery is probably better.
- Thrombolysis of occluded infrainguinal grafts may be attempted in patients aged under 80 years with critical ischaemia provided that limb viability is not severely threatened, that the patient has not undergone surgery within 3 months and that the occlusion is less than 14 days old.
- *Staphylococcus epidermidis* is the most frequent cause of low-grade graft infection. *Staphylococus aureus* and Gram-negative infections tend to present early and are more virulent. The incidence of MRSA infection is increasing.
- Any fluid around a graft after 3–6 months or gas beyond 7–10 days on CT or ultrasound suggests infection. Aspiration and culture of perigraft fluid pus can usually secure the diagnosis.
- Conservative measures, such as prolonged antibiotic therapy, drainage and irrigation, or covering exposed grafts with muscle or omental flaps are rarely curative. The same is true for partial graft excision.
- Simple graft excision without revascularisation usually causes severe ischaemia, leading to amputation or death.
- Extra-anatomical revascularisation has been the 'gold standard' in the past. In situ revascularisation with autologous vein (e.g. femoral vein) has better patency and recurrent infection is rare.
- Endoprostheses can buy time in cases of bleeding aortoduodenal fistulas, but recurrence of infection is high.
- True aneurysms can occur within prosthetic or vein grafts or adjacent to previous aneurysms.
- False aneurysms may result from anastomotic distraction or infection. Treatment of femoral false aneurysms is surgical. Endovascular treatment offers an excellent alternative in cases of non-infected iliac or aortic false aneurysms.
- Surgical conversion is rarely needed after endovascular treatment of abdominal aortic aneurysms. If necessary, surgery can be performed with excellent results.

## References


1. Dawson I, van Bockel JH. Reintervention and mortality after infrainguinal reconstructive surgery for leg ischaemia. Br J Surg 1999; 86:38–44.
2. Blankensteijn JD, de Jong SC, Prinssen M et al. Two year outcomes after conventional or endovascular repair of abdominal aortic aneurysms. N Engl J Med 2005; 352:2398–405.
3. Mills JL Sr, Wixon CL, James DC et al. The natural history of intermediate and critical vein graft stenosis: recommendations for continued surveillance or repair. J Vasc Surg 2001; 33:273–8.
4. Norgren L, Hiatt WR, Dormandy MR et al. Inter-Society Consensus for the Management of Peripheral Arterial Disease (TASC II). Eur J Vasc Endovasc Surg 2007; 33:S1–75.

   Authorative consensus view and guidelines for the treatment of vascular disease.
5. Klinkert P, Post PN, Breslau PJ et al. Saphenous vein versus PTFE for above-knee femoropopliteal bypass. A review of the literature. Eur J Vasc Endovasc Surg 2004; 27:357–62.

   A meta-analysis on the results of above-knee femoropopliteal bypass with superior results for saphenous vein bypass.
6. Wengerter KR, Veith FJ, Gupta SK et al. Prospective randomized multicenter comparison of in situ and reversed vein infrapopliteal bypasses. J Vasc Surg 1991; 13:189–97.

   A relatively small multicentre study (60 patients in each group) that failed to show any advantage for in situ infrapopliteal bypass.
7. Moody AP, Edwards PR, Harris PL. In situ versus reversed femoropopliteal vein grafts: long term follow-up of a prospective, randomized trial. Br J Surg 1992; 79:750–2.

   A prospective randomised trial including 226 patients which also showed no advantage of in situ vein bypass over reversed vein grafting.
8. Gibbons CP, Osman HY, Shiralkar S. The use of alternative sources of autologous vein for infrainguinal bypass. Eur J Vasc Endovasc Surg 2003; 25:93–4.
9. Stonebridge PA, Prescott RJ, Ruckley CV. Randomized trial comparing infrainguinal polytetrafluoroethylene bypass grafting with and without vein interposition cuff at the distal anastomosis. The Joint Vascular Research Group. J Vasc Surg 1997; 26:543–50.

   A randomised controlled trial with 130 patients in each group showing a significant advantage for interposition vein cuffs in below-knee but not above-knee PTFE femoropopliteal bypass.
10. 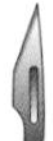 Albers M, Battistella VM, Romiti M et al. Meta-analysis of polytetrafluoroethylene bypass grafts to infrapopliteal arteries. J Vasc Surg 2003; 37:1263–9.

    A meta-analysis indicating moderate success for PTFE bypass grafts to infrapopliteal arteries, but the role of adjunctive procedures remans uncertain.
11. Panneton JM, Hollier LH, Hofer JM. Multicenter randomized prospective trial comparing a precuffed polytetrafluoroethylene graft to a vein cuffed polytetrafluoroethylene graft for infragenicular arterial bypass. Ann Vasc Surg 2004; 18:199–206.

    A small randomised trial (104 patients) that showed equivalent results on two types of femorodistal reconstructon.
12. Jackson MR, Belott TP, Dickason T et al. The consequences of a failed femoropopliteal bypass grafting: comparison of saphenous vein and PTFE grafts. J Vasc Surg 2000; 32:498–504.
13. Ulus AT, Ljungman C, Almgren B et al. The influence of distal runoff on patency of infrainguinal vein bypass grafts. Vasc Surg 2001; 35:31–5.
14. Nasr MK, McCarthy RJ, Budd JS et al. Infrainguinal bypass graft patency and limb salvage rates in critical limb ischemia: influence of the mode of presentation. Ann Vasc Surg 2003; 17:192–7.
15. Cheshire NJ, Wolfe JH, Barradas MA et al. Smoking and plasma fibrinogen, lipoprotein (a) and serotonin are markers for postoperative infrainguinal graft stenosis. Eur J Vasc Endovasc Surg 1996; 11:479–86.
16. Wolfle KD, Bruijnen H, Loeprecht H et al. Graft patency and clinical outcome of femorodistal arterial reconstruction in diabetic and non-diabetic patients: results of a multicentre comparative analysis. Eur J Vasc Endovasc Surg 2003; 25:229–34.
17. Albers M, Romiti M, Bragança Pereira CA et al. A meta-analysis of infrainguinal reconstruction in patients with end-stage renal disease. Eur J Vasc Endovasc Surg 2001; 22:294–300.
18. Watson HR, Schroeder TV, Simms MH et al. Association of sex with patency of femorodistal bypass grafts. Eur J Vasc Endovasc Surg 2000; 20:61–6.
19. Timaran CH, Stevens SL, Grandas OH et al. Influence of hormone replacement therapy on graft patency after femoropopliteal bypass grafting. J Vasc Surg 2000; 32:506–16.
20. Dorffler-Melly J, Koopman MM, Adam DJ et al. Antiplatelet agents for preventing thrombosis after peripheral arterial bypass surgery. Cochrane Database Syst Rev 2003; CD000535.

    An up-to-date systematic review concluding that aspirin has a slight beneficial effect on bypass patency.
21. The Dutch Bypass Oral Anticoagulants or Aspirin Study. Efficacy of oral anticoagulants compared with aspirin after infrainguinal bypass surgery: a randomised trial. Lancet 2000; 355:346–51.

    An important randomised controlled study of over 2500 patients showing that oral anticoagulation was better for the prevention of infrainguinal vein graft occlusion

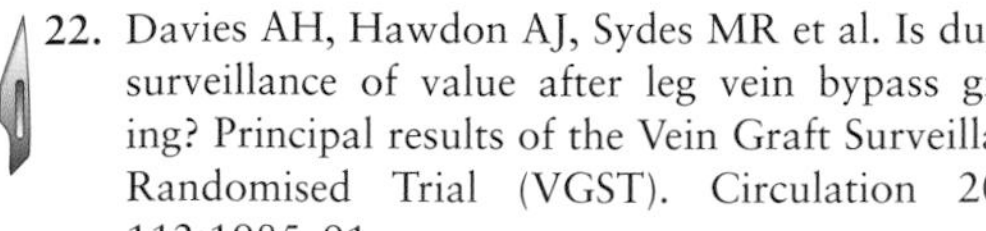
**and for lowering the rate of ischaemic events, whereas aspirin was better for the prevention of non-venous bypass graft occlusion and was associated with fewer bleeding episodes.**

22. Davies AH, Hawdon AJ, Sydes MR et al. Is duplex surveillance of value after leg vein bypass grafting? Principal results of the Vein Graft Surveillance Randomised Trial (VGST). Circulation 2005; 112:1985–91.

    **A multicentre, prospective, randomised, controlled trial (594 patients) that showed no benefit of duplex scan follow-up over clinical follow-up in patients with femorodistal venous bypass.**

23. Berceli SA, Hevelone ND, Lipsitz SR et al. Surgical and endovascular revision of infrainguinal vein bypass grafts: analysis of midterm outcomes from the PREVENT III trial. J Vasc Surg 2007; 46:1173–9.
24. Carlson GA, Hoballah JJ, Sharp WJ et al. Balloon angioplasty as a treatment of failing infrainguinal vein bypass grafts. J Vasc Surg 2004; 39:421–6.
25. Garvin R, Reifsnyder T. Cutting balloon angioplasty of autogenous infrainguinal bypasses: short-term safety and efficacy. J Vasc Surg 2007; 46:724–30.
26. Vikram R, Ross RA, Bhat R et al. Cutting balloon angioplasty versus standard balloon angioplasty for failing infra-inguinal vein grafts: comparative study of short- and mid-term primary patency rates. Cardiovasc Intervent Radiol 2007; 30:607–10.
27. Duda SH, Bosiers M, Lammer J et al. Drug-eluting and bare nitinol stents for the treatment of atherosclerotic lesions in the superficial femoral artery: long-term results from the SIROCO trial. J Endovasc Ther 206; 13:701–10.
28. Comerota AJ, Weaver FA, Hosking JD et al. Results of a prospective, randomized trial of surgery versus thrombolysis for occluded lower extremity bypass grafts. Am J Surg 1996; 172:105–12.
29. Braithwaite BD, Buckenham TM, Galland RB et al. Prospective randomized trial of high-dose bolus versus low-dose tissue plasminogen activator infusion in the management of acute limb ischaemia. Thrombolysis Study Group. Br J Surg 1997; 84:646–50.
30. Aburahma AF, Hopkins ES, Wulu JT Jr et al. Lysis/balloon angioplasty versus thrombectomy/open patch angioplasty of failed femoropopliteal polytetrafluoroethylene bypass grafts. J Vasc Surg 2002; 35:307–15.
31. Richards T, Pittathankal AA, Magee TR et al. The current role of intra-arterial thrombolysis. Eur J Vasc Endovasc Surg 2003; 26:166–9.
32. Tiek J, Foureneau I, Daenens K et al. The role of thrombolysis in acute infrainguinal bypass occlusion: a prospective nonrandomized controlled study. Ann Vasc Surg 2007 (Epub ahead of print).
33. Ricco JB, Probst H. French University Surgeons Association. Long-term results of a multicenter randomized study on direct versus crossover bypass for unilateral iliac artery occlusive disease. J Vasc Surg 2008; 47:45–53.
34. Beard JD, Nyamekye I, Earnshaw JJ et al. Intraoperative streptokinase: a useful adjunct to balloon catheter embolectomy. Br J Surg 1993; 80:21–4.
35. Jensen SL, Sandermann J. Compartment syndrome and fasciotomy in vascular surgery. A review of 57 cases. Eur J Vasc Endovasc Surg 1997; 13:48–53.
36. Yeager RA, Porter JM. Arterial and prosthetic graft infection. Ann Vasc Surg 1992; 5:485–91.
37. Naylor AR, Hayes PD, Darke S on behalf of the Joint Vascular Research Group. A prospective audit of complex wound and graft infections in Great Britain and Ireland: the emergence of MRSA. Eur J Vasc Endovasc Surg 2001; 21:289–94.
38. Earnshaw JJ, Whitman B, Heather BP on behalf of the Joint Vascular Research Group. Two-year results of a randomized controlled trial of rifampicin-bonded extra-anatomic Dacron grafts. Br J Surg 2000; 87:758–9.

    **A small, multicentre, randomised, controlled trial that failed to show any prophylactic effect of rifampicin bonding on subsequent graft infection.**

39. D'Addato M, Curti T, Freyrie A. Prophylaxis of graft infection with rifampicin-bonded Gelseal graft: 2-year follow-up of a prospective clinical trial. Italian Investigators Group. Cardiovasc Surg 1996; 4:200–4.

    **A randomised controlled trial that failed to show any effect of rifampicin bonding in Dacron grafts but the power of the study was low, with only 5 of 296 infections in the rifampicin group compared with 7 of 304 in the control group.**

40. Dunlop MG, Fox JN, Stonebridge PA et al. Vacuum drainage of groin wounds after vascular surgery: a controlled trial. Br J Surg 1990; 77:562–3.
41. Healy DA, Keyser J III, Holcomb GW III et al. Prophylactic closed suction drainage of femoral wounds in patients undergoing vascular reconstruction. J Vasc Surg 1990; 10:18–19.
42. Menawat SS, Gloviczki P, Serry RD et al. Management of aortic graft enteric fistulae. Eur J Vasc Endovasc Surg 1997; 14(Suppl A):74–81.
43. Hicks RJC, Greenhalgh RM. The pathogenesis of vascular graft infection. Eur J Vasc Endovasc Surg 1997; 14(Suppl A):5–9.
44. Becquemin JP, Qvarfordt P, Kron J et al. Aortic graft infection: is there a place for partial graft removal? Eur J Vasc Endovasc Surg 1997; 14(Suppl A):53–8.
45. Kieffer E, Gomes, Chiche L et al. Allograft replacement for infrarenal aortic graft infection: early and late results in 179 patients. J Vasc Surg 2004; 39:1009–17.
46. O'Connor S, Andres P, Batt M et al. A systematic review and meta-analysis of treatments for aortic graft infection. J Vasc Surg 2006; 44:38–45.
47. Clagett GP, Valentine RJ, Hagino RT. Autogenous aortoiliac/femoral reconstruction from superficial

femoral–popliteal veins: feasibility and durability. J Vasc Surg 1997; 25:255–70.

48. Verhelst R, Lavroix V, Vraux H et al. Use of cryopreserved arterial homografts for management of infected prosthetic grafts: a multicentric study. Ann Vasc Surg 2000; 14:601–7.
49. Batt M, Magne JL, Alric P et al. In situ revascularisation with silver-coated polyester grafts to treat aortic graft infection: early and midterm results. J Vasc Surg 2003; 38:983–9.
50. Nasim A, Hayes P, London N et al. Vascular Society of Great Britain and Ireland: in situ replacement of infected aortic grafts with rifampicin-bonded prostheses. Br J Surg 1999; 86:695.
51. Nevelsteen A, Lacroix H, Suy R. Autogenous reconstruction with lower extremity deep veins: an alternative treatment of prosthetic infection after reconstructive surgery for aortoiliac disease. J Vasc Surg 1995; 22:129–34.
52. Daenens K, Fourneau I, Nevelsteen A. Ten-year experience in autogenous reconstruction with the femoral vein in the treatment of aortofemoral prosthetic infection. Eur J Vasc Endovasc Surg 2003; 25:240–5.
53. Modrall JG, Sadjadi J, Ali AT et al. Deep vein harvest: predicting need for fasciotomy. J Vasc Surg 2004; 39:387–94.
54. Nevelsteen A, Baeyens I, DaenensK et al. Regarding "Deep vein harvest: predicting the need for fasciotomy." J Vasc Surg 2004; 40:403.
55. Gibbons CP, Ferguson CJ, Fligelstone LJ et al. Experience with femoro-popliteal veins as a conduit for vascular reconstruction in infected fields. Eur J Vasc Endovasc Surg 2003; 25:424–31.
56. Danneels MJ, Verhagen TJ, Teijink JA et al. Endovascular repair for aorto-enteric fistula: a bridge too far or a bridge to surgery? Eur J Vasc Endovasc Surg 2006; 32:27–33.
57. Ducasse E, CalistiA, Speziale F et al. Aortoiliac stent graft infection: current problems and management. Ann Vasc Surg 2004; 18:521–6.
58. Nevelsteen A, Smet G, Wilms G et al. Intravenous substraction angiography and duplex scanning in the detection of late human umbilical vein degeneration. Br J Surg 1988; 75:668–70.
59. Reipe G, Chafke N, Morlock M et al. Dilatation and durability of polyester grafts. In: Branchereau A, Jacobs M (eds) Complications in vascular and endovascular surgery, Part 1. Armonk, NY: Futura, 2000; pp. 35–43.
60. White GH, Donayre CE, Williams RA et al. Exertional disruption of axillofemoral graft anastomosis. 'The axillary pullout syndrome'. Arch Surg 1990; 125:625–7.
61. Jones WT, Hagino RT, Chiou AC et al. Graft patency is not the only clinical predictor of success after exclusion and bypass of popliteal artery aneurysms. J Vasc Surg 2003; 37:392–8.
62. Maleux G, Hendrickx S, Vaninbrouckx J et al. Percutaneous injection of human thrombin to treat iatrogenic femoral pseudoaneurysms: short- and midterm ultrasound follow-up. Eur Radiol 2003; 13:209–12.
63. Nevelsteen A, Wouters L, Suy R. Aortofemoral Dacron reconstruction for aorto-iliac occlusive disease: a 25-year survey. Eur J Vasc Surg 1991; 5:179–86.
64. Nevelsteen A. Anastomotic false aneurysms of the abdominal aorta and the iliac arteries. J Vasc Surg 1989; 10:595.
65. Derom A, Nout E. Treatment of femoral pseudoaneurysms with endograft in high-risk patients. Eur J Vasc Endovasc Surg 2005; 30:644–7.
66. Curti T, Stella A, Rossi C et al. Endovascular repair as the first-choice treatment for anastomotic and true iliac aneurysms. J Endovasc Ther 2001; 8:139–43.
67. Tielliu IF, Verhoeven EL, Zeebregts CJ et al. Endovascular treatment of iliac artery aneurysms with a tubular stent-graft: mid-term results. J Vasc Surg 2006; 43:440–5.
68. Mii S, MoriA, Sakata H et al. Para-anastomotic aneurysms: incidence, risk factors, treatment and prognosis. J Cardiovasc Surg (Torino) 1998; 39:259–66.
69. Mulder EJ, van Bockel JH, Maas J et al. Morbidity and mortality of reconstructive surgery of noninfected false aneurysms detected long after aortic prosthetic reconstruction. Arch Surg 1998; 133:45–9.
70. Sachdev U, Baril DT, Morissey NJ et al. Endovascular repair of para-anastomotic aortic aneurysms. J Vasc Surg 2007; 46:636–41.
71. Pifaretti G, Tozzi M, Lomazzi C et al. Endovascular treatment for para-anastomotic abdominal aortic and iliac aneurysms following aortic surgery. J Cardiovasc Surg (Torino) 2007; 48:711–17.
72. Gawenda M, Zaehringer M, Brunkwall J. Open versus endovascular repair of para-anastomotic aneurysms in patients who were morphological candidates for endovascular treatment. J Endovasc Ther 2003; 10:745–51.
73. Van Herwaarden JA, Waasdorp EJ, Bendermacher BL et al. Endovascular repair of paraanastomotic aneurysms after previous open aortic prosthetic reconstruction. Ann Vasc Surg 2004; 18: 280–6.
74. Becquemin JP, Kelley L, Zubilewicz T et al. Outcomes of secondary interventions after abdominal aortic aneurysm endovascular repair. J Vasc Surg 2004; 39:298–305.
75. Van Nes JG, Hendriks JM, Tseng LN et al. Endoscopic aneurysm sac fenestration as a treatment for growing aneurysms due to type II endoleak or endotension. J Endovasc Ther 2005; 12:430–4.
76. Kolvenbach R, Pinter L, Raghunandan M et al. Laparoscopic remodeling of abdominal aortic aneurysms after endovascular exclusion: a technical description. J Vasc Surg 2002; 36(6):1267–70.

77. Walschot LH, Laheij RJ, Verbaak AL. Outcome after endovascular abdominal aortic aneurysm repair: a meta-analysis. J Endovasc Ther 2002; 9:82–9.
78. Verzini F, Cao P, De Rango P et al. Conversion to open repair after endografting for abdominal aortic aneurysms: causes, incidence and results. Eur J Vasc Endovasc Surg 2006; 31:136–42.
79. Lifeline Registry of EVAR Publications Committee. Lifeline registry of endovascular aneurysm repair: long-term primary outcome measures. J Vasc Surg 2005; 42:1–10.
80. Lawrence-Brown MM, Hartley D, MacSweeney ST et al. The Perth endoluminal bifurcated graft system – development and early experience. Cardiovasc Surg 1996; 4:706–12.
81. Böckler D, Probst Th, Weber H et al. Surgical conversion after endovascular grafting for abdominal aortic aneurysms. J Endovasc Ther 2002; 9:111–18.

# 8

# Management of acute lower limb ischaemia

Jonothan J. Earnshaw
Peter A. Gaines
Jonathan D. Beard

## Introduction

There is no internationally accepted definition of acute leg ischaemia (ALI). The acutely bloodless limb with sensorimotor loss obviously falls within any definition but there is often a delay in the presentation and the ischaemia is not immediately limb-threatening. Chronic critical leg ischaemia is defined as rest pain of more than 2 weeks' duration (see Chapters 2 and 3).

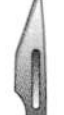

The revised (2007) TASC Inter-Society Consensus defines ALI as any sudden decrease in limb perfusion causing a potential threat to limb viability.[1]

Presentation is usually less than 2 weeks' duration. However, some overlap with chronic critical leg ischaemia is inevitable. The severity of ischaemia is often defined according to the SVS/ISCVS guidelines (Table 8.1),[2] although this classification seems difficult to use in clinical practice. It is simpler to group patients into the following categories:

- subcritical acute ischaemia (viable leg) where there is no neurological deficit and an audible arterial Doppler signal at the ankle;
- critical acute ischaemia (threatened leg) where there is no audible ankle Doppler signal and a partial neurological deficit;
- irreversible acute ischaemia where the leg has a complete neurological deficit, tense muscles, with absent capillary return and no arterial or venous Doppler signal.[3]

In the Gloucestershire community survey done in 1994, the incidence of ALI was 1 per 6000 of the population per year, which means that an average district general hospital serving approximately 250 000 people should see 30–40 cases annually.[4] The condition is on the increase and there is evidence that the outcome is improved when patients are managed by a vascular service providing 24-hour cover.[5] ALI is associated with a high cost to the community because of the risk of amputation and prolonged hospitalisation. Costs are minimised and outcome optimised by accurate clinical assessment and an understanding of the available therapeutic options.

## Aetiology

ALI is the result of occlusion of a native artery or bypass graft.The commonest causes are thrombosis of a atherosclerotic stenosis and embolim of cardiac orgin (Box 8.1).

### Embolism

Until about 30 years ago, embolism caused most ALI. Emboli large enough to occlude major vessels usually arise in the heart. Rheumatic mitral valve disease was the most common cause, with large emboli forming in a dilated left atrium. In 80% of patients, atrial fibrillation due to ischaemic heart disease is now the origin of cardiac embolism; mural thrombus following acute myocardial infarction causes most of the remainder.[6] Large emboli typically

Table 8.1 • Suggested classification of acute limb ischaemia

| Category | Description | Capillary return | Muscle paralysis | Sensory loss | Doppler signals | |
|---|---|---|---|---|---|---|
| | | | | | Arterial | Venous |
| I Viable | Not immediately threatened | Intact | None | None | Audible | Audible |
| IIa Threatened | Salvageable if promptly treated | Intact/slow | None | Partial | Inaudible | Audible |
| IIb Threatened | Salvageable if immediately treated | Slow/absent | Partial | Partial/ complete | Inaudible | Audible |
| III Irreversible | Primary amputation | Absent staining | Complete tense compartment | Complete | Inaudible | Inaudible |

Reprinted from Rutherford RB, Flanigan DP, Gupta SK et al. Suggested standards for reports dealing with lower extremity ischemia. J Vasc Surg 1986; 4:80–94. With permission from the Society for Vascular Surgery.

Box 8.1 • Aetiology of acute lower limb ischaemia

**Thrombosis**

Atherosclerosis
Popliteal aneurysm
Bypass graft occlusion
Thrombotic conditions

**Embolism**

Atrial fibrillation
Mural thrombosis
Vegetations
Proximal aneurysms
Atherosclerotic plaque

**Rare causes**

Dissection
Trauma (including iatrogenic)
External compression
Popliteal entrapment
Cystic adventitial disease
Compartment syndrome

lodge at an arterial bifurcation, particularly in the common femoral or popliteal arteries (**Fig. 8.1**). Patients with cardiac embolism may also suffer from peripheral vascular disease as a result of the underlying process of atherosclerosis. This increases the difficulty in establishing the cause of the ischaemia and in revascularisation, which may be one reason why the prognosis for this condition remains poor.

### Atheroembolism

Less common sources of emboli include proximal aneurysms on atherosclerotic plaques, usually located in the thoracic or abdominal aorta. Whereas cardiac embolism usually consists entirely of platelet thrombus, embolism from proximal arteries can include atherosclerotic plaque or cholesterol-rich emboli. This has a much worse prognosis than cardiac embolism because embolectomy is less effective. Small particles of atheroembolism can pass to very distal vessels in the foot. This digital embolism can result in the 'acute blue toe syndrome'. In this condition, the embolic source should be identified and treated if possible. Often this is a proximal arterial plaque with platelet thrombus that can be treated by balloon angioplasty (**Fig. 8.2**). Embolisation of cholesterol-rich atheroma can occur spontaneously, but also follows intravascular manipulation by radiological intervention, or occasionally surgery (trash foot). This can be disastrous, since both large and small arteries are occluded and cannot be reopened with either surgery or thrombolysis. This often results in limb or end-organ damage, and is often fatal (**Fig. 8.3**).

## Thrombosis

In situ thrombosis in a native artery is now the commonest cause of ALI. It is usually the result of critical flow arrest at the site of an atherosclerotic stenosis. The advancing age of the population and the commensurate increase in atherosclerosis explains the rising incidence of ALI. Acute native vessel arterial occlusion may be compounded by surgery (e.g. knee replacement destroying geniculate collateral vessels formed around a popliteal occlusion), heart failure or a thrombotic tendency (polycythaemia, dehydration, etc.). Acute thrombosis of a popliteal aneurysm poses the highest risk to the leg. Typically, this occurs in elderly men in association with aneurysms elsewhere (50% have an aortic aneurysm) or generalised arterial ectasia. Popliteal aneurysms usually

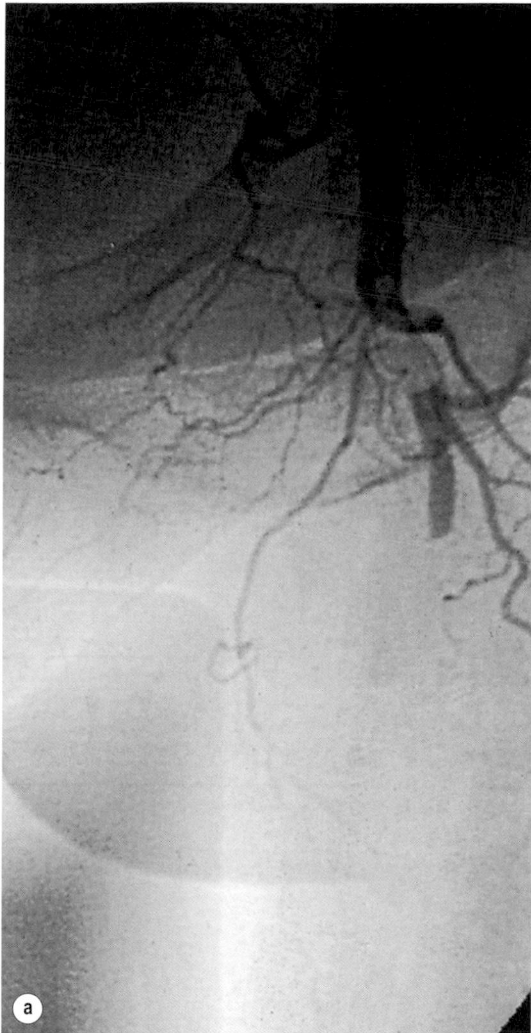


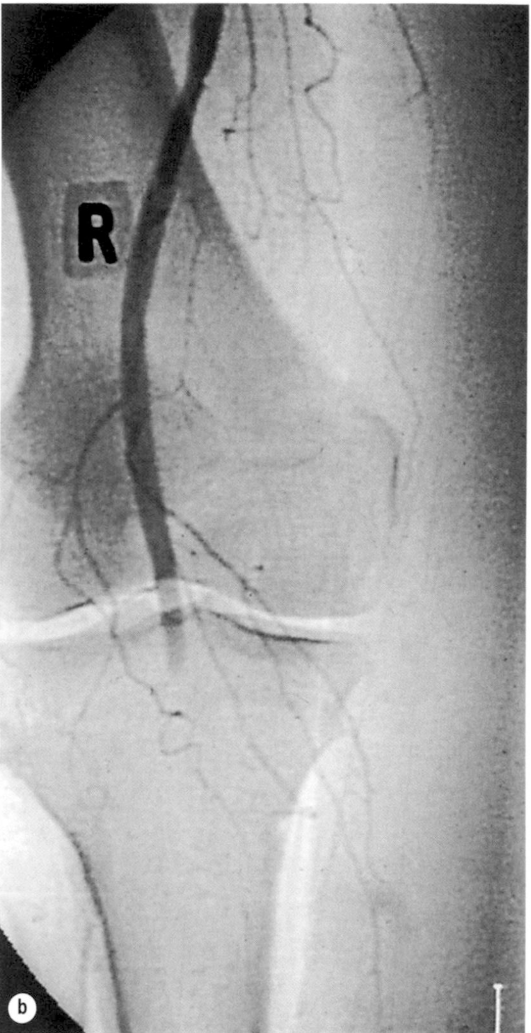


**Figure 8.1** • Arteriogram demonstrating an embolus lodged in the bifurcation of the common femoral artery **(a)** with further emboli occluding the distal profunda and popliteal artery **(b)**.

commence in the above-knee popliteal artery and extend distally to the tibial trifurcation. As they enlarge they can fill with lamellar thrombus, which may cause either acute thrombosis or distal embolisation that occludes the tibial vessels. The latter will place the leg in extreme jeopardy. In 20% of patients with ALI, a source for the embolus cannot be found.

## Other causes

The increasing use of bypass grafts for arterial insufficiency means that surgeons often have to deal with acute graft thrombosis. Grafts occlude for a variety of reasons. Graft occlusion within 1 month of insertion is usually the result of technical problems at the time of surgery or poor distal run-off. Graft occlusion within 1 year of placement is often caused by myointimal hyperplasia at an anastomosis or the development of stenoses within a vein graft. Occlusion after 1 year is usually due to progression of distal atherosclerosis. Prosthetic grafts have a higher occlusion rate than autogenous vein grafts (see Chapters 3 and 7).

Spontaneous native arterial thrombosis occasionally occurs without an underlying flow-limiting stenosis and these patients should be investigated for an intrinsic clotting abnormality, e.g. antiphospholipid syndrome, activated protein C deficiency (see Chapter 17), or malignancy.

Occasionally, acute arterial occlusion may be due to arterial dissection, trauma, extrinsic compression or compartment syndrome. In a young patient with acute popliteal artery occlusion, either popliteal entrapment or cystic adventitial disease should be considered.

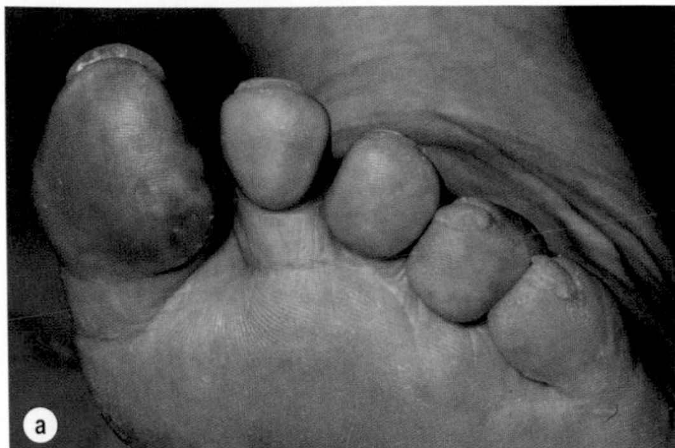


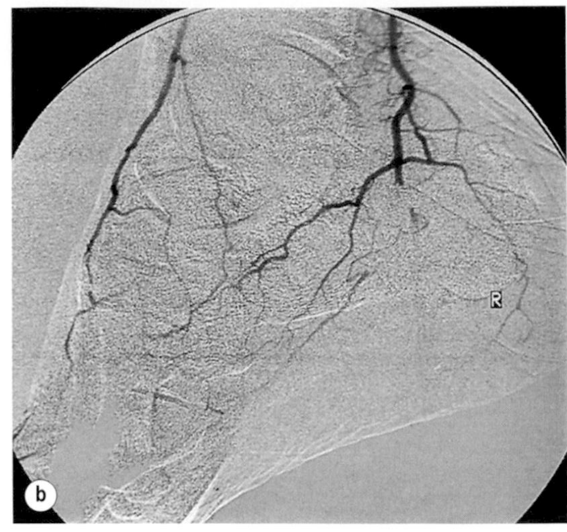


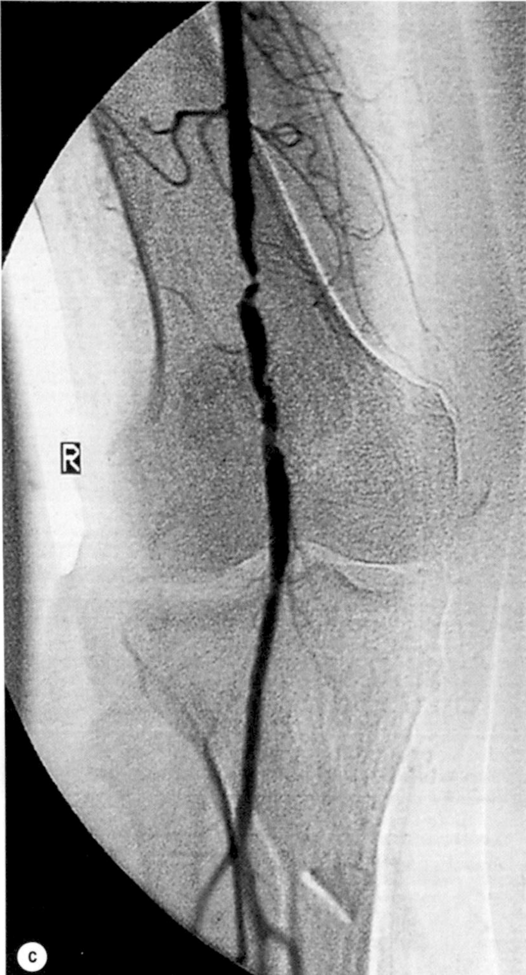


**Figure 8.2** • 'Blue toe syndrome' **(a)** due to digital and pedal arterial atheroembolism **(b)** from a proximal atherosclerotic stenosis **(c)**. Note the acute cut-off of the posterior tibial artery. Ultrasonography excluded a popliteal aneurysm and the lesion was treated by balloon angioplasty.

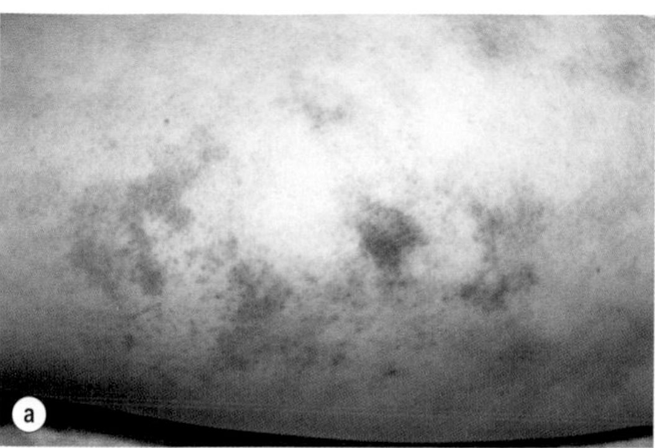

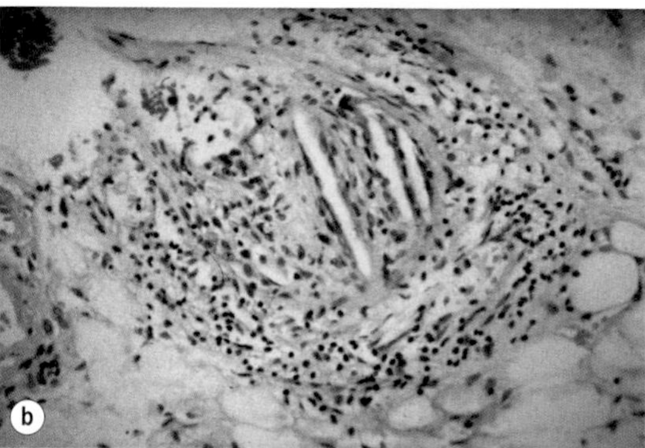

**Figure 8.3** • Livedo reticularis **(a)** caused by cholesterol embolism **(b)**. The skin has a typical mottled staining which is fixed.

## Recent changes

A number of factors may have changed the presentation of ALI. For example, many patients are now treated with risk factor-modifying drugs such as antiplatelet therapy and statins. It is not yet clear whether this has had a global effect, but there is a perception amongst vascular specialists that the rate of in situ thrombosis is falling. Similarly, many patients with atrial fibrillation are currently treated with prophylactic warfarin. Whilst this does not entirely prevent embolisation, it can make the acute ischaemia easier to deal with, since there is less secondary thrombosis, particularly affecting small distal arteries.

## Clinical features

The severity of ischaemia at presentation is the most important factor affecting outcome of the leg.[3,7] Complete occlusion of a proximal artery in the absence of preformed collateral vessels (as in cardiac embolism) results in the classical clinical presentation of pain, paralysis, paraesthesia, pallor, pulselessness and a perishingly cold leg. The pain is severe and frequently resistant to analgesia. Calf pain and tenderness with a tense muscle compartment indicates muscle necrosis and critical (often irreversible) ischaemia. Sensorimotor deficit including muscle paralysis and paraesthesia are indicative of muscle and nerve ischaemia with the potential for salvage with prompt treatment. Initially the leg is white with empty veins but after 6–12 hours vasodilatation occurs, probably caused by hypoxia of the smooth muscle. The capillaries then fill with stagnant deoxygenated blood, resulting in a mottled appearance that blanches on digital pressure (**Fig. 8.4**). If flow is not restored rapidly, the arteries distal to the occlusion fill with propagated thrombus and the capillaries rupture, resulting in a fixed blue staining of the skin that is a sign of irreversible ischaemia. These features are typical of an acute arterial occlusion in the absence of existing collaterals, and suggest an embolic cause. When arterial occlusion occurs as part of a chronic process where collaterals have developed, the leg is typically less severely ischaemic. Patients with peripheral atherosclerosis deteriorate in a stepwise fashion as thrombosis supervenes on an existing arterial plaque. Patients often report a sudden change in symptoms, which progress over a few days: the foot often has a dusky hue with slow capillary return. Previous claudication or absent pulses in the contralateral foot help make a clinical diagnosis of in situ thrombosis. Palpation of a mass in either popliteal fossa suggests thrombosis of a popliteal aneurysm.

## Initial management

Patients presenting with ALI are often in poor general health, which is one reason why the condition has such a high mortality rate from associated cardiovascular disease. Dehydration, cardiac failure, hypoxia and pain should all be managed in the standard way. An intravenous infusion is required for rehydration and is also often the best means of providing analgesia with an infusion pump. If thrombolysis is an option, intramuscular analgesia should be avoided because of the risk of bleeding. Intravenous unfractioned heparin (5000 units) should be given immediately followed by systemic heparinisation, principally to restrict propagation of thrombus, although there is also evidence that it improves the prognosis.[8] In many units low-molecular-weight heparins have replaced unfractioned heparin. The short half-life of the latter, however, is helpful in this situation. Anticoagulation should be deferred if regional anaesthesia is required. In order to improve oxygenation, 24% oxygen should be given by face mask.

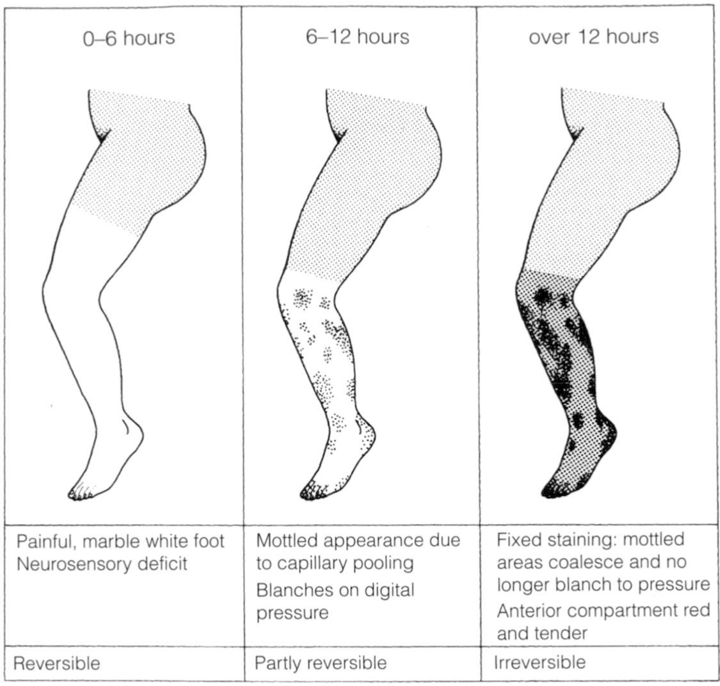


**Figure 8.4** • Clinical outcome after acute leg ischaemia.

Venous blood should be taken for full blood count, urea, electrolytes and glucose. An ECG and chest radiograph may be of value in diagnosing and managing cardiac arrhythmias and heart failure. If a primary thrombotic tendency is suspected, investigation of this should be delayed as the diagnostic tests are inaccurate in the face of fresh thrombus.

When clinical examination suggests that an aortic aneurysm or popliteal aneurysm may be the cause of ALI, then duplex ultrasound imaging is indicated.

# Revascularisation

The clinical assessment of the severity of limb ischaemia will largely dictate the most appropriate form of therapy (**Fig. 8.5**).

## Irreversible leg ischaemia

A small number of patients will present in a moribund state or with irreversible leg ischaemia (muscle paralysis, tense swollen fascial compartments, fixed skin staining). Terminal care may be the kindest option. For the irreversibly ischaemic leg revascularisation is, by definition, inappropriate and may be dangerous. This includes the patient who develops ALI while being treated for another condition, usually as an inpatient on an elderly care ward. Prognosis is particularly dismal in this group.[4] Surviving patients should be resuscitated and stabilised before considering amputation.

## Acute critical ischaemia

The acute white leg with sensorimotor deficit requires urgent intervention to prevent limb loss. Although the differentiation between thrombosis and embolus is often difficult, it is in this group of patients that embolism is more likely.

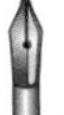

An acute white leg with no prior history of claudication, normal contralateral pulses and a probable embolic source, such as atrial fibrillation, would indicate that embolisation is the likely cause. Urgent surgery is indicated in these patients, after resuscitation, without the need for preoperative arteriography, which simply wastes time.

Many vascular surgeons are now experienced with the use of portable duplex ultrasound imaging, and valuable information can be achieved quickly with this investigation. Groin exploration with balloon catheter embolectomy and on-table arteriography is indicated (see below). There is some debate about whether preoperative investigation provides beneficial information when the femoral pulse is absent, as it may help to exclude alternative diagnoses,

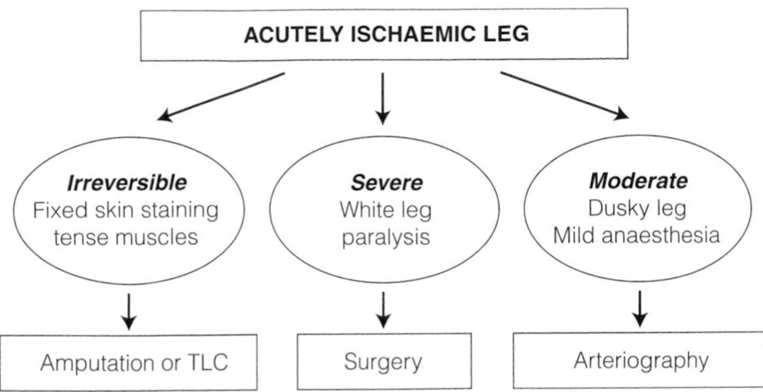


**Figure 8.5** • Clinical approach to the management of the acutely ischaemic leg.

such as aortic dissection, and may permit endovascular treatment of an iliac stenosis or occlusion. An alternative is to proceed directly to operation but to prepare both groins so that a femoral crossover graft can be inserted if adequate inflow cannot be achieved using an embolectomy catheter.

## Acute subcritical ischaemia

The majority of patients presenting with ALI have acute onset of rest pain but no paralysis and no, or only mild, sensory loss. The cause is often acute thrombosis of either an atherosclerotic artery or graft. Because the leg is not immediately threatened, time is available to plan appropriate intervention after investigation. Conventionally, acute leg ischaemia was investigated using arteriography (**Fig. 8.6**). The advantage was that imaging could be followed by therapeutic thrombolysis at the same sitting. There are now, however, non-invasive alternatives such as duplex imaging and computed tomography angiography, both of which can provide enough information on which to plan intervention. The method of investigation will depend on the time of presentation and the available facilities. The two main alternatives in these patients are intervention with surgery or percutaneous thrombolysis. Thromboembolectomy is unlikely to reopen an artery occluded by thrombus and atherosclerotic plaque; formal arterial bypass is more likely to be needed.

Thrombolysis is arguably less invasive than revascularisation surgery. It has the capacity to open small as well as large arteries. It may also uncover the cause of the in situ thrombosis, such as an arterial stenosis, which can be treated by angioplasty to produce a lasting outcome.

Some patients are admitted to hospital with acute thrombosis of a peripheral artery (usually the superficial femoral) but have only claudication and no ischaemic pain at rest. Thrombolysis might appear an attractive option to treat the claudication, but the risks are as high as in patients with limb-threatening ischaemia.[9] Reverting to the principles described by Blaisdell et al., i.e. initial anticoagulation followed by management depending on the progression of ischaemia, reduces the risk to both life and limb.[8]

## Choice between surgery and thrombolysis: the evidence

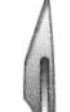

There remains considerable controversy about the individual roles of surgery and thrombolysis for ALI. A review of 42 studies (most non-randomised) by Diffin and Kandarpa[10] suggested that thrombolysis was associated with substantially better limb salvage and mortality rates than surgery. There are three major randomised studies from which to draw harder evidence.[11–16] The New York study was the first to show that thrombolysis improves survival in patients with limb-threatening ischaemia of less than 14 days.[11] This study was small and the advantage was due to the high incidence of cardiorespiratory deaths following emergency surgery. The STILE study was much larger and included patients with ischaemia for longer than 14 days.[12] This study has been much criticised because of the failure of one-third of the radiologists to insert a catheter successfully for peripheral thrombolysis. The study introduced the concept of amputation-free survival but failed to show any significant improvement in this primary end-point between the treatment groups. In the subgroup of patients with ischaemia for fewer than 14 days, thrombolysis reduced the rate of amputation. Subsequent analysis of patients from this study up to 1 year revealed that thrombolysis was better initial treatment for graft occlusions, whereas surgery was more effective and durable for native vessel occlusions.[13,14] However, few of the patients in the STILE study had critical ischaemia. The TOPAS trial was designed, using lessons learned from the above studies, to try to settle this debate. In the first phase, an optimal dose of thrombolytic therapy was selected (urokinase 4000 IU/hour)[15] and in phase II this was compared with urgent surgery in 544 patients.[16] Amputation-

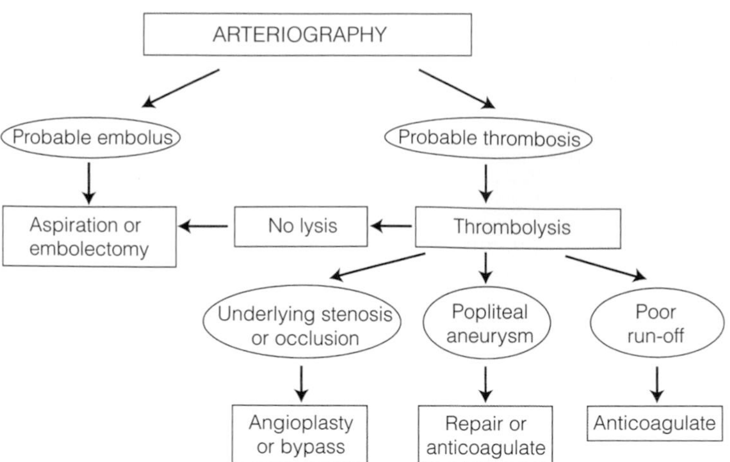


**Figure 8.6** • Treatment pathways following arteriography.

free survival was similar in both groups at 6 months and 1 year (72% and 65% for urokinase vs. 75% and 70% for surgery respectively), though thrombolysis reduced the need for open surgical procedures.

In conclusion, both surgery and thrombolysis seem effective and the choice should be made on an individual basis for each patient, taking into account the skills and experience available in the vascular unit.

## Peripheral arterial thrombolysis

Thrombus dissolution is achieved by stimulating the conversion of fibrin-bound plasminogen into the active enzyme plasmin. Plasmin is a non-specific protease capable of degrading fibrin and producing thrombus dissolution.

In contrast to the thrombolytic treatment of acute myocardial infarction, systemic infusion of thrombolytic agents for ALI results in a poor success rate and unacceptable complications. By selectively placing a catheter within the thrombus via the percutaneous route and delivering the thrombolytic agent locally, the concentration of agent is maximised and plasmin is less likely to be neutralised by circulating antiplasmins. The dose of thrombolytic agent can be optimised to the minimum level that results in a local effect without producing systemic thrombolysis and the attendant complications.

### Contraindications (Box 8.2)

Perhaps the only absolute contraindication to lysis is active internal bleeding. Most other contraindications are relative, where the risk of complications from thrombolysis must be weighed against the potential benefits of limb salvage. It is unwise to consider thrombolysis within 2 weeks of surgery or within 2 months of a stroke. Dacron grafts may take 3 months to seal, and if they do not become fully incorporated they may become porous if thrombolytic therapy is employed. Care should be exercised when using thrombolysis to open Dacron grafts within the abdomen where manual compression is not possible should bleeding occur. The presence of cardiac thrombus theoretically increases the likelihood of systemic embolisation during thrombolysis, but there is no evidence that patient selection based on echocardiography affects management or outcome.

**Box 8.2** • Contraindications to thrombolysis

- Active internal bleeding
- Known pregnancy
- Stroke within 2 months
- Transient ischaemic attack within 2 months
- Known intracerebral tumour, aneurysm or arteriovenous malformation
- Severe bleeding tendency
- Craniotomy within 2 months
- Vascular surgery within 2 weeks
- Abdominal surgery within 2 weeks
- Puncture of a non-compressible vessel or biopsy within 10 days
- Previous gastrointestinal haemorrhage
- Trauma within 10 days

### Technique

All patients should have adequate analgesia and a cannula inserted for venous access, analgesia and hydration. The extent of occlusive disease needs to be defined by arteriography or duplex imaging before intervention. The number of arterial punctures should be kept to a minimum to reduce the risk of puncture-site bleeding during treatment. The initial diagnostic approach is tailored to the distribution of disease. If there is an absent femoral pulse in the affected leg but a palpable femoral pulse on the contralateral side, then it is reasonable to anticipate an iliac artery occlusion. In this situation, a contralateral femoral puncture will provide access for the diagnostic arteriogram and subsequently the iliac thrombosis can be approached from the same puncture site using a crossover technique (**Fig. 8.7**). If there is a normal femoral pulse on the side of acute ischaemia, then initial diagnostic information may be provided by intravenous digital subtraction angiography or duplex imaging. As long as adequate inflow can be ensured using one of these methods, an antegrade puncture should be attempted to treat occlusions below the femoral bifurcation so that adjuvant procedures such as angioplasty or thrombus aspiration can be performed from the same side (Fig. 8.7). An occluded arterial bypass graft is optimally accessed from the native artery proximal to the graft so that any stenoses can be treated via the same puncture site. However, this is not always possible for technical reasons, although direct puncture of the most proximal accessible part of the graft results in a high success rate from thrombolysis. Once access has been achieved, a guidewire should be passed through the occlusion; indeed, the ability to do this implies the presence of soft thrombus and is a good predictor of success (guidewire traversal test). The catheter used to deliver the lytic agent is then placed within the thrombus.

Several techniques are described for delivering thrombolysis. The low-dose infusion method involves running the thrombolytic drug through the catheter over several hours. This may be combined with an initial high-dose bolus. More recently, high-dose techniques have been described that accelerate the rate of thrombus dissolution.[17] This may be achieved by administering a number of high-dose boluses sequentially or by using the 'pulse spray' technique.[18] The latter involves high-pressure injection of tiny pulses of lytic agent through a catheter with multiple side holes, and thus it combines enzymatic thrombolysis with mechanical disruption. The high-dose techniques accelerate thrombolysis and allow patients to be treated within the normal working hours of a radiology department.

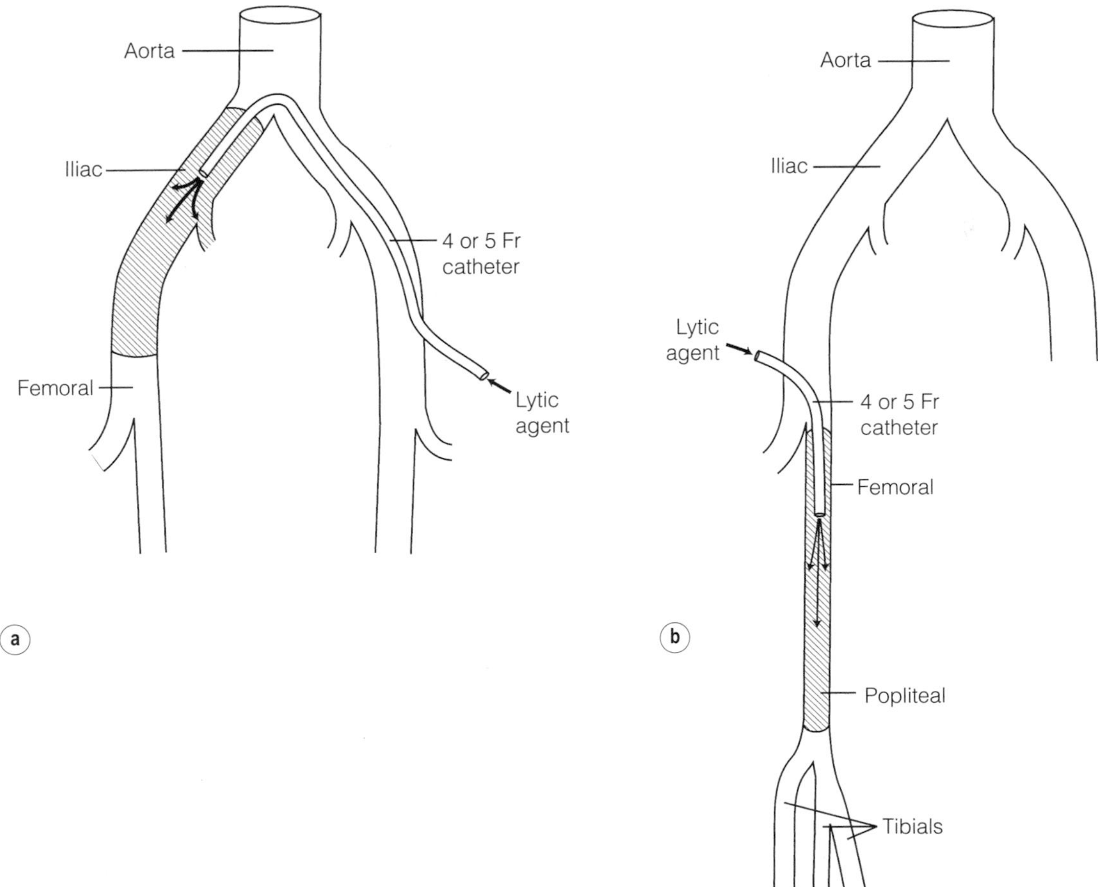


**Figure 8.7** • Technique of percutaneous thrombolysis: contralateral **(a)** and ipsilateral **(b)** transfemoral approaches.

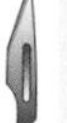

Several randomised trials comparing low-dose and accelerated methods of thrombolysis have found that limb salvage rate and complication rates appear similar, though accelerated methods are quicker.[17–20] Experienced radiologists use both high- and low-dose techniques to treat the majority of patients with ALI; the high-dose technique allows treatment of more severe ischaemia in patients where surgery is not possible and rapid revascularisation is required.

Three drugs are currently available for peripheral thrombolysis: streptokinase, urokinase and tissue plasminogen activator (t-PA). Appropriate dose regimens are shown in Box 8.3. There are very few high-quality trials to determine which drug is most effective, but most agree that t-PA and urokinase are superior to streptokinase.[22] t-PA is the agent of choice in the UK; in North America, many radiologists preferred urokinase, but it has not been widely available due to manufacturing difficulties in the past few years. The STILE trial suggested that urokinase and t-PA had equivalent activity,[12] and this was confirmed in unpublished manufacturers' data. Further randomised data would be helpful but cost considerations and availability largely determine the choice between urokinase and t-PA. A number of new agents such as staphylokinase and alfimeprase are under investigation, but as yet they have not been shown to be better than existing agents.

Heparin is often administered systemically before and after thrombolysis to counteract the associated prothrombotic tendency, although some data from trials of the thrombolytic treatment of acute stroke suggest that heparin may increase haemorrhagic complications. An alternative is concurrent administration of low-dose heparin (200 units/hour) via the proximal arterial sheath while delivering the thrombolytic agent via an end-hole catheter to an occlusion below the inguinal ligament. Heparin should be given routinely for 48 hours after completion of thrombolysis. Consideration will then be needed to determine whether individual patients need lifelong anticoagulation with warfarin. No data exist to guide appropriate therapy. Where contraindications exist to warfarin therapy, some clinicians use dual antiplatelet therapy, e.g. aspirin with clopidogrel, as an alternative. Thrombolysis should be considered a diagnostic process aimed at exposing the underlying flow-limiting lesion (**Fig. 8.8**). This should be found in the majority of patients using duplex ultrasonography of the suspect arterial segment. The majority of lesions can be managed by angioplasty or stent placement. Where the disease appears too extensive, surgical reconstruction may be required, particularly when an anastomotic stenosis results in graft occlusion.

**Box 8.3** • Suggested drug regimens for thrombolysis

**Slow infusion**

Streptokinase 5000 units/hour

Tissue plasminogen activator (t-PA) 0.5 mg/hour

Urokinase* 4000 IU/min for 2 hours, then 2000 IU/min for 2 hours, then 1000 IU/min

**Pulsed spray**

t-PA 0.3 mg per pulse every 30 seconds

Urokinase 5000 IU per pulse every 30 seconds

**High-dose bolus**

t-PA 5-mg bolus every 10 min three times, then 3.5 mg/hour for up to 4 hours, then (if required) as for slow infusion

*Urokinase is not currently available.

ALI due to a popliteal aneurysm remains a difficult clinical problem. The bulk of thrombus within the aneurysm restricts the use of thrombolysis because of the high risk of massive distal embolisation, the slow clearance and large amount of residual thrombus after recanalisation. If thrombolysis does have a role to play, then it is to open run-off vessels for distal bypass grafting. This is achieved by placing a catheter through the popliteal artery into a tibial vessel and then lysing it until a distal vessel becomes patent for bypass. Alternatively, urgent surgery may be performed with on-table angiography and thrombolysis to clear the run-off (see later).

## Percutaneous thrombectomy devices

Percutaneous mechanical thrombectomy (PMT) devices have been developed to hasten thrombus removal and either replace the need for thrombolytic drugs or reduce the dose required.[23] The devices may be classified according to their mode of action. The most basic technique involves simply aspirating the thrombus by applying suction to a wide-bore catheter. Some devices simply macerate thrombus into particles so small that they are removed by natural fibrinolysis (e.g. Amplatz Thrombectomy™ Device). Others include a clot aspiration system based on the Bernoulii or Venturi principle to remove fragments of thrombus and prevent distal embolisation (e.g. Angiojet™). Ultrasound catheters use ultrasound energy to lyse thrombus (e.g. the Acolysis™ catheter). Thrombolysis is often required as a supplement after mechanical thrombectomy: in the Trellis Thrombectomy System, the occluded segment of artery is isolated by proximal and distal balloons. An oscillating wire fragments the thrombus while a thrombolytic infusion helps to dissolve it before the liquefied material is aspirated from the isolated segment. These devices are all expensive and disposable, and there is little consensus about their use. Few are licensed for use in peripheral arteries; manufacturers usually seek approval for clotted dialysis fistulas

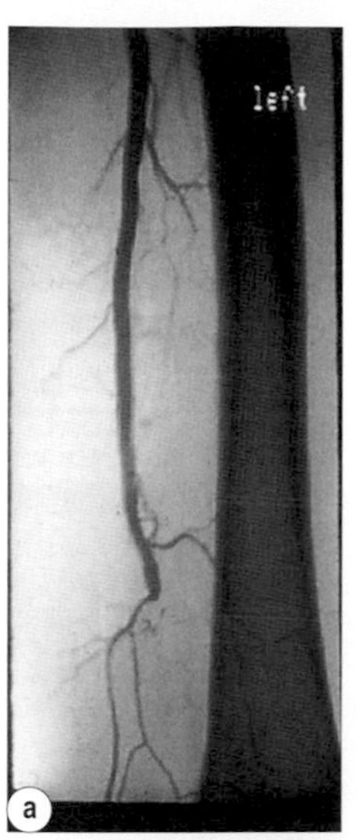

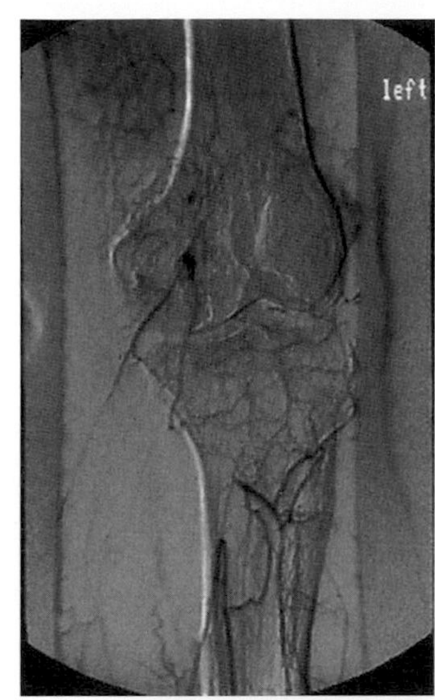

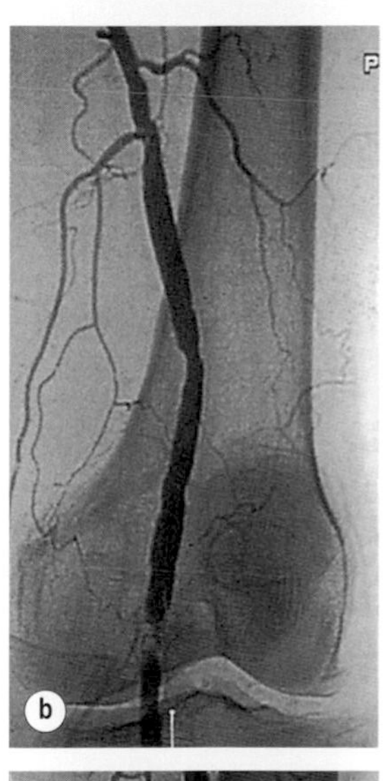

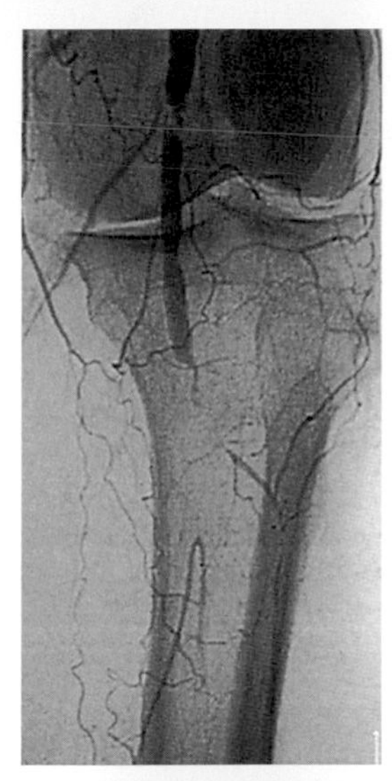

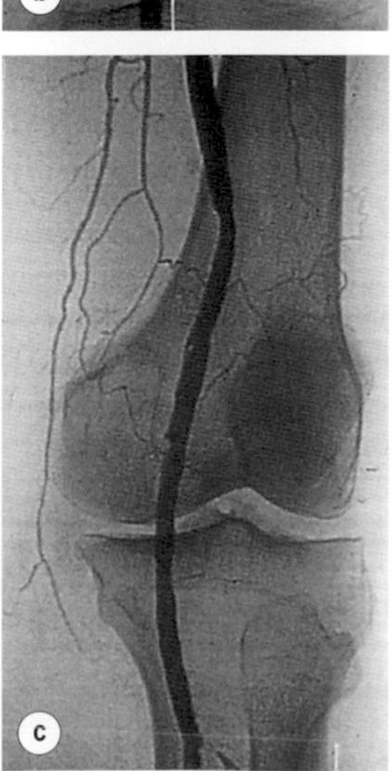

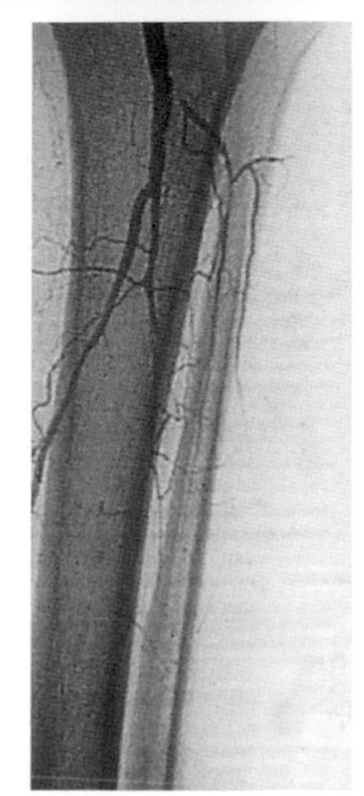

**Figure 8.8 • (a)** Arteriography demonstrates an occlusion of the popliteal artery extending into the tibial vessels. **(b)** Thrombolysis reveals a popliteal stenosis but persistent occlusion of the tibial trifurcation. **(c)** The stenosis was treated by balloon angioplasty and the thrombus aspirated from the tibial vessels using an aspiration catheter.

first. There is also the potential for further arterial damage during deployment, and large volumes of blood can be lost with the clot aspiration devices.

## Complications

There are significant risks associated with percutaneous thrombolytic therapy, most of which can be attributed to the fragile health of the patients and their advanced systemic atherosclerosis. Myocardial infarction and stroke are the commonest causes of death. The rate of reported adverse outcomes is variable, depending on the condition of the patients treated. In the review by Diffin and Kandarpa, principally of North American articles, the mortality rate after thrombolysis was 4% at 30 days.[10] The British Thrombolysis Study Group (TSG) database, which includes over 1100 episodes of thrombolysis (mostly for limb-threatening ischaemia), records a 12.4% mortality rate at 30 days.[24] Other large series report intermediate results.[23–26] Major haemorrhage occurs in approximately 9% of patients, usually at a groin puncture site but occasionally retroperitoneal or intra-abdominal. If major haemorrhage occurs during thrombolysis, aprotinin is an effective plasmin inhibitor and the administration of whole blood, fresh frozen plasma and, in particular, fibrinogen concentrate will replenish the clotting factors. Stroke is seen in approximately 3% of patients (2.3% in the TSG database). Most occur after thrombolysis, during therapeutic anticoagulation. About half are thrombotic rather than haemorrhagic. If a stroke occurs, cerebral haemorrhage should be excluded by urgent computed tomography. If haemorrhage is not the cause, then a clinical decision needs to be made whether to persist with thrombolysis to salvage the affected limb, with possible additional benefits to the intracerebral circulation.

Minor haemorrhage is common (approximately 40% of infusions) and usually occurs at the groin puncture site. It can be managed by direct compression or by exchanging the catheter system for a larger catheter or sheath. Distal embolisation during thrombolysis is a nuisance, occurring in 4% of patients, and is usually managed by either aspiration thromboembolectomy[21] or continued lysis. Reperfusion damage has been reported in 2% and pericatheter thrombosis in 1%.

## Outcome

Diffin and Kandarpa[10] report successful thrombolysis in 70% of treatments, with limb salvage in 93%, although many patients in the collected review did not have limb-threatening ischaemia. The TSG database records complete lysis in 45.5% and clinically useful lysis in a further 27.9% of infusions, leading to a limb salvage rate of 75.2%; 12.4% of patients required an amputation and 12.4% died.[24] Thrombolysis was similarly effective in bypass grafts and native vessels. The outcome seems dependent on the nature of the lesion treated and the clinical state of the patient. Patients with subcritical ischaemia appear less likely to need amputation than patients with critical ischaemia including a neurosensory deficit. In addition, the following are more likely to predict failure of thrombolysis: inability to traverse the occlusion with a guidewire or place a catheter within the thrombus, diabetes, multilevel disease, vein graft occlusion, advancing age and female sex.[25] In the long term, approximately 75% of successfully opened native vessels remain patent at 1 year and 55% at 2 years.[26,27] When an identifiable lesion is found after graft thrombolysis, the 2-year patency is approximately 85%. Long-term patency is less good where no underlying lesion is found in native vessels or grafts. In addition, successfully treated iliac occlusions and emboli have a better long-term outlook.[28,29]

There is currently great interest in trying to improve the results of peripheral thrombolysis. It is unlikely that advances in techniques will make a significant difference as no one method can be shown to be superior.

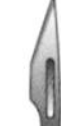

A consensus group has produced a document containing all the available evidence and made recommendations for thrombolytic treatment.[30] Other scoring systems may be used to try to identify patients unlikely to survive after thrombolysis.[31] Detailed analysis of available data and large databases may help identify patients at greater risk of a poor outcome from thrombolysis. A detailed statistical analysis of the TSG database has shown that the following factors were associated with reduced amputation-free survival: increasing patient age; increasing severity of ischaemia (Fontaine grade and presence of a sensorimotor deficit); shorter duration of ischaemia; and diabetes.[23] Being on warfarin at the time of the occlusion improved the chance of amputation-free survival. The risk of death after thrombolysis was highest in patients with an embolic occlusion, women, older patients and those with ischaemic heart disease. Amputation risk was highest in younger men, legs with a sensorimotor deficit, and graft and thrombotic occlusions.

# Surgical management

With the increasing age of the population, underlying atherosclerosis often complicates ischaemia even if the cause is primarily embolic. Consequently, complex secondary procedures may well be necessary if initial balloon catheter embolectomy fails (**Fig. 8.9**). It is therefore advisable that an experienced vascular surgeon performs or supervises the operation. Local

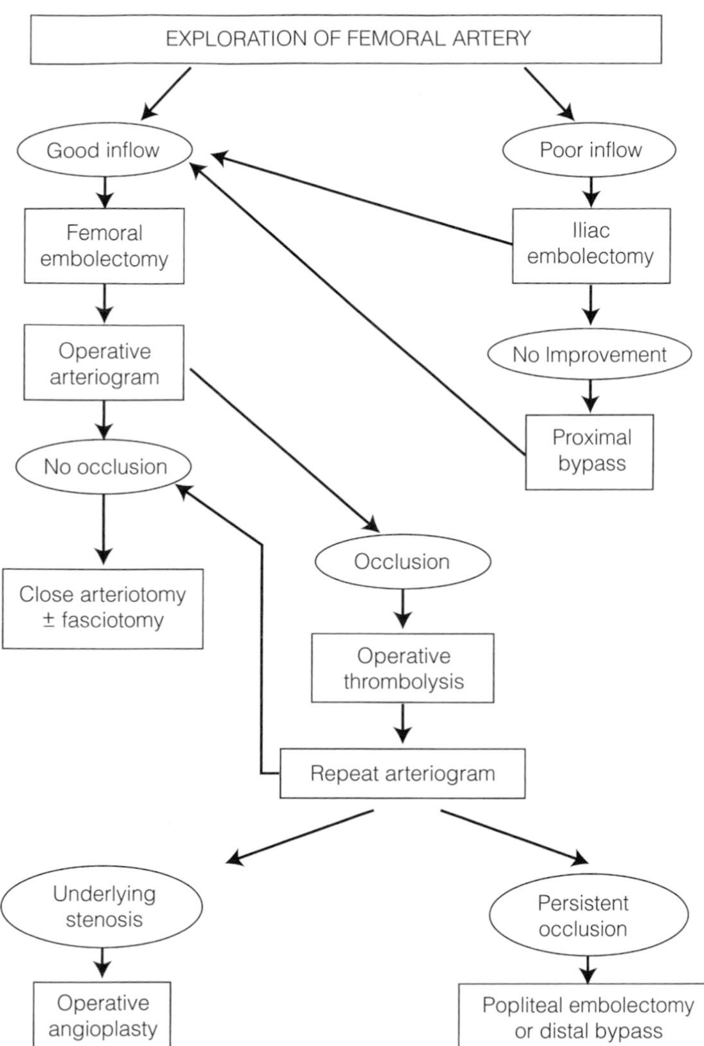


**Figure 8.9** • Possible treatment pathway required when exploring the femoral artery.

anaesthesia may be preferred in a slim patient with a clear-cut embolus and high cardiac risk. However, an anaesthetist should always be present to monitor the ECG and oxygen saturation, administer sedation or analgesia and convert to general anaesthesia if required. Obesity, patient confusion and the likelihood of additional procedures seem good reasons for general or regional anaesthesia.

## Balloon catheter embolectomy

Both groins and the entire leg should be prepared to permit surgical access and arteriography. The foot should be placed in a sterile transparent bag for easy inspection. The common femoral artery bifurcation is exposed via an oblique groin incision, which reduces wound-healing problems, and the vessels controlled with Silastic slings. Clamps should be avoided initially because they fragment thrombus that may otherwise be removed intact. A transverse arteriotomy is made in the common femoral artery proximal to the bifurcation, avoiding any obvious plaque (**Fig. 8.10**). A transverse arteriotomy is easier to close without narrowing and it can be converted to a diamond shape for proximal anastomosis if a bypass is required. Any thrombus at the bifurcation can be removed by gentle suction or forceps and momentary release of the sling or clamp.

If pulsatile inflow is not present, then a 4-Fr or 5-Fr balloon catheter is passed proximally up into the aorta, inflated and withdrawn. Pressure should be applied to the contralateral femoral artery during this procedure to prevent contralateral embolisation. If good inflow cannot be achieved, then a femoro-femoral or axillo-femoral bypass will be required. A saddle embolus can usually be retrieved by bilateral femoral embolectomy. Next, a 3-Fr

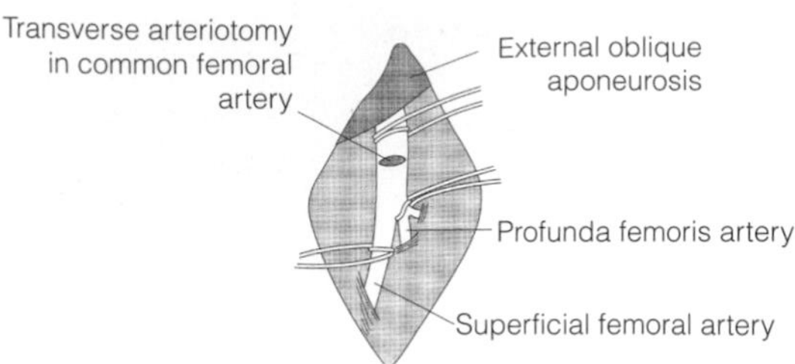


**Figure 8.10** • Exploration of the femoral artery using Silastic slings to control the vessels and a transverse arteriotomy proximal to the common femoral bifurcation.

or 4-Fr balloon catheter is passed as far distally as possible down both the profunda and superficial femoral arteries. Force should not be used if resistance is met as dissection or perforation may result. The balloon is inflated only as the catheter is withdrawn and the amount of inflation adjusted to avoid excessive intimal friction. The procedure is repeated until no more thromboembolic material can be retrieved. Conventional embolectomy is performed blind and the surgeon has no control over the direction of the catheter past the popliteal trifurcation. Use of an end-hole balloon catheter permits selective catheterisation of the tibial arteries, over a guidewire, under fluoroscopic control (**Fig. 8.11**).

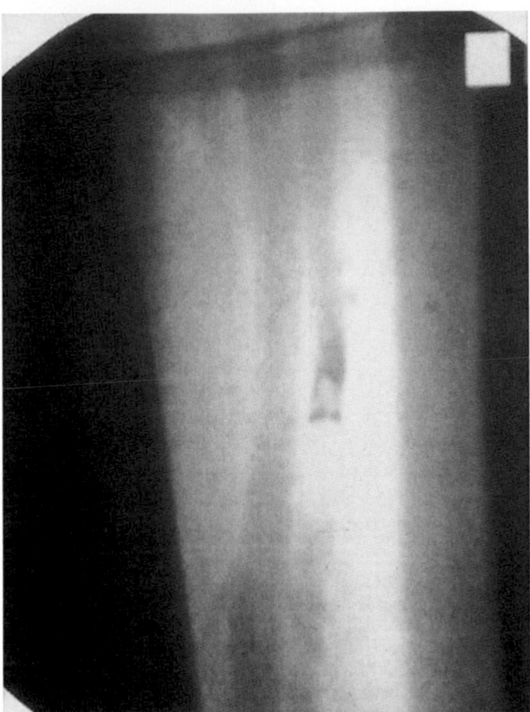

**Figure 8.11** • Angiographically controlled balloon catheter embolectomy. The balloon occluding the lumen and the thrombus above it can be seen as negative images against the contrast-filled artery.

### Completion arteriography

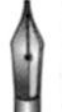

A completion arteriogram should always be performed because persistent thrombus may be present even if the catheter passes to the foot;[32] back-bleeding is of no prognostic value as it may arise from established proximal collaterals. Many theatres now have excellent fluoroscopic facilities capable of high-quality arteriography. If this is not available, place a radiography film cassette wrapped in a sterile towel under the leg and infuse 20 mL of contrast medium down the superficial femoral artery via an umbilical catheter before exposing the film. The distal arteries are irrigated with 100 mL of heparin saline and if no thrombus is present on the arteriogram, the arteriotomy is repaired with 5/0 prolene. On removing the clamps the foot should become pink with palpable pulses.

### Failed embolectomy

If the arteriogram shows persistent occlusion, then streptokinase 100 000 units or t-PA 15 mg in 100 ml heparin saline can be infused via an umbilical catheter over 30 minutes and the arteriogram repeated (**Fig. 8.12**). This often results in complete lysis and reduces the need for popliteal exploration.[33] The technique may also be used to lyse residual thrombus in the tibial arteries during bypass of a popliteal aneurysm.[34] If an underlying stenosis of the superficial femoral artery is revealed, then on-table angioplasty may be attempted. Persistent distal occlusion requires exploration of the below-knee popliteal artery and either popliteal embolectomy or distal bypass. The origins of the anterior tibial artery and tibioperoneal trunk should be controlled with slings and selective embolectomy performed via a longitudinal arteriotomy. The popliteal arteriotomy usually repair requires with a vein patch.

## Further management

Revascularisation of an ischaemic leg results in a sudden venous return of blood with low pH and a high potassium concentration. The anaesthetist must be prepared to correct these, as hypotension and arrhythmias may occur. Reperfusion of a large mass of ischaemic tissue results in a systemic inflammatory reaction caused by neutrophil activation. This may cause multiple organ dysfunction including renal and pulmonary failure. Renal function may be further impaired by myoglobinuria, which is helped by maintaining a good diuresis.

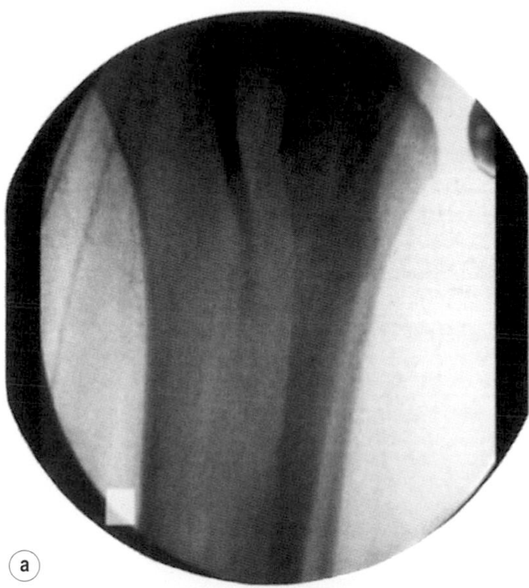

a

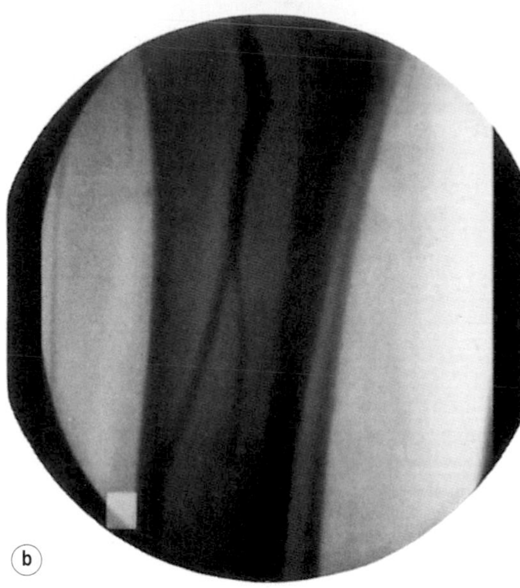

b

**Figure 8.12** • Completion angiogram after embolectomy showing persistent occlusion of the popliteal trifurcation **(a)** and complete lysis after intraoperative thrombolysis **(b)**.

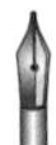

Revascularisation of ischaemic muscle can result in considerable swelling within the fascial compartments of the leg. This compartment syndrome will lead to further muscle and nerve damage if not relieved. All muscle compartments should be decompressed via full-length skin and fascial incisions from knee to ankle if any muscle tenseness is present at the time of embolectomy or subsequently.[35] The anterior fasciotomy should be made about two finger-breadths lateral to the anterior border of the tibia, which avoids the peroneal nerve. The posterior fasciotomy incision is done in a line about two finger-breadths posterior to the medial condyle of the femur and the medial malleolus, which avoids the long saphenous vein. A split-skin graft can be applied to the defects later.

After embolectomy, anticoagulation with heparin and then warfarin is continued as this reduces the risk of recurrent embolism, especially if atrial fibrillation is present.[36–38] There is little guidance about the role of anticoagulation in patients who are not fibrillating and have no other obvious cause. Results of a search for proximal sources of emboli using echocardiography and aortic ultrasound may indicate the need for lifelong anticoagulation, but in many patients an individual decision will need to be made based on the risks of warfarinisation and the state of the distal circulation.

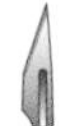

The addition of a 4- to 7-day infusion of iloprost after treatment by embolectomy was tested in a randomised trial that included 192 patients. The combined rate of death and/or amputation was reduced from 27.2% to 16.0% ($P$ = 0.03).[39]

## Overall prognosis

There has been little change in overall outcome from ALI because the improvements in radiological and surgical techniques have been balanced by increasing atherosclerotic arterial disease in ever older patients. A Swedish population study demonstrated that between 1965 and 1983 there was an increasing incidence of ALI, without any improvement in amputation rates or survival,[40] although outcome after treatment in a university hospital was better than in a district hospital.[41] A prospective survey by the Vascular Surgical Society of Great Britain and Ireland that included 539 episodes in 474 patients recorded a limb salvage rate of 70% and an overall mortality rate of 22%.[42] An analysis of patients taken from the National Inpatient Sample in the USA recorded an amputation rate of 12.7% and a mortality rate of 9%.[28] Patients with embolism have a higher mortality rate due to their underlying cardiac disease. In contrast, those with thrombosis are at increased risk of amputation. Patients with a high mortality rate after embolectomy are characterised by:[37]

- poor cardiac function;
- associated peripheral vascular disease;
- short duration of symptoms;
- the need for amputation.

The amputation risk appears higher in patients with a longer duration of ischaemia and poor preoperative and postoperative cardiac function.[43] Recently an analysis of preoperative cardiac troponin T has suggested it can be used to predict outcome after embolectomy.[44] Patients with ALI are often elderly and within this group there is a cohort of individuals whose leg problem heralds the end of life. It is important to recognise this group and to offer appropriate palliative care rather than aggressive intervention.[45]

## Conclusions

Although there have been huge changes in the therapeutic options for patients with ALI, there remains debate over the optimal management. Clinical trials in this area are difficult to organise and are often flawed by the great variation in the condition of the patients and their legs. However, further stratification of existing data could help define which occlusions are most suitable for thrombolysis or surgery. A clear comparison between the different drugs available and delivery techniques would help. New drugs will undoubtedly become available with improved safety profiles. In future, thrombolysis combined with other endovascular techniques may enhance its effectiveness.

### Key points

- Patients with ALI have high morbidity and mortality rates.
- Optimal management is based on the severity of the ischaemia at presentation.
- Randomised trials have failed to show superiority of thrombolysis or surgery as primary management for all cases.
- Current research is starting to show which patients benefit most from intra-arterial thrombolysis.
- The best results are achieved when management is agreed jointly by a team consisting of vascular surgeon and interventional radiologist using available expertise and local guidelines.

## References


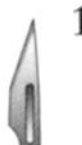

1. Norgeren L, Hiatt WR, Dormandy JA . Inter-Society consensus for the management of peripheral arterial disease. Eur J Vasc Endovasc Surg 2007; 33:S1–75.

   Latest definitive standards for scientific research.
2. Rutherford RB, Flanigan DP, Gupta SK et al. Suggested standards for reports dealing with lower extremity ischemia. J Vasc Surg 1986; 4:80–94.
3. Earnshaw JJ, Hopkinson BR, Makin GS. Acute critical ischaemia of the limb: a prospective evaluation. Eur J Vasc Surg 1990; 4:365–8.
4. Davies B, Braithwaite BD, Birch PA et al. Acute leg ischaemia in Gloucestershire. Br J Surg 1997; 84:504–8.
5. Clason AE, Stonebridge PA, Duncan AJ et al. Acute ischaemia of the lower limb: the effect of centralising vascular surgical services on morbidity and mortality. Br J Surg 1989; 76:592–3.
6. Earnshaw JJ. Demography and aetiology of acute leg ischaemia. Semin Vasc Surg 2001; 14:86–92.
7. Jivegard L, Holm J, Schersten T. Acute limb ischaemia due to arterial embolism or thrombosis: influence of limb ischaemia versus pre-existing cardiac disease on postoperative mortality rate. J Cardiovasc Surg (Torino) 1988; 29:32–6.
8. Blaisdell FW, Steele M, Allen RE. Management of lower extremity arterial ischaemia due to embolism and thrombosis. Surgery 1978; 84:822–34.
9. Braithwaite BD, Tomlinson MA, Walker SR et al. Peripheral thrombolysis for acute-onset claudication. Br J Surg 1999; 86:800–4.
10. Diffin DC, Kandarpa K. Assessment of peripheral intraarterial thrombolysis versus surgical revascularization in acute lower limb ischemia: a review of limb salvage and mortality statistics. J Vasc Intervent Radiol 1996; 7:57–63.
11. Ouriel K, Shortell CK, DeWeese JA et al. A comparison of thrombolytic therapy with operative revascularisation in the initial treatment of acute peripheral arterial ischaemia. J Vasc Surg 1994; 19:1021–30.

    Intra-arterial thrombolysis was associated with a reduction in cardiorespiratory complications and a corresponding increase in survival.
12. The STILE Investigators. Results of a prospective randomized trial evaluating surgery versus thrombolysis for ischaemia of the lower extremity. Ann Surg 1994; 220:251–68.

    There were similar outcomes at 30 days, but patients with ischaemia for less than 14 days had improved amputation-free survival after thrombolysis.

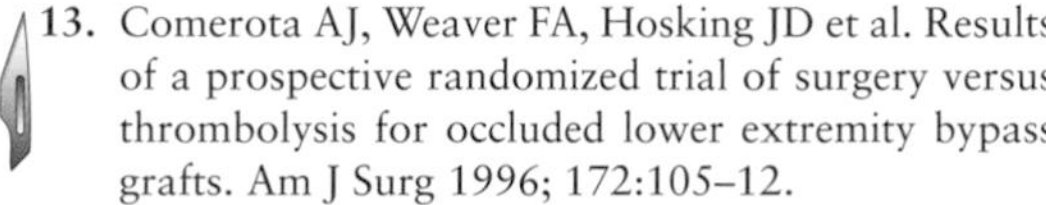

13. Comerota AJ, Weaver FA, Hosking JD et al. Results of a prospective randomized trial of surgery versus thrombolysis for occluded lower extremity bypass grafts. Am J Surg 1996; 172:105–12.

    Patients with ischaemia for less than 14 days did better after surgery, those with shorter-duration ischaemia did better after thrombolysis.

14. Weaver FA, Comerota AJ, Youngblood M et al. Surgical revascularisation versus thrombolysis for nonembolic lower extremity native artery occlusions: results of a prospective randomized trial. J Vasc Surg 1996; 24:513–23.

Surgical revascularisation was more effective and durable than lysis for native vessel occlusions.

15. Ouriel K, Veith FJ, Sasahara AA for the TOPAS investigators. Thrombolysis or peripheral arterial surgery: phase I results. J Vasc Surg 1996; 23:64–75.

This study was designed to find the optimum dose of urokinase for the second phase of the trial.

16. Ouriel K, Veith FJ, Sasahara AA for the TOPAS investigators. A comparison of recombinant urokinase with vascular surgery as initial treatment for acute arterial occlusion of the legs. N Engl J Med 1998; 338:1105–11.

This was the largest of the thrombolysis studies and included 544 patients; the results were similar up to 1 year in both groups.

17. Braithwaite BD, Buckenham TM, Galland RB et al. on behalf of the Thrombolysis Study Group. Prospective randomized trial of high-dose bolus versus low-dose tissue plasminogen activator infusion in the management of acute limb ischaemia. Br J Surg 1997; 84:646–50.

High-dose bolus therapy significantly accelerated thrombolysis without compromising outcome.

18. Yusuf SW, Whitaker SC, Gregson RHS et al. Prospective randomised comparative study of pulse spray and conventional local thrombolysis. Eur J Vasc Endovasc Surg 1995; 10:136–41.

Pulse spray lysis was quicker.

19. Kandarpa K, Chopra PS, Arung JE et al. Intraarterial thrombolysis of lower extremity occlusion: prospective randomized comparison of forced periodic infusion and conventional slow continuous infusion. Radiology 1993; 188:861–7.

There was no difference in success or complication rates but forced periodic infusion was quicker.

20. Plate G, Jansson L, Forssell C. Thrombolysis for acute lower limb ischaemia – a prospective, randomised multicenter study comparing two strategies. Eur J Vasc Endovasc Surg 2006; 31:651–60.

Success rates were similar in the two groups.

21. Cleveland TJ, Cumberland DC, Gaines P. Percutaneous aspiration thromboembolectomy to manage the embolic complications of angioplasty and as an adjunct to thrombolysis. Clin Radiol 1994; 49:549–52.

22. Berridge DC, Gregson RHS, Hopkinson BR et al. Randomized trial of intra-arterial recombinant tissue plasminogen activator, intravenous recombinant tissue plasminogen activator and intra-arterial streptokinase in peripheral thrombolysis. Br J Surg 1991; 78:988–95.

Intra-arterial t-PA was safer and more effective than streptokinase.

23. Haskal ZJ. Mechanical thrombectomy devices for the treatment of acute peripheral arterial occlusions. Rev Cardiovasc Med 2002; 3(Suppl 2):S45–52.

24. Earnshaw JJ, Whitman B, Foy C on behalf of the Thrombolysis Study Group. National Audit of Thrombolysis for Acute Leg Ischaemia (NATALI): clinical factors associated with early outcome. J Vasc Surg 2004; 39:1018–25.

25. Hess H, Mietaschk A, Bruckl R. Peripheral arterial occlusions: a 6-year experience with local low-dose thrombolytic therapy. Radiology 1987; 163:753–8.

26. Eliason JL, Wainess RM, Proctor MC et al. A national and institutional experience in the contemporary treatment of acute lower extremity ischaemia. Ann Surg 2003; 238:382–9.

27. Ouriel K, Shortell CK, Azodo MVU et al. Acute peripheral arterial occlusions: predictors of success in catheter-directed thrombolytic therapy. Radiology 1994; 193:561–6.

28. McNamara TO, Bomberger RA. Factors affecting initial and six month patency rates after intra-arterial thrombolysis with high dose urokinase. Am J Surg 1986; 152:709–12.

29. Durham JD, Rutherford RB. Assessment of long-term efficacy of fibrinolytic therapy in the ischaemic extremity. Semin Intervent Radiol 1992; 9:166–73.

30. Working Party on Thrombolysis in the Management of Limb Ischemia. Thrombolysis in the management of lower limb peripheral arterial occlusion: a consensus document. J Am Coll Cardiol 1998; 81:207–18.

Recommendations from expert surgeons and radiologists.

31. Neary B, Whitman B, Foy C et al. Value of POSSUM physiology scoring to assess the outcome after thrombolysis for acute leg ischaemia. Br J Surg 2001; 88:1344–5.

32. Bosma HW, Jorning PJG. Intraoperative arteriography in arterial embolectomy. Eur J Vasc Surg 1990; 4:469–72.

33. Beard JD, Nyamekye I, Earnshaw JJ et al. Intraoperative streptokinase: a useful adjunct to balloon catheter embolectomy. Br J Surg 1993; 80:21–4.

34. Thompson JF, Beard J, Scott DJA et al. Intraoperative thrombolysis in the management of thrombosed popliteal aneurysm. Br J Surg 1993; 80:858–9.

35. Ernst CB. Fasciotomy in perspective. J Vasc Surg 1989; 9:829–30.

36. Hammarsten J, Holm J, Shersten T. Positive and negative effects of anticoagulant treatment during and after arterial embolectomy. J Cardiovasc Surg 1978; 19:373–9.

37. Ljungman C, Adami H-O, Bergqvist D et al. Risk factors for early lower limb loss after embolectomy for acute arterial occlusion: a population-based case–control study. Br J Surg 1991; 78:1482–5.

38. Campbell, Ridler BM, Szymanska TH. Two year follow-up after acute thromboembolic leg ischaemia: the importance of anticoagulation. Eur J Vasc Endovasc Surg 2000; 19:169–73.

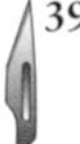
39. de Donato G, Gussoni G, de Donato G. Acute limb ischaemia in elderly patients: can iloprost be useful as an adjuvant to surgery? Results from the ILAILL Study. Eur J Vasc Endovasc Surg 2007; 34:194–8.

**Single trial suggesting that iloprost is beneficial, but may need confirming in other studies.**

40. Ljungman C, Adami H-O, Bergqvist D et al. Time trends in incidence rates of acute, non-traumatic extremity ischaemia: a population based study during a 19-year period. Br J Surg 1991; 78:857–60.

41. Ljungman C, Holmberg L, Bergqvist D et al. Amputation risk and survival after embolectomy for acute arterial ischaemia. Time trends in a defined Swedish population. Eur J Vasc Endovasc Surg 1996; 11:176–82.

42. Campbell WB, Ridler BMF, Symanska TH on behalf of the Vascular Surgical Society of Great Britain and Ireland. Current management of acute leg ischaemia: results of an audit by the Vascular Surgical Society of Great Britain and Ireland. Br J Surg 1998; 85:1498–503.

43. Dreglid EB, Stangeland LB, Eide GE et al. Patient survival and limb prognosis after arterial embolectomy. Eur J Vasc Surg 1987; 1:263–71.

44. Rittoo D, Stahnke M, Lindesay C et al. Prognostic significance of raised cardiac troponin T in patients presenting with acute limb ischaemia. Eur J Vasc Endovasc Surg 2006; 32:500–3.

45. Braithwaite BD, Davies B, Birch PA et al. Management of acute leg ischaemia in the elderly. Br J Surg 1998; 85:217–20.

# 9

# Vascular trauma

Jacobus van Marle
Dirk A. le Roux

## Introduction

Trauma is a major health and social problem and is the main cause of death in people up to the age of 38 years.[1] Fewer than 10% of patients with polytrauma have associated vascular injuries, but these injuries can cause significant morbidity and mortality.[2] The incidence and type of vascular trauma differs between various societies. In most European countries today the majority of vascular trauma is caused by blunt (traffic accidents) and iatrogenic injuries.[3] In South Africa and the USA, injuries are mostly penetrating and have also changed from predominantly stab wounds to injuries caused by firearms.[4]

Complex vascular injuries have a high morbidity and mortality, and a clear understanding of the pathophysiology of vascular trauma and a logical approach to the management of those injuries are essential for a favourable outcome.

## Mechanism of injury

Vascular injuries are classified according to the mechanism of the injury.

### Blunt trauma

Direct trauma to the artery accounts for the majority of blunt vascular injuries. Indirect trauma is usually the result of shearing and distraction forces following dislocation of major joints, displaced long-bone fractures and acceleration/deceleration injuries as seen with high-speed motor vehicle accidents and falls from a height. The usual result of blunt trauma to the arterial wall is disruption of the intima followed by thrombosis (**Fig. 9.1a,b**). The arterial intima is the least elastic layer of the arterial wall and gives way first. This intimal tear may cause immediate obstruction due to an intimal flap or may predispose to thrombosis and delayed obstruction. As the vessel is stretched further, progressive layers of the media are disrupted until the continuity of the vessel is maintained only by the elastic adventitia or there is complete disruption.

### Penetrating trauma

This results in either partial or complete transection of a vessel or penetrating or perforating wounds. Bleeding is often brisk and peripheral flow may be interrupted. The damage caused by stab and low-velocity missile injuries is localised and confined to the tract of the injury. High-velocity missiles cause a cavitation effect, with total tissue destruction around the missile tract surrounded by an area of doubtful tissue viability, all of which results in extensive associated soft-tissue trauma.[5] The shock wave of a high-velocity missile can also cause intimal injury. The vessel is macroscopically intact with minimal bruising, but on opening the vessel there is an intimal tear with superimposed thrombosis.[6] Shotgun injuries cause extensive local tissue destruction with often multiple sites of perforation. Bomb blasts cause complex injuries due to the combination of extensive local tissue trauma, high-velocity fragments and thermal injury.

Iatrogenic injuries are becoming increasingly important and account for more than 40% of vascular trauma in many European countries.[3]

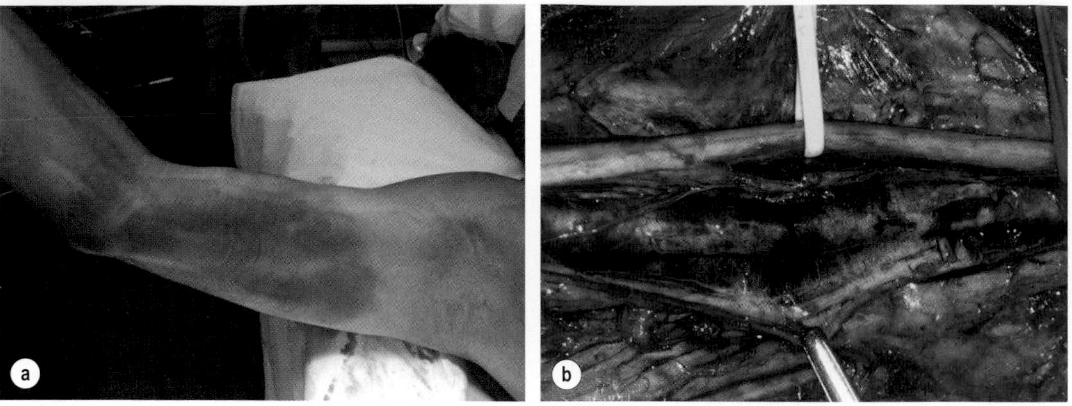

**Figure 9.1** • Blunt injury to the arm **(a)** causing contusion of the brachial artery **(b)**.

## Sequelae of vascular injuries

Vascular injuries have significant sequelae (Box 9.1, **Figs 9.2** and **9.3**). A contused artery may be patent initially but thrombose later. Propagation of clot may cause progressive ischaemia by obstructing essential collaterals. Acute ischaemia leads to nerve myelin degeneration and axial retraction within 4–6 hours, with discoid degeneration of muscle cells at 6 hours and marked impairment of contractility at 12 hours.[7] Most of the muscle impairment is irreversible after 12 hours (see Chapter 8).

Concomitant fractures, dislocations, injuries to accompanying veins and nerves, soft-tissue trauma and contamination of the wound with foreign material serve to compound vascular injury. Other determinants of the final outcome are the level of vascular injury, the quality of the collateral circulation and pre-existing occlusive arterial disease.

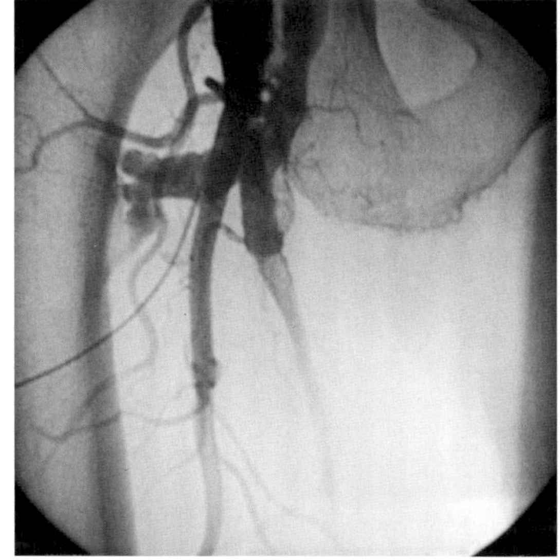

**Figure 9.2** • Arteriovenous fistula of the right femoral vessels following iatrogenic injury after diagnostic cardiac catheterisation.

Box 9.1 • Sequelae of vascular injuries

Acute haemorrhage
- Overt external bleeding
- Contained bleeding (e.g. in muscle compartment)
- Concealed bleeding (e.g. pleural cavity)

Hypovolaemia, shock
Haematoma with or without secondary infection
Delayed bleeding and rebleeding
Thrombosis: acute or delayed
Ischaemia: acute or delayed
Arteriovenous fistula (see Fig. 9.2)
Pseudoaneurysm formation (see Fig. 9.3)

## Clinical assessment

### History

Information regarding the mechanism of the trauma, blood loss prior to hospital admission and underlying vascular disease should be obtained.

### Examination

Initial assessment should be carried out according to advanced trauma life support (ATLS) principles

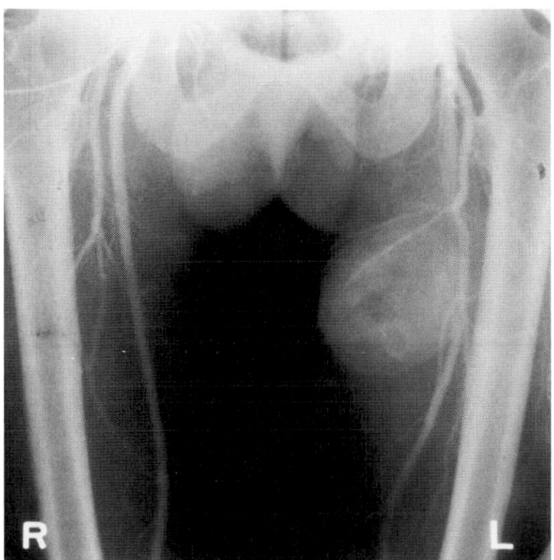


**Figure 9.3** • False aneurysm of the left thigh after gunshot wound.

and life-threatening conditions managed. Vascular injury may present with any of the sequelae listed in Box 9.1. Clinical signs of vascular injuries can be divided into hard and soft signs.

**Hard signs of vascular injury**

- Active pulsatile bleeding.
- Shock with ongoing bleeding.
- Absent distal pulses.
- Symptoms and signs of acute ischaemia.
- Expanding or pulsating haematoma.
- Bruits or thrill over the area of injury.

**Soft signs of vascular injury**

- History of severe bleeding.
- Diminished distal pulse.
- Injury of anatomically related structures.
- Small non-expanding haematoma.
- Multiple fractures and extensive soft-tissue injury.
- Injury in anatomical area of major blood vessel.

Distal pulses may be difficult to evaluate in patients with extensive soft-tissue trauma, swelling and multiple wounds. A diminished or absent pulse is due to arterial occlusion until proven otherwise and should not be attributed to vascular spasm, external compression or any other ill-defined factor.

Signs of acute arterial insufficiency (ischaemia) include pulse deficit (absent/diminished pulse), pain, pallor, paraesthesia and paralysis. Neurological deficit must be evaluated carefully in order to distinguish between ischaemic neuropathy and direct injury to the nerve.

## Diagnosis

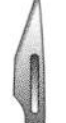

The value and accuracy of a thorough clinical examination in predicting significant vascular injury has been reported in various series.[8]

Arterial Doppler pressure measurement is a useful supplement to the clinical examination. The arterial pressure index (API; systolic arterial pressure in the injured limb divided by systolic pressure in an uninvolved arm) of more than 0.9 reliably excludes significant occult arterial injury.[9]

Special investigations should only be performed in patients who have been adequately resuscitated and who are haemodynamically stable. Haemodynamic instability, active bleeding and an expanding haematoma are indications for immediate surgery.

# Resuscitation and initial management

ATLS guidelines are followed, keeping in mind that the resuscitation of the unstable patient in urgent need of surgery may be best conducted in the operating room.

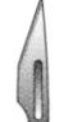

The amount and timing of fluid resuscitation is important. In uncontrolled haemorrhagic shock where bleeding has been temporarily stopped due to hypotension, vasoconstriction and thrombus formation, aggressive fluid resuscitation may lead to increased intravascular pressure, decreased blood viscosity and loss of the haemostatic plug, with resultant increased bleeding and mortality.[10]

Hypotensive resuscitation (permissive hypotension) aims at a systolic blood pressure of between 70 and 90 mmHg to maintain cerebral and renal perfusion until operative control of bleeding has been achieved.

Active bleeding is an indication for urgent exploration, but can usually be temporarily controlled by direct pressure. Blind clamping of vessels in the depth of a wound is contraindicated. Tourniquets should only be used under exceptional circumstances and then only for short periods.

Fractures must be stabilised during the period of resuscitation and diagnostic investigation in order to protect blood vessels and other soft tissue from further trauma. Preliminary reduction of a displaced fracture or dislocation may improve distal circulation.

## Special investigations

### Plain radiography

Plain radiographs are usually taken for associated skeletal injuries. A high index of suspicion for vascular trauma should exist with dislocations and displaced fractures (**Fig. 9.4**). Chest radiography is valuable in patients with chest trauma.

### Arteriography

Arteriography replaced mandatory surgical exploration for exclusion of vascular trauma in the 1980s.

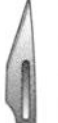

The routine use of arteriography for excluding vascular injury in the absence of hard clinical signs is no longer warranted, especially in extremity trauma.[11]

Arteriography is still indicated for the following conditions in haemodynamically stable patients: multiple fractures, extensive soft-tissue injury, shotgun injuries, zone 1 and 3 neck injuries, thoracic and abdominal injuries.

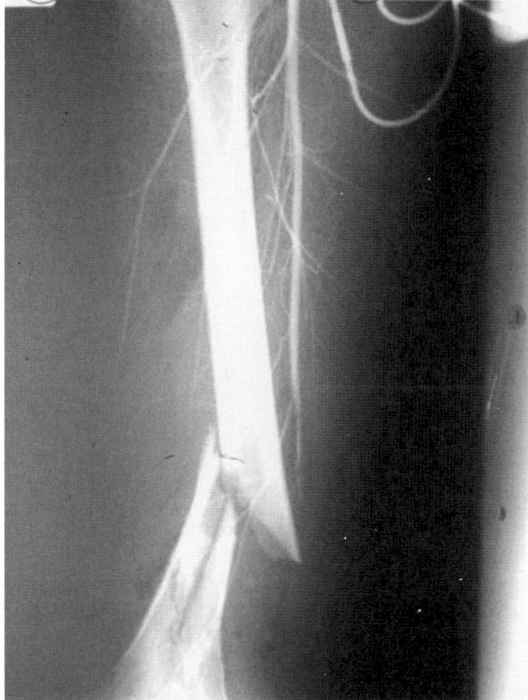

**Figure 9.4** • Displaced fracture of the femur with injury to the superficial femoral artery.

Surgical intervention should not be delayed by arteriography where vascular injury is evident and the patient unstable or the limb is at ischaemic risk. On-table arteriography in the operating room should be performed in vascular injuries to the extremity where surgery cannot be delayed and the additional information is considered valuable.[12]

### Ultrasound

Duplex Doppler examination has been described in the evaluation of extremity vascular trauma and neck and abdominal injuries. It is mostly used as a screening test in the absence of hard signs and for follow-up evaluation in patients managed expectantly.

### Axial imaging

Computed tomographic angiography is valuable in blunt cervical, abdominal and thoracic injuries. The use of magnetic resonance angiography (MRA) in trauma is limited due to time constraints and inaccessibility to the patient during the examination.

## General principles of management of vascular injury

Procedures are performed under general anaesthesia in a well-equipped theatre. Blood products should be available and arrangements for intraoperative autotransfusion should be made where further bleeding is expected. The value of prophylactic antibiotics in vascular surgery is established.

Adequate exposure is vital for obtaining proximal and distal control of injured vessels. This often requires inclusion of adjacent anatomical areas in the operative field, e.g. preparing the neck in thoracic injuries (and vice versa) and the abdomen in groin injuries. An uninjured leg is prepared for possible vein harvesting should bypass be required. Vascular control must be achieved proximally and distally before directly approaching the area of injury. Bleeding may be temporarily arrested by digital compression until clamps have been applied.

In blunt and high-velocity trauma there is often extensive intimal damage, and careful debridement of the vessel is necessary until normal-appearing intima is found (**Fig. 9.5**). Antegrade and retrograde flow should be evaluated. Arteries are cleared of clot by careful passage of embolectomy catheters followed by irrigation with heparin/saline solution.

Vascular repair/reconstruction is completed by a technique suitable to the specific lesion. Simple

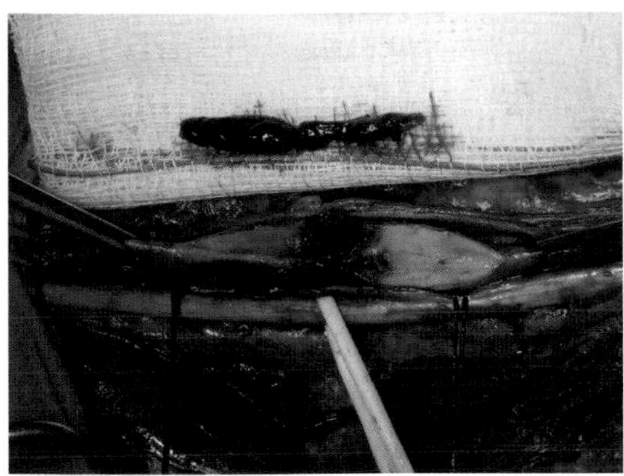

**Figure 9.5** • Intimal damage and thrombosis of the artery due to blunt trauma.

laceration of the vessel wall is repaired by lateral suture, provided it does not lead to stenosis, when patch graft angioplasty is indicated. Where more than 50% of the circumference of a vessel wall is damaged, this area should be excised followed by end-to-end anastomosis. This requires mobilisation of the proximal and distal arterial stumps to achieve approximation without tension. Failing this, an interposition graft is indicated. Although autogenous vein is the preferred conduit for reconstruction, prosthetic material may be used in exceptional circumstances.[13]

Where there is a mismatch in diameter between the vessel that needs to be repaired and the available autogenous vein, two techniques can be employed to manufacture a venous conduit of appropriate size:

1. **Panelled vein graft.** The vein is cut in segments of required length. These segments are opened longitudinally, placed alongside and sutured together using a polypropylene 70 continuous suture. The outer sides of this panel are now sutured together creating a tube of the required length and diameter.
2. **Spiral vein graft.** A length of vein is opened longitudinally and wrapped around a tubular structure of the required diameter (silicon tubing, syringe, etc.) in a spiral fashion with the endothelial surface of the vein on the inside. The sides of the vein are then sutured together.

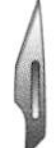

Where complex arterial repair is required resulting in delay in revascularisation, intraluminal shunts can be used to maintain antegrade flow during repair and thereby reduce ischaemic time.[14]

Completion angiography should be performed where possible to document a technically perfect repair and to assess the distal arterial tree. Associated injuries are addressed once vascular repair has been completed. Wound debridement should be performed, with removal of all devitalised and contaminated tissue. Contaminated wounds are left open but the vascular repair must be covered by soft tissue. Repeated wound inspections are performed, with delayed primary suture when the wound is clean.

## Venous injuries

Venous injuries found during exploration for associated arterial injury should be repaired, if the repair itself can be done simply (e.g. lateral suture repair) and only if it will not significantly delay treatment of associated injuries or destabilise the patient's condition. Complex venous repair or bypass should only be attempted if the patient is haemodynamically stable. All veins, including the inferior vena cava (IVC), can be tied off in cases of haemodynamic instability, but with the subsequent risk of venous hypertension, depending on the venous collateral network.

# Endovascular management of vascular trauma

Endovascular procedures have become an integral part of the elective treatment of peripheral vascular disease. The application of these techniques in the injured patient has many potential advantages. General anaesthesia is not required and surgical trauma, with further blood loss, hypothermia, etc., is avoided. It is not necessary to cross-clamp major vessels, preventing distal ischaemia and subsequent reperfusion injury. The main advantage is the option of approaching complex arterial lesions in anatomically challenging locations from a remote site. A difficult exploration in an injured area is avoided, with less potential damage to surrounding structures. Opening a contained haematoma, releasing the tamponade effect and inducing fresh bleeding is also avoided.

Endovascular techniques are increasingly applied in vascular trauma, but there are still certain limitations. These techniques are usually not applicable, mainly due to time constraints, in patients with active bleeding, in unstable patients or where there is end-organ ischaemia. Endovascular techniques should also not be used where there are compression symptoms, infected wounds or where concomitant injuries require open exploration, e.g. penetrating abdominal injuries. There are also technical restrictions, e.g. inability to traverse the lesion by guidewire, where intraluminal clot prevents the safe passage of a guidewire due to the danger of distal embolisation or where luminal discrepancy exists between the proximal and distal involved segments.

Endovascular/interventional techniques are used to manage vascular trauma in three ways:

1. **To obtain haemostasis.** Damaged vessels are embolised using a variety of substances including haemostatic agents (gel foam), coils and balloons. This technique for managing significant bleeding following pelvic fractures has become the standard treatment,[15] and is also a recognised option for treating lesions of non-essential, inaccessible vessels in the cervical, pelvic and limb regions.[16] It is also used to control bleeding due to penetrating and blunt trauma of the liver, kidneys and spleen.[17–19]
2. **To obtain vascular control.** A balloon placed in the damaged vessel at the time of diagnostic angiography can be used to temporarily occlude vessels. It is especially valuable in relatively inaccessible regions where temporary balloon occlusion limits the extent of the exposure to obtain surgical control.[20] This technique is also valuable in managing vascular injuries in zones 1 and 3 of the neck. Occlusion balloons can be placed in the abdominal aorta, proximal subclavian and iliac arteries to prevent exsanguinating bleeding until surgical control is achieved.
3. **For vascular repair.** Covered stentgrafts are used for repairing vessels in anatomically challenging locations to avoid major surgical exposures. Stentgrafts are therefore indicated for injuries of the thoracic aorta, thoracic outlet vessels, internal carotid and vertebral arteries (**Fig. 9.6**).[21–24] This will be discussed in more detail in the relevant sections. Abdominal vascular injuries are usually associated with haemodynamic instability or concomitant bowel injuries requiring laparotomy. Trauma to the extremity vessels are also best addressed by conventional open surgical techniques.

In-stent stenosis, graft migration, stent breakage and endoleaks are well-known complications of stentgraft repair. Durability is therefore of concern in the younger population who are the main victims of trauma. Although early results are promising, long-term follow-up and randomised prospective trials comparing standard surgery with endovascular grafting will be necessary before the generalised use of these devices can be recommended.

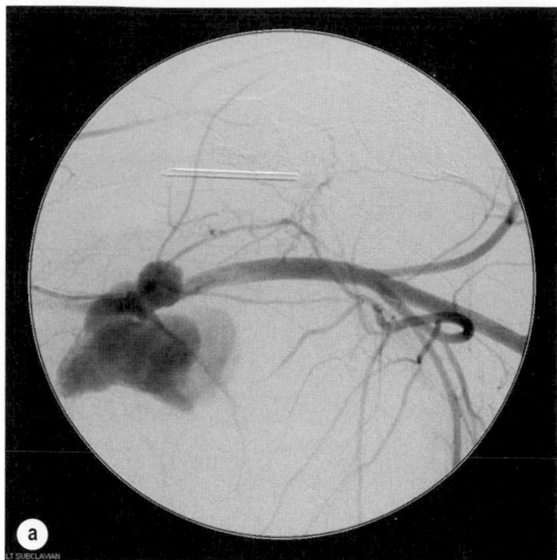


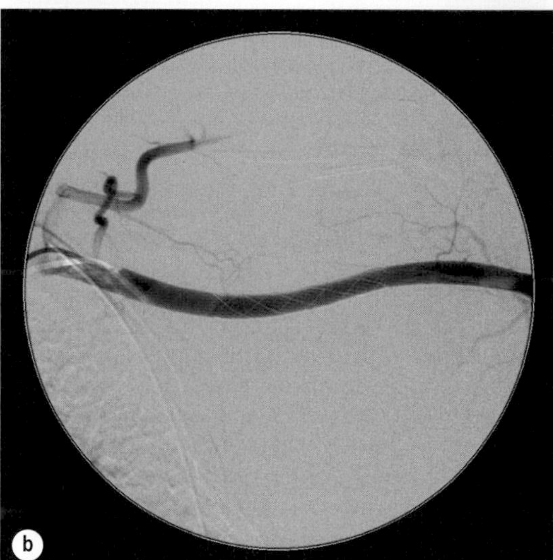


**Figure 9.6** • False aneurysm of left subclavian artery after infraclavicular stab wound **(a)** repaired by means of a covered stentgraft **(b)**.

## Cervical vascular injuries

The cervical vessels are involved in 25% of patients with head or neck trauma and carotid artery injury constitutes 5–10% of all arterial injuries.[25] The mortality and morbidity of these injuries remain high despite advances in diagnosis and treatment. Mortality for carotid injuries ranges from 10% to 31%, with permanent neurological deficit ranging from 16% to 60%.[26,27]

### Mechanism

More than 90% of carotid injuries are caused by penetrating trauma. Blunt trauma is caused by a direct blow to the artery, hyperextension, hyperrotation, or contusion by bone fragments associated with fractures of the mandible, temporal bone or cervical spine.

Penetrating injury may cause partial or complete transection with thrombosis of the vessel or pseudoaneurysm. Pseudoaneurysm may have an acute or delayed onset, with progressive enlargement causing compression of the aerodigestive tract or brachial plexus. An arteriovenous fistula develops where there is adjacent arterial and venous perforation (**Fig. 9.7**). Blunt trauma of the carotid and vertebral arteries may cause a variety of lesions: intimal flaps, intramural haematoma, dissection, complete disruption of arterial wall with pseudoaneurysms, arteriovenous fistulas and total occlusion (**Fig. 9.8**).

Neurological sequelae are caused by hypoperfusion (transected or thrombosed vessels) or embolisation from thrombus, pseudoaneurysm or arteriovenous fistula.

The neck has been divided into three anatomical zones in order to standardise diagnosis and management of cervical vascular injuries (**Fig. 9.9**).

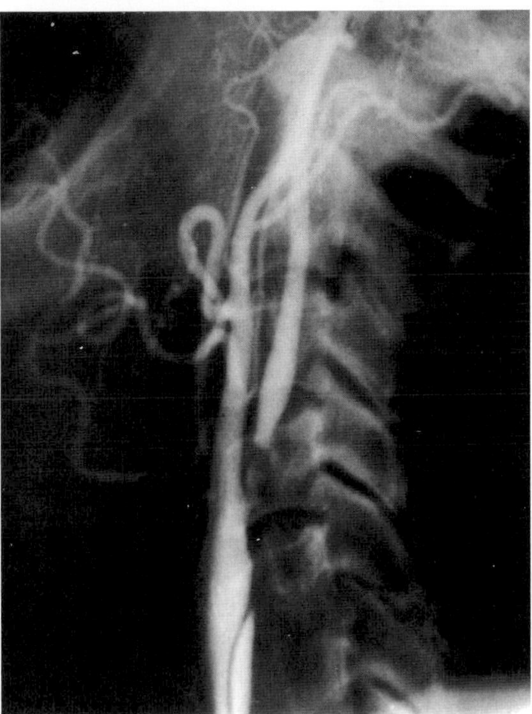

**Figure 9.8** • Dissection of the common carotid artery with blunt trauma to the neck following a motor vehicle accident.

## Clinical signs

Active external bleeding, rapidly expanding cervical haematoma, absent carotid pulse and a bruit or thrill are hard signs indicative of vascular injury. Soft signs that may indicate an associated vascular injury and which warrant further investigation include bleeding from wounds of the neck or the pharynx, a deficit of the superficial temporal artery pulse, ipsilateral Horner's sign, dysfunction of cranial nerves IX–XII, a widened mediastinum, fractures of the skull base and temporal bone, and fractures and dislocation of the cervical spine. Neurological deficit may be present but obscured due to concomitant head injury, shock or the use of alcohol or drugs. About 50% of patients with established blunt injury to the carotid and vertebral arteries could initially be asymptomatic, but 43–58% of these will eventually develop neurological signs after hospital admission.[28]

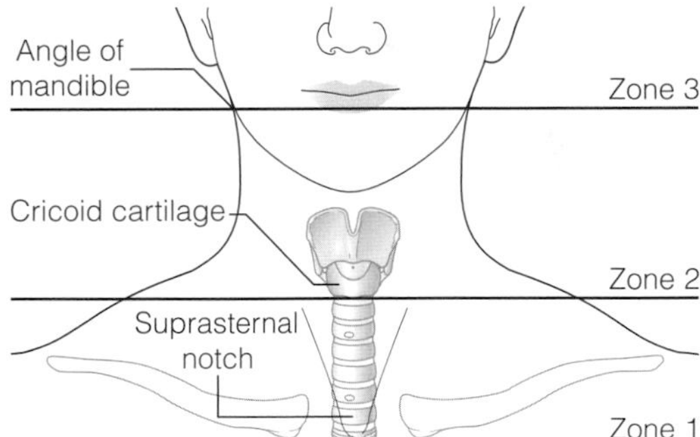


**Figure 9.9** • Zones of the neck.

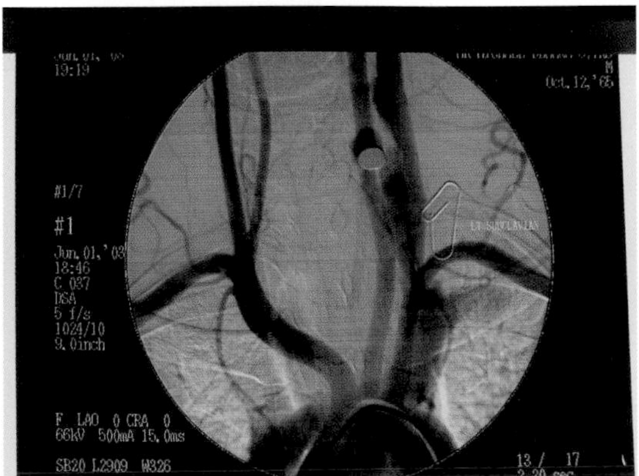


**Figure 9.7** • Arteriovenous fistula between the carotid artery and internal jugular vein caused by gunshot wound.

## Diagnosis

Patients with active bleeding and a compromised airway require immediate exploration, while those who are haemodynamically stable and have a patent airway should undergo further appropriate investigations.

Anteroposterior chest radiography can provide valuable information regarding associated haemothorax or pneumothorax, widening of the mediastinum, surgical emphysema of the neck with concomitant aerodigestive tract injuries, etc.

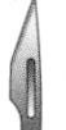

Duplex Doppler examination is extremely useful for investigating zone 2 vascular injuries and is now the preferred diagnostic modality.[29,30]

Duplex scanning has limitations in zones 1 and 3 where arch angiography remains the gold standard for the diagnosis of vascular injuries. It is also important for proper planning of the surgical procedure and evaluation for possible endovascular treatment. Routine angiography is not indicated in asymptomatic patients. It has been shown to offer no benefit over clinical examination and other non-invasive investigations.[31]

Computed tomography (CT) of the brain should be used to investigate patients with associated head trauma, bone injuries of the spine and skull, and neurological deficit. CT of the brain is a good predictor of outcome: patients who have an infarct on initial CT on admission have a high mortality with poor chance of neurological recovery compared with those who have a normal CT on admission. MRA may be valuable in carotid artery and vertebral artery dissection.[32]

## Management

Active external bleeding may be controlled in the emergency room by direct digital compression (a gloved finger in the wound). Where this is not successful, a Foley catheter can be inserted into the wound tract and inflated to obtain balloon tamponade.[33]

Mandatory exploration of all penetrating neck injuries has been replaced by a selective approach.[34] Active pulsatile haemorrhage, expanding cervical haematoma and airway compromise are indications for urgent surgical exploration. Some low-velocity penetrating injuries may be managed expectantly with careful observation, provided there is no active bleeding and the distal circulation is normal. These injuries include intimal defects, small pseudoaneurysms (<5 mm) and non-obstructive intimal flaps. This selective non-operative management is advocated by Stain et al.[34] and Frykberg et al.[35] Robbs, however, recommends that all perforations, as well as small pseudoaneurysms, should be dealt with as the consequences of late haemorrhage are highly significant in terms of morbidity.[36]

The majority of penetrating carotid artery injuries are best managed by primary arterial repair, regardless of contralateral neurological status.[27,37] Neurological deficit is only a contraindication to surgical repair in a deeply comatose patient with a dense neurological deficit, arterial occlusion and a huge infarct on cerebral CT; these patients have poor outcome regardless of treatment.[36] All other patients with associated neurological deficit would benefit from arterial repair, with improved mortality and final neurological status.

Most blunt injuries of the carotid and vertebral arteries result in intimal disruption, with dissection and/or thrombosis, and the immediate goal of management is to restore cerebral perfusion and to prevent embolisation. Systemic anticoagulation is therefore the treatment of choice, because it limits the formation, propagation and/or embolisation of the thrombus. Intravenous heparin is administered in the acute phase, followed by oral anticoagulation for at least 3 months.[38]

## Operative technique

Detailed description of operative technique falls outside the scope of this chapter and the reader is referred to the standard textbooks on operative surgery.[39] The general principles of management include the following:

- The patient should be in a supine position with a bolster between the scapulae and with the neck extended and the head rotated to the contralateral side. The patient must be draped to allow access from the base of the skull to the xiphisternum.
- Zone 2 injuries are explored by the standard carotid incision overlying the anterior border of the sternocleidomastoid muscle.
- Zone 1 injuries may require a median sternotomy.
- Various techniques have been described to improve exposure of the distal internal carotid artery in zone 3 injuries, including subluxation of the mandible, mandibular osteotomy, excision of the styloid process, etc.
- Some authors recommend routine shunting to maintain antegrade flow. We only make use of intraluminal shunts during complicated repairs requiring a graft.
- Where simple repair, i.e. lateral suturing or patch angioplasty, is not feasible, a bypass should be performed. Saphenous vein should preferably be used in the internal carotid artery whereas polytetrafluoroethylene (PTFE) is used to repair the common carotid artery.

- The external carotid artery can be safely ligated if the internal carotid artery is patent. Internal carotid artery ligation is only allowed when the distal vessel is thrombosed with no back-bleeding following extraction of thrombus.
- Minor venous injuries can be managed by lateral suture repair, but complex venous repair is not indicated as there is a high occlusion rate and it increases the magnitude of the operative procedure. Ligation of the jugular vein can be performed without significant sequelae.[40]
- In the presence of associated injuries to the trachea and oesophagus, the vascular repair should be protected by soft-tissue interposition (sternocleidomastoid muscle).

## Vertebral artery injuries

The occurrence of vertebral artery injury is low, with the reported incidence in penetrating neck trauma ranging from 1% to 7.4%. Gunshot wounds are the most common mechanism of injury.[41] Blunt injury of the vertebral artery is even less common and is caused by fractures of the lateral mass of the cervical vertebrae involving the foramen transversarium, vertebral fractures, ligamentous cervical spine injury, or severe and sudden rotation and/or hyperextension of the head. These injuries are seen with motor vehicle accidents and near-hanging injuries and have also been described during extreme chiropractic manipulation.[42]

The majority of patients with vertebral artery injuries have associated injuries of the cervical spine, spinal cord and other vascular structures in the neck or aerodigestive tract.[43] Helical CT angiography has a high sensitivity and specificity for detecting injury of the vertebral artery and is being used increasingly in penetrating neck trauma.[44]

Angiographic embolisation is the treatment of choice in the majority of patients with vertebral artery injuries.[24] Operative management is only indicated for severe active bleeding or when embolisation has failed. Haemodynamically stable patients with a thrombosed vertebral artery do not need any intervention.

A detailed description of surgical approaches to, and management of, vertebral artery injuries is given by Hatzitheofilou et al.[45]

## Endovascular management of cervical injuries

Endovascular therapies are used in two ways in the management of cervical vascular trauma:

1. **Angiographic embolisation.** This is indicated for (a) persistent bleeding from external carotid artery branches (face, oro- and nasopharynx) and (b) injury to the vertebral artery in the osseus vertebral canal.
2. **Covered stentgrafts.** These are indicated for penetrating wounds, arteriovenous fistulas and pseudoaneurysms in (a) surgically inaccessible regions, e.g. distal carotid artery, and (b) in patients where extensive surgical exploration is to be avoided due to multiple trauma, local aggravating factors or high surgical risk due to medical comorbidities. This includes injuries to the brachiocephalectic trunk, and proximal common carotid and subclavian arteries.

# Thoracic vascular injuries

Penetrating trauma is responsible for more than 90% of thoracic vascular injuries.[46] Blunt aortic injuries account for 10–15% of motor vehicle accident fatalities;[47] 70–90% of patients sustaining these injuries will die before reaching a hospital. The site of insertion of the ligamentum arteriosum, just distal to the origin of the left subclavian artery, is the typical point of injury. Frontal deceleration is the most common mechanism causing blunt thoracic injury, but recent studies have also implicated side-impact collisions.[48] Deceleration or compression injury may also involve the brachiocephalic trunk, the pulmonary veins and the vena cava.

## Clinical presentation and initial management

Patients with penetrating thoracic vascular trauma are usually haemodynamically unstable, often with continuing haemorrhage into the pleural cavity or the mediastinum and should be taken for urgent thoracotomy. A precise diagnosis of vascular injury is only made intraoperatively. Patients with blunt thoracic trauma may initially be haemodynamically stable and the injury may not be immediately apparent due to the high incidence of concomitant trauma. The following clinical findings may be associated with underlying thoracic great vessel injury:[49]

- shock/hypotension;
- difference in blood pressure or pulses between the two upper extremities (brachiocephalic trunk or subclavian artery injury);
- difference in blood pressure between upper and lower extremities (pseudocoarctation syndrome);
- expanding haematoma at the thoracic outlet;

- left flail chest;
- infrascapular murmur;
- palpable fracture of the sternum;
- palpable fracture of the thoracic spine;
- external evidence of major chest trauma;
- history indicating deceleration or compression injury to the chest.

## Diagnostic studies

The number and type of diagnostic studies performed will be determined by the patient's haemodynamic stability and general status as well as the type of aortic lesion and concomitant injuries.

### Chest radiography

A frontal chest radiograph is an important screening tool and should be obtained in all patients with penetrating and suspected blunt thoracic trauma. Radio-opaque markers are useful for identifying entrance and exit sites.

A widened mediastinum on chest radiography is associated with more than 90% of thoracic aortic injuries, with a 90% sensitivity and 95% negative predictive value.[50] Other radiographic findings associated with blunt injuries of the descending aorta include the following:[49]

1. Mediastinal findings:
   (a) widening of the mediastinum greater than 8 cm;
   (b) obliteration of the aortic knob contour;
   (c) depression of the left main stem bronchus greater than 140°;
   (d) loss of the paravertebral pleural line;
   (e) lateral displacement of the trachea;
   (f) deviation of a nasogastric tube;
   (g) calcium layering of the aortic knob.
2. Fractures of sternum, first and second ribs and thoracic spine. Scapular and clavicular fractures in a polytrauma patient.
3. Other findings on (a) anteroposterior chest radiograph: apical pleural haematoma (apical cap), massive left haemothorax/effusion, ruptured diaphragm; (b) lateral chest radiograph: anterior displacement of trachea, loss of the aorto-pulmonary window.

Positive findings on chest radiography are indications for further advanced diagnostic studies, mainly angiography and helical CT.

### Angiography

Angiography is indicated in penetrating thoracic trauma for suspected injury to the innominate, carotid or subclavian arteries, but only if the patient is haemodynamically stable.

It provides important information that may influence operative strategy as different thoracic incisions may be required for different injuries. The proximity of a missile trajectory to the brachiocephalic vessels may in itself be an indication for arteriography even without any physical findings of vascular injury.[49]

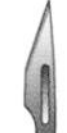

CT angiography/helical CT is no longer used just as a screening procedure to select patients for angiography but is considered a definitive diagnostic procedure that recognises aortic injury and rupture.[51]

CT is less invasive, faster to obtain and more readily available compared with angiography, and has a further advantage that it can provide important information regarding associated lesions. However, the relative inaccessibility to the patient during examination limits its use in unstable patients.

### Other imaging modalities

Transoesophageal echocardiography and intravascular ultrasound may be used as complementary modalities in selected patients, but routine use of these techniques is limited.

## Treatment

Indications for urgent surgery are haemodynamic instability, increasing haemorrhage from chest tubes and radiographic evidence of an expanding haematoma. An initial large volume of blood drained from a chest tube (>1500 mL) or ongoing haemorrhage of more than 200–300 mL/hour may indicate great vessel injury which requires thoracotomy.

The current indications for delayed aortic repair are haemodynamically stable patients with trauma to the central nervous system and coma, respiratory failure from lung contusion, body surface burns, blunt cardiac injury, visceral injury that will undergo non-operative management, retroperitoneal haematoma, contaminated wounds, hypothermia, coagulopathy and other conditions that can be corrected to improve the outcome of operative repair, age 50 years or older and medical comorbidities.[52,53]

Certain minimal aortic lesions, for example intimal defects, small intimal flaps and pseudoaneurysms, may be managed non-operatively with close observation.[54] Patients selected for initial non-operative management should be closely monitored, with systolic blood pressure kept below 120 mmHg or mean arterial pressure below 80 mmHg. Intravenous beta-blockade, titrated to heart rate, was shown to be beneficial in patients with a blunt aortic injury and is currently included in many protocols.[55]

## Surgical repair

Adequate exposure for proximal and distal control of the great vessels is mandatory. Skin preparation should include the anterior neck, thorax, abdomen and a lower extremity. There are four basic surgical approaches:

1. Left anterolateral thoracotomy is indicated for hypotensive unstable patients with an undiagnosed injury. The patient is placed in the supine position and a left anterior thoracotomy performed through the fourth intercostal space. If wider exposure is needed, the incision may be extended medially across the sternum or posteriorly.
2. Left posterolateral thoracotomy through the fourth intercostal space or bed of the fifth rib gives excellent exposure to most of the left hemithorax. The incision may be extended across the sternum or into the abdomen for further exposure to manage accompanying injuries.
3. A median sternotomy is indicated for injuries to the ascending aorta, transverse aortic arch, innominate and proximal carotid and right subclavian arteries. The incision may be extended into the neck to improve exposure of the arch and the brachiocephalic branches.
4. The proximal left subclavian artery is approached via an anterolateral thoracotomy in the third intercostal space with a separate supraclavicular incision to provide distal control if required.

The main controversial issue in the repair of thoracic aortic injuries is whether distal circulatory support should be used. Many authors still advocate a simple clamp-and-sew repair technique without the use of systemic anticoagulation or shunts.[56] However, others advocate the use of distal circulatory support, of which left heart bypass between the left atrium and distal aorta or femoral artery seems to be the most promising.[57] Regardless of the technique used, paraplegia occurs in approximately 8% of patients and no prospective randomised trial has as yet identified the superiority of any single method.[49]

## Endovascular repair

Endovascular stentgrafts have been successfully applied in traumatic aortic injuries, with a high technical success rate and significantly lower morbidity and mortality than open surgery[21] (**Fig. 9.10a,b**).

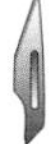

The short-term results of endovascular repair are superior to those reported after open surgery, but long-term results are required to establish whether endovascular repair is a definitive treatment for traumatic aortic rupture.[58]

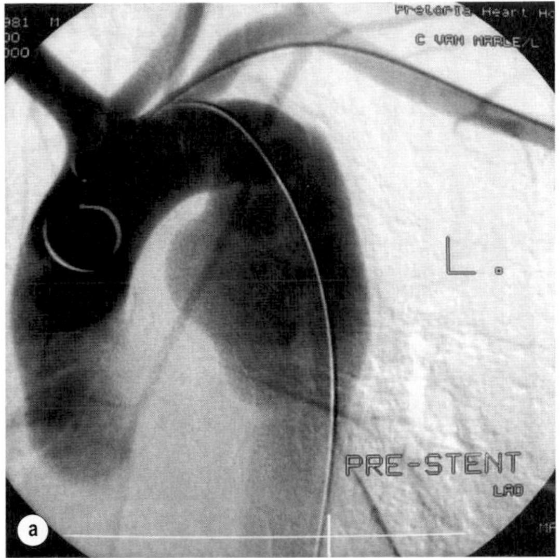


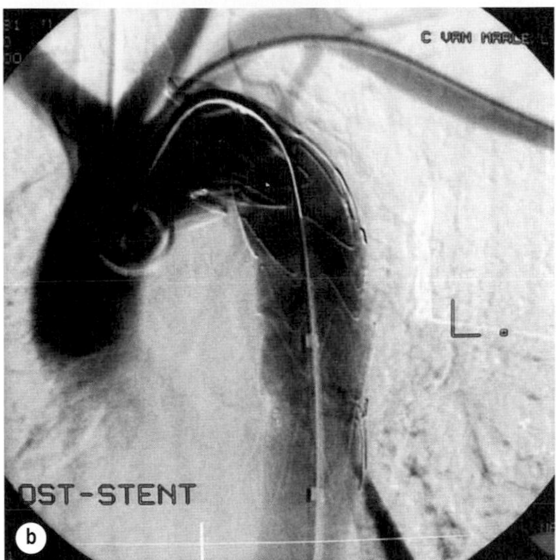


**Figure 9.10** • Thoracic aneurysm after blunt injury to the chest **(a)** treated with a covered aortic stentgraft **(b)**.

# Abdominal vascular injuries

Penetrating trauma accounts for 90–95% of abdominal vascular injuries (**Fig. 9.11**), with a high mortality due to the nature of these injuries as well as associated injuries to other intra-abdominal organs. It is important to consider intra-abdominal injury with all penetrating injuries from the nipples to the upper thighs.

## Diagnosis

The unstable patient with a possible abdominal vascular injury requires immediate surgery. The stable patient should be investigated according to the

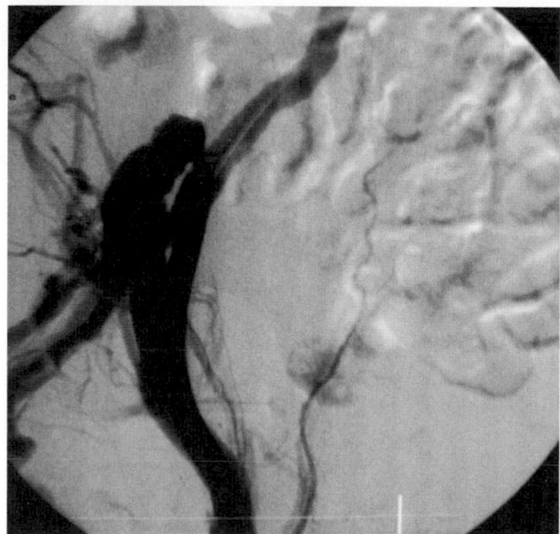

**Figure 9.11** • Fistula of left common iliac artery after a penetrating injury (gunshot wound to the abdomen).

injuries. Plain abdominal radiography using radio-opaque markers is of value in establishing the trajectory of missiles in penetrating injuries. Arteriography and CT have little if any role in the diagnosis of penetrating abdominal vascular injury.[59]

## Management

The abdominal cavity should be entered rapidly at induction of anaesthesia. A generous laparotomy incision is required from xiphisternum to suprapubis. Four-quadrant packing of the abdomen is performed immediately and the proximal aorta is controlled at the diaphragmatic crus. Once the vascular injury is controlled, resuscitation with blood products is started. Bowel injuries are temporarily controlled until vascular repair is effected.

The retroperitoneum is divided into three anatomical zones for purposes of treatment. Central retroperitoneal haematomas (zone 1) are formally explored due to the high incidence of associated major vascular, pancreatic or duodenal injuries, and the high morbidity and mortality if these are overlooked. Flank/perinephric haematomas (zone 2) caused by penetrating injuries should routinely be explored, whilst haematomas caused by blunt trauma can be left alone if they are not expanding and the urogram on contrast-enhanced CT scan is normal. Zone 3 injuries, which are confined to or originate from the pelvis, are most often associated with pelvic fractures. Retroperitoneal haematomas following penetrating injuries are usually explored to exclude major vascular injuries. Haematomas secondary to blunt trauma usually have associated pelvic fractures; exploration can be hazardous and is usually avoided.

Different surgical exposures are used for specific injuries:

- Medial visceral rotation of the left-sided viscera (Mattox manoeuvre), i.e. spleen, tail of the pancreas, left colon and kidney allows access to the supracoeliac aorta, coeliac axis with its branches to the left, superior mesenteric artery (SMA), inferior mesenteric artery, left renal artery and left iliac vessels.
- The Cattell–Braasch or extended Kocher manoeuvre (right-sided medial visceral rotation) allows access to infrahepatic inferior vena cava, right renal vein, portal system and right iliac vessels.
- The infrarenal aorta and IVC are exposed by reflecting the transverse colon superiorly and the small intestine to the right and then dividing the midline retroperitoneum.
- The iliac arteries are exposed via separate incisions lateral to the caecum and sigmoid respectively, avoiding injury to the ureters as they cross the common iliac arteries. The iliac veins may only be accessible after dividing the arteries that lie anterior to them.

### Aortic injury

Direct repair is used for simple lacerations; this should be done transversely to avoid narrowing. An interposition polyester or PTFE graft may be necessary where there is extensive destruction, but should be avoided in a contaminated field.

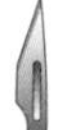

In the 'damage control' scenario, a temporary shunt using a sterile thoracostomy tube can be placed. Definitive repair is performed once the patient is stable and all physiological parameters are normal.[60]

In severe contamination, a graft made of panelled saphenous vein may be used, or the aorta is ligated and an extra-anatomical bypass (e.g. axillo-femoral) performed.[59]

### Iliac injury

These injuries can be repaired using primary suturing or interposition grafting. In the case of severe contamination, ligation and femoro-femoral bypass is an accepted technique.[59] The internal iliac artery may be ligated.

### Visceral artery injury

Injuries to the coeliac trunk and its branches are usually dealt with by primary ligation.[59]

Fullen et al.[61] divided the superior mesenteric artery into four zones; injuries to the first two zones (i.e. SMA trunk to the origin of the middle colic artery) should be repaired. Where primary repair is not possible due to extreme damage, bypass with saphenous vein or PTFE should be performed to maintain midgut viability. Injuries to the inferior mesenteric artery can usually be ligated.

### Renal artery injury

Blunt injury, usually caused by acceleration/deceleration, results in intimal disruption with subsequent thrombosis of the vessels. These injuries should be repaired within 12 hours, since renal viability after this period is very slim.[59] Proximal injuries are approached from the midline through the base of the mesentery, while distal injuries are approached laterally. Repair is performed by either primary repair or interposition grafting using saphenous vein.

### Inferior vena cava and iliac vein injury

The IVC consists of four parts: infrarenal, suprarenal, retrohepatic and intrapericardial. The retrohepatic and intrapericardial portions are usually affected by blunt trauma. Approximately 50% of patients die before reaching hospital and the in-hospital mortality ranges between 20% and 57%.[62]

Wounds in the infrahepatic IVC can be temporarily controlled by means of digital pressure or intraluminal balloon catheters. When clamps are applied, one should be aware of the abundant lumbar collateral circulation. Repair is effected by means of lateral suture or, when there are large defects, even prosthetic material. The anterior laceration in a through-and-through lesion may need to be extended so that the posterior defect can be repaired first. In dire attempts to save an exsanguinating patient this part of the IVC may be ligated. The same treatment algorithm applies to injuries to the common and external iliac veins.

The retrohepatic IVC should be approached with extreme caution and if haemorrhage can be controlled with packing this should be the method of treatment. Various strategies to repair these injuries have been described but the prognosis is still dismal, with a reported mortality of 70–90%.[63] The Shrock shunt, which is inserted through the right atrium, can be used to control these injuries temporarily. We use a modified technique by inserting an endotracheal tube through the infrahepatic IVC and inflating the balloon in the right atrium. Total hepatic isolation (Heany manoeuvre) is associated with a high mortality, especially in an exsanguinated patient. Venous repair is by means of ligation of hepatic veins or direct repair.

### Pelvic vascular injury

Haemorrhage is the primary cause of death in patients with pelvic fractures. The major sources of bleeding are branches of the internal iliac artery and vein, bone and soft tissues. Bleeding can usually be controlled by external stabilisation of the pelvic ring and then packing. Persistent bleeding from branches of the internal iliac artery can be treated with transcatheter embolisation.[15]

# Extremity vascular trauma

The incidence of peripheral vascular injury depends on the extent and type of trauma, ranging from 0.6–3.6% for isolated extremity fractures to 25–30% for all penetrating injuries of the extremities.[2] The risk of limb loss is greatest following blunt trauma and injuries from high-velocity missiles or close-range shotgun wounds.

## Diagnosis

Any extremity injury warrants a complete physical examination of the injured extremity and distal vessels. The absence of hard signs of vascular injury reliably excludes surgically significant arterial injury and does not require arteriography.[64] Arteriography for proximity injury is indicated only in patients with shotgun injuries and multiple fractures (**Fig. 9.12**).[65]

Although ischaemia may not be present initially, it may develop rapidly if thrombosis supervenes. The occurrence of delayed thrombosis stresses the importance of regular reassessment of the peripheral circulation for at least 24 hours after orthopaedic injury. There may be a role for duplex Doppler studies in patients with soft signs of vascular injury or with proximity injuries.[66]

## General principles of management

- Restoration of perfusion to an extremity with an arterial injury should generally be performed in less than 6 hours in order to maximise limb salvage.
- Non-operative observation of asymptomatic non-occlusive arterial injuries is acceptable. These injuries can be defined as small pseudoaneurysms, intimal flaps or irregularities, small arteriovenous fistulas, and haemodynamic insignificant narrowings of the vessels. Should subsequent repair of these injuries be required, it can be done without significant increase in morbidity.[8]
- Simple arterial repairs do better than grafts. If complex repair is required, vein grafts appear to be the best choice.[67] PTFE is an acceptable conduit when no vein is available and may even be used in a contaminated field.[13] Effort should be made to cover the graft with soft tissue.

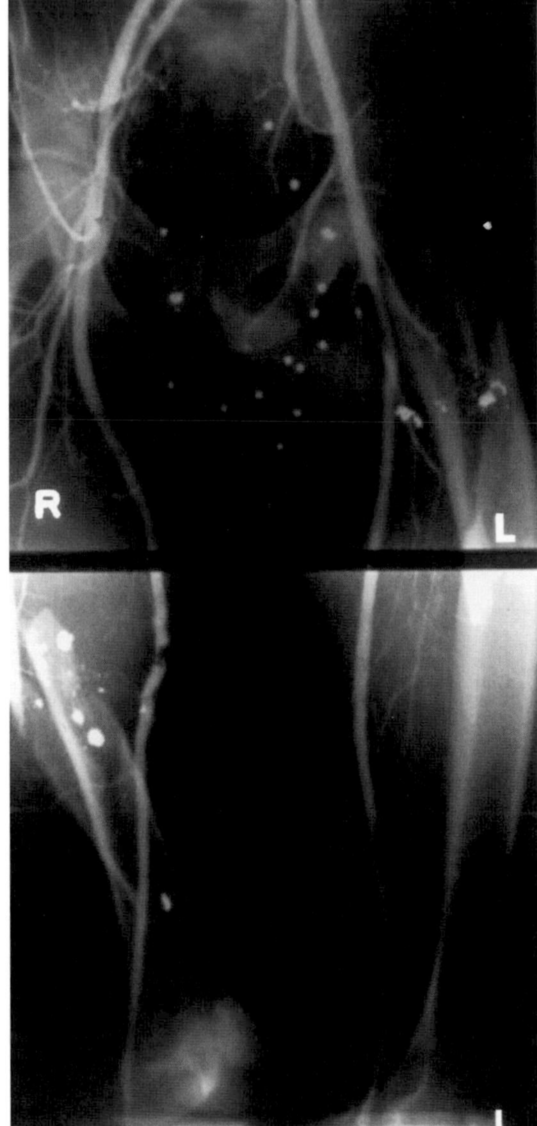


**Figure 9.12** • Arteriogram of the pelvis and thighs to assess level of arterial injury after shotgun wound.

- Temporary shunting is valuable for maintaining antegrade flow in order to allow stabilisation of unstable fractures and/or dislocations prior to definitive arterial repair (**Fig. 9.13**).[14]
- Early four-compartment lower leg fasciotomy should be applied liberally. Indications for fasciotomy include (i) ischaemic time greater than 4–6 hours, (ii) signs of acute ischaemia, (iii) extensive soft-tissue injuries, (iv) combined arterial and venous injuries, (v) intracompartmental bleeding and (vi) increased compartmental pressure.

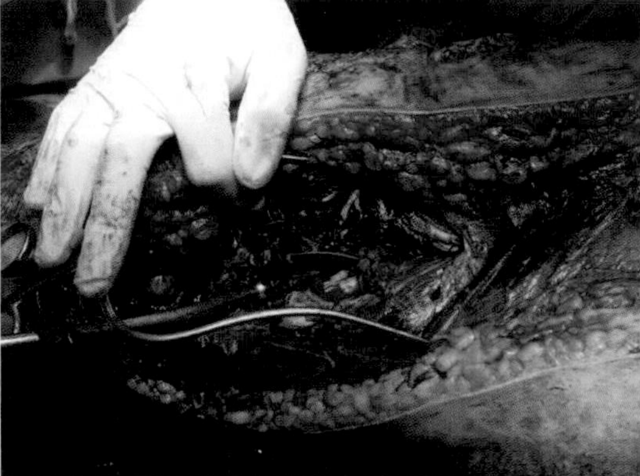

**Figure 9.13** • Temporary shunt in right superficial femoral artery, allowing distal perfusion while external fixator is applied to the femur, following a motorcycle accident.

Measurement of compartment pressures is an important adjunct, and must be done in all compartments. Pressures should be interpreted in the context of each individual patient, because tissue perfusion is a balance between compartment pressure and blood pressure. Acceptable compartment pressures have been defined as absolute compartment pressures of less than 20 mmHg and at least 30 mmHg less than mean arterial pressure.[68]

- Completion arteriogram should be performed after arterial repair to assess patency and technical perfection of the repair.
- Although amputation rates increase with longer ischaemia times, quantifying the relationship is difficult, because amputation rates also depend on other factors such as extent of soft-tissue damage, the capacity of collaterals, pre-existing arterial disease and the vessels injured.[69]
- In certain cases primary amputation may be considered. Scoring systems such as the mangled extremity severity score (MESS) have been developed to help predict outcome of limb salvage procedures.[70] A MESS score of 7 or more has a predicted amputation rate of 100%. Given the significance of amputation, delaying the procedure even by a day or two is preferred as it allows careful examination of the limb and discussion with the patient and family.
- Measures should be taken to protect against the systemic effects of reperfusion injury and subsequent renal damage. A diuresis of at least 1.5–2 mL/kg per hour is maintained with the administration of adequate volumes of

normal saline. Mannitol, which has a diuretic as well as a radical scavenger effect, is added. Urine is alkalinised by administering 8.5% sodium bicarbonate to prevent precipitation of myoglobin crystals in the renal tubuli. Measures to treat hyperkalaemia may be required. Serum myoglobin levels should be monitored regularly.

## Vascular injuries to the upper extremity (Fig. 9.14)

The majority of injuries are to the brachial artery, and 90% of injuries are due to penetrating trauma.[71] Upper extremity vascular injuries are usually not life-threatening but significant morbidity may occur. Return of function is often related to associated nerve injury. Venous injuries to the arm rarely require repair and even injuries to the brachial and axillary veins may be ligated because the collateral venous network is extensive.

### Subclavian and axillary injuries

All patients with periclavicular trauma should be evaluated for possible vascular injury. Most of these injuries are caused by penetrating trauma. The presence of a peripheral pulse does not reliably exclude significant proximal arterial injury. A difference in blood pressure of more than 20 mmHg between the upper limbs or an API of less than 0.9 warrants further investigation. The brachial plexus is injured in about one-third of patients with subclavian or axillary artery injuries due to the anatomical proximity of the neurovascular structures. A thorough neurological assessment should be performed.

Duplex ultrasound reliably assesses arterial and venous injuries but has certain limitations, for example visualising the origin of the subclavian artery.[72] Arteriography has a diagnostic role in evaluating superior mediastinal injuries or where duplex is inconclusive, and also has a therapeutic role in embolisation or stentgraft repair.

Where surgical repair is required, the neck and chest should be included in the operative field. The patient is placed supine and the arm is draped free and abducted to 30°. The head is turned to the other side. The standard incision starts at the sternoclavicular joint and extends over the medial half of the clavicle, curving over the deltopectoral groove. For proximal right subclavian injuries this incision can be combined with a median sternotomy. The proximal left subclavian artery is approached via a left anterior thoracotomy through the third intercostal space. The so-called 'trapdoor' incision (supraclavicular incision, upper third median sternotomy and left anterior thoracotomy) is not recommended due to significant postoperative morbidity.

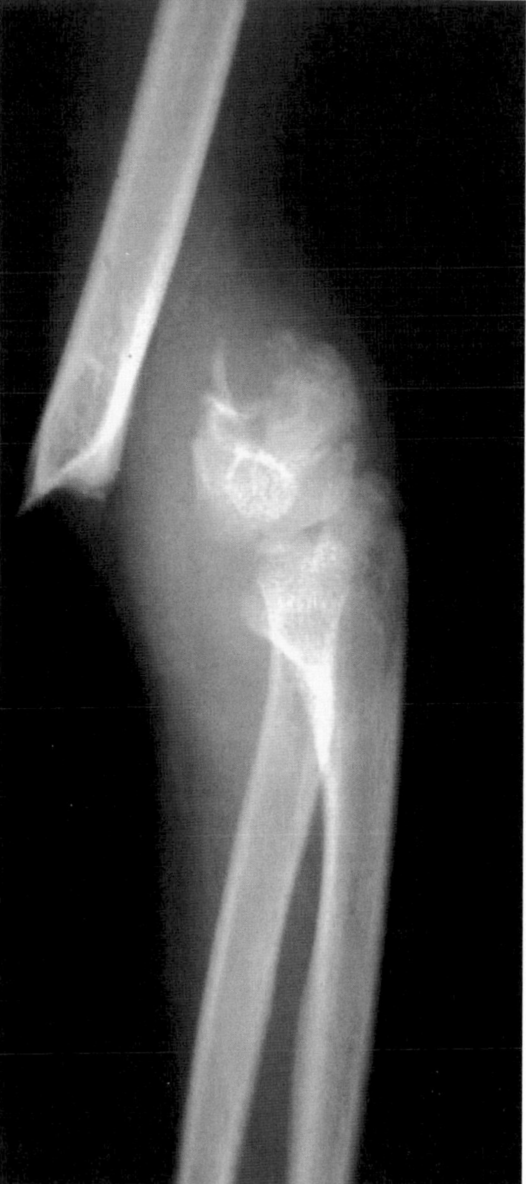

**Figure 9.14** • Fractures of the supracondylar humerus are often associated with vascular injuries and should alert the physician to the possibility of a vascular injury.

The axillary artery is exposed through an infraclavicular incision between the clavicular and sternal parts of the pectoralis major muscle. Dividing the clavicle should be avoided whenever possible due to postoperative morbidity.

Promising results have been obtained with endovascular repair of pseudoaneurysms and arteriovenous fistulas in selected patients[22] (**Fig. 9.15a,b**).

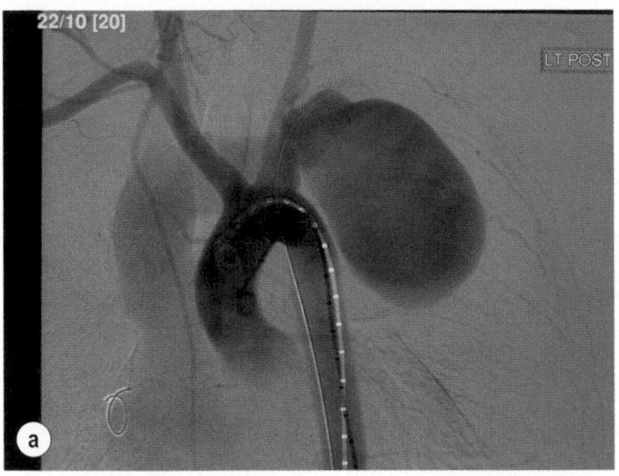


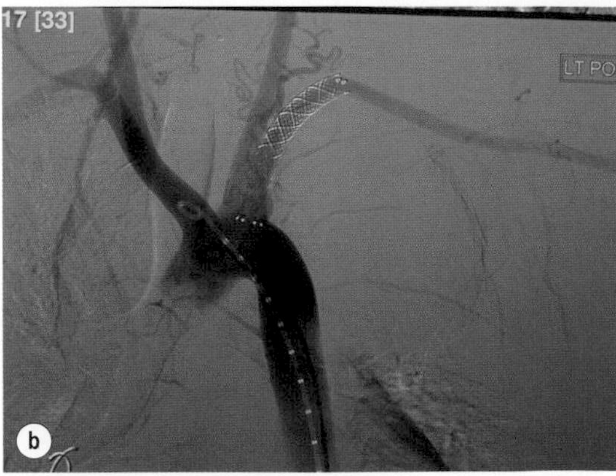


**Figure 9.15** • Arteriovenous fistula of the subclavian artery **(a)** repaired by stentgraft **(b)**.

## Vascular injuries to the lower limb

These injuries are often associated with skeletal injuries, of which posterior dislocation of the knee, proximal tibial fractures and supracondylar femur fractures are the most common. Immediate arterial repair should be performed when the skeletal injury is stable and not significantly displaced. When there is instability or severe displacement or where extreme orthopaedic manipulation is anticipated, a temporary shunt should be placed to restore blood flow while the orthopaedic repair is completed, after which definite arterial repair is performed.

Injuries to the femoral artery are usually clinically apparent and tend to result from penetrating trauma. Patients may have significant exsanguination from arterial injuries, which should be controlled with direct pressure.

### Femoral vascular injuries

Bleeding from the femoral triangle can be difficult to control, particularly if both the artery and vein are injured. Blind clamping in this area is strongly discouraged because of the danger of injuring adjacent nerves and vessels. The suprainguinal region can be entered through a separate incision above the inguinal ligament to obtain proximal control of vessels.

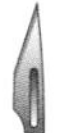

Common femoral artery injuries should always be repaired as ligation has a 50% amputation rate.[69]

Effort should be made to also repair the common femoral vein.

### Popliteal vascular injury

The lower leg is almost totally dependent on the popliteal artery. An amputation rate of up to 16% after popliteal artery injury has been reported in a recent series.[69] The association between posterior knee dislocation and popliteal artery disruption is well known (**Fig. 9.16**). All patients with posterior knee dislocations should have a complete neurovascular examination of the affected limb. Most popliteal artery injuries present with hard signs of arterial injury. The absence of hard signs is usually sufficient to rule out injuries to the popliteal artery.[73]

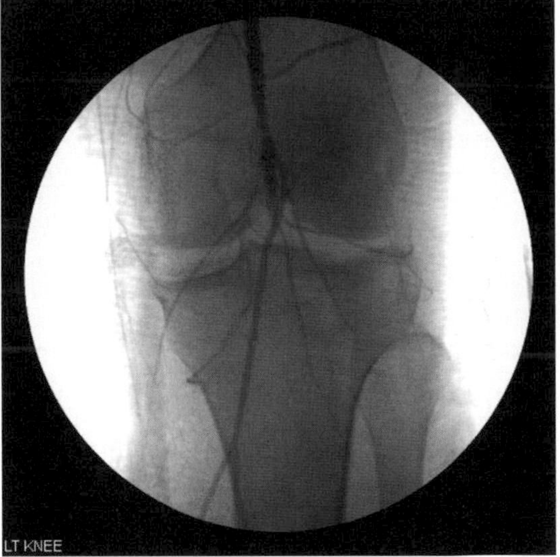


**Figure 9.16** • Popliteal artery injury after posterior dislocation of the left knee.

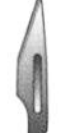

Selective arteriography following knee dislocation is safe as there is a strong correlation between results of serial physical examinations and the need for arteriography. Patients who are managed expectantly should be closely observed, with regular reassessment of the peripheral circulation.[74]

Injury to popliteal veins should be repaired in order to minimise postoperative swelling and compartment syndrome and to improve the patency of arterial repairs.

Compartment syndrome is a major risk factor for amputation following popliteal artery injury.[70] There is evidence that fasciotomy performed at the time of arterial repair, but before the development of compartment syndrome (prophylactic fasciotomy), may lower amputation rates, particularly in patients with long preoperative delays, extensive injuries, injuries of the artery and vein, and venous injuries treated with ligation.[75]

Single tibial vessels may be ligated if there is documented collateral flow distally.

## Key points

- A high index of suspicion should be maintained regarding possible vascular injuries in the trauma patient.
- A thorough clinical examination is accurate in predicting significant vascular injury.
- Special investigations should only be performed in adequately resuscitated and haemodynamically stable patients.
- Haemodynamic instability, active bleeding and an expanding haematoma are indications for immediate surgery.
- The absence of hard signs of arterial injury justifies an expectant non-operative approach with careful observation.
- Restoration of arterial blood supply should be achieved as soon as possible; temporary intra-arterial shunts are valuable in this regard.
- Adequate surgical exposure is vital for proper management of vascular injuries.
- Fasciotomy should be applied liberally in lower-extremity vascular trauma.
- Endovascular treatment is useful in managing arterial lesions in anatomically challenging locations and is currently indicated for injuries of the descending thoracic aorta, proximal aortic arch branches, and distal internal carotid and vertebral arteries.

## References


1. Trunkey DD. Overview of trauma. Surg Clin North Am 1982; 62:3–7.
2. Herberer G, Becker HM, Ditmer H et al. Vascular injuries in polytrauma. World J Surg 1983; 7:68–79.
3. Fingerhut A, Leppäniemi AK, Androulakis GA et al. The European experience with vascular injuries. Surg Clin North Am 2002; 82:175–88.
4. Bowley DMG, Degiannis E, Goosen J et al. Penetrating vascular trauma in Johannesburg, South Africa. Surg Clin North Am 2002; 82:221–36.
5. Levien LJ. Ballistics of bullet injury. In: Champion HR, Robbs JV, Trunkey D (eds) Robb and Smith's operative surgery, 4th edn. London: Butterworths, 1989; pp. 106–10.
6. Robbs JV. Basic principles in the surgical management of vascular trauma. In: Greenhalgh RM (ed.) Vascular and endovascular techniques, 4th edn. London: WB Saunders, 2001; pp. 455–65.
7. Malan E, Taltoni G. Physio- and anatomo-pathology of acute ischaemia of the extremity. J Cardiovasc Surg (Torino) 1963; 4:212–25.

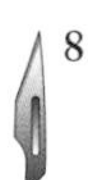

8. Dennis JW, Frykberg ER, Veldenz HC et al. Validation of non-operative management of occult vascular injuries and accuracy of physical examination alone in penetrating extremity trauma: 5–10 year follow up. J Trauma 1998; 44:243–53.

**A prospective study with 10-year follow-up proving the accuracy of clinical assessment and conservative management of occult vascular trauma.**

9. Johansen K, Lynch K. Non-invasive vascular tests reliably exclude occult arterial trauma in injured extremities. J Trauma 1991; 31:515–22.

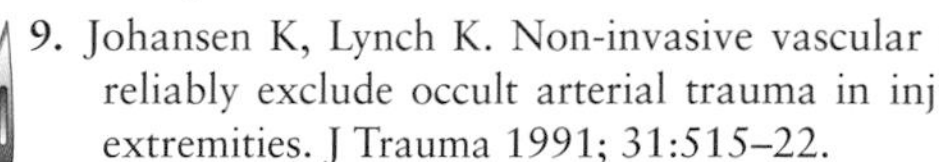

**In this prospective study it was shown that an API of more than 0.9 has a negative predictive value of 99% for excluding significant arterial trauma. Reserving arteriography for limbs with an API of less than 0.9 is safe, accurate and cost-effective.**

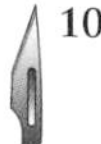

10. Bickell WH, Wall MJ, Pepe PE et al. Immediate vs delayed fluid resuscitation for hypotensive patients with penetrating torso injuries. N Engl J Med 1994; 331:1105–9.

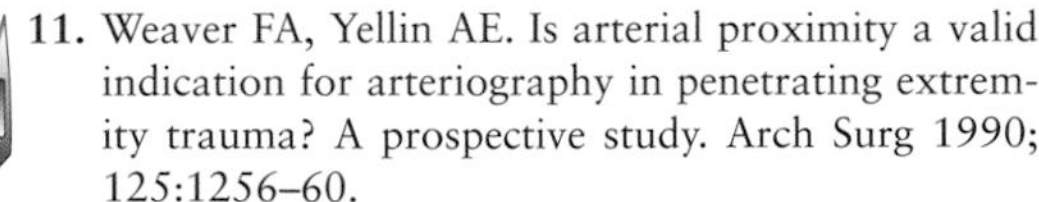

In a randomised controlled trial of patients with penetrating torso injuries, reduced mortality and complications were seen when fluid resuscitation was delayed until haemorrhage was controlled.

11. Weaver FA, Yellin AE. Is arterial proximity a valid indication for arteriography in penetrating extremity trauma? A prospective study. Arch Surg 1990; 125:1256–60.

    In this prospective study of 373 patients with penetrating extremity trauma it was found that arteriography rarely identified significant arterial injury in the absence of clinical signs, and that its routine use was not justified.

12. O'Gorman RB, Feliciano DV. Emergency centre arteriography in the evaluation of suspected peripheral vascular injuries. Arch Surg 1984; 119:568–73.
13. Shah DM, Leather RP, Carson JD et al. Polytetrafluoro-ethylene grafts in the rapid reconstruction of acute contaminated peripheral vascular injuries. Am J Surg 1984; 148:229–33.
14. Barros D'Sa AAB. Complex vascular and orthopedic injuries. J Bone Joint Surg 1992; 74:176–8.

    This paper discusses the problems encountered with, and management of, complex vascular and orthopaedic injuries, advocating the use of temporary arterial and venous shunts for improving outcome.

15. Panetta T, Sclafani SJA, Goldstein AS et al. Percutaneous transcatheter embolization for massive bleeding from pelvic fractures. J Trauma 1985; 25:1021–9.
16. Coldwell DM, Stokes KR, Jakes WF. Embolotherapy: agents, clinical applications and techniques. Radiographics 1994; 14:623–43.
17. Mervis SE, Pais SO. Trauma radiology: part 3. Diagnostic and therapeutic angiography in trauma. Intensive Care Med 1994; 9:244–56.
18. Carrillo EH, Spain DA, Wohltmann D et al. Interventional techniques are useful adjuncts in nonoperative management of hepatic injuries. J Trauma 1999; 46:619–22.
19. Sclafani SJ, Shafton GW, Scalea TM et al. Non-operative salvage of CT diagnosed splenic injury: utilization of angiography for triage and embolization for hemostases. J Trauma 1995; 39:818–25.
20. Scalea TM, Sclafani SJ. Angiographically placed balloons for arterial control: a description of a technique. J Trauma 1991; 31:1671–77.
21. Lachat M, Phammatter T, Witzke H et al. Acute traumatic aortic rupture: early stentgraft repair. Eur J Cardiothorac Surg 2002; 21:956–63.
22. Du Toit DF, Strauss DC, Blaszczyk M et al. Endovascular treatment of penetrating thoracic outlet arterial injuries. Eur J Vasc Endovasc Surg 2000; 19:489–95.

    The authors give an overview of the clinical problem and discuss the technique used.

23. Gomez CR, May AK, Terry JB et al. Endovascular therapy of traumatic injuries of the extracranial cerebral arteries. Crit Care Clin 1999; 15:789–809.
24. Demetriades D, Theodorou D, Asensio J. Management options in vertebral arteries injuries. Br J Surg 1996; 83:83–86.
25. Kumar SR, Weaver FA, Yellin AE. Cervical vascular injuries: carotid and jugular venous injuries. Surg Clin North Am 2001; 81:1331–44.
26. McKevitt EC, Kirkpatrick AW, Vertisi L et al. Blunt vascular neck injuries: diagnosis and outcomes of extra-cranial vessel injury. J Trauma 2002; 53:-472–6.
27. Weaver FA, Yellin AE, Wagner WH et al. The role of arterial reconstruction in penetrating carotid injuries. Arch Surg 1988; 123:1106–11.
28. Biffl WL, Moore EE, Offner PJ et al. Blunt carotid and vertebral arterial injuries. World J Surg 2001; 25:1036–43.
29. Fry WR, Dot JA, Smith RS et al. Duplex scanning replaces arteriography and operative exploration in the diagnosis of potential cervical vascular injury. Am J Surg 1994; 168:693–5.
30. Corr P, Abdool-Carim AT, Robbs J. Colour-flow ultrasound in the detection of penetrating vascular injuries of the neck. S Afr Med J 1999; 80:644–6.

    This prospective study demonstrates the sensitivity of colour-flow ultrasound as a screening investigation to detect vascular injuries following penetrating neck trauma.

31. Demetriades D, Charalambides D, Lakhoo M. Physical examination and selective conservative management in patients with penetrating injuries of the neck. Br J Surg 1993; 80:1534–36.
32. Levy C, Laissy JP, Raveau V et al. Carotid and vertebral artery dissections: three-dimensional time-of-flight MR angiography and MR imaging vs conventional angiography. Radiology 1994; 190:97–103.
33. Gilroy D, Lakhoo M, Sharalambides D et al. Control of life-threatening haemorage from the neck: a new indication for balloon tamponade. Injury 1992; 23:557–9.
34. Stain SC, Yellin AE, Weaver FA et al. Selective management of non-occlusive arterial injuries. Arch Surg 1989; 124:1136–1140.
35. Frykberg ER, Crump JM, Dennis JW et al. Nonoperative observation of clinically occult arterial injuries: a prospective evaluation. Surgery 1991; 109:85–96.
36. Robbs JV. Penetrating injury to the blood vessels of the neck and mediastinum. In: Branchereai A, Jacobs M (eds) Vascular emergencies. New York: Futura, 2003; pp. 39–48.
37. Robbs JV, Human RR, Rajaruthnam P et al. Neurologic deficit and injuries involving the neck arteries. Br J Surg 1983; 70:220–2.
38. Fabian TC, Pattern JH Jr, Croce MA et al. Blunt carotid injury. Importance of early diagnosis and anticoagulation therapy. Ann Surg 1996; 223:513–25.

39. Robbs JV. Injuries to the vessels of the neck and superior mediastinum. In: Champion HR, Robbs JV, Trunky D (eds) Robb and Smith's operative surgery, 4th edn. London: Butterworths, 1989; pp. 529–38.

40. Nair R, Robbs JV, Muckart D. Management of penetrating cervico-mediastinal venous trauma. Eur J Vasc Endovasc Surg 2000; 19:65–9.

41. Demetriades D, Theodorou D, Cornwill E et al. Evaluation of penetrating injuries of the neck: prospective study of 223 patients. World J Surg 1997; 21:41–8.

42. Nadgir RN, Loevner LA, Ahmed T et al. Simultaneous internal carotid and vertebral artery dissection following chiropractic manipulation: case report and review of the literature. Neuroradiology 2003; 45:311–14.

43. Biffl WL, Moore E, Elliot J et al. The devastating potential of blunt vertebral artery injuries. Ann Surg 2000; 231:672–81.

44. Munera F, Solo J, Palacio D et al. Diagnosis of arterial injuries caused by penetrating trauma to the neck: comparison of helical CT angiography and conventional angiography. Radiology 2000; 216:556–62.

45. Hatzitheofilou C, Demetriades D, Melissas J et al. Surgical approaches to vertebral artery injuries. Br J Surg 1988; 75:234–7.

46. Mattox KL, Feliciano DV, Burch J et al. Five thousand seven hundred and sixty cardiovascular injuries in 4459 patients. Epidemiologic evolution 1958–1978. Ann Surg 1989; 209:698–707.

47. Williams JS, Graff JA, Uku JM et al. Aortic injury in the vehicular trauma. Ann Thorac Surg 1994; 57:726–30.

48. Katyal D, McLellan BA, Brenneman FD et al. Lateral impact motor vehicle collisions: significant cause for blunt traumatic rupture of the thoracic aorta. J Trauma 1997; 42:769–72.

49. Wall MJ, Hirshberg AH, Le Maire SA et al. Thoracic aortic and thoracic vascular injuries. Surg Clin North Am 2001; 81:1375–93.

50. Patel NH, Stephens KE, Mirvis SE et al. Imaging of acute thoracic aortic injury due to blunt trauma: a review. Radiology 1998; 209:335–48.

51. Gavant ML, Menke PG, Fabian T et al. Blunt traumatic aortic rupture: detection with helical CT of the chest. Radiology 1995; 197:125–33.

Helical CT is compared to conventional arteriography in a series of 1518 patients with blunt chest trauma. CT sensitivity and specificity were 100% and 82% respectively vs. 94% and 96% for conventional arteriography.

52. Magissano R, Nathens A, Alexandrova NA et al. Traumatic rupture of the thoracic aorta: should one always operate immediately? Ann Vasc Surg 1995; 9:44–52.

53. Walker WA, Pate JW. Medical management of acute traumatic rupture of the aorta. Ann Thorac Surg 1990; 50:965–7.

54. Fischer RG, Oria RA, Mattox KL et al. Conservative management of aortic lacerations due to blunt trauma. J Trauma 1990; 30:1562–6.

55. Aronstam EN, Domez AC, O'Connell J et al. Recent surgical and pharmacological experience with acute dissecting and traumatic aneurysms. J Thorac Cardiovasc Surg 1970; 59:231–8.

56. Sweeney MS, Young DH, Frasier OH et al. Traumatic aortic transsections: eight year experience with a 'clamp-sew' technique. Ann Thorac Surg 1997; 64:384–9.

57. Read RA, Moore EE, Moore FA et al. Partial left heart bypass for thoracic aortic repair. Arch Surg 1993; 128:746–52.

58. Arnofsky AG, Moll FL, Verhagen HJM. Thoracic endovascular aneurysm repair (TEVAR) for traumatic injuries. In: Greenhalgh RM (ed.) More vascular and endovascular challenges. London: PIBA Publishing, 2007; pp. 266–75.

A review of the current literature, technique and results.

59. Asensio JA. Abdominal vascular injuries. Surg Clin North Am 2001; 81:1395–416.

60. Aucar JA, Hirshberg A. Damage control for vascular injuries. Surg Clin North Am 1997; 77:853–62.

A good review of the different techniques in vascular damage control.

61. Fullen WD, Hunt J, Altemeier WA. The clinical spectrum of penetrating injury to the superior mesenteric arterial circulation. J Trauma 1972; 12:656–64.

62. Burch JM, Feliciano DV, Mattox KL. Injuries to the inferior vena cava. Am J Surg 1998; 156:548–52.

63. Buckman RF, Bradley M. Injuries to the inferior vena cava. Surg Clin North Am 2001; 81:1431–48.

64. Frykberg ER, Dennis JW, Bishop K et al. The reliability of physical examination in the evaluation of penetrating extremity trauma for vascular injury: results at one year. J Trauma 1991; 31:502–11.

65. Frykberg ER, Crump JM, Vines FS et al. A reassessment of the role of arteriography in penetrating proximity trauma: a prospective study. J Trauma 1989; 29:1041–52.

66. Schwartz M, Weaver F, Yellin A et al. The utility of color flow Doppler examination in penetrating extremity arterial trauma. Am Surg 1993; 59:375–8.

67. Keen RR, Meyer JP, Durham JR et al. Autogenous vein graft repair of injured extremity arteries: early and late results with 134 consecutive patients. J Vasc Surg 1991; 13:664–8.

68. Mabee JR, Bostwick TL. Pathophysiology and mechanisms of compartment syndrome. Orthop Rev 1993; 22:175–81.

69. Hafez HM, Woolgar J, Robbs JV. Lower extremity arterial injury: results of 550 cases and review of risk factors associated with limb loss. J Vasc Surg 2001; 33:1212–19.

The authors review the factors associated with limb loss in their extensive experience of more than 500 cases.

70. Johansen K, Daines M, Howey T et al. Objective criteria accurately predict amputation following lower extremity trauma. J Trauma 1990; 30:568–72.

71. Hunt CA, Kingsley JR. Upper extremity trauma. South Med J 2000; 93:466–8.

72. Demetriades D, Ascensio JA. Subclavian and axillary vascular injuries. Surg Clin North Am 2001; 81:1357–73.

73. Miranda FE, Dennis JW, Frykberg ER et al. Confirmation of the safety and accuracy of physical examination in the evaluation of knee dislocation for injury of the popliteal artery: a prospective study. J Trauma 2000; 49:247–52.

74. Stannard JP, Shiels TM, Lopez-Ben RR et al. Vascular injuries in knee dislocations: the role of physical examination in determining the need for arteriography. J Bone Joint Surg 2004; 86:910–14.

A prospective study including 138 patients with multiligamentous knee injuries.

75. Fainzilber G, Roy-Shapira A, Wall MJ Jr et al. Predictors of amputation for popliteal artery injuries. Am J Surg 1995; 170:568–70.

# 10

# Extracranial cerebrovascular disease

A. Ross Naylor
Sumaira MacDonald

## Introduction

Stroke is the third commonest cause of death after heart disease and cancer and the principal cause of neurological disability. It is defined as an acute loss of focal cerebral function (occasionally global in coma or subarachnoid haemorrhage) with symptoms exceeding 24 hours (or leading to death), with no apparent cause other than that of a vascular origin. A transient ischaemic attack (TIA) has the same definition but a time scale of <24 hours. In the UK, the annual incidence of stroke is 2 per 1000 and 125 000 patients will suffer their first stroke each year.[1] Half of all strokes affect patients >75 years of age, but 25% affect patients <65 years. Stroke patients use 10% of hospital bed-days and 5% of annual healthcare expenditure.[2] Although mortality has diminished by about 20%, attributed to improved survival rather than a decline in incidence, the overall incidence of stroke could increase by 30% by 2033 because of the ageing population.[3] Community studies suggest that about 36 000 patients will suffer a TIA each year, giving an annual UK incidence of 0.5 per 1000. The incidence of TIA increases with age, from 0.9 per 1000 for those aged 55–64 years to 2.6 per 1000 for those aged 75–84 years.[4]

## Aetiology and risk factors

About 80% of strokes are ischaemic, the remainder haemorrhagic (intracerebral/subarachnoid). Approximately 80% of ischaemic strokes affect the carotid territory. Risk factors include increasing age, smoking, hypertension (50%), ischaemic heart disease (38%), cardioembolic source (20%), previous TIA (15%), diabetes (10%), peripheral vascular disease, high plasma fibrinogen and hypercholesterolaemia.[5] The principal causes of ischaemic carotid territory infarction are detailed in Box 10.1.

### Large-vessel thromboembolism

The commonest cause of ischaemic stroke is thromboembolism of the internal carotid artery (ICA) and/or middle cerebral artery (MCA), while haemodynamic failure accounts for <2% of all strokes. Stenoses develop at the origin of the ICA because of a complex region of low shear stress, flow stasis and flow separation that predisposes to atherosclerotic plaque formation. Should the plaque undergo acute disruption (rupture, ulceration, intraplaque haemorrhage), the inner core of thrombogenic subendothelial collagen is exposed, predisposing towards thrombus formation and onset of symptoms.

### Small-vessel disease

Occlusion of penetrating end-arterioles causes lacunar infarcts, so named after the cavity/hole that remains after macrophages have removed the infarcted tissue. Autopsy studies suggest that the occlusive process follows fibrinoid necrosis (associated with hypertensive encephalopathy), lipohyalinosis and microatheroma (associated with chronic hypertension) or microcalcinosis (associated with diabetes). The commonest sites for lacunar infarction include the basal ganglia, thalamus and internal capsule.

**Box 10.1** • Aetiology of carotid territory infarction

Thromboembolism of internal carotid artery/middle cerebral artery (50%)
Small-vessel disease (25%)
Cardiogenic brain embolism (15%)
Haematological disease (5%)
Non-atheromatous disease (5%)

Data derived from Dennis MS, Bamford JM, Sandercock PAG et al. Incidence of transient ischaemic attacks in Oxfordshire, England. Stroke 1989; 20:333–9.

### Cardiogenic brain embolism

Sources of cardiac embolism include ventricular mural thrombus (post-myocardial infarction, cardiomyopathy), left atrial thrombus (atrial fibrillation) and valvular lesions (vegetations, prostheses, calcified annulus, endocarditis).

### Haematological disorders

Myeloma, sickle-cell disease, polycythaemia, the oral contraceptive pill and related prothrombotic disorders predispose towards stroke.

## Non-atheromatous carotid diseases

### Fibromuscular dysplasia (FMD)

FMD is a rare disorder of unknown aetiology (<1% of all carotid angiograms) that primarily affects the renal and carotid arteries in young women up to middle age. FMD is subclassified as intimal fibroplasia, medial fibroplasia, medial hyperplasia and perimedial dysplasia. The commonest is medial fibroplasia, which is characterised by alternating stenotic webs and dilatation/aneurysm formation (**Fig. 10.1**). In up to 60% of patients, FMD is bilateral. Patients may be asymptomatic or symptomatic (TIA, stroke, dissection, false aneurysm). Although management tends to be conservative in asymptomatic individuals, they should be kept under regular clinical/duplex surveillance to identify aneurysm formation. Once symptomatic, patients should be treated with the same policy as for symptomatic atherosclerotic disease. Options include resection and interposition bypass, open graduated internal dilatation or (more commonly) percutaneous angioplasty.

### Arteritis

The inflammatory process in Takayasu's arteritis (TA) is transmural, granulomatous and ultimately causes occlusion through fibrosis. TA predominantly affects younger females (female to male ratio 7:1) and the initial presentation may be a relatively innocuous illness comprising malaise, fever and arthralgia/myalgia. In the acute phase, there is a granulomatous vasculitis with medial disruption followed later by transmural fibrosis. Occasionally, focal aneurysms form as a consequence of disruption of the internal elastic lamina and media.

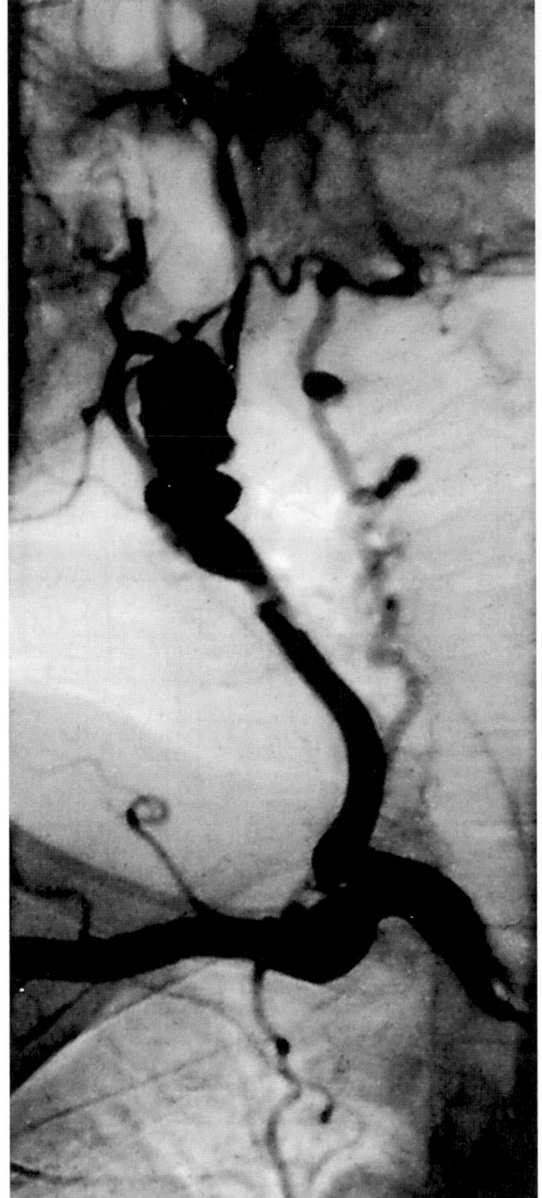

**Figure 10.1** • Example of fibromuscular dysplasia causing early aneurysm formation in the carotid artery.

Neurological symptoms develop as a consequence of occlusion or via renovascular hypertension. Type I disease (aortic arch and arch branches including subclavian, carotid and vertebral) occurs in 8% of cases and presents with cerebral vascular/ocular symptoms or asymptomatic stenoses. Type III TA (arch vessels plus abdominal aorta and its branches) accounts for 65% of cases and is characterised by stroke, renovascular hypertension and mesenteric ischaemia.

The mainstay of management is steroid therapy with cyclophosphamide/methotrexate as alternatives. Surgery should be avoided in the acute phase. Neither endarterectomy nor angioplasty is really an option with involvement of the carotid vessels because of the long segments of fibrotic disease. If surgery becomes necessary, bypass is the preferred option and the inflow should be taken from the ascending aorta (as opposed to the subclavian artery) as the latter may be involved in the disease process.

Giant-cell arteritis is another chronic granulomatous arteritis that primarily affects the older female population (female to male ratio 4:1). It is a systemic disorder, affecting any large artery, although branches of the carotid artery tend to predominate with bilateral symmetrical involvement. The intracranial vessels are unaffected. The commonest presentation is generalised malaise, headache and myalgic pain. Jaw claudication is present in up to 50%, while 50% will develop pain over the temporal artery. Stroke is a rare presentation, the commonest being transient or permanent blindness. Ocular symptoms (blindness, corneal ulcers and cataracts) can occur up to 6 months after the initial presentation. Treatment is with corticosteroid therapy.

## Carotid aneurysm

Carotid aneurysms are rare, comprising <4% of all peripheral aneurysms. The currently accepted definition is a diameter >150% of that of the common carotid artery (CCA) or twice the diameter of the distal ICA. The aetiology is usually atherosclerosis but may follow trauma, infection or trauma.

Clinical presentation includes pulsatile swelling (with or without pain), thrombosis, dissection, rupture or embolisation. Treatment consists of exclusion and either primary reanastomosis or interposition vein bypass. Endovascular intervention is the preferred option in patients with aneurysms affecting the distal ICA.

## Carotid dissection

Carotid dissection accounts for 2% of all strokes, increasing to 20% in young adults. One-fifth of trauma patients with an unexplained neurological deficit will have suffered a dissection and 25% will be bilateral. Dissection can be spontaneous (fibromuscular dysplasia), can follow iatrogenic dissection (angioplasty), can be part of a central dissection (type A thoracic dissection) or follow blunt trauma (direct crushing, forced hyperextension or forced rotation) with crushing of the ICA between the mastoid process and the transverse process of C2.

Dissections are classed as type I if there is irregularity but no significant stenosis on angiography, type II if there is a 70–99% stenosis and/or a >50% dilatation, or type III in the presence of a characteristic 'flame'-shaped occlusion about 2–3 cm distal to the bifurcation. The latter appearance is due to compression of the true lumen by thrombus in the false channel.

The commonest presentation is ipsilateral head/neck pain (70%) that usually precedes onset of neurological symptoms. Between 50% and 75% of patients with spontaneous dissection will present with TIA or stroke (usually embolic), pulsatile tinnitus, syncope, ocular signs or cranial nerve palsies (III, IV, VI, VII, IX, X, XII). Cranial nerve signs probably follow mechanical compression from mural haematoma or stretching. Up to 60% of patients with spontaneous dissection will have ocular signs, comprising oculo-sympathetic paresis, amaurosis fugax (aggravated by sitting/standing), hemianopia, ischaemic optic neuropathy and painful Horner's syndrome. The latter follows segmental ischaemia of the postganglionic fibres distal to the superior cervical ganglion and may persist in 50%.

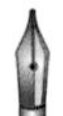

Recognition of ocular symptoms in patients with suspected dissection is important as up to 25% will suffer a stroke within 7 days.

Following duplex scanning, patients suspected of having a dissection should undergo angiography. This typically shows the dissection to start 2–3 cm beyond the origin of the ICA. The distal limit is variable (occasionally as high as the petrous segment) with varying combinations of stenosis, dilatation, intimal flaps and occlusion in the intervening segment.

The majority are managed conservatively (heparinisation then warfarinisation), with the aim being to reduce the risk of thrombosis and embolism. Surgery (or endovascular interventions) is reserved for complex trauma cases (usually type II), but may be indicated in patients with recurrent cerebral events despite medical therapy. Overall, dissection carries a 20% mortality and a 30% rate of persisting disability.

## Carotid body tumour

The carotid body is a discrete structure within the adventitia of the posterior aspect of the carotid bifurcation and is responsible for monitoring blood gases and pH. A carotid body tumour (CBT) is derived from cells originating from the neural crest ectoderm (chemoreceptor cells), is typically located in

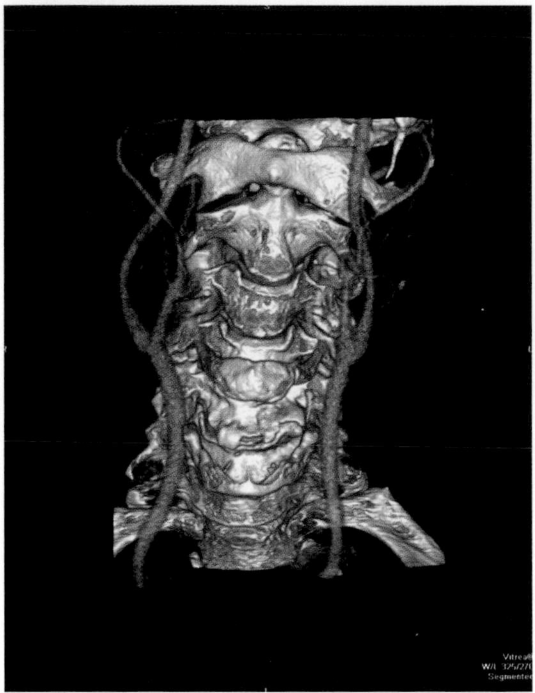

**Figure 10.2** • 3-D reconstruction of a CT angiogram of a highly vascular right carotid body tumour causing splaying of the bifurcation. In addition to providing information about the size and location of the tumour, this type of imaging is useful to exclude bilateral involvement (present in 5%). Note that the majority of the tumour circulation arises from branches of the ECA.

the space between the internal and external carotid arteries, and consists of nests of neoplastic epithelioid chief cells. As the tumour enlarges, the bifurcation splays (**Fig. 10.2**) and the patient becomes aware of a neck swelling. Other presentations include pain, local invasion/compression causing hoarseness, cranial nerve palsies and Horner's syndrome. CBTs rarely present with cerebral ischaemia, but can present as a hormonally mediated syndrome comprising flushing, dizziness, arrhythmias and hypertension.

Diagnosis requires awareness (all too often the neck has already been explored) supplemented by angiography, computed tomography (CT)/magnetic resonance imaging (Fig. 10.2) or radionuclide imaging as appropriate. Overall, 5% of CBTs are bilateral, metachronous tumours may appear and 5% are locally and 5% systemically malignant. Treatment consists of excision, although a more conservative approach might be appropriate in elderly patients with small asymptomatic tumours. The role of preoperative embolisation remains controversial, but may reduce intraoperative bleeding. Another aid to minimising blood loss is to line the external carotid artery (ECA) with a covered stent preoperatively,[6] as the majority of the blood supply to a CBT is derived from the ECA. This approach is not necessary in all patients, but could be very useful in very large lesions.

Important differential diagnoses for CBT include glomus vagale and glomus jugulare tumours. The glomus vagale tumour is a paraganglionoma arising from chemoreceptor cells within the vagus nerve. It can be differentiated from a CBT because the bifurcation is not splayed. Instead, the tumour causes deviation of the ICA *above* the bifurcation. It is important to consider a glomus vagale tumour preoperatively as resection leads to swallowing problems (injury to motor fibres) and hoarseness (recurrent laryngeal nerve) and the patient has to be warned of this possibility.

# Presentation of carotid disease

## Asymptomatic cerebrovascular disease

This is usually discovered as a consequence of detecting a cervical bruit or as an incidental finding in the ICA contralateral to that under investigation. Overall, 4% of patients over 45 years old will have a bruit, increasing to 12% in patients over 60 years.[7] Approximately 30% of patients with a symptomatic ICA stenosis of 70–90% will not have a bruit, increasing to 60% for those with a 90–99% stenosis. Paradoxically, up to 30% of patients with an ICA occlusion will still have an audible bruit. If no bruit is present at the time of examination, 1% of patients over the age of 65 years will develop a bruit each year thereafter.[8] The commonest reasons for a false-positive bruit (i.e. not due to ICA disease) are systolic cardiac murmurs, haemodynamic causes and bruits arising from the vertebral and external carotid arteries.

There is no evidence that either the presence or absence of a bruit or the quality of the bruit correlates with the degree of stenosis.

## Symptomatic cerebrovascular disease

### Carotid

'Classical' carotid territory symptoms include: (1) hemimotor/sensory signs, (2) transient monocular blindness (amaurosis fugax) and (3) higher cortical dysfunction (Box 10.2). Transient monocular blindness usually develops over a few seconds and clears within a few minutes. Failure to resolve within 24 hours is analogous to a stroke. A clear-cut history of amaurosis in the absence of a carotid/cardiac

**Box 10.2** • 'Classical' carotid and vertebrobasilar features

**Carotid territory**

Hemimotor/hemisensory signs
Monocular visual loss (amaurosis fugax)
Higher cortical dysfunction (dysphasia, visuospatial neglect etc.)

**Vertebrobasilar**

Bilateral blindness
Problems with gait and stance
Hemi- or bilateral motor/sensory signs
Dysarthria
Homonymous hemianopia
Diplopia, vertigo and nystagmus (provided it is not the only symptom)

source of embolisation should prompt referral to an ophthalmologist to exclude anterior ischaemic optic neuropathy (microvascular disease of the posterior ciliary arteries), which causes acute ischaemia of the optic nerve head.

The main differential diagnoses for carotid territory events include epilepsy, tumour, giant aneurysm, hypoglycaemia and migraine. It is often not possible to differentiate embolic from haemodynamic events. However, where TIAs are precipitated by a heavy meal, hot bath or exercise, a haemodynamically critical ICA stenosis should be suspected.

Conventional teaching has been that the risk of stroke after a TIA/minor stroke is only about 1–2% at 7 days and 2–4% at 30 days,[9,10] implying that there was no real urgency regarding referral and investigation. However, evidence suggests that these data dangerously underestimate the true risk. In a recent review of 524 stroke patients who had suffered a preceding TIA, the TIA occurred on the day of stroke in 17%, on the day before in 9%, while 43% of strokes (overall) occurred within 7 days of the index TIA.[11] Further data supportive of the need for prompt investigation and treatment come from a systematic review of 18 studies (10 126 TIA patients) which showed that the 2-day stroke risk after TIA was 3.1%, increasing to 5.2% at 7 days.[12]

As a consequence of increasing awareness that TIAs should be treated more urgently, attention has been directed towards developing scoring systems capable of identifying cohorts of TIA patients who would benefit from really urgent evaluation. The 'ABCD' system (Table 10.1) allocates a score to four parameters (A = age, B = blood pressure, C = clinical features, D = duration of symptoms), with '6' being the maximum. In this series, no patient with an 'ABCD' score of <3 suffered a stroke within 7 days of presenting with their TIA. An ABCD score of 4 was associated with a 2% 7-day risk, inceasing to 16% in patients scoring 5 and 35% in those scoring 6. All strokes occurring within 7 days happened in patients presenting with focal weakness or speech impairment.[13]

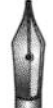

The early risk of stroke in patients presenting with a carotid territory TIA (especially those with speech or motor symptoms) is much greater than previously thought. TIA patients should now be considered on a par with 'heart attack' sufferers, with provision for urgent evaluation and treatment. The decision to refer should never be influenced by the presence or absence of a carotid bruit.

## Vertebrobasilar

Vertebrobasilar symptoms (Box 10.2) include bilateral blindness, problems with gait and stance, hemilateral/bilateral motor or sensory impairment (N.B. 10% will have hemisensory/motor signs), dysarthria, homonymous hemianopia, nystagmus, dizziness, diplopia and vertigo (provided the latter three are not isolated). Patients with dizziness associated with neck rotation are more likely to have inner ear pathology.

**Table 10.1** • ABCD scoring system for predicting the 7-day risk of stroke after TIA

| Parameter | | Score | Max. score |
|---|---|---|---|
| Age >60 years | | 1 | 1 |
| Systolic >140 mmHg or diastolic >90 mmHg | | 1 | 1 |
| Clinical features | Unilateral weakness | 2 | |
| | Speech disturbance, no weakness | 1 | 2 |
| | Other | 0 | |
| Duration of symptoms | >60 min | 2 | |
| | 10–59 min | 1 | 2 |
| | <10 min | 0 | |

Data derived from Rothwell PM, Giles MF, Flossman E et al. A simple score (ABCD) to identify individuals at high early risk of stroke after transient ischaemic attack. Lancet 2005; 366:29–36.

### Non-hemispheric

The term 'non-hemispheric' is allocated to patients with isolated syncope (blackout, drop attack), presyncope (faintness), isolated dizziness, isolated double vision (diplopia) and isolated vertigo.

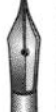

'Non-hemispheric' symptoms should never be considered to be carotid or vertebrobasilar in origin unless other more 'classical' symptoms are present. It is very important to exclude a cardiac or inner ear pathology.

# Investigation of carotid disease

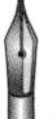

The UK Department of Health's National Stroke Strategy was released in November 2007[14] and recommended that 'carotid imaging should ideally be performed at initial assessment and should not be delayed for >24 hours after the first clinical assessment in TIA/minor stroke patients at higher risk of stroke (e.g. ABCD score ≥4)'.

This recommendation focuses attention on three important issues. (i) What is the best single and/or combination imaging strategy? (ii) How do imaging strategies for carotid artery stenting (CAS) and carotid endarterectomy (CEA) differ? (iii) Can these imaging strategies be provided within a 24-hour window in symptomatic patients?

## Duplex ultrasound

The degree of stenosis is usually first evaluated using duplex ultrasound, which combines B-mode (real-time) imaging with waveform analysis using pulsed-wave Doppler. Advantages include: (i) low cost, (ii) accessibility, especially in 'single-visit' clinics, and (iii) being non-invasive. There are, however, a number of recognised limitations to duplex, most relating to the expertise of the practitioner. With highly experienced sonographers, however, duplex can identify up to 95% of lesions responsible for carotid territory symptoms. Experience and reproducibility does, however, vary between centres.

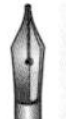

The Society of Radiologists in Ultrasound Consensus Conference[15] noted that duplex 'is often performed inconsistently within a given laboratory and there is non-uniformity in practice from one laboratory to the next. In many settings, interpretive criteria for carotid stenosis are either indiscriminately applied or the interpreters are uncertain about exactly how to make the diagnosis of carotid stenosis.'

Duplex can only insonate the cervical portion of the extracranial carotid artery and is therefore relatively unreliable at excluding disease elsewhere. In diabetic patients, the incidence of tandem distal ICA stenoses varies between 14% and 21.3%, while 17–24% will have tandem intracranial disease.[16] Suspicion of additional lesions therefore requires alternative imaging (e.g. magnetic resonance angiography, MRA).

The Society of Radiologists in Ultrasound Consensus Conference[16] has developed consensus ultrasound criteria for diagnosing the severity of carotid disease based on the North American Symptomatic Carotid Endarterectomy Trial (NASCET) measurement method (Table 10.2).

The identification of the 'vulnerable plaque', i.e. those more likely to cause thromboembolic complications

Table 10.2 • Society of Radiologists in Ultrasound Consensus Conference on ultrasound criteria for measuring carotid stenosis using the NASCET measurement method

| | Primary parameters | | Additional parameters | |
|---|---|---|---|---|
| Degree of stenosis (%) | ICA PSV (cm/s) | Plaque estimate (%)* | ICA/CCA PSV ratio | ICA EDV (cm/s) |
| Normal | <125 | None | <2.0 | <40 |
| <50 | <125 | <50 | <2.0 | <40 |
| 50–69 | 125–230 | >50 | 2.0–4.0 | 40–100 |
| ≥70 but less than near occlusion | >230 | >50 | >4.0 | >100 |
| Near occlusion | High, low, or undetectable | Visible | Variable | Variable |
| Total occlusion | Undetectable | Visible, no detectable lumen | Not applicable | Not applicable |

Reproduced from Grant EG, Benson CB, Moneta GL et al. Carotid artery stenosis: gray-scale and Doppler US diagnosis – Society of Radiologists in Ultrasound Consensus Conference. Radiology 2003; 229:340–6. With permission from the Radiological Society of North America.

has proved difficult to achieve with ultrasound. The Gray–Weale classification[17] allocates according to whether they are echolucent (type 1), predominantly echolucent (type 2), predominantly echogenic (type 3) or echogenic (type 4). Unfortunately, correlation with histology and clinical risk is variable.[18] An objective ultrasound parameter, the grey-scale median (GSM), has been shown to reliably differentiate between plaques associated with retinal and cerebrovascular symptomatology and asymptomatic status.[19] There are conflicting reports in the literature regarding the correlation between those plaques considered to be vulnerable on the basis of a GSM ≤25 and increased procedural risk during CAS.[20,21]

## Catheter angiography

In the modern era of sophisticated non-invasive imaging and multiplanar reconstructions from multidectector row CT (MDCT) and MRA, some have challenged the place of catheter angiography as being the 'gold standard'. However, it must be remembered that selective carotid angiography formed the basis of measuring the degree of stenosis in the Asymptomatic Carotid Atherosclerosis Study (ACAS), NASCET and European Carotid Surgery (ECST) Trials. All other forms of carotid imaging are essentially surrogates of this invasive imaging assessment.

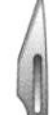

In ACAS, selective catheter angiography incurred a stroke/death risk of 1.5%. This accounted for >50% of the overall surgical risk.[22] It is no longer considered part of the routine work-up of a carotid patient.

Arch angiography is currently employed in some CAS centres as a means of reliably assessing anatomic suitability for CAS and the status of the aortic arch/arch origins of the great vessels. It is associated with a much lower rate of stroke than selective angiography.[23]

There are currently three methods for measuring stenosis, each using the residual luminal diameter at the point of maximum stenosis as the numerator (**Fig. 10.3**). Stenoses measured using the ECST method generate higher grades than those generated using the NASCET method (Table 10.3); however, the CCA method may be the most reproducible.

## Magnetic resonance angiography

MRA uses either flowing blood (time of flight) or gadolinium (contrast-enhanced MRA, CEMRA) as the contrast agent. CEMRA is not so dependent on vessel orientation and therefore the field of view can be extended to include the arch of aorta and intracranial vessels (**Fig. 10.4**). This is now the technique of choice.

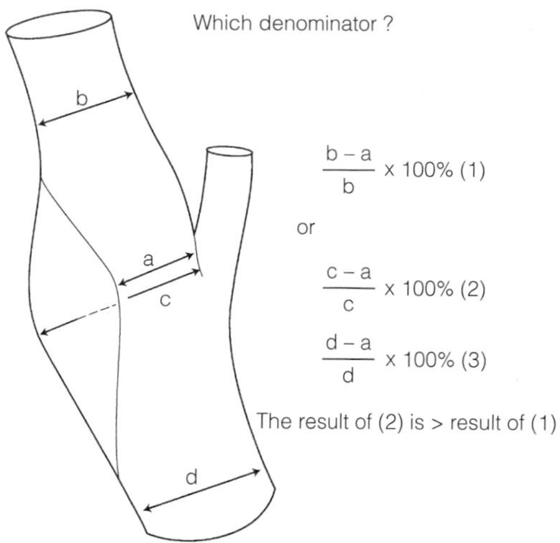


**Figure 10.3** • Measurement of carotid stenosis by the ECST, NASCET and common carotid methods.

Table 10.3 • Correlation between ECST and NASCET measured carotid stenoses

| NASCET (%) | ECST (%) |
|---|---|
| 30 | 65 |
| 40 | 70 |
| 50 | 75 |
| 60 | 80 |
| 70 | 85 |
| 80 | 90 |
| 90 | 95 |

Although many studies comparing MRA with catheter angiography are methodologically flawed, a few are worthy of mention. One compared 71 carotid bifurcations in 39 symptomatic patients with ultrasound, CEMRA and digital subtraction angiography (DSA).[24] For the detection of 'surgically appropriate' lesions, CEMRA was found to have a sensitivity of 95% and a specificity of 79%, with 10% false-positive and 2.5% false-negative rates. Ultrasound has similar accuracy. However, if ultrasound and CEMRA were concordant (80% of cases), then all 70–99% stenoses were correctly identified and there were only 8.4% false-positive results. These 'false positives' were in the 60–65% category of stenoses which some might still consider for surgical intervention. A second study in 50 patients found that CEMRA misclassified 24% of surgically amenable lesions (ultrasound misclassified 36%), but when CEMRA and ultrasound were concordant (48% of lesions) there was 100% sensitivity and only 17% of lesions were misclassified.[25]

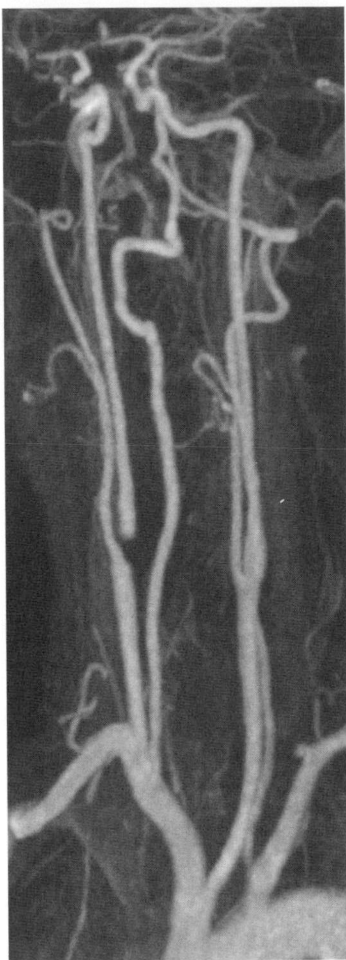

**Figure 10.4** • CEMRA in the right anterior oblique orientation providing overview anatomical imaging, i.e. from the arch origin to the circle of Willis. There is an extremely tight stenosis (>95%) at the right carotid bulb/proximal internal carotid artery.

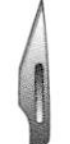

Non-invasive imaging modalities for the evaluation of carotid stenosis were compared with DSA in a recent systematic review.[25] As more data were available for analysis of patients categorised as operable (70–99% stenosis) versus non-operable (0–69% or occluded) than in possibly operable (50–69%) or definitely not operable (0–49% or occluded) groups, the study focused on the accuracy for detection of 70–99% stenosis. CEMRA had the highest sensitivity (0.94, 95% CI 0.88–0.97), followed by ultrasound (0.89, 95% CI 0.85–0.92).

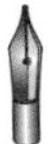

If MRA is to be used to non-invasively image the carotid arteries, current data would suggest that this is best done in conjunction with ultrasound. There are no studies describing the accuracy of MRA in assessing arch disease.

Whilst MRA is non-invasive and does not involve the use of ionising radiation, gadolinium has recently been identified as the cause of nephrogenic systemic fibrosis (NSF).

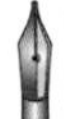

NSF is a systemic scleroderma-like condition which affects 3–5% of patients with pre-existing renal impairment exposed to gadolinium-based compounds. Five percent of affected individuals exhibit a rapidly progressive course.

### Computed tomography angiography (CTA)

MDCT angiography, i.e. up to (and shortly beyond) 64 detectors, permits the rapid acquisition of large amounts of cross-sectional data that can be reformatted into any plane. Contrast-enhanced MDCT is used routinely to assess abdominal aortic aneurysms but very few studies have yet assessed its use in carotid disease.

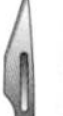

In a recent systematic review on the performance of non-invasive imaging modalities in the assessment of a 70–99% stenosis, CTA had the highest specificity (0.94, 95% CI 0.91–0.97), followed by CEMRA (0.93, 95% CI 0.89–0.96), then ultrasound (0.84, 95% CI 0.77–0.89).[25] Unfortunately only single-detector row CT was evaluated in this review.

The principal advantages of CTA include: (i) minimally invasive (i.v. injection of iodinated contrast), (ii) overview anatomical imaging possible (particularly for MDCT – short scan times and thinner 'slices' mean less artefact from patient movement/breathing and from the patients' shoulders at the arch origins), (iii) more accessible than MRA and (iv) generally well tolerated. Disadvantages include: (i) requirement for iodinated contrast load, (ii) radiation burden (but 2–3 times lower than for DSA), (iii) inability to impart dynamic information, i.e. 'trickle flow' not reliably identified and (iv) heavy calcification can increase the difficulty of reliable estimates of degree of stenosis.

## Guidelines for imaging

There are a variety of (sometimes conflicting) national and 'consensus' guidelines for imaging carotid arteries. Each should be interpreted in the context of which professional body published them and also the availability/rapidity of access (and experience) of the varying imaging modalities in individual units.

## The National Clinical Guideline for Stroke 2004[27]

This recommends that duplex findings be confirmed by MRA (or a second duplex), although the evidence base for this is limited.[26] If a centre prefers the 'second' duplex option, it is good practice to ensure that this is performed by a second practitioner in a vascular laboratory or radiology department that has validated its duplex findings against the 'gold standard'. This is not an easy undertaking as it essentially means auditing each new member of staff against catheter angiography or an intact endarterectomy specimen. In reality, this rarely happens.

## The Society of Radiologists in Ultrasound Consensus[16]

This panel recommended that: (i) all vascular laboratories should have a system for quality assurance and (ii) the NASCET measurement method was preferred to all others (hardly surprising as it was a North American group of clinicians).

## The Health Technology Assessment exercise[27]

The recent Health Technology Assessment exercise observed that the net benefit of stroke prevention clinics was ultimately dependent on the speed with which patients were investigated and treated. The current provision of services in the UK, where patients are unlikely to undergo a carotid intervention within 40 days of presentation, has to be improved. This delayed approach (regardless of imaging strategy) is failing to prevent up to 100 strokes per 1000 patients within the first month of suffering a TIA/minor stroke.

# Management of cerebrovascular disease

## 'Best medical therapy'

All patients with cerebrovascular disease benefit from optimisation of risk factors, antiplatelet/statin therapy and exclusion of important comorbidity. Everyone should undergo an ECG to exclude occult cardiac pathology. Baseline blood tests will exclude diabetes, arteritis, polycythaemia, anaemia, thrombocytosis, sickle-cell disease and hyperlipidaemia.

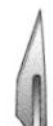

Table 10.4 summarises the main recommendations from the European Stroke Initiative[28] regarding what should now constitute 'best medical therapy' in patients with symptomatic and asymptomatic carotid disease. Angina therapy must be optimised because the principal cause of late death is cardiac. Blood pressure (BP) should be maintained below 150/90 mmHg, although some would reasonably argue that 140/85 mmHg is a better target. Systematic overviews suggest that reducing the diastolic BP by 5 mmHg lowers the relative risk of stroke by 35%, while the relative risk of myocardial infarction (MI) will also fall by 25%.[29]

**Table 10.4** • European Stroke Initiative[28] recommendations for what constitutes 'best medical therapy' in patients with asymptomatic and symptomatic carotid disease

| Treatment | Level of evidence | |
|---|---|---|
| | Asymptomatic | Symptomatic |
| BP <140/90 mmHg or <130/80 mmHg in diabetics | Level I | Level I |
| Glycaemic control to prevent other diabetic complications | Level III | Level III |
| Statin therapy | Level I | Level I |
| Stop smoking | Level II | Level II |
| Avoid heavy consumption of alcohol | Level I | Level I |
| Regular physical activity | Level II | Level II |
| Low salt, low saturated fat, high fruit and vegetable diet rich in fibre | Level II | Level II |
| If BMI elevated, reduce weight | Level II | Level II |
| HRT should not be used for stroke prevention in women | Level I | Level I |
| Aspirin | To prevent MI level IV | Level I |
| Aspirin and dipyridamole | Not recommended level IV | Level I |
| Clopidogrel | Not recommended level IV | Level I |

BMI, body mass index; BP, blood pressure; HRT, hormone replacement therapy; MI, myocardial infarction.

However, evidence suggests that only 60% of patients with known hypertension will be receiving treatment prior to suffering their first stroke and only half of these will have a documented diastolic blood pressure below 90 mmHg.[30]

The Heart Protection Study[31] has provided level 1, grade A evidence for the role of statin therapy in patients with cerebrovascular disease. Accordingly, the European Stroke Initiative[28] recommends that all patients (symptomatic and asymptomatic) should take a statin unless contraindicated.

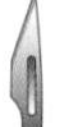

In the British Heart Protection Study (which randomised 20 000 patients with angina, stroke/TIA, diabetes or claudication to 40 mg simvastatin or placebo daily), patients randomised to statin had an average 25% relative risk reduction (RRR) in: (i) any major coronary event, (ii) any stroke and (iii) the need for revascularisation at 5 years. This benefit was irrespective of age, gender or presenting cholesterol level.[31]

Antiplatelet therapy should be commenced in all patients unless contraindicated.

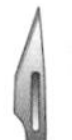

Aspirin remains the first-line antiplatelet agent and meta-analyses suggest that it will reduce the long-term risk of stroke by 25%.[32]

But what dose? NASCET reported that patients receiving high-dose aspirin (650–1300 mg) had a lower perioperative risk than patients taking 0–325 mg aspirin daily.[33] This was an unplanned analysis and a randomised trial of 2849 patients undergoing CEA subsequently showed that the risks of stroke, MI and death within 30 and 90 days of CEA were significantly lower in patients receiving 80–325 mg as opposed to 650–1300 mg.[34] This suggests greater evidence for prescribing low-dose aspirin. Dipyridamole and clopidogrel are ADP inhibitors (aspirin is a cyclo-oxygenase pathway inhibitor). Although dipyridamole is a weak ADP inhibitor, randomised trials suggest that the combination of aspirin plus dipyridamole confers a significant reduction in late stroke risk as compared with either agent alone.[35]

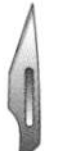

The National Institute for Health and Clinical Excellence (NICE) recommends combination aspirin/dipyridamole therapy for 3 years in patients with stroke/TIA who are not undergoing CEA. After 3 years, the patient should continue with aspirin. However, following CEA, NICE recommends that only aspirin need be taken.[36]

Clopidogrel significantly reduced the composite end-point of ischaemic stroke, MI or vascular death as compared with aspirin alone (absolute risk reduction (ARR) 0.51%, RRR 8.7%, $P = 0.043$).[37] However, the risk of stroke was not reduced and clopidogrel has not been adopted into widespread clinical practice in the UK, largely because of its cost.

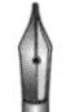

Clopidogrel (75 mg daily) is the second-line agent in patients who are unable to take aspirin because of side-effects, intolerance or resistance.

As stated previously, the early risk of stroke after suffering a TIA is higher than was previously thought. This led to a review of practice regarding the timing of surgery (see later), but also regarding the benefit of very early implementation of 'best medical therapy'. The EXPRESS study evaluated early stroke risk in two cohorts of patients presenting with TIA or minor stroke. In the first cohort (634 patients recruited from 2002 to 2004), patients were seen in a dedicated daily TIA clinic (appointment based, usual referral delays, etc.) with recommendations being made to the referring physician/primary care doctor regarding what constituted 'best medical therapy'. In the second cohort (644 patients recruited from 2004 to 2007), patients did not have to make appointments (i.e. it was a 'walk-in' service) and treatment (statin, antiplatelet therapy, etc.) was started in the outpatient clinic.[38] The 90-day risk of stroke fell from 10.3% in the first cohort to 2.1% in the second. This reduction in risk was independent of age and gender, and rapid commencement of therapy was not associated with an increased risk of haemorrhagic stroke.

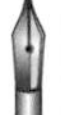

Rapid institution of 'best medical therapy' is associated with a significant reduction in the risk of early stroke and should be started in a dedicated 'walk-in' clinic. The responsibility for prescribing and starting therapy should not simply be delegated to the referring doctor.

# Surgical management of carotid disease

## Symptomatic carotid artery disease

The Carotid Endarterectomy Trialists Collaboration (CETC) have combined data from ECST, NASCET and the Veteran's Affairs (VA) trials having remeasured the pre-randomisation angiograms using the NASCET measurement method. This unique database[39–41] includes 5-year outcomes in >6000 patients (Table 10.5).

**Table 10.5** • Carotid Endarterectomy Trialists Collaboration: 5-year risk of any stroke (including 30-day stroke/death) from the combined VA, ECST and NASCET trials

| Trial | Stenosis | *n* | 30-day CEA risk | 5-year risk | | ARR | RRR | NNT | Strokes prevented per 1000 CEAs |
|---|---|---|---|---|---|---|---|---|---|
| | | | | Surgery | Medical | | | | |
| CETC | <30% | 1746 | No data | 18.36% | 15.71% | −2.6% | N/b | N/b | None at 5 years |
| CETC | 30–49% | 1429 | 6.7% | 22.80% | 25.45% | +2.6% | 10% | 38 | 26 at 5 years |
| CETC | 50–69% | 1549 | 8.4% | 20.00% | 27.77% | +7.8% | 28% | 13 | 78 at 5 years |
| CETC | 70–99% | 1095 | 6.2% | 17.13% | 32.71% | +15.6% | 48% | 6 | 156 at 5 years |
| CETC | String | 262 | 5.4% | 22.40% | 22.30% | −0.1% | N/b | N/b | None at 5 years |

ARR, absolute risk reduction; N/b, no benefit conferred by CEA; NNT, number needed to treat; RRR, relative risk reduction; strokes prevented per 1000 CEAs, number of strokes prevented at 5 years by performing 1000 CEAs.
Data derived from the CETC[39–41] with all pre-randomisation angiograms remeasured using NASCET method.

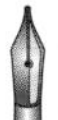

Notwithstanding criticisms of the 'historical' nature of these trials, the 5-year CETC should now be quoted in preference to the constituent studies.

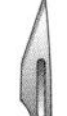

CEA is not indicated in symptomatic patients with a 0–50% NASCET stenosis.

CEA confers modest (but significant benefit) in recently symptomatic patients (<6 months) with NASCET 50–69% stenoses (ARR in stroke = 7.8% at 5 years, number needed to treat (NNT) to prevent 1 stroke at 5 years = 13). This is equivalent to an ECST 70–85% stenosis.

CEA confers maximum benefit in recently symptomatic patients (<6 months) with NASCET 70–99% stenoses but not including those with the 'string sign' (ARR = 15.6% at 5 years, NNT to prevent 1 stroke at 5 years = 6).

CEA does not confer any long-term benefit in patients with near-occlusion (string sign).

Following the 1991 publication of ECST and NASCET, there were concerns that the results may not be generalisable into clinical practice. For example, <0.5% of patients undergoing CEA in North America in 1988–1989 were randomised into NASCET. At present, 94% of CEAs in the USA are performed in non-NASCET hospitals with a mortality significantly higher than observed in NASCET.[42,43] The controversial issue regarding the relationship between hospital volume and outcome has been addressed in a systematic review of death/stroke after 936 436 CEAs.[44]

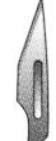

This meta-analysis concluded that there was a significant relationship between volume and outcome, with the critical volume threshold (per hospital) being 79 CEAs per annum.[44]

Interestingly, low-volume surgeons had similar results to higher-volume surgeons provided they worked in higher-volume centres. The question as to who and where CEA should be performed has always been a provocative subject, but the evidence from this meta-analysis, together with the growing drive for faster (and perhaps more risky) surgery, means that surgeons cannot simply ignore this controversial issue in the future.

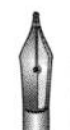

Surgeons must know and quote their own results rather than simply justifying practice on the basis of ECST and NASCET.

ECST and NASCET have now published over 50 papers since 1991, most being secondary analyses that have increased knowledge about the role of CEA in patients with symptomatic cerebral vascular disease.[45] These data should probably not be used to *exclude* patients from intervention, but rather to identify clinical and imaging predictors of increased risk of stroke on 'best medical therapy' (Box 10.3) and also who derives the 'least' and 'greatest' benefit from CEA (Table 10.6).

One of the most topical issues facing practitioners of both CEA and CAS is the effect of delay to intervention upon overall long-term benefit. Previously, there was no great impetus for expediting intervention other than recommending that CEA should be performed 'as soon as reasonably possible'.

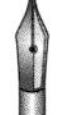

This approach has now been called into question because of indisputable evidence that: (a) the most vulnerable patients are probably suffering strokes before they can undergo surgery and (b) the long-term benefit of surgery diminishes rapidly following onset of the index event.

**Figure 10.5** details the cumulative risk of stroke following onset of a TIA or minor stroke in 174 patients where follow-up was commenced in

**Box 10.3** • Which patients with symptomatic 70–99% stenoses are at higher risk of suffering a stroke on 'best medical therapy'?

**Clinical features**

Male versus female gender
Increasing age (especially >75 years)
Hemispheric versus ocular symptoms
Cortical versus lacunar stroke
Recurrent symptoms for >6 months
Increasing medical comorbidity
Symptoms within 1 month

**Imaging features**

Irregular versus smooth plaques
Increasing stenosis but not near occlusion
Contralateral occlusion
Tandem intracranial disease
No recruitment of intracranial collaterals

Adapted from Naylor AR, Rothwell PM, Bell PRF. Overview of the principal results and secondary analyses from the European and the North American randomised trials of carotid endarterectomy. Eur J Vasc Endovasc Surg 2003; 26:115–29. With permission from Elsevier.

primary care. At 7 days, the incidence of stroke was 8% in patients initially presenting with a TIA as compared with 11.5% in patients presenting with a minor stroke. At 30 days, the incidence of stroke was 11.5% and 15% respectively.[6]

In parallel, the CETC published compelling (and uncomfortable) evidence that 'delay to surgery' significantly reduced benefit to the patient.[10,39–41] By implication, the same applies to CAS. Table 10.7 presents a reanalysis of CETC data in patients with NASCET 50–99% stenoses (i.e. ECST 70–99%) undergoing CEA, specifically: (i) the ARR in ipsilateral stroke conferred by CEA stratified for delay to surgery, (ii) the NNT to prevent one ipsilateral stroke at 5 years, (iii) the number of ipsilateral strokes prevented per 1000 CEAs at 5 years and (iv) the number of 'uneccessary' procedures per 1000 CEAs at 5 years.

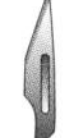

Maximum benefit, regarding late stroke prevention, was observed when surgery was performed within 2 weeks. If surgery was delayed beyond 12 weeks, only eight ipsilateral strokes were prevented at 5 years by performing 1000 CEAs.[11,40–42]

Only Vancouver has documented a median of 14 days from index event to surgery.[10] The 1997 UK Audit of CEA practice reported that the median time from event to surgery was 189 days. In the contemporary GALA trial, the median delay was 80 days (M. Gough, personal communication). In the 2007 UK CEA Audit (>3000 patients) the median delay from referral to surgery was 45 days.

**Table 10.6** • Predictors of relative benefit conferred by CEA

| 'Lower' benefit conferred by CEA | | 'Higher' benefit conferred by CEA | |
|---|---|---|---|
| **Clinical: imaging parameter** | **CVA/1000** | **Clinical: imaging parameter** | **CVA/1000** |
| Symptomatic female (50–69%)+ CEA >4 weeks | 0 at 5 years | Symptomatic, 70–99%, aged >75 years | 333 at 2 years |
| Symptomatic + string sign (subocclusion) | 0 at 5 years | Symptomatic, 70–99%, high comorbidity | 333 at 2 years |
| 'All' asymptomatic females | 2 at 5 years | Symptomatic, 70–99%, recurrent TIAs >6 months | 333 at 2 years |
| Asymptomatic (anyone) with op. risk 6% | 22 at 5 years | Symptomatic, 70–99%, operation < 2 weeks | 333 at 3 years |
| Asymptomatic (anyone) with op. risk 2.8% | 53 at 5 years | Symptomatic, 80–99%, + intracranial disease | 333 at 3 years |
| Symptomatic (all) 50–69% stenosis | 67 at 3 years | Symptomatic, 90–99%, no string sign | 370 at 3 years |
| Symptomatic (female) 70–99%, op 2–4 weeks | 67 at 3 years | Symptomatic, 70–99%, female + CEA <2 weeks | 417 at 3 years |
| Symptomatic (all) 70–99% + lacunar stroke | 91 at 3 years | Symptomatic, 70–99%, + contralateral occlusion | 500 at 2 years |
| Symptomatic (all) 70–99% + age <65 years | 100 at 2 years | Symptomatic, 90–99% + plaque ulceration | 500 at 2 years |

CVA/1000, number of strokes prevented per 1000 patients treated.
Derived from secondary analyses from ECST, NASCET, ACAS, ACST and CETC.

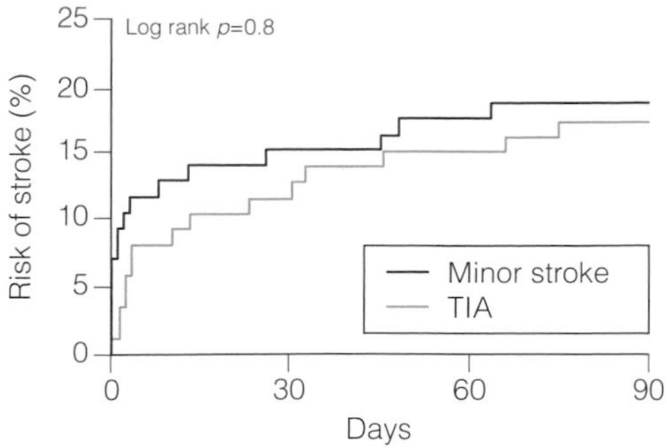


**Figure 10.5** • Cumulative early risk of stroke in 174 patients presenting with either a TIA ($n$ = 87) or minor stroke ($n$ = 87). Note that the maximum risk of stroke is within the first 7–14 days after onset of the index event. Reproduced from Coull AJ, Lovett JK, Rothwell PM. Population based study of early risk of stroke after transient ischaemic attack or minor stroke: implications for public education and organization of services. Br Med J 2004; 328:326–8. With permission form the BMJ Publishing Group Ltd.

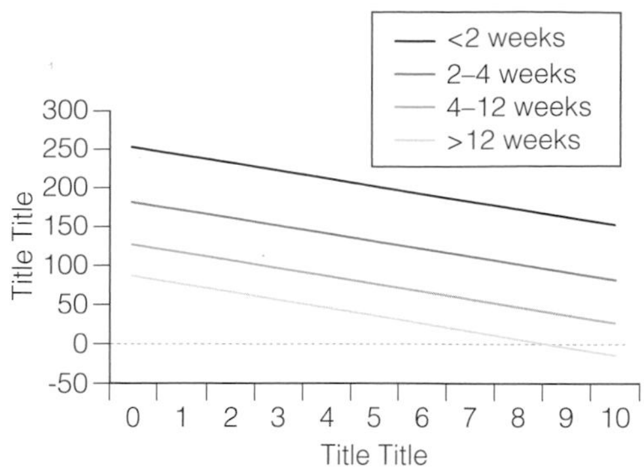


**Figure 10.6** • Strokes prevented per 1000 CEAs at 5 years stratified for: (i) delay from last event to randomisation and (ii) 30-day death/stroke risk. Reproduced from Naylor AR. Time is brain! The Surgeon 2007; 5:23–30. With permission from the Royal College of Surgeons of Edinburgh and Ireland.

While this represents an improvement upon 1997, a simple review of **Fig. 10.5** and Table 10.7 suggests that there is still considerable room for improvement.

However, this is only one side of a complex argument. It is also important to consider that early CEA might be associated with increased procedural risk. In a retrospective review of 1046 symptomatic patients undergoing CEA in New York, the 30-day death/stroke rate was three times higher (5.1%) if CEA was performed within 4 weeks as compared with 1.6% if surgery was deferred for >4 weeks.[46]

Paradoxically, an alternative interpretation of the CETC data used in Table 10.7 may be used to generate a solution to this problem. In addition to providing data on outcomes relative to the delay to surgery, CETC also provided 30-day death/stroke rates following CEA in each time category as well. This enables modelling of the effect of different procedural risks upon outcome (**Fig. 10.6**).

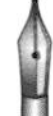

Figure 10.6 suggests that even if a surgeon operated <2 weeks with a 10% procedural risk, he/she was likely to prevent more strokes than by waiting >12 weeks and then operating with a 0% risk! Future guidelines must therefore consider whether it is reasonable to accept a slightly higher procedural risk if the operation is carried out early.

More controversial is the effect of 'delay to surgery' relative to gender. **Figure 10.7** now separates CETC data for males and females.[10,41] As can be seen, males gain considerable (and durable) benefit irrespective of the delay to surgery and the degree of stenosis. However, the CETC data suggest that the benefit conferred in women diminishes very rapidly after 4 weeks. Once again, these data reinforce the need for expedited investigation and treatment.

## Asymptomatic carotid artery disease

Of the population aged >65 years, 5–10% will have an asymptomatic 50–99% stenosis, increasing to 12% in those with peripheral vascular disease and 25% in patients with hypertension.[47,48] Although five randomised trials have compared CEA + 'best medical therapy' (BMT) with BMT alone, only two (the ACAS and the Asymptomatic Carotid Surgery Trial (ACST)) have influenced practice.[22,49]

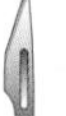

The principal results from ACAS and ACST are summarised in Table 10.8. Note that ACAS reported 5-year risks of 'ipsilateral' and 'any stroke', while ACST only reported 5-year risks of 'any stroke'.

ACAS (1995) attracted considerable criticism, in particular: (i) the 30-day death/stroke rate was 2.3% (half due to angiographic stroke) and not considered generalisable into routine practice, (ii) the 5-year risk was projected (median follow-up was only 2.7 years), (iii) there was no benefit in women (even when the procedural risk was excluded),[50] (iv) CEA did not prevent disabling stroke, and (v) there was an *inverse* relationship between late stroke risk and stenosis severity in medically treated patients. ACST reported in 2004 having randomised 3120 patients with asymptomatic 60–99% carotid stenoses.[49] The headlines were that: (i) CEA significantly reduced the

**Table 10.7** • Effect of 'delay to CEA' on 5-year prevention of ipsilateral stroke in patients with NASCET 50–99% stenoses

| | < 2 weeks | 2–4 weeks | 4–12 weeks | >12 weeks* |
|---|---|---|---|---|
| ARR conferred by CEA at 5 years | 18.5% | 9.8% | 5.5% | 0.8% |
| NNT | 5 | 10 | 18 | 125 |
| Strokes prevented per 1000 CEAs | 185 | 98 | 55 | 8 |
| 'Unnecessary' procedures | 815 | 902 | 945 | 992 |

* Delay refers to time from randomisation to CEA. In the constituent studies, the average time from randomisation to CEA was about 7 days (P.M. Rothwell, personal communication).
Data derived from a reanalysis of the CETC data.[39–41]

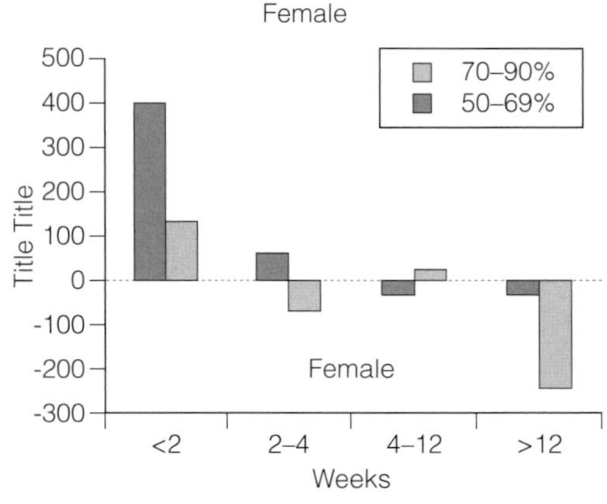


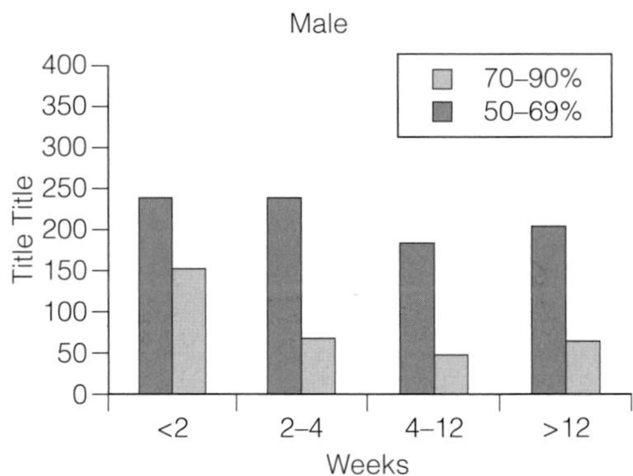


**Figure 10.7** • Strokes prevented per 1000 CEAs at 5 years stratified for stenosis severity and gender. Reproduced from Naylor AR. Time is brain! The Surgeon 2007; 5:23–30. With permission from the Royal College of Surgeons of Edinburgh and Ireland.

risk of fatal and disabling stroke, and (ii) significant benefit was only present in patients aged <75 years.

ACAS and ACST showed that CEA conferred a small but significant benefit over deferred endarterectomy in asymptomatic patients. The key is to identify high-risk patient subgroups that will gain most benefit so as to optimise resources and minimise unnecessary risk.

ACST did not resolve the issue regarding gender and a 6-year update in 2004 (which now included the operative risk) shows a definite (but still non-significant) trend favouring surgery in women.[51]

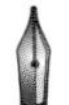

Future guidelines must recognise that asymptomatic women gain less benefit from CEA than men.

## CEA and synchronous coronary bypass

The role of prophylactic CEA in patients undergoing coronary artery bypass grafting (CABG) with an asymptomatic carotid stenosis remains an enduring controversy.

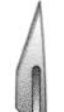

In a meta-analysis of 190 449 patients undergoing CABG,[52] the risk of stroke was 1.7% (95% CI 1.5–1.9).

Most post-CABG strokes (62%) occur after more than 24 hours has elapsed. The meta-analysis observed that three 'carotid' factors were significantly predictive of post-CABG stroke: (i) carotid bruit, (ii) a prior history of stroke or TIA and (iii) the presence of a severe carotid stenosis or occlusion.[52]

The stroke risk in 4674 duplex-screened patients undergoing CABG was 1.8% in patients with no significant carotid disease, 3.2% in those with unilateral 50–99% stenoses, 5.2% in those with bilateral 50–99% stenoses and 7–11% in patients with carotid occlusion.[52]

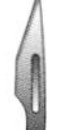

A number of factors emerged from the meta-analysis to suggest that carotid disease (alone) was not the principal cause of post-CABG stroke.[53] (i) Most occurred after 24 hours had

**Table 10.8** • Primary end-points from ACAS and ACST

| 30-Day death/stroke after CEA: | ACAS $n$ = 1662 2.3% | | ACST $n$ = 3120 2.8% | |
|---|---|---|---|---|
| **5-Year risk of:** | **BMT** | **CEA** | **BMT** | **CEA** |
| Ipsilateral stroke + any perioperative stroke/death | 11.0% | 5.1% ($P$ = 0.004) | No data | No data |
| Major ipsilateral stroke + any perioperative stroke/death | 6.0% | 3.4% ($P$ = 0.12) | No data | No data |
| Any stroke + any perioperative stroke/death | 17.5% | 12.4% ($P$ = 0.09) | 11.8% | 6.4% ($P$ < 0.0001) |
| Any major stroke + any perioperative stroke/death | 9.1% | 6.4% ($P$ = 0.26) | 6.1% | 3.5% ($P$ = 0.004) |
| **Clinical implications** | | | | |
| NNT to prevent one 'any stroke' at 5 years | 20 | | | 19 |
| No. of 'any strokes' prevented at 5 years per 1000 CEAs | 50 | | | 53 |
| NNT to prevent one ipsilateral stroke at 5 years | 17 | | | No data |
| No. of ipsilateral strokes prevented at 5 years/1000 CEAs | 59 | | | No data |

elapsed. This is the opposite of that observed in NASCET and ECST. (ii) Although the risk of stroke increased with stenosis severity (see above), 85% of strokes occurring in the 4674 duplex-screened patients were not associated with any significant carotid artery disease. (iii) At least 60% of stroke victims had areas of ischaemic infarction at autopsy/CT with no ipsilateral carotid disease.

It is now increasingly accepted that while carotid disease is an important predictor for post-CABG stroke, the single most important cause is atheroembolism from the aortic arch.

Two meta-analyses (Table 10.9) examined the results of staged and synchronous CEA in 8972 patients undergoing CABG.[53,54] Mortality was highest following synchronous procedures, stroke was highest during reverse-staged procedures (CABG–CEA), while MI was most prevalent after a staged CEA–CABG operation. However, when the cumulative cardiovascular risk was calculated, 11.5% (95% CI 8.9–14%) of synchronous patients either died or suffered a non-fatal stroke or MI. This compares with 9.4% (95% CI 6.4–12.4%) for patients undergoing either of the staged strategies. There was no statistically significant difference between staged/synchronous interventions, but there was considerable bias. Synchronous procedures tended to include more neurologically symptomatic and unstable patients, while staged procedures tended to include more patients with asymptomatic stenoses.

## Emergency CEA

In the 1960s, emergency CEA for acute stroke was associated with significant mortality and morbidity, mainly due to haemorrhagic transformation of ischaemic infarction. This led to the abandonment of this strategy and a recommendation that any patient suffering a stroke should wait at least 6 weeks before undergoing CEA in order to allow the area of infarction to stabilise. This is clearly at odds with earlier recommendations to expedite carotid interventions and a meta-analysis of published studies suggests that procedural risks for early surgery in patients with minor stroke are similar to those in whom surgery is deferred.[55]

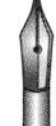

At present, emergency CEA (i.e. immediate) should be reserved for patients who suffer a thrombotic stroke in the early postoperative period after CEA or CAS. Urgent CEA (within 24 hours) is recommended in patients with stroke in evolution, stuttering hemiplegia or crescendo

Table 10.9 • Operative risk following staged, reverse staged or synchronous CEA in patients undergoing CABG

| | | Stroke (%) | MI (%) | Death (%) |
|---|---|---|---|---|
| Synchronous CEA + CABG | $n = 7863$ | 4.6 | 3.6 | 4.6 |
| CEA then staged CABG | $n = 917$ | 2.7 | 6.5 | 3.9 |
| CABG then staged CEA | $n = 302$ | 6.3 | 0.9 | 2.0 |

Adapted from Naylor AR, Mehta Z, Rothwell PM et al. Stroke during coronary artery bypass surgery: a critical review of the role of carotid artery disease. Eur J Vasc Endovasc Surg 2002; 23:283–94. With permission from Elsevier.

TIAs. There remains no evidence that patients with extensive neurological deficits should be considered for early intervention.

## Vertebral artery reconstruction

The vertebrobasilar territory is affected in 15–25% of all ischaemic strokes, but there have been no randomised trials similar to ECST or NASCET to guide practice. In contrast to the primarily embolic aetiology of carotid stroke, vertebrobasilar events tend to be haemodynamic.

For patients with symptomatic lesions at the origin of the vertebral artery, surgical options include short vein bypass or transposition of the vertebral artery onto the CCA. However, angioplasty with or without stenting is now assuming an increasing role in this situation. The latter may also have an important role in patients with more distal disease as surgical access to the upper two-thirds of the vertebral artery is difficult.

An occlusion or severe stenosis at the origin of the subclavian artery may result in reversed flow down the ipsilateral vertebral artery to perfuse the arm (subclavian steal). Arm exercise may therefore result in vertebrobasilar ischaemia. Classical symptoms include forearm claudication, coexistent vertebrobasilar symptoms are less common. In practice, intervention is recommended in patients with symptomatic lesions, especially involving the dominant arm. Both surgery and endovascular intervention carry a small risk of procedural stroke. A similar syndrome exists (coronary steal) in patients who have undergone coronary bypass using the internal mammary artery. Should a proximal subclavian stenosis have been missed preoperatively, or subsequently develop, angina can be precipitated by arm exercise. In this situation, the angina can be treated by carotid–subclavian bypass or angioplasty. There is no evidence that either strategy is preferable.

## Surgical management of carotid disease–Carotid endarterectomy

### Anaesthesia

CEA can be performed under local or general anaesthesia. Local anaesthesia (superficial and deep cervical plexus blockade supplemented by local infiltration) has been used during CEA since the 1960s. CEA under regional anaesthesia is currently the only method for accurately predicting who needs a shunt, but it will not prevent complications due to thromboembolism (which is the principal cause of intraoperative stroke).

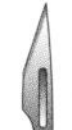

The GALA trial randomised >3500 CEAs to loco-regional or general anaesthesia. There was no difference in 30-day outcomes. Surgeons may therefore use either anaesthetic strategy according to their own preserence.[56]

## Surgical technique

CEA is usually performed using loupe magnification with the extended head turned away from the side of operation and placed on a rubber ring. An incision is made over the anterior border of sternomastoid and dissection continued down to the carotid bifurcation, which is exposed after division of the common facial vein. The CCA and ECA are controlled with slings; some prefer not to sling the ICA because of the potential for dislodging thrombus. Some surgeons infiltrate the carotid sinus with 1% lidocaine (lignocaine) to prevent reflex hypotension and bradycardia. Four RCTs have addressed this question and none have found any evidence of benefit regarding this practice.

The distal ICA should be mobilised 1 cm beyond the upper limit of the plaque and this is facilitated by ligation and division of the sternomastoid artery and vein (which tethers the hypoglossal nerve) with/without division of digastric. If surgeons are worried about the need to proceed high in the neck, access can be facilitated preoperatively by nasolaryngeal intubation or temporomandibular subluxation. The latter must be planned in advance as it cannot be performed once the operation has started.

The principal cranial nerves (hypoglossal, vagus) are identified and preserved. With high dissections, the glossopharyngeal nerve is also at risk. Contrary to classical teaching, however, most postoperative swallowing problems do not follow glossopharyngeal nerve injury. These usually follow damage to the small motor branches of the vagus nerve which cross the ICA anteriorly, just distal to the hypoglossal nerve.

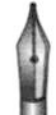

Any patient who has undergone a contralateral CEA, neck dissection or thyroidectomy must undergo a preoperative check of recurrent laryngeal and hypoglossal nerve function. Bilateral injuries to either can be fatal.

Following systemic heparinisation (5000 units), soft clamps are applied to the distal ICA, CCA and ECA. A longitudinal arteriotomy is made from the distal CCA across the plaque and into the ICA beyond the stenosis. If a shunt is to be deployed it is inserted now (**Fig. 10.8**). The endarterectomy plane is entered using a Watson–Cheyne dissector and it is conventional to divide the plaque first at the CCA aspect and then carefully mobilise it up towards the ICA. The distal end usually feathers off smoothly but can be tacked down with interrupted fine prolene sutures. Loose intimal fragments are removed in a radial, as opposed to axial, direction. An alternative technique to that described is 'eversion' endarterectomy. Here the origin of the ICA is transected and reimplanted after eversion of the atheromatous core.

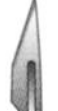

There is no evidence from systematic reviews that eversion endarterectomy confers any benefit over traditional endarterectomy provided the arteriotomy is closed with a patch.

The arteriotomy can be closed primarily or with a patch (see below). Flow is restored first up the ECA and then the ICA. There is no compelling evidence that reversal of anticoagulation with protamine is beneficial and it may increase the risk of postoperative thrombosis. However, all patients should receive long-term antiplatelet therapy. There is no evidence that anticoagulation reduces the risk of restenosis or late stroke.

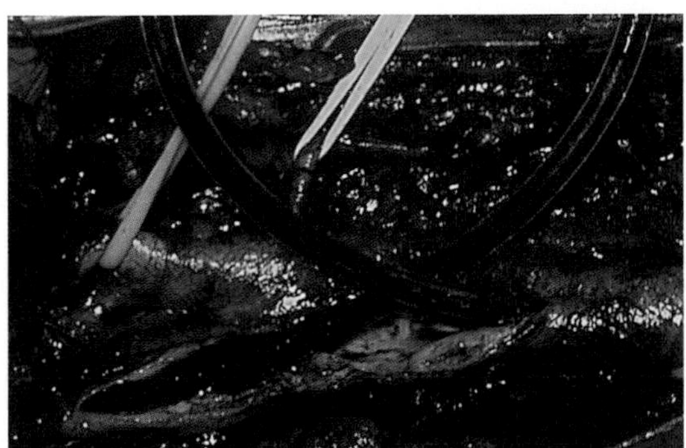

**Figure 10.8** • An arteriotomy has been made across the carotid stenosis and a Pruit–Inahara shunt inserted. This type of shunt is held in place with balloons.

### Patch or primary closure?

The rationale underlying patch closure is that it reduces the risk of early postoperative thrombosis and late restenosis. Early carotid thrombosis complicates 2–3% of CEAs and is a major cause of perioperative stroke. Recurrent stenosis affects about 13% of patients but very few develop symptoms.[57,58] Critics of patching argue that it increases clamp or shunt times by 15–20 minutes, that a vein patch is susceptible to rupture, while a prosthetic patch is susceptible to infection.

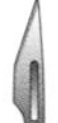

The 2004 Cochrane Review of seven RCTs[59] showed that a policy of routine patching was preferable to routine primary closure with a threefold reduction in perioperative stroke, thrombosis and late restenosis. No RCT has compared routine patching with selective patching and there is no evidence that patch type (polytetrafluoroethylene, Dacron, vein) influences stroke rate, mortality or arterial restenosis.

### Shunt deployment

A temporary shunt may be used never, selectively or routinely and again there is no consensus amongst surgeons. Supporters of shunting argue that its routine use allows time for a more thorough endarterectomy, facilitates safer training of young surgeons and ensures familiarity with shunt insertion, which is useful when a difficult situation (e.g. high dissection) arises. Non-shunters claim that there is an increased risk of intimal injury and embolisation and that the shunt physically interferes with the procedure. As a consequence, many deploy a shunt selectively on the basis of intraoperative monitoring. The most commonly used shunts are the Javid shunt (which has higher flow rates but requires an external retaining clamp, i.e. you need to mobilise even more of the distal ICA) and the double-ballooned Pruitt–Inahara shunt (which is more flexible).

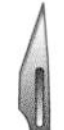

Few RCTs are available but a recent overview of the available data suggests that routine shunting does not alter outcome.[60] However, the Cochrane meta-analysis must be interpreted in the knowledge that in one of the biggest contributory studies, patients randomised to no shunt were then shunted if EEG abnormalities occurred during clamping.[61]

## Perioperative monitoring

The aim of monitoring is to correct and/or prevent cerebral ischaemia before permanent neurological injury occurs. The simplest assessment of intracranial flow is a subjective assessment of ICA backflow or ICA stump pressure, but this may bear little relation to intracranial blood flow in the presence of circle of Willis anomalies or stenoses.

Transcranial Doppler (TCD) is probably the most versatile and practical of the available monitoring methods and uses a low-frequency (2 MHz) pulsed-wave ultrasound beam directed through the temporal bone. This permits insonation of the MCA, which receives 80% of ICA inflow. The quality of the signal depends on the thickness of the cranium and an inaccessible window may be present in about 10% of patients.

A single monitoring modality is no guarantee of global protection. During CEA, TCD fulfils only four roles: (i) to diagnose particulate embolisation during carotid mobilisation (i.e. warning of an unstable plaque), (ii) to ensure mean middle cerebral blood flow velocity remains >15 cm/s, (iii) to ensure the shunt is working and (iv) to identify the very rare case of on-table thrombosis following flow restoration.

Neurological activity can be evaluated directly by performing CEA under local anaesthesia and this is the 'gold standard' for determining who needs a shunt. However, it will not prevent thromboembolic complications. Neurological activity can be evaluated indirectly by EEG or sensory-evoked potential (SEP) measurement. The principle underlying the use of EEG is that once perfusion falls below 18 mL/100 g brain per minute there is loss of high-frequency activity, whereas below 15 mL/100 g brain per minute the EEG becomes isoelectric.[62]

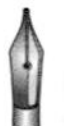

The surgeon must be aware that just because the EEG is flat, it does not mean that a neurological injury is inevitable, as this only tends to occur once perfusion falls below 10 mL/100 g brain per minute.[62] Thus loss of EEG function is a warning that insertion of a shunt or elevation of systemic blood pressure may be beneficial.

The main problem with conventional EEG monitoring is that it is generally oversensitive to the superficial cortex and data can be complex to interpret. Centres using EEG usually require the support of experienced neurophysiological technicians. The advantage of SEP measurement is that it reflects the function of the entire afferent pathway from peripheral nerve (usually the median nerve) to the somatosensory cortex. Ischaemia causes a reduction in the amplitude of the primary cortical wave and prolongation of central conduction time.

## Quality control assessment

Although most vascular surgeons undertake some form of quality control (QC) assessment following peripheral reconstructions, the same does not generally apply following CEA. This is despite the fact that most neurological complications follow inadvertent technical error. The role of QC is to identify incomplete endarterectomy, distal intimal flaps, adherent luminal thrombus, residual stenoses and wall irregularities. The most important, however, is exclusion of residual luminal thrombus which originates from bleeding from endarterectomised vasa vasorum.[63]

QC techniques include TCD, angiography, colour duplex ultrasound, continuous-wave Doppler and angioscopy. TCD ensures optimal shunt function and it is the only method capable of diagnosing on-table carotid thrombosis and early postoperative occlusion. Angiography (which must be biplanar) provides easily interpretable anatomical data but requires ionising radiation and can only be performed after restoration of flow (i.e. any thrombus could be swept distally). The latest colour duplex probes are smaller and more accessible because of the development of L-shaped probes but usually require the presence of a technician in theatre.

At the Leicester Royal Infirmary, there is experience of using completion angioscopy in over 1500 patients. The principal advantage over all other QC techniques is that it is performed *prior* to restoration of flow. Its main role is to identify the 3% of patients with residual luminal thrombus and the 1–2% with large intimal flaps. Since introducing this technique, the intraoperative stroke rate has fallen from 4% to 0.2% and it has contributed significantly towards a 60% reduction in the 30-day risk.[63]

## Operative complications

### Cranial nerve injuries

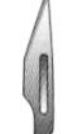

Cranial nerve injury is rarely discussed before CEA, but is an important source of morbidity. In a detailed review, Forsell et al.[64] have shown that up to 50% of patients will suffer some degree of cranial nerve injury.

In NASCET, the incidence of injury to the mandibular branch of the facial nerve was 2.2%, to the vagus 2.5%, to the spinal accessory nerve 0.2% and to the hypoglossal 3.7%. The overall rate of cranial nerve injury was 8.6%,[65] although 92% were minor and fully recovered within 4 weeks. Studies using indirect laryngoscopy or video fluoroscopy reveal a much higher incidence of occult cranial nerve injury.[65] In the ECST, 6.4% of CEA patients suffered a cranial nerve injury.[45] In only nine patients was the injury permanent.

### Wound complications

In NASCET, 132 CEA patients (9.3%) developed wound complications, of which 76 (58%) were minor, 52 (39%) moderate, while only 4 (3%) were classed as severe.[65] Early vein patch rupture complicates <1% of CEAs and is virtually abolished if saphenous vein is harvested from the groin.

### Perioperative stroke

Neurological events are classed as intraoperative if the patient recovers from anaesthesia with a new deficit and postoperative if the event occurs thereafter. In historical series, intraoperative stroke predominated and was more likely to affect patients with a combination of cerebral infarction and partial or total haemodynamic compromise. This suggests that high-risk patients are more vulnerable to otherwise minor changes in perfusion pressure or emboli, so that the margin for technical error is reduced or possibly non-existent.

Intraoperative stroke has been virtually abolished at the Leicester Royal Infirmary (0.3% in 1500 cases), a feature attributed to removing luminal thrombus (identified by angioscopy) prior to flow restoration. The commonest causes of postoperative stroke are: (i) ICA thrombosis (especially in the first six postoperative hours), (ii) hyperperfusion syndrome and (iii) intracranial haemorrhage (ICH). ICH and the hyperperfusion syndrome complicate 1–2% of CEAs and are more common in patients with severe bilateral extracranial disease in association with impaired cerebral vascular reserve, defective autoregulation and poor collateral flow patterns.[66]

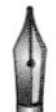

It is essential that emergency medical units recognise the absolute importance of early treatment in the CEA patient who presents with seizures, usually 5–7 days after surgery. These patients have a high risk of suffering an ICH and the mainstay of management is control of seizures and aggressive control of blood pressure.[66]

The strategy for managing perioperative events depends on: (i) timing (intraoperative or postoperative), (ii) whether it follows thrombosis, embolism or haemorrhage, and (iii) the severity of the neuro-logical deficit. In general, the more extensive the deficit, the more likely that the ICA or MCA has occluded. For those without access to TCD and duplex, the surgeon has to assume that any deficit occurring following recovery from anaesthesia or in the first 24 hours is thromboembolic and the patient re-explored. Although re-exploration will not benefit patients with focal embolism or haemodynamic stroke, this cannot currently be avoided.

For those with access to TCD and duplex, decision-making is easier. The immediate priority is to identify patients with ICA thrombosis, as they require immediate exploration. Provided flow is restored within 1 hour, good neurological recovery can be expected.

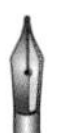

TCD features of early carotid thrombosis include flow reversal in the ipsilateral anterior cerebral artery, enhanced flow in the ipsilateral posterior cerebral artery and, most importantly, flow velocities in the ipsilateral MCA that mimic those observed during carotid clamping.

However, it would be preferable to *prevent* thrombosis from happening. Evidence from three continents has now conclusively shown that early postoperative carotid thrombosis (POCT) is preceded by 1–2 hours of increasing embolisation, which can be diagnosed using TCD,[67] and that 50–60% of patients with sustained embolisation will progress to a thrombotic stroke.[67] At the Leicester Royal Infirmary, Dextran 40 is administered to the 5% of patients with high rates of embolisation (>25 emboli in any 10-minute period). Since this protocol was implemented in October 1995, more than 1300 CEAs have been performed and no patient has suffered a stroke due to POCT. This represents a major change to previous practice, where 2–3% suffered a stroke due to carotid thrombosis in the first six postoperative hours.

## Long-term follow-up and restenosis

The final results from the ECST showed that the average annual risk of late ipsilateral stroke after CEA was 1–2%.[68] The risk of stroke in the contralateral, non-operated ICA territory is 1.4% per annum.[69]

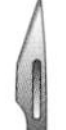

Meta-analyses suggest that the average annual risk of recurrent stenosis (50–100%) is 1.5–4.5%,[57,58] although the risk is highest in the first 12 months. The association between recurrent stenosis and ipsilateral stroke is tenuous.

Some surgeons recommend serial clinical and duplex ultrasound surveillance with the intention of performing repeat CEA in patients with recurrent stenoses >70%. However, there is little if any evidence to support this practice. A recent review suggests that the risk of late ipsilateral stroke in patients with recurrent stenoses >50% is about 2% per annum, falling to 1% per annum in those with no recurrent disease or a stenosis <50%.[70] Moreover, 11–20% of treated patients will develop a second recurrent stenosis after either repeat CEA or carotid angioplasty.

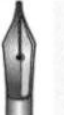

If one focuses solely on outcomes from RCTs (usually independent neurological verification and a pre-planned follow-up strategy), there is no evidence that recurrent stroke correlates with recurrent stenosis. In ACAS, the risk of late stroke was unrelated to the presence of a recurrent stenosis and only one patient (0.15%) suffered a stroke and had a severe recurrent stenosis.[71]

Thus there seems to be little clinical or cost-based evidence for recommending a policy of long-term surveillance. For the most part, patients can be safely discharged at 6 weeks and told to report back should they develop further symptoms. The only exception to this practice is patients who have undergone a vein bypass graft as they have a higher 20% incidence of recurrent stenosis within 3 years. The Leicester policy is to survey these patients with duplex and treat any severe recurrent lesions with angioplasty, especially if middle cerebral artery flow velocities during carotid clamping had been <15 cm/s.

## Patch infection

Late patch infection complicates <1% of all CEAs and can be very difficult to manage.[73]

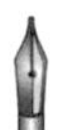

A fundamental rule should be that no abscess overlying a CEA wound is incised before the patient has been seen by a vascular surgeon.

If infection is suspected, the CCA must be controlled well below the original incision. The prosthetic patch should be removed and replaced (where appropriate with a saphenous vein patch). If this is not possible, a reversed vein graft should be considered. Distal ligation should only be considered as a last resort (uncontrollable haemorrhage) and preferably if some form of monitoring (e.g. TCD, awake neurological testing at the original procedure) suggests that collateral flow is satisfactory.[72]

# Endovascular treatment of carotid disease

Over the last 10 years, the role of endovascular therapy in the management of carotid disease has received growing attention with the emergence of dedicated systems, refinement of cerebral protection strategies and perhaps most importantly the performance of RCTs. There is no doubt that CAS has emerged as a viable alternative to open surgery but, as with CEA, care must be taken to select patients appropriately, to ensure appropriate pharmacological management before, during and after stenting, and to perform the procedure with meticulous attention to technique.

## Assessing suitability for CAS

Careful case selection is an absolute requirement for safe practice. All patients being considered for CAS require 'overview' anatomical imaging, i.e. from the arch origins of the great vessels to the circle of Willis (see earlier).

Absolute contraindications to CAS include an occluded ICA or visible thrombus and a difficult origin to the brachiocephalic artery or left CCA making selective catheterisation difficult or impossible. In addition, any severe tortuosity of the brachiocephalic artery or CCA is a relative contraindication to CAS. Tortuosity of the ICA above the stenosis (**Fig. 10.9**) may prevent use of a cerebral protection system other than reverse flow devices. This tortuosity could be turned into a kink or occlusion by a stent.

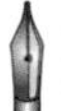

Once anatomical suitability for CAS is confirmed, the decision to intervene by CAS is best made in a multidisciplinary environment.[73]

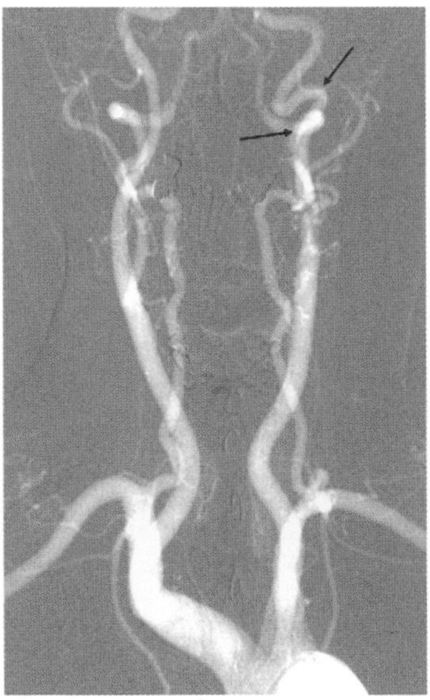

**Figure 10.9** • Tortuosity of the distal left ICA may preclude the use of distal protection devices (filters and distal balloons), but the neuroprotection system from Gore (Flagstaff, Arizona) which causes flow reversal could be used.

## Dual antiplatelet therapy

It is now routine practice to employ dual antiplatelet therapy; 75 mg of clopidogrel is commenced 1 week prior to intervention in addition to 75 mg aspirin daily. In recently symptomatic patients, 300–600 mg clopidogrel (depending on body weight) is given at least 15 hours pre-intervention. The dual antiplatelet regime should be continued for 28 days post-stent placement, i.e. the presumed time-frame for endothelialisation of the stent.

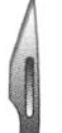

A randomised trial comparing aspirin plus clopidogrel versus aspirin plus 24-hour anticoagulation in patients undergoing CAS showed a significant and dramatic benefit regarding procedural adverse events and stent patency in favour of dual antiplatelet therapy.[74]

## Summary of CAS procedure

Femoral access is obtained in the usual manner. Brachial (or radial) approaches are alternatives if there is a difficult arch (i.e. either 'type III' or 'bovine'). In a type III arch, the origin of the brachiocephalic is significantly lower than a horizontal line drawn across the highest point of the arch (by as much as 2 cm). In the 'bovine' arch (a misnomer as this is not seen in cattle), there is a conjoint origin to the brachiocephalic and left CCA. A loading dose of unfractionated heparin (5000–7500 units) is administered at the time of arterial access, with repeat boluses to maintain an activated clotting time >200 seconds.

The CCA is catheterised (Headhunter 1, Sidewinder, Vitek) and a support (stiff) wire placed in the ECA, over which a suitable guiding catheter or long sheath is placed with the tip 2–3 cm below the bifurcation. The size of the guiding catheter or sheath is dependent on the diameter of the stent delivery system.

Calibrated angiography is performed to assess the sizes of the ICA and CCA. The size of the ICA will determine the size of the protection device; the size of the CCA will determine the diameter of the stent.

Atropine (0.6–1.2 mg) or glycopyrrolate (a synthetic derivative with less cardioaccelerator effects than atropine) at a dose of 0.6 mg is delivered into the CCA to block the carotid sinus baroreceptors.

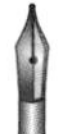

The administration of atropine/glycopyrrolate will cause short-term unilateral mydriasis. Staff looking after the patient upon return to the ward should be notified about this harmless finding as it is otherwise likely to cause alarm.

The ICA stenosis is crossed either with a 0.014 wire onto which a filter is later loaded ('bare wire' system) or with the cerebral protection device itself (a wire-mounted filter or occlusion balloon). This is then deployed. The lesion should be crossed only once and movement of the guidewire once the tip has been placed below the base of skull should be minimised.

Stent delivery systems are now 5-Fr compatible (i.e. just under 2 mm in diameter). Occasionally it may be possible to cross the lesion with the delivery system without predilatation, but care must be taken to avoid 'snow-ploughing' the plaque during passage of the delivery system. The severity of the stenosis may be underestimated on single-plane angiography and it is therefore recommended to predilate all lesions to 3 mm in order to allow safe passage of the stent-delivery system through potentially vulnerable plaque.

The stent is delivered across the stenosis using road-mapping (real-time digital subtraction). Once deployed, the stent is usually gently dilated with a balloon to ensure good apposition against the arterial wall. It is probably not necessary to aggressively dilate, and many practitioners are comfortable leaving some residual stenosis rather than overdilating the lesion.

Angiography is performed in at least two planes after completion of the procedure with specific attention being paid to the following details. First there is no prolapse of plaque material into the lumen through stent interstices (**Fig. 10.10**). This requires gentle re-ballooning and often 'double scaffolding', i.e. placement of a second stent inside the first. Second is to exclude significant spasm around the filter. This is usually evident early in the procedure and the slow administration of boluses of diluted nitroglycerine (100–200 μg) into the long sheath and/or prompt completion of the procedure and retrieval of the filter is likely to resolve the problem. Spasm is usually well tolerated. Third is that the filter (if used) is not completely occluded by material, a situation which might require aspiration through a large-bore catheter prior to filter retrieval. Fourth is to ensure that there is no obvious loss of intracranial vessels as a result of embolisation.

A closure device is used to close the femoral puncture. The procedure should take less than 1 hour. Generally, CAS procedures are rendered lengthy due to difficult anatomy making access more challenging. The longer it takes to engage the great vessel origin and secure access with a long sheath/guiding catheter, the greater the potential for cerebral embolisation due to excessive manipulation of catheters/guidewires along the aortic arch. A recent evaluation of 627 protected CAS procedures yielded important findings regarding the timing of procedural complications.[75] The procedure

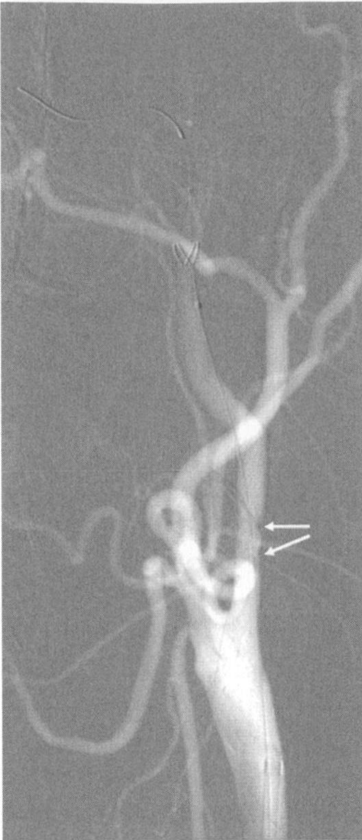

**Figure 10.10** • Plaque prolapse through the interstices of a closed-cell stent (the Abbott XAct; white arrows). This was treated by placing a second stent inside the first, i.e. 'double scaffolding'.

was subdivided arbitrarily into five major stages. At 30 days there were 10 major strokes (two of which were fatal) and one cardiac death, for an overall major stroke/death rate of 1.75%. Eighteen minor strokes (2.9%) were also recorded. Four major strokes occurred in phase 1 (catheterisation of the arch, target vessel and CCA) and six in phase 3 (stent deployment, pre- and postdilatation). It was concluded that a large proportion of major strokes (4/10) during CAS occurred during catheterisation and that these could not have been prevented by the use of a protection device.

## Cerebral protection devices

Perhaps the most feared complication of stent placement is plaque embolisation. Three strategies have been proposed in order to avoid this.

### Distal balloon occlusion

Theron positioned a distal protection balloon in the ICA above the stenosis, prior to stent placement, and commercial variations on distal balloon protection are now available. Although the basic principle is simple, there are a number of disadvantages. Angulated lesions may be difficult to cross, the balloon can inflict damage to the arterial wall, up to 10% of patients are intolerant of ICA occlusion, and the stenosis cannot be imaged while the ICA is occluded.

### Distal filters

These are currently used in up to 95% of cases. All require that the lesion be crossed with a constrained filter that is then deployed above the stenosis or crossed with a 0.014-inch guidewire onto which the filter is subsequently loaded. The filter prevents the majority of emboli passing to the brain during manipulation of the stenosis, and is retrieved following final dilatation of the stent. There is the potential for filter through-flow (relating to the pore size of the filtration element) and filter peri-flow. Self-limiting spasm of the ICA is relatively common (**Fig. 10.11**a–c).

### Flow reversal

A third variation involves the establishment of reverse flow within the ICA prior to any intervention. This is achieved by occluding flow in the CCA using a balloon on the guide-catheter and another in the ECA using a separate balloon occlusion system. The side arm of the guide-catheter is then connected percutaneously to the common femoral vein, effectively producing reverse flow through an arteriovenous fistula.

## Do cerebral protection systems make a difference?

There are, as yet, no randomised trials. The world registry,[76,77] a systematic review of the literature[78] and data from individual units[79,80] suggest that protection devices do reduce stroke and death, although each of these studies are limited scientifically. Interestingly, in the SPACE and EVA-3S trials, there was no difference in outcome relative to whether a protection device was used or not.[81,82]

# Periprocedural haemodynamic problems

## Haemodynamic depression

Haemodynamic instability is common during CAS and is baroreceptor mediated. The early CAS literature suggested that without anticholinergic prophylaxis, the incidence of intraprocedural hypotension was 17–22%, while 28–71% develop intraprocedural bradycardia.

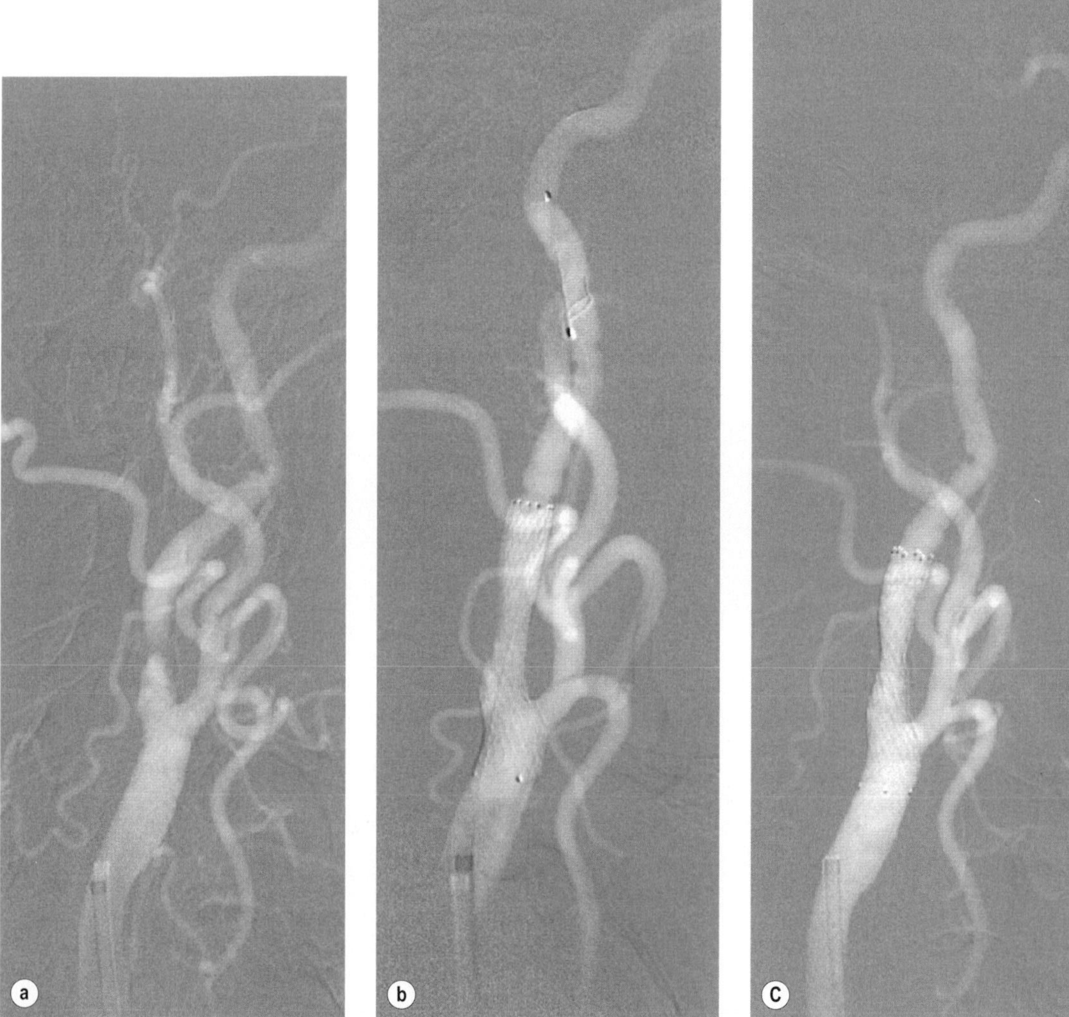


**Figure 10.11** • An example of non-flow-limiting spasm. **(a)** Pre-stenting appearance of the lesion. **(b)** Post-stenting appearances (EV3 Protégé) with a filter in place (EV3 SpideRx). Spasm extends from the leading stent struts to the base of the filter. The patient remained asymptomatic. **(c)** Appearance after retrieval of the filter and the administration of 250 µg of isosorbide dinitrate into the arterial sheath.

Intraprocedural haemodynamic instability is an important but often ignored cause of stroke. Baseline systolic BP >180 mmHg is an independent risk factor for haemodynamic compromise during CAS, resulting in an increased incidence of intra- and periprocedural hypotension and hypertension. If hypotension ensues, the degree of drop in BP correlates linearly with the severity of subsequent neurological insult.[83]

By comparison, postprocedural hypotension is common but usually benign. Treatment is reserved for symptomatic patients or those in whom sustained hypotension may cause cardiovascular compromise (patients awaiting coronary artery bypass grafting or aortic valve replacement). Postprocedural hypotension commonly lasts around 24 hours.

Pharmacotherapy for haemodynamic depression in symptomatic or 'at-risk' patients includes antimuscarinic and/or selective alpha agonists. A recent study evaluated the use of vasopressors in the critical care unit (CCU) for treatment of persistent post-CAS hypotension in 623 patients.[84] The authors concluded that compared with the the mixed alpha/beta agonist dopamine, the more selective alpha agonists (norepenephrine and phenylephrine) were associated with a shorter infusion time and reduced CCU length of stay and fewer major adverse events.

## Hyperperfusion

A total of 54 cases of CAS-associated ICH have been reported and a pooled analysis suggests that the incidence of ICH is 0.63% (95% CI 0.38–0.97%) in studies reporting >100 cases. This is significantly lower ($P < 0.0001$) than that observed in studies reporting <100 cases (2.69%; 95% CI 1.75–3.94%).[86] The incidence of ICH is 2.01% (9/448; 95% CI 0.98–3.65%) in patients treated with glycoprotein IIb/IIIa inhibitors.[85]

Features predictive of an increased risk of ICH include symptomatic lesions, severe stenosis (≥90%) and pre-existing cerebral infarction. The interval between CAS and ICH ranges from immediately after the procedure to 6 days. In 33 of 47 reported cases (70%), the interval between CAS and ICH was ≤24 hours. In 13 cases, the interval was ≤1 hour. In two cases, there was sustained hypotension prior to suffering the ICH (contrary to expectation) and in 9 of 21 patients (43%) there were no prodromal symptoms. Prophylactic pharmacotherapy (e.g. short-acting beta-blockers) is considered in patients considered to be at high risk, and may reduce the incidence of hyperperfusion syndrome and ICH.[86]

## Post-CAS care

Following CAS, patients should be monitored closely to ensure that they remain free of neurological, haemodynamic and puncture-site complications. BP monitoring should continue after discharge for at least 2 weeks following CAS and patients should be advised to return immediately should severe headache develop within the first few weeks of intervention. Patients should also undergo independent review following carotid intervention. Self-audit of outcomes following CEA is notoriously unreliable and the same will undoubtedly apply to CAS.

## Achievement and maintenance of competence

Not so very long ago, CEA was a procedure almost solely performed by consultants and this is still very much the case regarding CAS in the UK. Accordingly, the issue of generalisability has still to be evaluated.

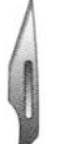

NICE[73] recommends that clinicians undertaking CAS 'should have adequate training before performing this procedure' and they refer the reader to the Royal College of Radiologists (RCR) guidelines.[87]

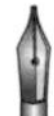

The RCR[87] recommends the following as being indicative of 'competence':

- a minimum number of 30 diagnostic cervicocerebral angiograms;
- 100 diagnostic angiograms;
- 50 non-neurological selective angiograms;
- 25 peripheral or coronary stents;
- Microcatheter techniques;
- Neuroimaging (carotid Doppler, MRA, CTA, catheter angiography).

## Results of CAS

The first human carotid angioplasty was performed by Mathias in 1980, the first dedicated carotid stent systems became available in 1997 and the first commercially available protection devices appeared in 2000. The first RCT comparing CAS and CEA reported just 1 year after dedicated stents became available.[88]

Eight randomised trials have now reported, although only three[88–91] ran to completion (CAVATAS, Lexington symptomatic and Lexington asymptomatic). Five were stopped early, three[82,88,92] for reasons of safety (Wallstent, published in abstract form only, the 'Leicester trial' and EVA-3S), one for futility and financial reasons (SPACE[81]) and one because of resistance on the part of patients or referring clinicians to continue randomisation (SAPPHIRE[93]). These eight trials fell short of their planned recruitment targets by around 1800 patients, leading to a high likelihood of bias and little chance of achieving any statistically meaningful outcome.[94]

The early trials are now largely historical; the later trials continue to arouse considerable criticism and controversy. SAPPHIRE[93] demonstrated 'non-inferiority' for CAS for 'high surgical risk' patients, though many of these were (in fact) asymptomatic. Most were deemed 'high risk' because of cardiac comorbidities, but 25% had post-CEA restenosis as the indication for treatment. In short, many of these patients may have been 'high risk for CEA', but they were not necessarily high risk for stroke. Overall, there was less clinically driven reintervention in the stent group ($P = 0.06$). However, of great concern was the fact that CEA and CAS carried a 5–6% risk of death/stroke at 30 days in patients with asymptomatic disease. At these levels of risk, there is no evidence that either treatment strategy confers any long-term benefit over 'best medical therapy'.

EVA-3S[82] (the French national trial) demonstrated superiority for CEA in recently symptomatic, low operative risk patients, but has faced many detractors. Some have argued that the relatively poor outcomes following CAS (30-day death/stroke 9.3%) may simply reflect what happens in the 'real world', but it is also clear that 85% of the interventionists had performed ≤50 cases and some were performing their first ever procedures within the trial (albeit proctored). The learning curve for CAS is considered to be around 80 cases,[95] but could be higher, especially in 'classically trained' vascular surgeons performing CAS.[95] A further, and often ignored, fact is that almost 50% of the CAS patients in EVA-3S underwent their intervention within 28 days of presentation. At this time, 66% of patients will still have thrombus on the plaque, thus inevitably increasing the possibility of procedural stroke. However, as was shown in Fig. 10.6, these practitioners were preventing more strokes than by waiting >4 weeks and then intervening with a 0% risk.

SPACE[82] (the German national trial) failed to show 'non-inferiority' for CAS as the upper confidence interval for the observed difference in the primary end-point for both intention to treat and per-protocol analyses was >2.5%. However, because the upper and lower confidence intervals crossed 'zero' this also indicated that there was no statistically significant difference.[94]

The Cochrane Collaboration published their latest systematic review in October 2007.[96] Data were available from 12 trials (3227 patients), but not all contributed to all of the analyses. The primary outcome comparison of 'any stroke or death' within 30 days of treatment significantly favoured surgery (odds ratio (OR) 1.39, 95% CI 1.05–1.84). There was a very highly significant reduction in the risk of cranial nerve injury favouring CAS (OR 0.07, 95% CI 0.03–0.20). The following outcomes showed no significant difference between CAS and CEA: (i) 30-day death (OR 0.99, 95% CI 0.50–1.97), (ii) 30-day death/disabling stroke (OR 1.22, 95% CI 0.83–1.79) and (iii) late stroke (OR 1.13, 95% CI 0.80–1.58). The Cochrane Collaboration concluded that the available data were limited and conflicting. The overall estimates of effect were considered imprecise and difficult to interpret because of substantial heterogeneity among the trials due to different patient populations, changes in the technique of endovascular procedures and duration of follow-up.

Two large RCTs (ICSS and CREST) are nearing completion and should inform the debate considerably. Until then, the Cochrane Group have concluded that the available data continue to support the inclusion of patients within ongoing RCTs. However, the 2004 National Clinical Guidelines for Stroke Working Party have conceded that in those units where there are experienced operators and independent audit showing outcomes equivalent to CEA, CAS for symptomatic atherosclerosis can be considered a suitable alternative to CEA.[27] There is, however, no evidence to support the role of CAS in asymptomatic patients outwith the protection of randomised trials and all CAS procedures performed outside trials in the UK should be submitted to the Endovascular Carotid Registry held by the British Society for Interventional Radiology and the Vascular Society of Great Britain and Ireland.[73]

### Key points

- Best medical therapy is indicated in all patients and includes risk factor prevention. It should not be delegated to junior team members. Best medical therapy depends on rapid access to cerebrovascular clinic and is not an alternative to consideration for carotid surgery.
- The beneficial role of CEA is supported by level 1 evidence in selected asymptomatic and sympotomatic patients. It is dependent on being performed early with a low operative risk, and requires surgeons to quote their operative risk rather than trial data.
- Carotid stenting is emerging as an alternative to CEA and is being evaluated in a number of randomised trials. It cannot be justified in units with an excessive interventional risk, and requires interventionists to quote their procedural risk rather than trial data.

## References


1. Bamford J, Sandercock P, Dennid M et al. A prospective study of acute cerebro-vascular disease in the community. The Oxfordshire Community Stroke Project 1981–1986. (I) Methodology, demography and incident cases of first ever stroke. J Neurol Neurosurg Psychiatry 1988; 51:1373–80.
2. Dunbabin D, Sandercock P. Stroke prevention. Hosp Update 1992; July:540–5.
3. Malmgren R, Bamford J, Warlow CP et al. Projecting the number of patients with first ever strokes and patients newly handicapped by stroke in England and Wales. Br Med J 1989; 298: 656–60.
4. Dennis MS, Bamford JM, Sandercock PAG et al. Incidence of transient ischaemic attacks in Oxfordshire, England. Stroke 1989; 20:333–9.

5. Sandercock PAG, Warlow CP, Jones LN et al. Predisposing factors for cerebral infarction: the Oxfordshire Community Stroke Project. Br Med J 1989; 298:75–80.
6. Tripp HF, Fail PJ, Beyer MG et al. New approach to preoperative vascular exclusion for carotid body tumor. J Vasc Surg 2003; 38:389–91.
7. Hammond JH, Eisinger RP. Carotid bruits in 1000 normal subjects. Arch Intern Med 1962; 109:563–5.
8. Wolf PA, Kannel WB, Sorlie P et al. Asymptomatic carotid bruit and risk of stroke: the Framingham Study. JAMA 1981; 245:1442–5.
9. Giles MF, Rothwell PM. The need for emergency treatment of transient ischaemic attack and minor stroke. Expert Rev Neurother 2005; 5:203–10.
10. Naylor AR. Time is brain! The Surgeon 2007; 5:23–30.
11. Rothwell PM, Warlow CP. Timing of TIAS preceding stroke: time window for prevention is very short. Neurology 2005; 64:817–20.
12. Giles MF, Rothwell PM. Risk of stroke early after transient ischaemic attack: a systematic review and meta-analysis. Lancet Neurol 2007; 6:1063–72.
13. Rothwell PM, Giles MF, Flossman E et al. A simple score (ABCD) to identify individuals at high early risk of stroke after transient ischaemic attack. Lancet 2005; 366:29–36.
14. The National Stroke Strategy; www.dh.gov.uk/stroke
15. Grant EG, Benson CB, Moneta GL et al. Carotid artery stenosis: gray-scale and Doppler US diagnosis – Society of Radiologists in Ultrasound Consensus Conference. Radiology 2003; 229:340–6.
16. Vidak V, Hebrang A, Brkljacic B et al. Stenotic occlusive lesions of internal carotid artery in diabetic patients. Coll Antropol 2007; 31:775–80.
17. Gray-Weale AC. Carotid artery atheroma: comparison of pre-operative B-mode ultrasound appearance with carotid endarterectomy specimen pathology. J Cardiovasc Surg 1988; 29:676–81.
18. Gaunt ME, Brown L, Hartshorne T et al. Unstable carotid plaques: pre-operative identification and association with intra-operative embolisation detected by transcranial Doppler. Eur J Vasc Endovasc Surg 1996; 11:78–82.
19. Tegos TJ, Sohail M, Sabetai MM et al. Echomorphic and histopathologic characteristics of unstable carotid plaques. Am J Neuroradiol 2000; 21: 1937–44.
20. Biasi GM, Froio A, Diethrich EB et al. Carotid plaque increases the risk of stroke in carotid stenting: the Imaging in Carotid Angioplasty and Risk of Stroke (ICAROS) study. Circulation 2004; 110:756–62.
21. Reiter M, Bucek RA, Effenberger I et al. Plaque echolucency is not associated with the risk of stroke in carotid artery stenting. Stroke 2006; 37:2378–80.
22. Executive Committee for the Asymptomatic Carotid Atherosclerosis Study. Endarterectomy for asymptomatic carotid artery stenosis. JAMA 1995; 273:1421–61.
23. Berczi V, Randall M, Balamurugan R et al. Safety of arch aortography for assessment of carotid arteries. Eur J Vasc Endovasc Surg 2006; 31:3–7.
24. Borisch I, Horn M, Butz B et al. Preoperative evaluation of carotid artery stenosis: comparison of contrast-enhanced MR angiography and duplex sonography with digital subtraction angiography. Am J Neuroradiol 2003; 24:1117–22.
25. Johnston DC, Eastwood JD, Nguyen T. Contrast-enhanced magnetic resonance angiogrophy of carotid arteries. Utility in routine clinical practice. Stroke 2002; 33:2834–8.
26. Intercollegiate Stroke Working Party. National clinical guidelines for stroke, 2nd edn, Section 3.5.6f, 2004.
27. Wardlaw JM, Chappell FM, Stevenson M et al. Accurate, practical and cost-effective assessment of carotid stenosis in the UK. Health Technol Assess 2006; 10:iii–iv, ix–x, 1–182.
28. The European Stroke Initiative Executive Committee and the EUSI Writing Committee. European Stroke Initiative recommendations for stroke management – Update 2003. Cerebrovasc Dis 2003; 16:311–37.
29. MacMahon S. Antihypertensive drug treatment: the potential, expected and observed effects on vascular disease. J Hypertens 1990; 8(Suppl):S239–44.
30. Kalra L, Perez I, Melbourn A. Stroke risk management: changes in mainstream practice. Stroke 1998; 29:53–7.
31. Heart Protection Study Collaborative Group. MRC/BHF Heart Protection Study of cholesterol lowering with simvastatin in 20536 high-risk individuals: a randomised placebo controlled trial. Lancet 2002; 360:7–22.
32. Antiplatelet Trialists Collaboration. Secondary prevention of vascular disease by prolonged anti-platelet treatment. Br Med J 1988; 296:320–31.
33. North American Symptomatic Carotid Endarterectomy Trial Collaborators. Beneficial effect of carotid endarterectomy in symptomatic patients with high grade stenosis. N Engl J Med 1991; 325:445–53.
34. Taylor DW, Barnett HJM, Haynes RB et al. Low dose and high dose acetylsalicylic acid for patients undergoing carotid endarterectomy: a randomised trial. Lancet 1999; 353:2179–84.
35. Diener H, Cunha L, Forbes C et al. European Stroke Prevention Study (ESPS) 2. Dipyridamole and acetylsalicylic acid in the secondary prevention of stroke. J Neurol Sci 1996; 143:1–13.
36. NICE Technology Appraisal Guidance 90, Vascular disease – clopidogrel and dipyridamole: quick reference guide, 25 May 2005.
37. CAPRIE Steering Committee. A randomised blinded trial of clopidogrel versus aspirin in patients at risk of ischaemic events. Lancet 1996; 348:1329–39.

38. Rothwell PM, Giles MF, Chandratheva A et al. Effect of urgent treatment of transient ischaemic attack and minor stroke on early recurrent stroke (EXPRESS Study): a prospective population based sequential comparison. Lancet 2007; 370:1–11.
39. Rothwell PM, Eliasziw M, Gutnikov SA. for the Carotid Endarterectomy Trialists Collaboration. Analysis of pooled data from the randomised controlled trials of endarterectomy for symptomatic carotid stenosis. Lancet 2003; 361:107–16.
40. Rothwell PM, Eliasziw M, Gutnikov SA. for the Carotid Endarterectomy Trialists Collaboration. Endarterectomy for symptomatic carotid stenosis in relation to clinical subgroups and timing of surgery. Lancet 2004; 363:915–24.
41. Rothwell PM, Eliasziw M, Gutnikov SA. Sex difference in the effect of time from symptoms to surgery on benefit from carotid endarterectomy for transient ischaemic attack and minor stroke. Stroke 2004; 35:2855–61.
42. Wennberg DE, Lucas FL, Birkmeyer JD et al. Variation in carotid endarterectomy mortality in the Medicare population. JAMA 1998; 279: 1278–81.
43. Karp HR, Flanders D, Shipp CC et al. Carotid endarterectomy among Medicare beneficiaries: a statewide evaluation of appropriateness and outcome. Stroke 1998; 29:46–52.
44. Holt PJE, Poloniecki J, Loftus IM. The relationship between hospital case volume and outcome from carotid endartectomy in England from 2000 to 2005. Eur J Vasc Endovasc Surg 2007; 34:646–54.
45. Naylor AR, Rothwell PM, Bell PRF. Overview of the principal results and secondary analyses from the European and the North American randomised trials of carotid endarterectomy. Eur J Vasc Endovasc Surg 2003; 26:115–29.
46. Rockman CB, Maldonado T, Jacobowitz GR et al. Early endarterectomy in symptomatic patients is associated with poorer perioperative outcomes. J Vasc Surg 2006; 44:480–7.
47. Klop RBJ, Eikelboom BC, Taks ACJM. Screening of the internal carotid arteries in patients with peripheral vascular disease by colour-flow Duplex scanning. Eur J Vasc Surg 1991; 5:41–5.
48. Sutton-Turrell KC, Alcorn HG, Wolfson SK et al. Prediction of carotid stenosis in older adults with and without isolated systolic hypertension. Stroke 1987; 18:817–22.
49. Halliday A, Mansfield A, Marro J et al. Prevention of disabling and fatal strokes by successful carotid endarterectomy in patients without recent neurological symptoms: randomized trial. Lancet 2004; 363:1491–502.
50. Young B, Moore WS, Robertson JT et al. An analysis of peri-operative surgical mortality and morbidity in the Asymptomatic Carotid Atherosclerosis Study. Stroke 1996; 27:2216–24.
51. ACST Writing Committee. Author's reply. Lancet 2004; 364:1125–6.
52. Naylor AR, Mehta Z, Rothwell PM. Stroke during coronary artery bypass surgery: a critical review of the role of carotid artery disease. Eur J Vasc Endovasc Surg 2002; 23:283–94.
53. Naylor AR, Cuffe R, Rothwell PM et al. A systematic review of outcomes following staged and synchronous carotid endarterectomy and coronary artery bypass. Eur J Vasc Endovasc Surg 2003; 25:380–9.
54. Naylor AR, Cuffe R, Rothwell PM et al. A systematic review of outcomes following synchronous carotid endarterectomy and coronary artery bypass. Influence of patient and surgical variables. Eur J Vasc Endovasc Surg 2003; 26:230–41.
55. Bond R, Rerkasem K, Rothwell PM. Systematic review of the risks of carotid endarterectomy in relation to the clinical indication for and timing of surgery. Stroke 2003; 34:2290–301.
56. GALA Trial Collaborative Group. General anaesthesia versus local anaesthesia for cartoid surgery (GALA): a multicentre randomised controlled trial. Lancet 2008; 372:2132–45.
57. Latimer CR, Burnand KG. Recurrent carotid stenosis after carotid endarterectomy. Br J Surg 1997; 84:1206–19.
58. Frericks H, Kievit J, van Baalen JM . Carotid recurrent stenosis and risk of ipsilateral stroke. A systematic review of the literature. Stroke 1998; 29:244–50.
59. Bond R, Rerkasem K, Naylor AR. Patch angioplasty versus primary closure for carotid endarterectomy. Cochrane Database Syst Rev 2004; 2:CD000160.
60. Bond R, Rerkasem K, Counsell C. Routine or selective carotid artery shunting for carotid endarterectomy (and different methods of monitoring in selective shunting). Cochrane Database Syst Rev 2002; 2:CD000190.
61. Sandmann W, Willeke F, Kolvenbach R. Shunting and neuromonitoring: a prospective randomised study. In: Greenhalgh RM, Hollier LH (eds) Surgery for stroke. London: WB Saunders, 1993; pp. 287–96.
62. Astrup J, Siesjo BK, Symon L. Thresholds in cerebral ischaemia: the ischaemic penumbra. Stroke 1981; 12:723–5.
63. Naylor AR, Hayes PD, Allroggen H et al. Reducing the risk of carotid surgery: a seven year audit of the role of monitoring and quality control assessment. J Vasc Surg 2000; 32:750–9.
64. Forsell C, Bergqvist D, Bergentz SE. Peripheral nerve injuries in carotid artery surgery. In: Greenhalgh RM, Hollier LH (eds) Surgery for stroke. London: WB Saunders, 1993; pp. 217–34.
65. Ferguson GG, Eliasziw M, Barr HWK et al. The North American Symptomatic Carotid Endarterectomy Trial: surgical results in 1415 patients. Stroke 1999; 30:1751–8.

66. Naylor AR, Evans J, Thompson MM et al. Seizures after carotid endarterectomy: hyperperfusion, dysautoregulation or hypertensive encephalopathy? Eur J Vasc Endovasc Surg 2003; 26:39–44.

67. Laman DM, Wieneke GH, van Duijn H et al. High embolic rate after carotid endarterectomy is associated with early cerebrovascular complications. J Vasc Surg 2002; 36:278–84.

68. European Carotid Surgery Trialists' Collaborative Group. Randomised trial of endarterectomy for recently symptomatic carotid stenosis: final results of the MRC European Carotid Surgery Trial (ECST). Lancet 1998; 351:1379–87.

69. Naylor AR, John T, Howlett J et al. Fate of the non-operated carotid artery after contralateral endarterectomy. Br J Surg 1995; 82:44–8.

70. Horrocks M. When should I re-operate for recurrent carotid stenosis. In: Naylor AR, Mackey W (eds) Carotid artery surgery: a problem based approach. London: Harcourt, 2000; pp. 371–4.

71. Moore WS, Kempczinski RF, Nelson JJ et al. Recurrent carotid stenosis: results of the Asymptomatic Carotid Atherosclerosis Study. Stroke 1998; 29:2018–25.

72. Naylor AR, Payne D, Thompson MM et al. Prosthetic patch infection after carotid endarterectomy. Eur J Vasc Endovasc Surg 2002; 23:11–16.

73. National Institute for Clinical Excellence (NICE). Carotid artery stent placement for carotid stenosis, September 2006, IPG 191.

74. McKevitt FM, Randall MS, Cleveland TJ. The benefits of combined anti-platelet treatment in carotid artery stenting. Eur J Vasc Endvasc Surg 2005; 29:522–7.

75. Verzini F, Cao P, De Rango P et al. Appropriateness of learning curve for carotid artery stenting: an analysis of periprocedural complications. J Vasc Surg 2006; 44:1205–11.

76. Wholey MW, Mathias K, Roubin G et al. Global experience in cervical carotid artery stent placement. Catheter Cardiovasc Interv 2000; 50:160–7.

77. Wholey MH, Al-Mubarak N. Updated review of the global carotid stent registry. Catheter Cardiovasc Interv 2003; 60:259–66.

78. Kastrup A, Groschel K, Krapf H et al. Early outcomes of carotid angioplasty and stenting with and without cerebral protection devices. A systematic review of the literature. Stroke 2003; 34:813–19.

79. Castriota F, Cremonesi A, Manetti R et al. Impact of cerebral protection devices on early outcome of carotid stenting. J Endovasc Ther 2002; 9:786–92.

80. McKevitt FM, Macdonald S, Venables GS et al. Complications following carotid angioplasty and carotid stenting in patients with symptomatic carotid artery disease. Cerebrovasc Dis 2004; 17:28–34.

81. SPACE Collaborators. Stent Protected Angioplasty versus Carotid Endarterectomy in symptomatic patients: 30 days results from the SPACE Trial. Lancet 2006; 368:1239–47.

82. Mas J-L, Chatellier G, Beyssen B et al. Endarterectomy versus stenting in patients with severe symptomatic stenosis N Engl J Med 2006; 355:1660–71.

83. Howell M, Krajcer Z, Dougherty K et al. Correlation of periprocedural systolic blood pressure changes with neurological events in high-risk carotid stent patients. J Endovasc Ther 2002; 9:810–16.

84. Nandalur MR, Cooper H, Satler LF. Vasopressor use in the critical care unit for treatment of persistent post-carotid artery stent induced hypotension. Neurocrit Care 2007; 7:232–7.

85. Hyun-Seung K, Han MH, Kwon O-Ki et al. Intracranial hemorrhage after carotid angioplasty: a pooled analysis. J Endovasc Ther 2007; 14:77–85.

86. Abou-Chebl A, Reginelli J, Bajzer CT et al. Intensive treatment of hypertension decreases the risk of hyperperfusion and intracerebral hemorrhage following carotid artery stenting. Catheter Cardiovasc Interv 2007; 69:690–6.

87. Advice from the Royal College of Radiologists concerning training for carotid artery stenting (CAS). Ref. No. BFCR (06)6.

88. Naylor AR, Bolia A, Abbott RJ et al. Randomized study of carotid angioplasty and stenting versus carotid endarterectomy: a stopped trial. J Vasc Surg 1998; 28:326–34.

89. CAVATAS investigators. Endovascular versus surgical treatment in patients with carotid stenosis in the Carotid and Vertebral Artery Transluminal Angioplasty study (CAVATAS): a randomized trial. Lancet 2001; 357:1729–37.

90. Brooks WH, McClure RR, Jones MR et al. Carotid Angioplasty and Stenting versus Carotid Endarterectomy: randomized trial in a community hospital. J Am Coll Cardiol 2001; 38:1589–95.

91. Brooks WH, McClure RR, Jones MR et al. Carotid Angioplasty and Stenting Versus Carotid Endarterectomy for the treatment of asymptomatic carotid stenosis: a randomized trial in a community hospital. Neurosurgery 2004; 54:318–24.

92. Alberts MJ. Results of a multicenter prospective randomized trial of carotid artery stenting vs. carotid endarterectomy. Stroke 2001; 32:325.

93. Yadav J, Wholey MH, Kuntz RE et al. Protected carotid-artery stenting versus endarterectomy in high-risk patients. NEngl J Med 2004; 351(15):1493–501.

94. Naylor AR. Where next after SPACE and EVA3S: "the good, the bad and the ugly". Eur J Vasc Endovasc Surg 2007; 33:44–7.

95. Ahmadi R, Willfort A, Lang W et al. Carotid artery stenting: effect of learning curve and intermediate-term morphological outcome. J Endovasc Ther 2001; 8:539–46.

96. Ederle J, Featherstone RL, Brown MM. Percutaneous transluminal angioplasty and stenting for carotid stenosis. Cochrane Database Syst Rev 2007; 4:CD000515.

# 11

# Vascular disorders of the upper limb

Jean-Baptiste Ricco
Etienne Marchand

## Introduction

Arterial diseases of the upper limb are relatively rare in comparison with those involving the lower extremity. The good collateral supply around the shoulder and elbow explains why chronic occlusive disease is commonly asymptomatic, but acute occlusion due to embolism can result in limb-threatening ischaemia. In addition, thoracic outlet syndrome, axillo-subclavian vein thrombosis and occupational vascular problems need to be considered. In this chapter we do not review vasospastic disorders, connective tissue disease, vasculitis and Raynaud's disease, as these are covered in Chapter 12, nor vascular trauma (covered in Chapter 9). The main causes of upper limb vascular disease are summarised in Box 11.1.

## Clinical examination

Vascular assessment of the upper limb should include the thoracic outlet. Palpation and auscultation of the supraclavicular region may help to detect a cervical rib, a subclavian stenosis or aneurysm. The arm pulses should be examined with the arm placed in the neutral position and then in abduction and external rotation (surrender position) in order to detect arterial thoracic outlet compression. Pulse palpation is important and must include the axillary, brachial, radial and ulnar pulses. The blood pressure should be measured in both arms, preferably using a hand-held Doppler. A difference of more than 15% is abnormal.

Examination of hand ischaemia is not complete unless Allen's test is performed. The examiner compresses the radial and ulnar arteries at the wrist. The examiner then asks the subject to clench the fist in order to empty the hand of blood. The radial artery is then released and the hand is observed for return of colour. The test is then repeated for the ulnar artery. The test is normal if refilling of the hand is complete within less than 10 seconds from either side. Any portion of the hand that does not blush is an indication of incomplete continuity of the palmar arch. The nail folds should be examined for infarcts and splinter haemorrhages.

## Occlusive disease

Occlusive lesions of the brachiocephalic and subclavian arteries occur in relatively young patients with mean ages ranging from 50 to 60 years. These lesions are much less frequent than those involving the carotid bifurcation.[1] Atherosclerosis is the predominant cause in Europe, with Buerger's disease and Takayasu's arteritis far behind. The symptoms of occlusive disease of the upper extremities include muscle fatigue and ischaemic rest pain. Digital necrosis or atheroembolisation is less common than in the lower extremities, accounting for no more than 5% of patients with limb ischaemia.[2]

### Brachiocephalic artery

Stenotic lesions of the brachiocephalic artery are uncommon and may be asymptomatic in 13–22%

**Box 11.1** • Causes of upper limb vascular diseases

**Arterial obstruction**
***Large artery***
Atherosclerosis
Radiotherapy
Thoracic outlet syndrome
Arteritis (giant cell, Takayasu's)
***Small artery***
Atherosclerosis
Connective tissue disease
Myeloproliferative disease
Buerger's disease
Vibrating tools

**Arterial vasospasm**
***Large artery***
Ergot-containing medications and other pharmacological causes
***Small artery***
Raynaud's disease
Vibrating tools
***Embolism: proximal sources***
Heart
Ulcerated arterial plaques (aortic arch, brachiocephalic and subclavian arteries)
Aneurysm (brachiocephalic, subclavian, axillary, brachial, ulnar arteries)
Thoracic outlet syndrome
***Subclavian–axillary vein thrombosis***
Primary: Paget–Schroetter syndrome (thoracic outlet syndrome)
Secondary: catheter, hypercoagulable states
***Hypercoagulable states***
Heparin antibodies
Deficiencies of antithrombin III, proteins C and S
Antiphospholipid syndrome
Malignancy
Cryoglobulinaemia
***Aneurysms***

of patients.[3,4] Symptomatic patients (53.8% and 76.9% respectively in the Mayo Clinic experience[5]) may present with ischaemia of the right upper extremity, carotid territory symptoms or vertebrobasilar symptoms. The diagnosis is suspected by physical examination (i.e. right supraclavicular/cervical bruit, absent right subclavian or axillary pulse) and confirmed by duplex scanning, conventional angiography or computed tomography (CT) or magnetic resonance angiography (MRA). Most patients (61–84%) with brachiocephalic artery occlusion have multiple lesions of the aortic arch vessels.[6] This should be kept in mind when planning treatment. Stenotic lesions of the brachiocephalic artery may be approached by median sternotomy with direct bypass grafting from the aortic arch, or indirectly by extra-anatomical bypass such as subclavian–subclavian, contralateral carotid–carotid or subclavian–carotid bypass.

## Aorto-brachiocephalic bypass

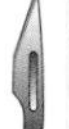

Extra-anatomical bypasses have a lower morbidity and mortality but direct bypasses from the aortic arch are more durable. In total, the combined postoperative death and stroke rate for direct reconstruction of the supra-aortic trunks ranges from 2.6% to 16% (Table 11.1). The primary patency is about 90% with a 72% survival rate at 10 years.[7]

A median sternotomy is used with extension into the neck to allow exposure of the subclavian and common carotid arteries. The left brachiocephalic vein is identified with division of the inferior thyroid and internal mammary vein (**Fig. 11.1**a). A partial occluding clamp or two curved clamps are applied to the ascending aorta proximal to the brachiocephalic artery in order to avoid the risk of fracturing atheromatous plaque (Fig. 11.1b). An 8–10 mm polyester or polytetrafluoroethylene (PTFE) prosthetic graft is anastomosed at this site with deep suture placement in the aortic wall (Fig. 11.1c). Once the anastomosis is completed, a clamp is applied across the graft and systemic heparin is given. The brachiocephalic artery is clamped, sectioned and the proximal stump oversewn. The patent distal artery is spatulated and the graft attached in an end-to-end fashion (Fig. 11.1d). Air is evacuated from the graft by back-bleeding the subclavian artery, then flow is released into the arm and then into the carotid artery. The mortality of direct bypass ranges from 5.8% to 8% in Kieffer's and Berguer's series with a primary patency rate at 5 years of 94% in both series.

## Brachiocephalic endarterectomy

This operation also has good results, although the proximal location of the disease with extension into the aortic arch makes this technique hazardous in some patients. Attempts to remove an orifice lesion may initiate an aortic dissection or distal embolisation. For this reason bypass is preferred for all brachiocephalic lesions except for those located in the distal segment.

## Endovascular treatment

Percutaneous transluminal angioplasty (PTA) or stenting of the brachiocephalic artery is being performed with increased frequency. The approach may be percutaneous from either the femoral

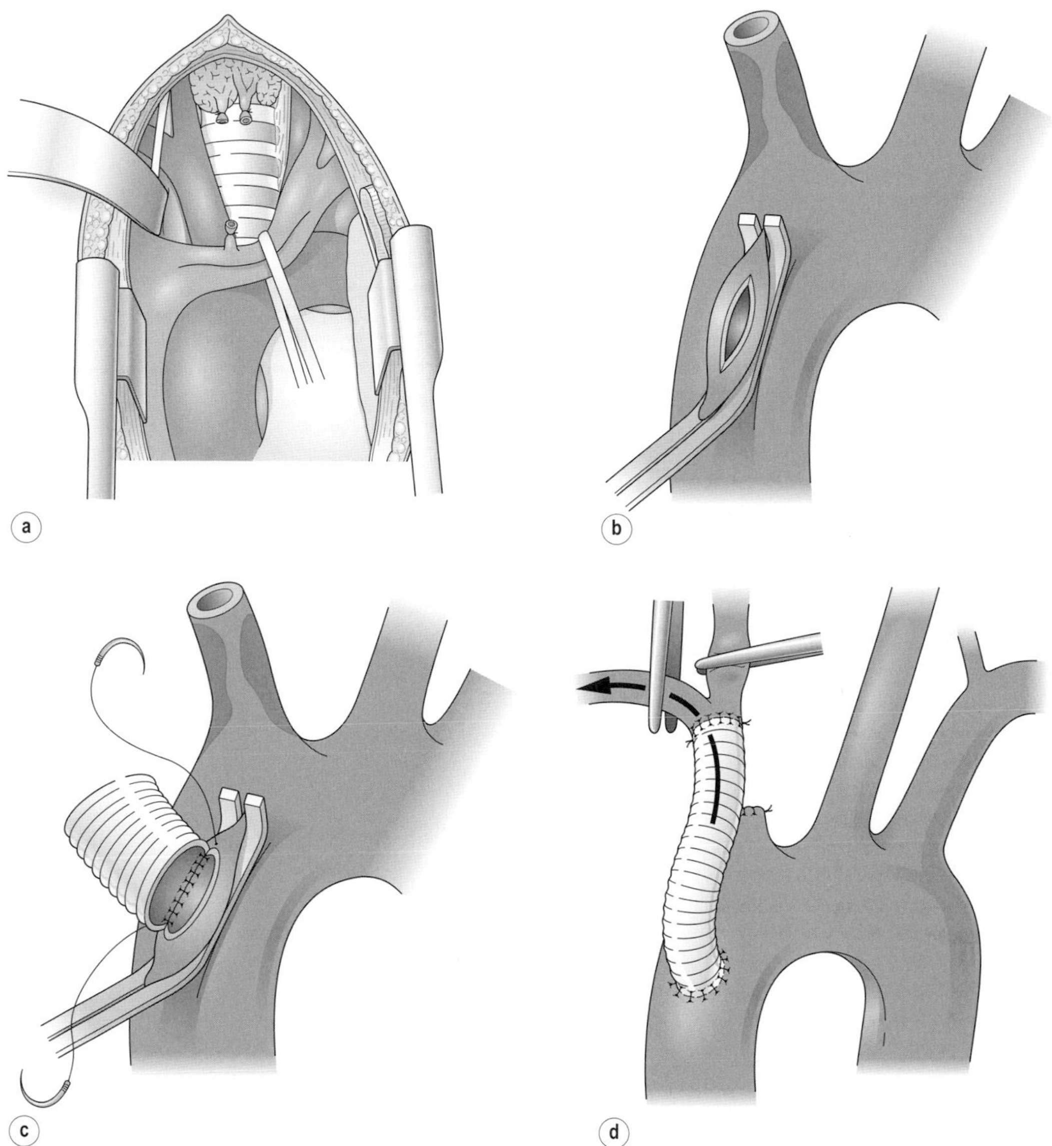


**Figure 11.1 • (a)** The left brachiocephalic vein is retracted to expose the brachiocephalic artery. **(b)** A clamp is applied laterally to the ascending aorta. **(c)** A polyester graft is implanted on the ascending thoracic aorta proximal to the brachiocephalic artery. **(d)** Completed bypass. Flow is released into the arm and then into the common carotid artery.

or brachial artery or through an anterolateral cervical approach with clamping of the right common carotid artery to avoid atheroembolisation during the angioplasty. Because of a relatively small number of cases, most papers concerning the angioplasty of the brachiocephalic artery include results of the subclavian artery. Only one series reports the PTA of brachiocephalic artery alone in 89 patients[9] (Table 11.2). The results of brachiocephalic PTA are therefore difficult to establish. Open surgery gives better mid-term results but angioplasty is less invasive.

## Subclavian artery

Symptomatic lesions of the subclavian artery are associated in 72% of cases with concomitant lesions of carotid and vertebral vessels.[1] The indications for intervention are those of vertebrobasilar insufficiency and upper extremity ischaemia. Atheroembolisation is quite common in this location.[12] If surgery is contemplated and the ipsilateral common carotid artery is healthy, carotid–subclavian bypass or carotid–subclavian transposition is the method of choice.

**Table 11.1** • Direct reconstruction of the supra-aortic vessels: complications and late patency

| Authors, year | Patients | Mean follow-up (months) [range] | Complications (%) | Primary patency (%) |
|---|---|---|---|---|
| Takach et al.,[8] 2005 | 113 | 61.2 ± 6<br>[3–264] | Death: 2.7<br>Stroke: 2.7<br>MI:* 1.8 | 10 years:† 94.4 ± 4 |
| Berguer et al.,[4] 1998 | 100 | 51 ± 4.8<br>[1–184] | Stroke + death: 16<br>Morbidity: 27 | 5 years:‡ 94 ± 3 |
| Uurto et al.,[7] 2002 | 76 | 158 [6–136] | Death: 2.6<br>Morbidity: 19.7 | 1 year: 95<br>5 years:§ 91 15 years:§ 89 |

*MI, myocardial infarction.
†22 patients were followed at 10 years.
‡34 patients followed at 5 years.
§54 patients followed at 5 years and 25 at 15 years.

**Table 11.2** • Angioplasty of the brachiocephalic artery: postoperative complications and late patency

| Authors, year | Patients | Mean follow-up (months) [range] | Complications (%) | Primary patency (%) | Secondary patency (%) |
|---|---|---|---|---|---|
| Hüttl et al.,[9] 2002 | 89 | Not available<br>[1–117] | Neurological: 5.6<br>Local: 3.0 | 6 months: 98 ± 2<br>1 year: 95 ± 3 | 100 98 ± 2 |
| Sullivan et al.,[10] 1998 | 7 | 14.3 [1–49] | Total: 20.7<br>Death: 4.8<br>Stroke: 2.3 | Not available | Not available |
| Brountzos et al.,[11] 2004 | 10 | 16.7 [0.3–68.2] | Total: 8.1<br>Death: 4.1 | 1 year: 91.7<br>2 years: 77 | 86.5<br>91.7 |

## Carotid–subclavian bypass

Access is achieved by a horizontal supraclavicular incision with division of both heads of the sternomastoid muscle. Scalenus anterior and phrenic nerves are exposed, and then scalenus anterior is sectioned near its insertion into the first rib (**Fig. 11.2**a). The internal jugular vein is freed to allow retraction in either direction. On the left side, take care to protect the thoracic duct or ligate it. The carotid sheath is opened, safeguarding the vagus nerve. After heparinisation, the common carotid artery is clamped as low as possible. A vein or PTFE graft is then attached to the lateral aspect of the common carotid artery in an end-to-side

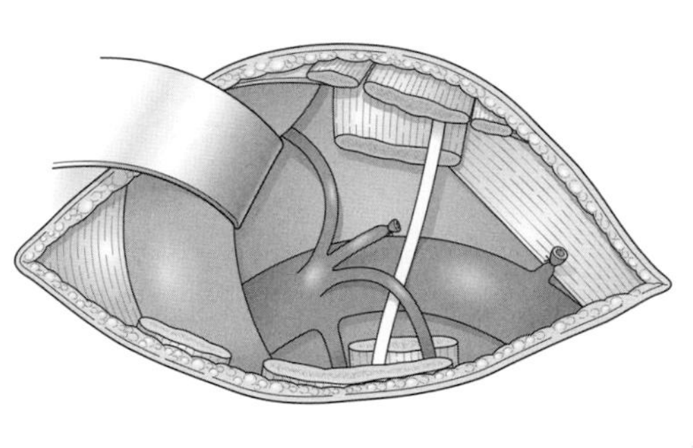

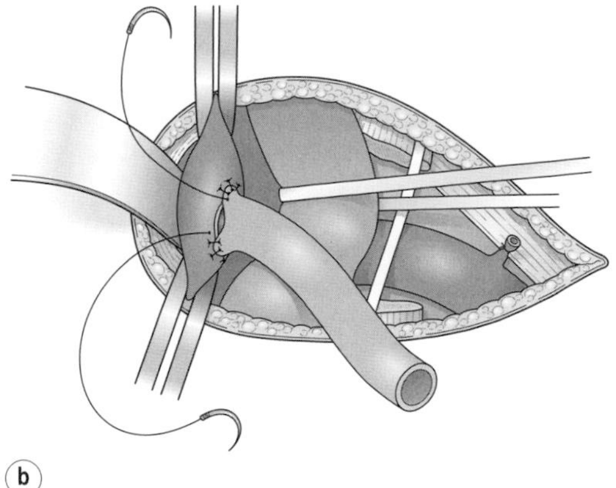

**Figure 11.2** • **(a)** Cervical approach for carotid–subclavian bypass. The sternomastoid muscle is divided and the subclavian artery is exposed by sectioning the scalenus anterior. **(b)** A PTFE graft is anastomosed to the lateral aspect of the left common carotid artery.

fashion (Fig. 11.2b). Use of a prosthetic graft seems to give better results than the vein graft in this location.[13] The graft under arterial tension is then passed behind the jugular vein. Graft length should be cautiously estimated and the graft attached end-to-side to the superior aspect of the distal subclavian artery. If the proximal subclavian lesion is ulcerated, it should be excluded by proximal ligation. If the distal subclavian artery is too diseased for distal implantation, the graft should be passed behind the clavicle and implanted on the axillary artery exposed via a short infraclavicular incision.

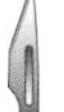

Prosthetic carotid–subclavian bypass has an excellent patency. Postoperative mortality is less than 1%, with a primary patency of 95% at 10 years.[14,15]

## Carotid transposition

Reimplantation of the subclavian artery into the common carotid artery is an alternative that avoids graft material but requires a more extensive cervical dissection. Dissection should avoid the recurrent laryngeal nerve, which is closely related to the posterior aspect of the subclavian artery. Systemic heparin is given and a curved clamp is applied across the left subclavian artery as close as possible to the aortic arch. The subclavian artery is transected and the proximal stump oversewn. The site of anastomosis to the common carotid artery should be chosen to avoid kinking and angulation of the vertebral artery. The clamps on the common carotid artery should be rotated anteriorly to present the posterolateral surface for anastomosis with the subclavian artery (**Fig. 11.3**). An ellipse is excised from this wall and the subclavian artery anastomosed in end-to-side fashion.

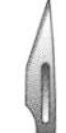

Subclavian–carotid reimplantation is an excellent technique that seems to give better results than the subclavian–carotid bypass in the series of Cinà et al.[16] (Table 11.3). Postoperative mortality is less than 1%, with a long-term patency of 100% in the series of Sandmann et al.[17] and Kretschmer et al.[18]

## Crossover grafts

Subclavian revascularisation may also be achieved by crossover subclavian–subclavian or axillo-axillary bypass. These grafts are relatively simple

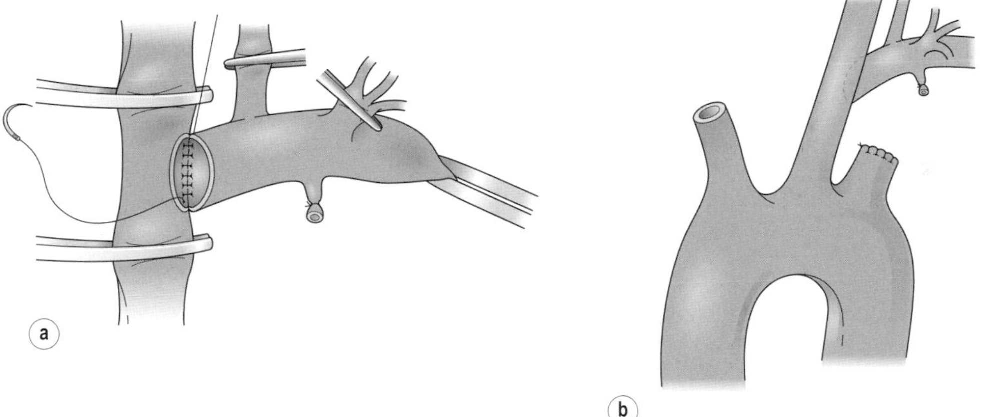


**Figure 11.3** • Carotid–subclavian transposition: **(a)** clamps on the common carotid artery are rotated anteriorly to present the posterolateral surface for anastomosis with the subclavian artery; **(b)** end-to-side anastomosis completed.

Table 11.3 • Carotid transposition: postoperative complications and late patency

| Authors, year | Patients | Mean follow-up (months) [range] | Complications (%) | Primary patency (%) at mean follow-up |
|---|---|---|---|---|
| Cinà et al.,[16] 2002 | 27 | $25 \pm 21$ | Morbidity: 11.1 | 100 |
| Schardey et al.,[13] 1996 | 108 | 70 [1–144] | Stroke: 1.8<br>Morbidity: 15 | 100* |

*84 patients followed.

to construct, although their greater length and reversed angle of take-off may reduce durability. Furthermore, problems may arise if subsequent median sternotomy is needed for coronary bypass. The donor and recipient arteries are exposed by a short supraclavicular incision on either side (**Fig. 11.4**). A tunnel is created from one side of the neck to the other passing behind the sternomastoid muscles and anterior to the carotid vessels. Crossover axillo-axillary bypass is easier to perform but the graft has to pass subcutaneously over the sternum with risks of compression or erosion. The postoperative death rate for crossover axillo-axillary bypass is 1.6% with a 5-year primary patency of 86.5% in the series of Mingoli et al.[19]

### Endovascular treatment

PTA of subclavian artery stenosis is a relatively safe and often simple procedure to perform. Access is usually obtained from the femoral artery or from the brachial artery and the lesion dilated to 5–8 mm (**Fig. 11.5**). Because there is usually retrograde flow in the vertebral artery, stroke is rare. When there is not retrograde flow, an occlusion balloon may be placed in the vertebral artery from the arm while the stenosis is dilated. Simple stenoses are adequately dilated by balloon. Occlusions are more difficult to cross and less frequent in most endovascular series;[20,21] they often require catheterisation from the brachial artery with the use of balloon or self-expandable stents.

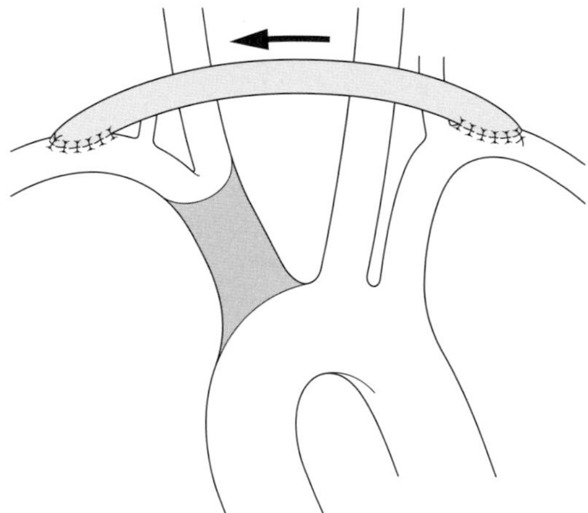

**Figure 11.4** • Brachiocephalic artery occlusion. Revascularisation by a cross-subclavian PTFE graft. Tunnelisation is done behind the sternomastoid muscles and anterior to the carotid vessels.

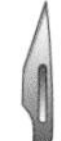

PTA with or without stenting is an appropriate treatment for symptomatic patients with localised subclavian artery stenosis with a 2-year primary patency of 90% in most series[20,21] (Table 11.4), but a long-term patency inferior to that obtained with carotid–subclavian bypass or transposition.

## Upper arm arteries

Patients with chronic atherosclerotic occlusion of the axillary or brachial arteries usually present with fatigue on using the arm. Many of these patients have radiation-induced occlusive disease. More severe ischaemia with rest pain or digital necrosis is uncommon unless there have been repeated episodes of embolism due to proximal ulceration or aneurysmal lesion. Direct reconstructive surgery is feasible since the occlusive lesions tend to be segmental with preserved distal patency. Axillobrachial occlusions are managed by a bypass procedure if symptoms justify it. These sites can usually be approached by limited incisions and the bypass tunnelled subcutaneously between the two (**Fig. 11.6**). Autogenous saphenous vein is the preferred graft material. When unavailable, the basilic or cephalic vein may be considered. Upper limb bypass using saphenous vein has a 5-year patency rate of 60–90%.[22] PTFE has a lower patency rate at this level.

## Lower arm and hand arteries

The causes of chronic occlusion in the forearm or hand vessels include atherosclerosis, Buerger's disease, immunological and connective tissue disorders (see Chapter 12), and occupational trauma. Arch angiography, to exclude proximal embolising disease, and selective arteriography are essential in evaluating these patients with distal disease. Most patients with distal disease and severe digital ischaemia can be managed conservatively. Avoidance of cold and abstinence of tobacco are essential. Vasodilator or sympatholytic agents may also be employed. Patients with digital necrosis may require local debridement or amputation if gangrene is extensive. Some patients with radial, ulnar or palmar arch occlusion and critical ischaemia may be managed, if run-off is present, by vein graft bypass using microsurgical techniques. Cervicodorsal sympathectomy by thoracoscopy may also be considered in patients with severe distal forearm ischaemia. However, results of sympathectomy have often been disappointing, particularly in patients with diffuse arteritis.

# Aneurysmal disease

True aneurysms of the upper limb arteries are uncommon. The subclavian artery is the most frequent site, usually caused by thoracic outlet compression, These patients may present with distal ischaemia,

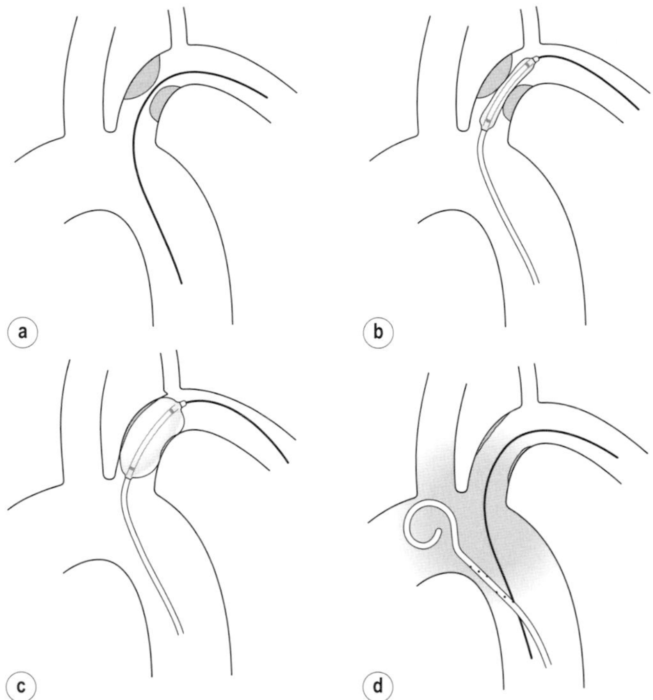


**Figure 11.5** • Retrograde approach from the brachial artery by percutaneous puncture, or cut-down if stenting is necessary: **(a)** the guidewire is placed through the subclavian stenosis; **(b)** balloon is advanced over the guidewire and balloon angioplasty performed; **(c)** arteriography completed by withdrawing the balloon with the same catheter; **(d)** more accurate arteriographic control can be achieved by using a second transfemoral pigtail catheter positioned in the aortic arch. Schneider PA (2003) Endovascular Skills 2003. Reproduced by permission of Informa Healthcare.

Table 11.4 • Angioplasty of the subclavian artery: postoperative complications and late patency

| Authors, year | Patients | Mean follow-up (months) [range] | Complications (%) | Primary patency (%) |
|---|---|---|---|---|
| De Vries et al.,[20] 2005 | 110 | 34<br>[3–120] | Stroke + death: 4.5<br>Local: 3.6 | 2 years:* 89<br>3 years:† 89 |
| Takash et al.,[21] 2005 | 162 | 39.6 ± 2.4<br>[3–139.2] | Death: 0.6 | 2 years:‡ 90<br>5 years:§ 83.9 |

*64 patients followed at 2 years.
†36 patients followed at 3 years.
‡80 patients followed at 2 years.
§9 patients followed at 5 years.

embolisation or acute thrombosis. False aneurysms from trauma or infection often produce motor or sensory impairment as a result of brachial plexus compression. Subclavian artery aneurysms are best managed by a combined supraclavicular and infraclavicular approach (see later). Aneurysms of the brachiocephalic artery are rare. In the series of Kieffer et al.[23] the perioperative death rate was 11%, most deaths occurring in patients operated in emergency.

An aberrant right subclavian artery arising from the descending thoracic aorta is a common anomaly. Rarely, the artery compresses the oesophagus against the trachea, producing a condition described as dysphagia lusoria. Aneurysmal degeneration, known as Kommerell's diverticulum, may also occur. The largest experience has been reported by Kieffer et al.;[24] their 33 patients with aberrant right subclavian arteries included 13 cases of Kommerell's diverticulum. Because of the possibility of rupture, resection of the aneurysmal artery with aortic prosthetic reconstruction via a thoracic approach is recommended. As this technique carries a high

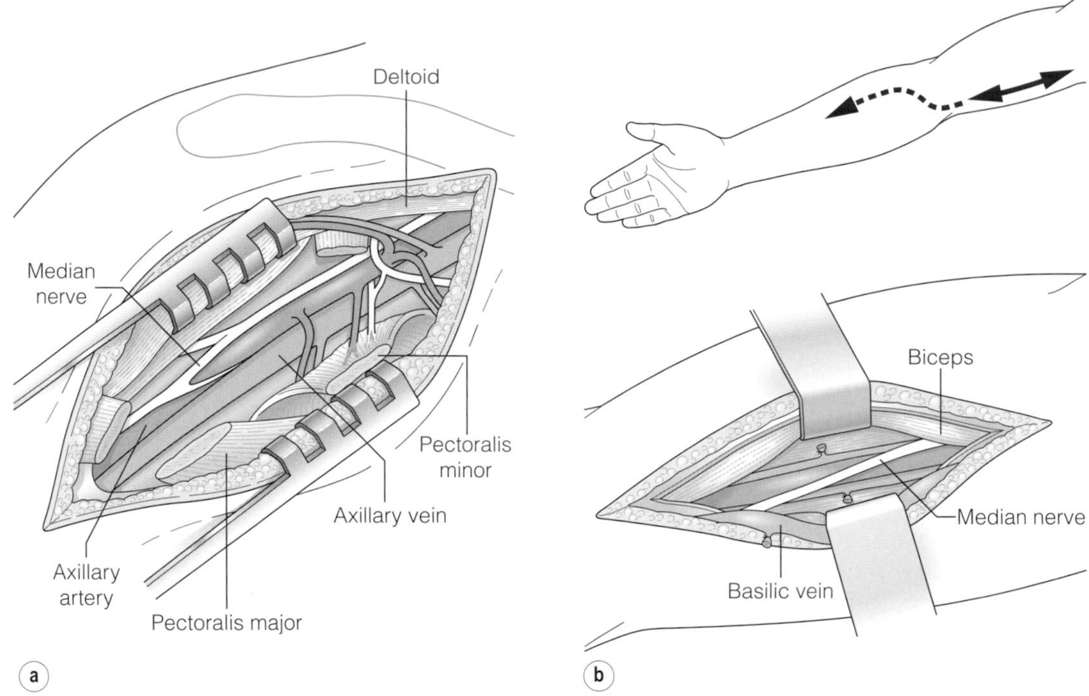


**Figure 11.6 • (a)** Axillary artery approach. The pectoralis minor muscle is divided and the neurovascular bundle is exposed. If access to the axillobrachial junction is needed, pectoralis major tendon should also be resected. **(b)** Brachial artery approach. Incision along the medial border of the biceps. If necessary, the bicipital aponeurosis is divided to expose the brachial artery division.

postoperative mortality, aortic stentgrafts have been tried in this location with limited success.

## Upper arm artery aneurysms

Axillary artery aneurysms are usually caused by blunt or penetrating trauma. Degenerative or congenital aneurysms are rare in this location. False aneurysms of the axillary artery occur with humeral fractures and anterior dislocation of the shoulder. These aneurysms can lead to neurological complications because of compression of the brachial plexus. Duplex scan and arteriography allow an accurate diagnosis. The axillary artery is exposed by a deltopectoral incision with section of pectoralis minor. The aneurysm is resected followed by interposition of a reversed saphenous vein. Stentgrafts have been used for emergency control of upper limb aneurysms but their long-term integrity is aften compromised by compression between the first rib and clavicle or by excessive arterial flexion.[25]

## Lower arm and hand artery aneurysms

Radial artery aneurysms are usually due to inadequate compression or infection following removal of intra-arterial blood pressure cannulas. If the Allen test shows good filling of the hand from the ulnar artery, then the radial artery can simply be ligated above and below the aneurysm. If not, reconstruction using a vein graft will be required.

### Ulnar artery aneurysm or hypothenar hammer syndrome

It is important to recognise an ulnar artery aneurysm because it may lead to digital necrosis. The condition known as hypothenar hammer syndrome develops in workers who suffer repetitive trauma to their hands, i.e. carpenters and pipe fitters. Those who play sports such as volleyball or karate are also at risk. The pathophysiology is related to the vascular anatomy of the hand. The distal ulnar artery is vulnerable to external trauma between the distal margin of Guyon's canal and the palmar aponeurosis. Over this short distance, the artery lies anterior to the hook of the hamate bone and is covered only by the palmaris brevis muscle and the skin. Trauma of the ulnar artery at this level causes thrombosis or aneurysm formation and distal embolisation in the fourth and fifth fingers, with pain, coldness and cyanosis. The thumb is always spared because of its radial blood supply. Angiography with magnification is essential in these patients.

When the ulnar artery is chronically thrombosed, calcium channel blockers may be helpful. In all cases, patients should avoid further hand trauma.

Surgical therapy includes microsurgical arterial reconstruction with or without adjunctive pre-operative thrombolytic therapy to restore patency to digital arteries. Resection of the aneurysm with placement of an interposition vein graft is the treatment of choice. Satisfactory long-term results have been reported by Vayssairat et al. using this approach.[26]

## Upper limb embolism

Embolic arterial occlusion is the major cause of acute upper limb ischaemia; upper limb emboli represent 20–32% of major peripheral emboli.[27] A cardiac origin is found in 90% of the cases and is related to arrhythmia, myocardial infarction, valvular disorder or ventricular aneurysm. Non-cardiac sources include ulcerative atherosclerotic plaques or aneurysms in the arch or subclavian–axillary arteries and thoracic outlet compression. The brachial bifurcation is the most frequently involved site for an embolus to lodge. Clinical examination and duplex scan can locate the level of the arterial occlusion. Preoperative conventional angiography or CT angiography is indicated in order to exclude a proximal arterial embolic lesion if a cardiac source is not evident or if the subclavian pulse is either absent (due to dissection or occlusion) or unduly prominent (due to a subclavian aneurysm or underlying cervical rib). Immediate systemic heparinisation is essential to limit the propagation of thrombus and to prevent recurrent embolism.

Most emboli can be retrieved through a distal brachial transverse arteriotomy. This site has the advantage that both forearm arteries can be directly cannulated. An S-shaped incision is made under local anaesthesia in the antecubital fossa and the brachial artery division exposed by dividing the bicipital aponeurosis. A transverse arteriotomy is made proximal to the bifurcation. It is important to clear both forearm vessels with a 2-Fr Fogarty catheter (**Fig. 11.7**). Heparin saline is then instilled distally, and after confirming proximal patency the arteriotomy is closed with 6/0 prolene interrupted sutures. At this time, on-table angiography should be performed. If there is retained distal thrombus, the ulnar and radial artery can be opened at the wrist and a 2-Fr Fogarty catheter passed distally. Alternatively, intraoperative thrombolysis can be used (see Chapter 8). Emboli in the axillary or subclavian arteries may also be removed by the same approach using transbrachial retrograde catheterisation. However, sometimes a large proximal embolus cannot be removed via the brachial arteriotomy, in which case an axillary or subclavian embolectomy will be required. Percutaneous thrombectomy via a femoral approach has also been used in this situation.

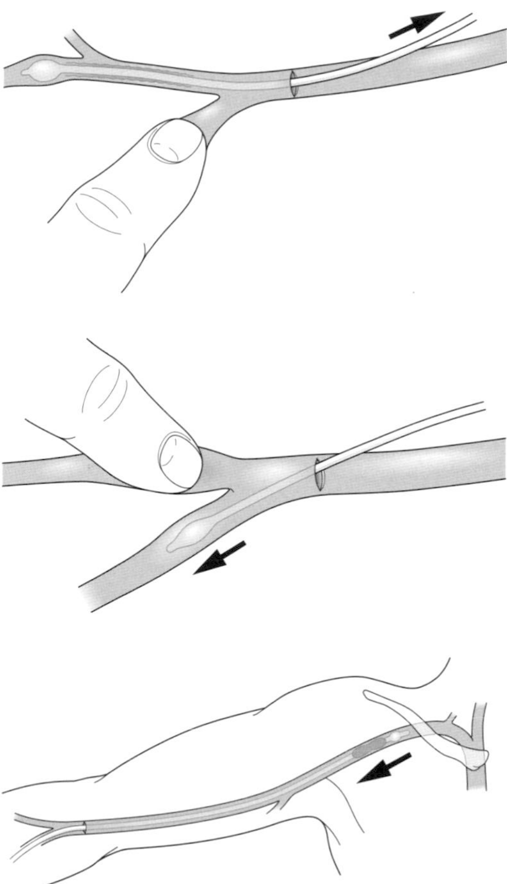

**Figure 11.7** • Brachial artery embolectomy. A transverse arteriotomy is performed. A Fogarty catheter is directed into the radial and ulnar arteries in turn using alternate digital compression. A subclavian–axillary embolectomy is carried out by retrograde catheterisation from the antecubital fossa.

## Other causes of acute ischaemia

The pharmacological causes of upper extremity ischaemia are summarised in Box 11.2. Inadvertent arterial injection by drug abusers often results in intense vasospasm due to particulate microembolism. Intra-arterial infusion of prostacyclin analogues such as iloprost or other vasodilators may help. Forearm compartment syndrome is rare except in this situation and requires fasciotomy. Limb loss is common.

**Box 11.2 • Upper extremity ischaemia due to pharmacological agents**

Ergot poisoning
Beta-blockers
Drug abuse, cocaine use
Dopamine overdose
Cytotoxic drugs

# Thoracic outlet syndrome

Thoracic outlet syndrome describes a variety of symptoms caused by compression of the brachial plexus or subclavian vessels at the thoracic outlet. In more than 90% of all thoracic outlet syndrome,[28] symptoms are neurological with pain and weakness resulting from C8 or T1 root compression. Arterial or venous symptoms resulting from compression are uncommon, accounting for 5% of cases in large published series.[29]

## Neurogenic thoracic outlet compression syndrome (N-TOCS)

The neurovascular bundle may be compressed between the first rib and the clavicle as a result of a low-lying shoulder girdle or loss of muscle tone. Other anatomical factors include congenital fibromuscular bands crossing the thoracic outlet that tent up the brachial plexus, and abnormalities/hypertrophy of the scalene muscles. Bony lesions may also be the cause. These include cervical ribs, a broad first rib, and fracture or exostoses of the first rib or clavicle. The scalene triangle is the commonest site of nerve compression. It contains the brachial plexus and the subclavian artery. N-TOCS probably represents a repetitive stress injury as there are well-defined at-risk occupations (e.g. typists) and sports (e.g. swimming). Most patients with N-TOCS are in the 25- to 45-year age group and 70% of them are women. The symptoms are arm pain, paraesthesia and weakness, with involvement of all the nerves of the brachial plexus or with specific patterns related to the upper plexus (median nerve) or lower plexus (ulnar nerve).

### Diagnosis

Positive findings on clinical examination include supraclavicular tenderness and paraesthesia in the ipsilateral upper extremity in response to pressure over the scalene muscles. Rotating the head and tilting the head away from the involved side often produces radiating pain in the upper arm. Abducting the arm to 90° in external rotation and repeated slow finger clenching in this position often reproduces the symptoms (Roos' test). Diagnostic tests include a scalene muscle block, and a good response to this test correlates well with successful surgical decompression.[30] Neurophysiology testing is helpful in excluding other sites of nerve compression, e.g. cervical root and carpal tunnel. There is a reduction in the sensory action potential of the medial cutaneous nerve of the forearm, prolonged F-wave conduction and the EMG shows motor unit drop-out in the thenar muscles. Duplex scanning is a useful surrogate marker if it shows arterial compression in the stress position. Cervical spine films may detect cervical or abnormal first ribs but will not detect non-bony causes of compression. Magnetic resonance imaging is more useful for excluding cervical disc lesions than confirming N-TOCS.

### Treatment

Therapy for N-TOCS should always begin with non-operative treatment, including postural exercises and physiotherapy. Patients should avoid heavy lifting and working with the arm above shoulder level. Conservative treatment should be continued for several months. The majority of patients will improve significantly and will not require surgery. Indications for surgery include failure of conservative therapy after several months and persisting disabling symptoms that interfere with work and activities of daily living. The goal of surgery is to decompress the brachial plexus. A cervical rib can usually be removed via a supraclavicular approach. In the absence of a cervical rib, a transaxillary first rib resection is required.

#### Transaxillary resection of first rib

The technique described by Roos[31] is indicated for neurogenic complications of N-TOCS and can be summarised as follows. The patient is placed in the lateral position leaving the arm free. The assistant elevates the shoulder by applying upward traction on the upper arm. This manoeuvre opens up the costoclavicular space and pulls the neurovascular bundle away from the first rib. A horizontal skin incision is made at the lower border of the axillary line over the third rib (**Fig. 11.8**). From here the dissection extends proximally toward the apex of the axilla. The intercostal nerve emerging from the second intercostal space should be preserved. The fascial roof of the axilla is opened to expose the anterior portion of the first rib. Scalenus anterior is separated from the artery with a right-angled forceps and sectioned at its attachment to the first rib (**Fig. 11.9**). The tendon of the subclavius muscle is divided with care because of its close relation with the subclavian vein. The scalenus medius is then pushed off the rib using a blunt elevator. The intercostal muscles are similarly detached from the lower part of the rib and the pleura is dropped back from the operative zone. The rib is then sectioned at the chondrocostal junction and maintained by bone-holding forceps to distance it from the neurovascular bundle (**Fig. 11.10**).

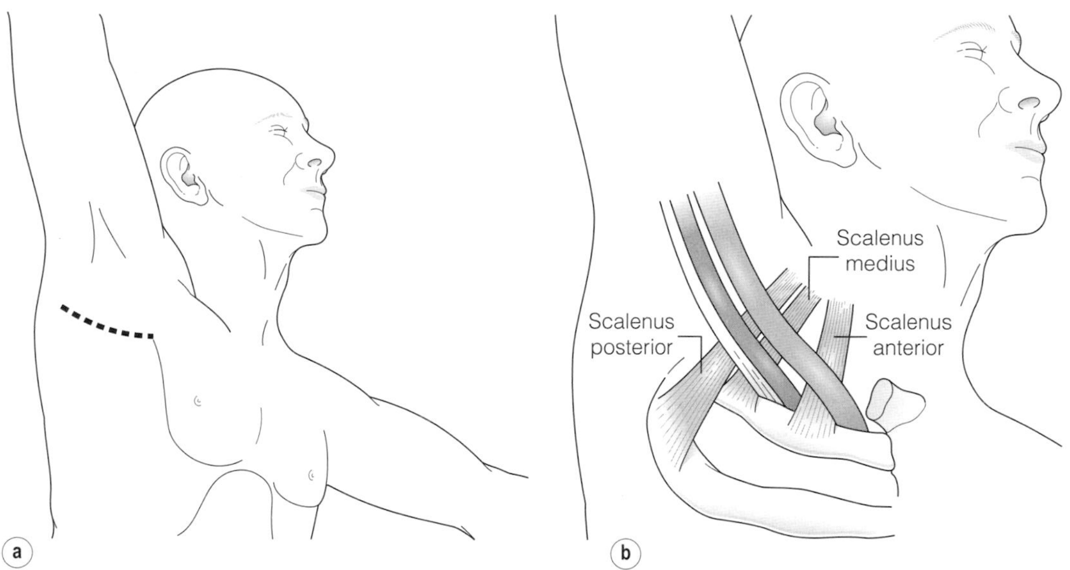


**Figure 11.8 •** Transaxillary resection of the first rib: **(a)** operative position and skin incision; **(b)** the neurovascular bundle is pulled away from the first rib by traction on the arm.

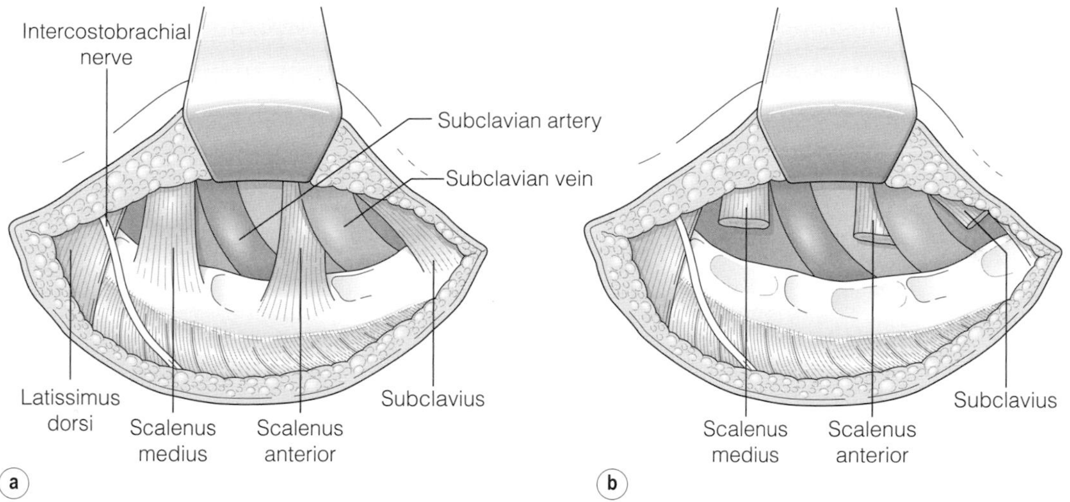


**Figure 11.9 •** Transaxillary resection of the first rib: **(a)** exposure of the first rib, scalene muscles and subclavian–axillary vessels; **(b)** detachment of the scalenus anterior, medius and subclavius muscles from the first rib.

With the arm elevated, the T1 root is identified at the neck of the first rib. The T1 root is displaced medially with care and an angled rib shear is set as far posteriorly as possible. The rib is then sectioned. This section is completed to within 1–2 cm of the vertebral transverse process using rongeurs. The stump must be smooth since sharp bony spicules may lacerate the plexus. Any remaining fibrous bands around the plexus or vessels should be resected. In the same way, the scalenus anterior is pulled down between the subclavian vessels and resected. Serum saline is then injected in the wound to ensure that the pleura is intact. The wound is closed in the usual way with suction drainage.

Complications of transaxillary rib resection include subclavian vein or artery injury, extrapleural haematoma or brachial plexus injury. The most serious complication is brachial plexus injury. Traction of the arm or damage to the T1 root by the rib shear or by retraction can be responsible for this complication.

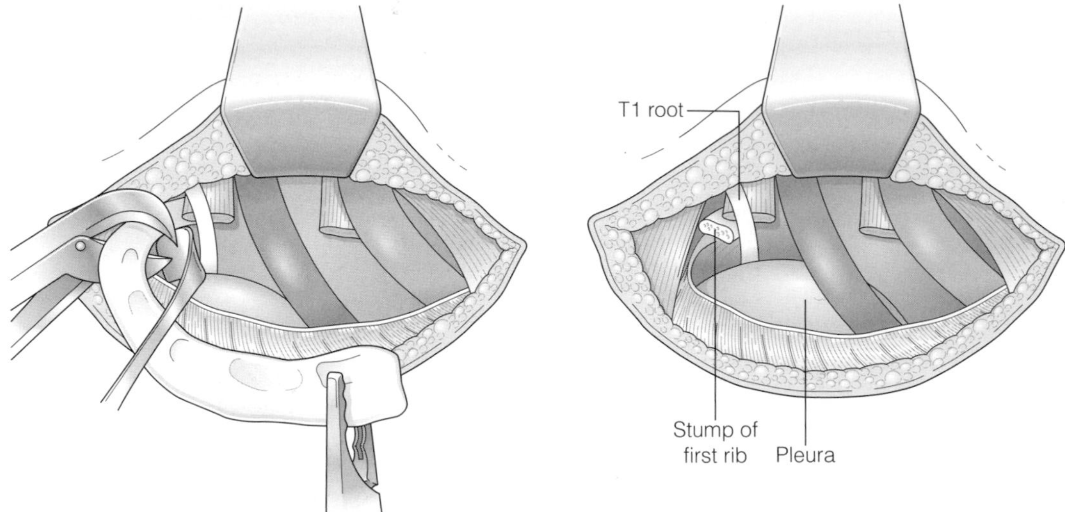


**Figure 11.10** • Transaxillary resection of the first rib. **(a)** Exposure of the first rib. The rib has been disarticulated at the chondrocostal junction. T1 root is protected by a retractor. **(b)** Extraperiosteal resection of the first rib is complete.

To avoid this, the T1 root should always be in view during posterior rib manipulation.

Other operative techniques for N-TOCS include a supraclavicular approach. Axelrod et al.[32] reported the results of surgery in 170 patients operated for N-TOCS. No major operative complication occurred in these patients who underwent decompression via a supraclavicular approach. Only 11% of patients experienced minor complications, most commonly the need for chest tube placement as a result of pneumothorax. At short-term follow-up (10 months), most patients had improved pain levels (80%) and range of motion (82%). However, at long-term follow-up (47 months), residual symptoms were present in 65% of patients, and 35% took medication for pain. Nonetheless, 64% said they were satisfied with the result. Lepantalo et al.[33] performed a long-term follow-up after first rib resection (average 6.1 years) in which the examiners were independent from the surgeons. One month postoperatively, 77% were improved whereas at long-term follow-up this improvement was only found in 37% of patients. Gordobes-Gual et al.[34] show the importance of a precise questionnaire (DASH) to evaluate the functional recovery after N-TOCS surgery.

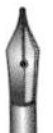

Controversy still exists concerning the surgical treatment of N-TOCS, and a randomised study of thoracic outlet surgery versus conservative treatment is lacking in this indication.

## Arterial thoracic outlet compression syndrome

Arterial complications are often associated with bony abnormalities, including a complete cervical rib or fracture callus of the first rib or clavicle. The initial arterial lesion is fibrotic thickening with intimal damage and poststenotic dilation, leading to aneurysmal degeneration with mural thrombus and the risk of embolisation. Most emboli are small and localised in the hand vessels, with pallor, paraesthesia and coldness suggestive of Raynaud's syndrome. If unrecognised, severe digital ischaemia with gangrene may occur. Early recognition of this condition is essential and a duplex scan should be performed in all patients with unilateral Raynaud's syndrome and asymptomatic patients with a cervical bruit. Loss or reduction of the radial pulse during Adson's manoeuvre (abduction and external rotation of the shoulder) is not very reliable as it is found in 9–53% of healthy volunteers.[28] The arteriographic changes may be obvious but sometimes minimal, with moderate dilation beyond a bony abnormality at the thoracic outlet and radiological evidence of distal embolisation (**Fig. 11.11**). Subclavian stenosis is not always evident on anteroposterior view and oblique stress views are often necessary.

### Surgical management

Subclavian lesions associated with cervical ribs can usually be repaired via a supraclavicular approach, after excision of the cervical rib. For more extensive arterial lesions, the transclavicular approach allows wide exposure of the supraclavicular and axillary

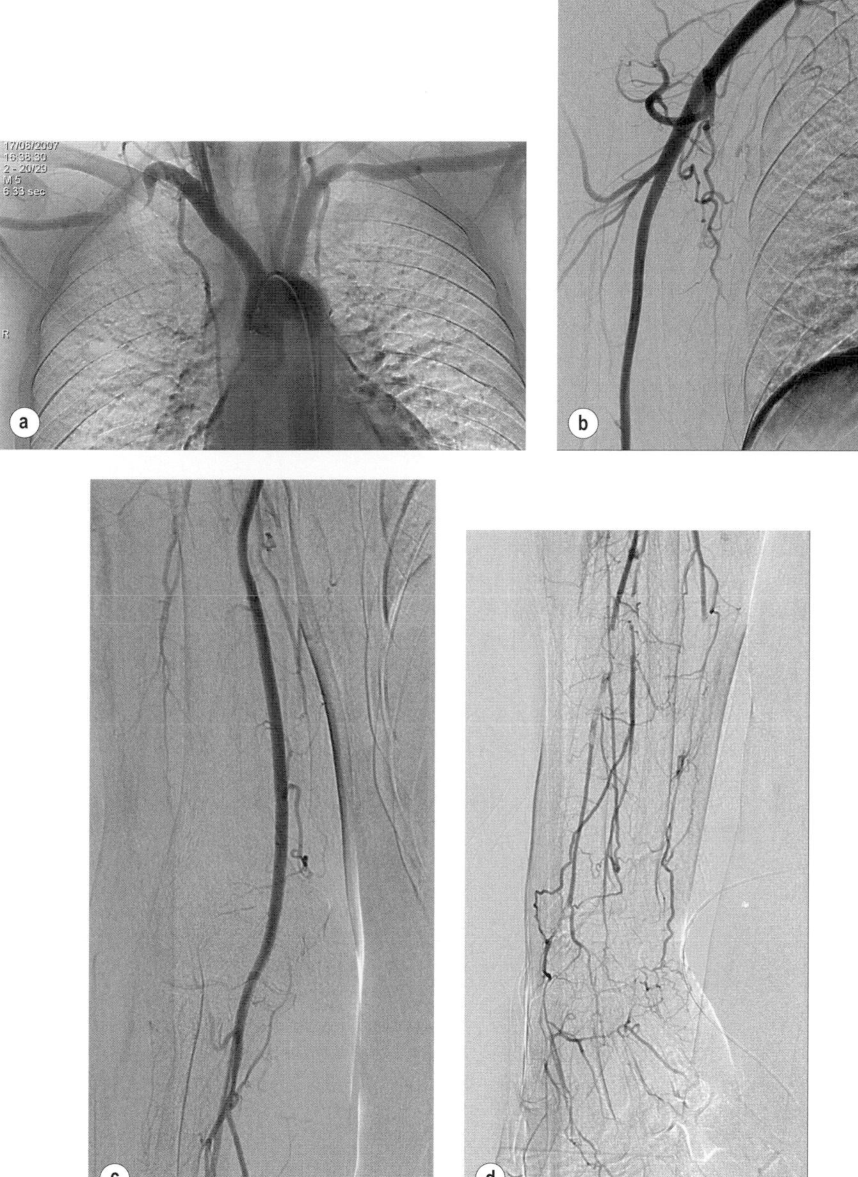


**Figure 11.11** • Angiography of a thoracic outlet compression syndrome with arterial compression. **(a)** Right subclavian artery compression when the arm is abducted to 90° in external rotation. **(b)** Poststenotic dilatation of the right subclavian artery. **(c)** Right brachial artery. **(d)** Distal arterial embolisation.

region but causes significant cosmetic and functional impairment. The same surgical procedure can be done without dividing the clavicle using a combined supraclavicular and infraclavicular approach. The only indications for clavicular resection are arterial complications due to malunion or hypertrophic callus of the clavicle.

### Combined supraclavicular and infraclavicular approach

The combined supraclavicular and infraclavicular approach offers a complete exposure. The infraclavicular dissection is commenced first with an S-shaped incision. Pectoralis major is detached from the upper sternum and clavicle (**Fig. 11.12**).

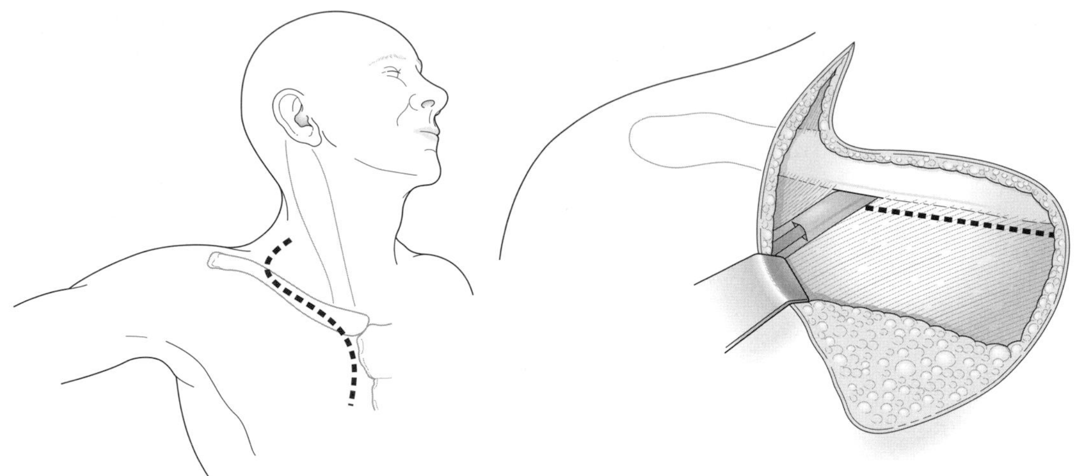

**Figure 11.12 •** Combined supraclavicular and infraclavicular approach for first rib resection when extensive arterial or venous reconstruction is required. Skin incision and section of the pectoralis major from the clavicle.

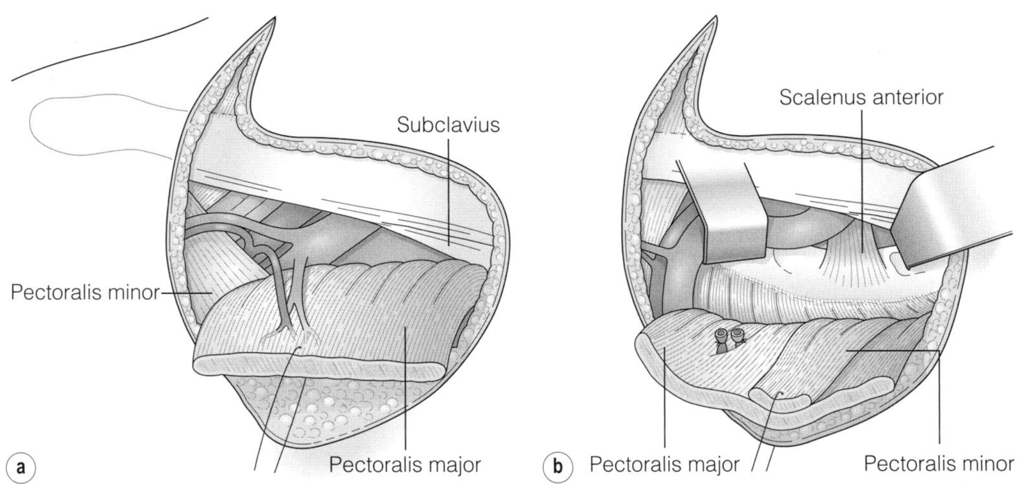


**Figure 11.13 •** Combined supraclavicular and infraclavicular approach. **(a)** Exposure of the proximal axillary vessels. The axillary vessels are held aside with a retractor to show the first rib and insertion of the scalenus anterior. **(b)** The infraclavicular dissection with detachment of the intercostal muscles from the first rib. The anterior portion of the rib will be removed and the first rib stump will be shortened via the supraclavicular exposure, not shown here.

Pectoralis minor is then sectioned and the clavipectoral fascia opened to expose the subclavius and the anterior segment of the first two ribs. The subclavius is resected and the artery and the axillary vein are then freed behind the clavicle. Via a supraclavicular incision, the clavicular head of the sternomastoid and the external jugular vein are divided to expose the scalenus anterior and the phrenic nerve. The scalenus anterior is then sectioned near the first rib. The subclavian artery and vein are freed (**Fig. 11.13**). The intercostal muscles are detached from the lower border of the first rib and the rib is disarticulated at the costochondral junction. The rib is then sectioned without attempting to reach the posterior segment. Access to the rib stump is achieved via the supraclavicular exposure by reflecting the brachial plexus laterally and the artery medially. The scalenus medius is then detached from the first rib and, after protecting the T1 root, the rib is sectioned near the transverse process. If a complete cervical rib is present, the tip is disarticulated via the infraclavicular exposure, the remaining part being removed above the clavicle with the stump of the first rib.

In patients with aneurysm or poststenotic dilation secondary to first rib or cervical rib, there is often sufficient length of artery to permit resection of the arterial lesion and direct anastomosis (**Fig. 11.14**). When arterial lesions are more extensive, graft replacement is required using reversed great saphenous vein or PTFE if no vein is available. Intraoperative angiography is recommended in all cases. In patients with a recent distal embolic event, catheter embolectomy should be attempted through a transverse brachial arteriotomy or, if ineffective, through a radial or ulnar arteriotomy at the wrist using a No. 2 Fogarty catheter. If embolectomy is impossible, a distal bypass using the great saphenous vein may be needed in an attempt to revascularise one of the forearm arteries including the interosseous artery. Additional sympathectomy may also be considered where there is extensive long-standing distal embolic occlusion. Difficulty in clearing the distal arterial bed accounts for the incomplete revascularisation observed in advanced cases with disabling ischaemic sequelae.

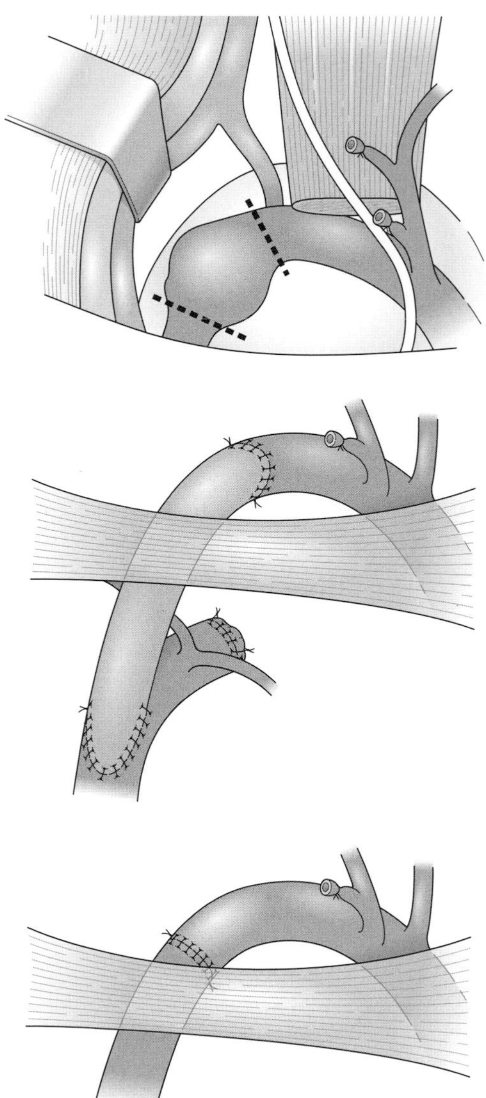

**Figure 11.14** • Combined supraclavicular and infraclavicular approach. Exposure of the subclavian and axillary vessels. Depending on the extent of arterial resection, end-to-end anastomosis or graft replacement is done.

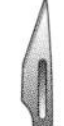

Arterial reconstruction and first rib or cervical rib resection are indicated in all patients with arterial complications of thoracic outlet syndrome.

## Subclavian–axillary vein thrombosis

Spontaneous or effort-related thrombosis in a fit young patient is known as Paget–Schroetter syndrome, the first cases being published separately by these two authors over a century ago. Hughes, who in 1949 collected 320 cases and recognised the distinct entity, coined the eponym. As the indications for central venous access have increased, so has the incidence of catheter-related subclavian–axillary vein thrombosis (SVT).[35]

Acute deep venous thrombosis (DVT) of the upper limb has many causes, with treatment and prognosis depending on the specific cause. SVT can be divided into two groups, primary and secondary. Primary SVT (Paget–Schroetter syndrome) is due to anatomical venous compression in the thoracic outlet during exercise (V-TOCS) and comprises about 25% of all cases. Secondary SVT is the result of multiple aetiological factors, although in most series trauma due to central venous catheters dominates this category (40% of all cases of SVT). SVT is responsible for 1–4% of all cases of DVT. Monreal et al.[36] reported a 15% incidence of pulmonary emboli in 30 consecutive patients with SVT who were investigated with ventilation-perfusion scanning.

### Primary SVT

In a review of the literature, Hurlbert and Rutherford[37] reported a male to female ratio of 2:1, with an average age of 30 years for patients with primary SVT that represents only 3.5% of all cases of thoracic outlet compression syndrome (TOCS). Venous thrombosis is seen three times more frequently in the right than the left upper limb, but bilateral venous compression also occurs frequently. Thrombosis is probably caused by repetitive trauma from compression. Virtually every patient with primary SVT has some degree of upper extremity swelling associated with pain that worsens with exertion. Some patients may have cyanosis of the arm. Unlike lower-extremity DVT, symptoms in the upper extremity are more related to venous obstruction than reflux. Venous outflow through the collateral vessels is limited, resulting in venous hypertension, swelling and even venous claudication. Venous gangrene is an extremely rare complication of SVT.

## Diagnosis

Clinically, the arm may be swollen and cyanosed with dilated shoulder girdle collateral veins. Duplex is the first-line investigation and has a sensitivity of 94% and a specificity of 96% compared with venography.[38] MRA has poor sensitivity for non-occlusive thrombi and short-segment occlusion. CT has been used to diagnose upper-extremity DVT but its specificity and sensitivity are undetermined. Venography is still considered as the reference in evaluating SVT (**Fig. 11.15**). The basilic vein is the preferred site for injection, with the arm abducted at 30°. The catheter used for the venogram should be left in position as it can be used for subsequent thrombolysis and/or heparin infusion. The cephalic vein is not used because it joins directly with the subclavian vein and may miss an axillary vein thrombosis.

## Treatment

For many years, treatment of SVT relied on rest and elevation of the upper limb with anticoagulant therapy. However, the morbidity associated with this conservative treatment is high. More recently, investigators have realised that many patients with SVT have compression at the thoracic outlet. Initially, in patients with primary SVT, subclavian vein patency was restored by open thrombectomy associated with first rib resection.[39] Although now supplanted by thrombolysis, open thrombectomy has proved effective and should be considered in patients with contraindications or failure of thrombolysis therapy. Catheter-directed techniques of thrombolysis allow for immediate venous evaluation and assess extrinsic compression with positional venography after thrombolysis.[40] However, Sheeran et al.[41] have shown that recanalisation of the vein by thrombolysis without decompression of the thoracic outlet has poor outcome, with 55% of patients remaining symptomatic. Conversely, Machleder[42] reported the success of combined treatment, with 86% of 36 patients becoming asymptomatic. The appropriate time interval between thrombolysis and thoracic outlet decompression is still under discussion. Machleder waited 3 months, whereas Lee et al.[43] recommended immediate first rib resection within 4 days after thrombolysis. Waiting too long risks rethrombosis, whereas operating immediately risks bleeding due to the thrombolytic agent.

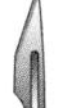

Patients with thoracic outlet syndrome and SVT should have early treatment with thrombolysis followed by first rib resection.[44]

Specific problems may arise in some patients after thrombolysis. In a small group, no residual lesion or compression is seen on positional venography after thrombolysis. In these cases, anticoagulation therapy is recommended without thoracic outlet decompression. In other patients, intrinsic stenosis is seen on venography after thrombolysis (Fig. 11.15). In these cases operative vein bypass or patch angioplasty with first rib resection is needed and should be performed in the days after thrombolysis

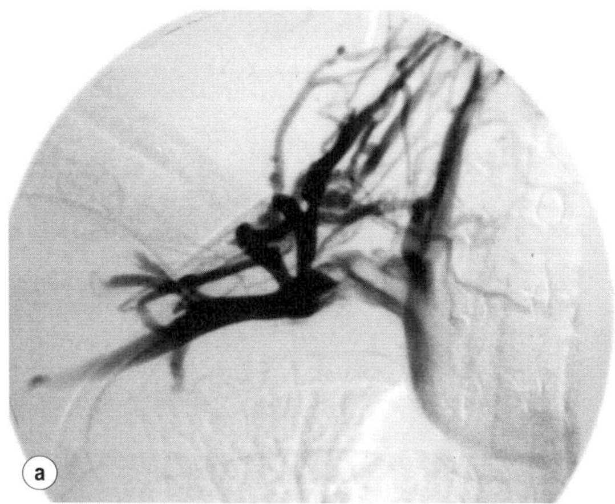


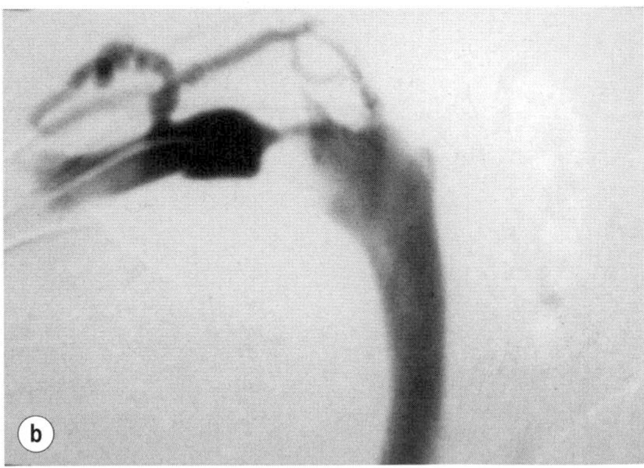


**Figure 11.15 • (a)** Venogram via basilic vein demonstrating SVT with collaterals. **(b)** Thombolysis revealed an underlying stenosis of the subclavian vein. This was treated by excision of the first rib and vein patch.

because the risk of rethrombosis appears to be quite high. In this setting, percutaneous balloon angioplasty with or without stenting has been suggested. The results of this technique without thoracic outlet decompression are poor, with a primary patency of 35% at 1 year.[45] Obviously, this technique does not obviate the need for surgery because thoracic outlet decompression is still needed. Even after thoracic outlet decompression, some venous stenoses are resistant to dilation or present intrinsic elastic recoil. Various types of stents have been used to treat residual stenoses, but acceptable results have been seen only in patients who had thoracic outlet decompression. In addition, venous stents underneath the clavicle are known to fracture.[46]

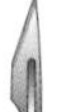

Stenting in primary SVT is not appropriate. As surgery is always needed for thoracic outlet decompression, it seems logical to repair the subclavian vein with patch angioplasty or a short autogenous bypass at the same time.

In a significant number of patients, seen more than 10 days after the onset of primary upper-limb DVT, late thrombolysis fails. Most of these patients should be treated conservatively with anticoagulation unless the occlusion is short. In these cases, open thrombectomy with vein reconstruction and first rib resection can be done with acceptable results.[47] The technique involves internal jugular vein transposition or cephalic vein bypass with a temporary arteriovenous fistula. Prosthetic bypass has shown inferior results in this location.

## Secondary SVT

The main cause of secondary SVT is central venous catheterisation. Overall, one-third of patients with central-line catheters develop SVT, although only 15% of them are symptomatic. The aetiology of catheter-associated thrombosis is multifactorial, but may be related to the fibrin sheath that forms around the catheter. The method of insertion, size, composition and duration of use of the catheter are also important. A reduced rate of thrombosis has been found with soft and more flexible catheters. Large catheters used for haemodialysis have a higher incidence of SVT. Another risk factor is the type of fluid infused through the catheter. Cancer chemotherapeutic agents are aggressive to vascular endothelium and may increase the risk of thrombosis. Furthermore, many patients with central-line catheters also have systemic risk factors for thrombosis, i.e. malignancy, sepsis, congestive heart failure and prolonged bed rest.

Symptomatic patients have oedema and distended veins around the shoulder. Pulmonary embolism is not uncommon, with 16% of patients positive on ventilation–perfusion scan.[48] Therapy guidelines are based on observational reports as no controlled studies are available. In all cases, anticoagulation using intravenous heparin via the affected arm is indicated to prevent clot extension until the catheter is removed. Thrombolytic therapy has a role in reopening thrombosed catheters. Prevention of thrombus formation has been emphasised, and for high-risk patients it may be advantageous to administer low-dose coumadin[49] or low-molecular-weight heparin to reduce the risk of catheter-associated thrombosis.

## Key points

- Vascular diseases of the upper limb are rare in comparison to those involving the lower limbs, with the exception of arterial embolism.
- Clinical examination, including the Allen test, is important.
- There are good mid-term results of endovascular treatment of supra-aortic trunk stenoses.
- The long-term results of carotid bypass or carotid transposition are excellent.
- It is important to consider arterial disease in the work environment, e.g. hypothenar hammer syndrome.
- There is controversy concerning the diagnosis and treatment of N-TOCS.
- The combined supraclavicular and infraclavicular approach for first rib resection and arterial bypass is of value in the treatment of patients with arterial thoracic outlet compression syndrome.
- Early thrombolytic therapy followed by surgical thoracic outlet decompression is indicated in patients with primary SVT.

# References


1. Fields WS, Lemak NA. Joint study of extracranial artery occlusion. Subclavian steal. A review of 168 cases. JAMA 1972; 222:1139–43.

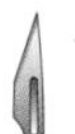

2. McCarthy WJ, Flinn WR, Yao JST. Results of bypass grafting for upper limb ischemia. J Vasc Surg 1986; 3:741–6.

   Between 1978 and 1984, the authors performed 33 bypass grafts to relieve hand and forearm ischaemia in 27 patients. A reversed saphenous vein graft was used in 22 cases and PTFE in the remaining 11 procedures. Follow-up of 31 grafts from 6 to 72 months (mean 35.5 months) revealed an overall patency rate of 73% at 2 years and 67% at 3 years. More proximal grafts fared better: the 2-year patency rate was 83% for grafts at or above the brachial artery but only 53% for bypass distal to the brachial bifurcation.

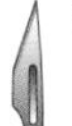

3. Kieffer E, Sabatier J, Koskas F. Atherosclerotic innominate artery occlusive disease: early and long term results of surgical reconstruction. J Vasc Surg 1995; 20:326–37.

   During a 20-year period (1974–93), the authors operated on 148 patients with brachiocephalic (innominate) artery atherosclerotic occlusive disease. Approach was through a median sternotomy in 135 (91%) patients. Endarterectomy was performed in 32 (22%) patients, whereas 116 (78%) patients underwent bypass. Eight (5.4%) patients died in the perioperative period. There were five (3.4%) perioperative strokes. Mean follow-up was 77 months. Survival was 51.9% at 10 years. The probability of freedom from ipsilateral stroke was 98.6% at 10 years. The primary patency rate was 98.4% at 10 years. In conclusion, surgical reconstruction of brachiocephalic artery atherosclerotic occlusive disease yields acceptable rates of perioperative complications with excellent long-term patency and freedom from neurological events and reoperation.

4. Berguer R, Morasch M, Kline R. Transthoracic repair of innominate and common carotid artery disease. Immediate and long-term outcome of 100 consecutive surgical reconstructions. J Vasc Surg 1998; 27:34–8.
5. Cherry KJ, McCullough JL, Hallett JW et al. Technical principles of direct innominate artery revascularization. A comparison of endarterectomy and bypass grafts. J Vasc Surg 1989; 9:718–24.
6. Reul GL, Jacobs MJHM, Gregoric ID et al. Innominate artery occlusive disease. Surgical approach and long-term results. J Vasc Surg 1991; 14:405–12.
7. Uurto IT, Lautamati V, Zeitlin R et al. Long-term outcome of surgical revascularization of supra-aortic vessels. World J Surg 2002; 26:1503–6.
8. Takach TJ, Reul GJ, Cooley DA et al. Brachiocephalic reconstruction I: Operative and long-term results for complex disease. J Vasc Surg 2005; 42:47–54.
9. Hüttl K, Nemes B, Simonffy A et al. Angioplasty of the innominate artery in 89 patients: experience over 19 tears. Cardiovasc Intervent Radiol 2002; 25:109–14.
10. Sullivan TM, Gray BH, Bacharach JM et al. Angioplasty and primary stenting of the subclavian, innominate, and common carotid arteries in 83 patients. J Vasc Surg 1998; 28:1059–65.
11. Brountzos EN, Petersen B, Binkert C et al. Primary stenting of subclavian and innominate artery occlusive disease: a single centers's experience. Cardiovasc Intervent Radiol 2004; 27:616–23.
12. Rapp JH, Reilly LM, Goldstone J et al. Ischemia of the upper extremity. Significance of proximal arterial disease. Am J Surg 1986; 152:122–6.
13. Schardey HM, Meyer G, Rau HG et al. Subclavian carotid transposition: an analysis of a clinical series and a review of the literature. Eur J Vasc Endovasc Surg 1996; 12:431–6.
14. Vitti MJ, Thompson BW, Read RC. Carotid–subclavian bypass. A twenty-two years experience. J Vasc Surg 1994; 20:411–18.

    A retrospective review of 124 patients who underwent carotid–subclavian bypass from 1968 to 1990 was done to assess primary patency and symptom resolution. Graft conduits were PTFE in 44 (35%) and Dacron in 80 (65%) cases; 30-day mortality was 0.8%, 30-day primary patency was 100%. Primary patency rate was 95% at 10 years. Survival rate was 59% at 10 years. Symptom-free survival rate was 87% at 10 years. Carotid–subclavian bypass appears to be a safe and durable procedure for relief of symptomatic occlusive disease of the subclavian artery.

15. AbuRahma AF, Robinson PA, Jennings TG. Carotid–subclavian bypass grafting with polytetrafluoroethylene grafts for symptomatic subclavian artery stenosis or occlusion: a 20-years experience. J Vasc Surg 2000; 32:411–19.
16. Cinà CS, Safar HA, Langanà A et al. Subclavian carotid transposition and bypass grafting: consecutive cohort study and systematic review. J Vasc Surg 2002; 35:422–9.
17. Sandmann W, Kniemeyer HW, Jaeschock R et al. The role of subclavian–carotid transposition in surgery for supra-aortic occlusive disease. J Vasc Surg 1987; 5:53–8.
18. Kretschmer G, Teleky B, Marosi L et al. Obliterations of the proximal subclavian artery. To bypass or to anastomose? J Cardiovasc Surg (Torino) 1991; 32:334–9.
19. Mingoli A, Sapienza P, Felhaus RJ et al. Long-term results and outcomes of crossover axillo-axillary bypass grafting: a 24-year experience. J Vasc Surg 1999; 29:894–901.
20. De Vries JPPM, Jagger LC, van den Berg JC et al. Durability of percutaneous transluminal angioplasty for obstructive lesions of proximal subclavian artery: long-term results. J Vasc Surg 2005; 41:19–23.

21. Takach TJ, Duncam JM, Livesay JJ et al. Brachiocephalic reconstruction II: Operative and endovascular management of single-vessel disease. J Vasc Surg 2005; 42:55–61.

22. Brunkwall J, Berqvist D, Bergentz SE. Long term results of arterial reconstruction of the upper extremity. Eur J Vasc Surg 1994; 8:47–53.

23. Kieffer E, Chiche L, Koskas F et al. Aneurysms of the innominate artery: surgical treatment of 27 patients. J Vasc Surg 2001; 34:222–8.

24. Kieffer E, Bahnini A, Koskas F. Aberrant subclavian artery: surgical treatment in thirty-three adult patients. J Vasc Surg 1994; 19:100–10.

The authors reviewed their experience with surgery for aberrant subclavian arteries (ASA). During a 16-year period they surgically treated 33 adult patients with ASA. Twenty-eight patients had a left-sided aortic arch with a right ASA, whereas five had a right-sided aortic arch with a left ASA. Eleven patients had dysphagia caused by oesophageal compression, five patients had ischaemic symptoms, 10 patients had aneurysms of the ASA and seven patients had an ASA arising from an aneurysmal thoracic aorta. In all cases the distal subclavian artery was revascularised, most often by direct transposition into the ipsilateral common carotid artery. The cervical approach was combined with a median sternotomy or a left thoracotomy in 17 patients. Aortic cross-clamping was required in 12 patients to perform the transaortic closure of the origin of the ASA with patch angioplasty or prosthetic replacement of the descending thoracic aorta. Cardiopulmonary bypass was used in six patients. Four patients died after operation. Satisfactory clinical and anatomical results were obtained in the remaining 29 patients. Provision should be made for cardiopulmonary bypass in patients with aneurysm of ASA or associated aortic aneurysm.

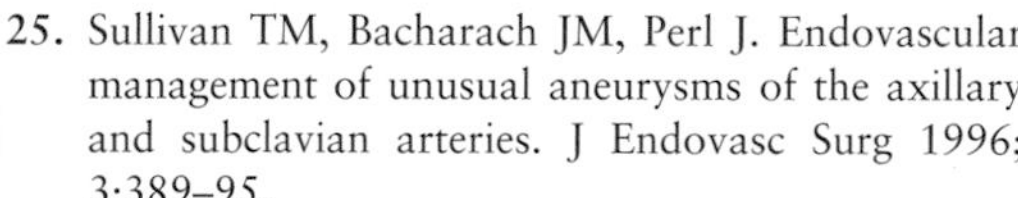

25. Sullivan TM, Bacharach JM, Perl J. Endovascular management of unusual aneurysms of the axillary and subclavian arteries. J Endovasc Surg 1996; 3:389–95.

Aneurysms of the upper extremity arteries are uncommon and may be difficult to manage in emergency with standard surgical techniques. The authors report the exclusion of three axillary–subclavian aneurysms with covered stents. Palmaz stents were covered with either PTFE (two cases) or brachial vein and deployed to exclude pseudoaneurysms in one axillary and two left subclavian arteries. Endovascular exclusion of axillary and subclavian aneurysms with covered stents may offer a useful alternative to operative repair in patients with ruptured aneurysm or significant comorbidities.

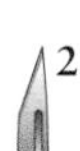

26. Vayssairat M, Debure C, Cormier J-M . Hypothenar hammer syndrome. Seventeen cases with long-term follow-up. J Vasc Surg 1987; 5:838–42.

The authors report 17 patients who had either ulnar thrombosis or ulnar aneurysm; most also had embolic occlusions of the digital arteries. Main pathological findings were thrombosis on the intima and fibrosis in the media. The authors adopted a surgical procedure

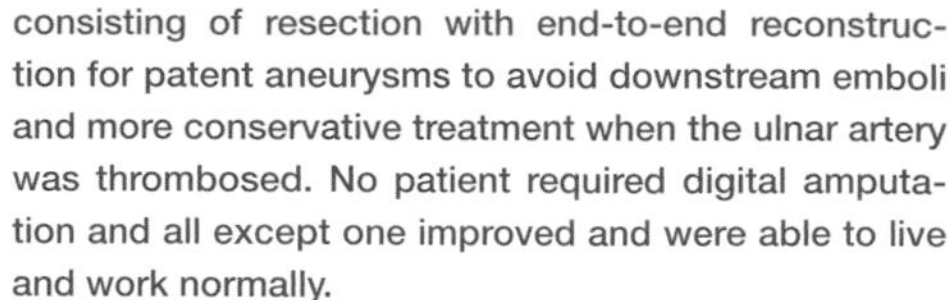

consisting of resection with end-to-end reconstruction for patent aneurysms to avoid downstream emboli and more conservative treatment when the ulnar artery was thrombosed. No patient required digital amputation and all except one improved and were able to live and work normally.

27. Haimovici H. Cardiogenic embolism of the upper extremity. J Cardiovasc Surg (Torino) 1982; 23:209–15.

28. Sanders RJ, Hammond SL, Rao NM. Diagnosis of thoracic outlet syndrome. J Vasc Surg 2007; 46:601–4.

29. Sanders RJ, Cooper MA, Hammond SL et al. Neurogenic thoracic outlet syndrome. In: Rutherford RB (ed.) Vascular surgery, 5th edn. Philadelphia: WB Saunders, 2000; pp. 1184–99.

30. Sanders RJ, Haug CE. Thoracic outlet syndrome: a common sequela of neck injuries. Philadelphia: JB Lippincott, 1991; p. 93.

31. Roos DB. Thoracic outlet and carpal tunnel syndrome. In: Rutherford RB (ed.) Vascular surgery, 2nd edn. Philadelphia: WB Saunders, 1984; pp. 708–24.

32. Axelrod DA, Proctor MC, Geisser ME. Outcomes after surgery for thoracic outlet syndrome. J Vasc Surg 2001; 33:1220–5.

This study determined whether there is an association between psychological and socio-economic characteristics and long-term outcome of operative treatment for patients with sensory N-TOCS. Multivariate logistic regression models were developed as a means of identifying independent risk factors for postoperative disability. Operative decompression of the brachial plexus via a supraclavicular approach was performed for upper extremity pain and paraesthesia, with no mortality and minimal morbidity in 170 patients. After an average follow-up period of 47 months, 65% of patients reported improved symptoms and 64% of patients were satisfied with their operative outcome. However, 35% of patients remained on medication and 18% of patients were disabled. Preoperative factors associated with persistent disability include major depression, being unmarried and having less than a high-school education. Operative decompression was beneficial for most patients. The impact of the preoperative treatment of depression on the outcome of TOCS decompression should be studied prospectively.

33. Lepantalo M, Lindgren KA, Leino E et al. Long-term outcome after resection of the first rib for thoracic outlet syndrome. Br J Surg 1989; 76:1255–6.

34. Gordobes-Gual J, Lozano-Vilardell P, Torreguitart-Mirada N et al. Prospective study of the functional recovery after surgery for thoracic outlet syndrome Eur J Endovasc Surg 2008; 35:79–83.

35. Rutherford RB, Hurlbert SN. Primary subclavian–axillary vein thrombosis. Consensus and commentary. Cardiovasc Surg 1996; 4:420–3.

Fifteen multiple-choice questions concerning options in the management of primary subclavian–axillary vein


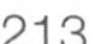

thrombosis were discussed by a panel of experts and then voted upon by 25 attending vascular surgeons with experience in subclavian–axillary vein thrombosis. The large majority favoured or agreed upon: (i) early clot removal for active healthy patients with a need/desire to use the involved limb in work or sport; (ii) catheter-directed thrombolysis as initial therapy; (iii) further therapy based on follow-up positional venography; (iv) surgical relief of demonstrated thoracic outlet compression after a brief period of anticoagulant therapy; (v) conservative therapy if post-lysis venogram showed either no extrinsic compression or a short residual occlusion; and (vi) intervention for residual intrinsic lesions with over 50% narrowing.

36. Monreal M, Lafoz E, Ruiz J. Upper extremity deep venous thrombosis and pulmonary embolism. Chest 1991; 99:280–3.

The authors prospectively evaluated the prevalence of pulmonary embolism in 30 consecutive patients with proved DVT of the upper extremity. Ten patients had primary DVT and 20 patients had catheter-related DVT. Ventilation–perfusion lung scans were routinely performed at the time of hospital admission in all but one patient. Lung scan findings were normal in 9 of 10 patients with primary DVT. In contrast, perfusion defects were considered highly suggestive of pulmonary embolism in four patients with catheter-related DVT. The authors conclude that pulmonary embolism is not a rare complication in upper-extremity DVT and that patients with catheter-related DVT seem to be at higher risk.

37. Hurlbert SN, Rutherford RB. Subclavian–axillary vein thrombosis. In: Rutherford RB (ed.) Vascular surgery, 5th edn. Philadelphia: WB Saunders, 2000; pp. 1208–21.

38. Koksoy C, Kuzu A, Kutlay J et al. The diagnostic value of colour Doppler ultrasound in central venous catheter related thrombosis. Clin Radiol 1995; 50:687–9.

39. DeWeese JA, Adams JT, Gaiser DL. Subclavian venous thrombectomy. Circulation 1970; 42:158–63.

40. Lokanathan R, Salvian AJ, Chen JC et al. Outcome after thrombolysis and selective thoracic outlet decompression for primary axillary vein thrombosis. J Vasc Surg 2001; 33:783–8.

41. Sheeran SR, Hallisey MJ, Murphy TP et al. Local thrombolytic therapy as part of a multidisciplinary approach to acute axillo-subclavian vein thrombosis (Paget–Schroetter syndrome). J Vasc Intervent Radiol 1997; 8:253–60.

42. Machleder HI. Evaluation of a new treatment strategy for Paget–Schroetter syndrome: spontaneous thrombosis of the axillary–subclavian vein. J Vasc Surg 1993; 17:305–17.

43. Lee MC, Grassi CJ, Belkin M. Early operative intervention following thrombolytic therapy for primary subclavian vein thrombosis. An effective treatment approach. J Vasc Surg 1998; 27:1101–8.

The authors conducted a study to determine an acceptable treatment approach to primary subclavian vein thrombosis. A retrospective review evaluated 11 patients in an 8-year period. All patients with occlusion received urokinase therapy and underwent surgical decompression within 5 days of thrombolytic therapy. Five percutaneous transluminal angioplasties were attempted before operative intervention. Eleven decompressions were performed. All patients received coumadin for 3–6 months after the operation. Urokinase therapy established wide venous patency in 9 of 11 extremities treated, with the remaining two requiring thrombectomy. One patient who underwent transluminal angioplasty before the operation had rethrombosis, and the remaining four showed no improvement in venous stenosis after the intervention. Eight of nine extremities treated by first rib resection and one of two treated by scalenectomy were free of residual symptoms at follow-up. The authors conclude that preoperative use of percutaneous balloon angioplasty is ineffective and should be avoided in this setting. Surgical intervention within days of thrombolysis enables patients to return to normal activity sooner.

44. Urschel HC, Razzuk MA. Paget–Schroetter syndrome: what is the best management? Ann Thorac Surg 2000; 69:1663–9.

The authors evaluated the results of 312 extremities in 294 patients with Paget–Schroetter syndrome to provide the basis for optimal management. Group I (35 extremities) was initially treated with anticoagulants only. Twenty-one developed recurrent symptoms after returning to work, requiring transaxillary resection of the first rib. Thrombectomy was necessary in eight. Group II (36 extremities) was treated with thrombolytic agents initially, with 20 requiring subsequent rib resection after returning to work. Thrombectomy was necessary in only four. Of the most recent 241 extremities (group III), excellent results accrued using thrombolysis plus prompt first rib resection for those evaluated during the first month after occlusion (199). The results were only fair for those seen later than 1 month (42). The authors conclude that early diagnosis (less than 1 month), expeditious thrombolytic therapy and prompt first rib resection are critical for the best results.

45. Glanz S, Gordon DH, Lipkowitz GS et al. Axillary and subclavian vein stenosis. Percutaneous angioplasty. Radiology 1988; 168:371–3.

46. Lee JT, Kawowski JK, Harris EJ et al. Long-term thrombotic recurrence after nonoperative management of Paget–Schroetter syndrome. J Vasc Surg 2006; 43:1236–43.

47. Sanders RJ, Cooper MA. Surgical management of subclavian vein obstruction, including six cases of subclavian vein bypass. Surgery 1995; 118: 856–63.

48. Monreal M, Raventos A, Lerma R et al. Pulmonary embolism in patients with upper extremity DVT associated with venous central lines. A prospective study. Thromb Haemost 1994; 72:548–50.

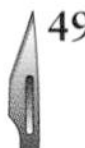

49. Bern MM, Lokich JJ, Wallach SR . Very low doses of warfarin can prevent thrombosis in central venous catheters. Ann Intern Med 1990; 112:423–8.

The goal of this study was to determine whether very low doses of warfarin are useful in thrombosis prophylaxis in patients with central venous catheters. Patients at risk for thrombosis associated with chronic indwelling central venous catheters were prospectively and randomly assigned to receive, or not to receive, 1 mg of warfarin beginning 3 days before catheter insertion and continuing for 90 days. Subclavian, innominate and superior vena cava venograms were done at onset of thrombosis symptoms or after 90 days in the study. A total of 121 patients entered the study and 82 patients completed the study. Of 42 patients completing the study while receiving warfarin, four had venogram-proven thrombosis. All four had symptoms from thrombosis. Of 40 patients completing the study while not receiving warfarin, 15 had venogram-proven thrombosis and 10 had symptoms from thrombosis ($P < 0.001$). In conclusion, very low doses of warfarin can protect against thrombosis without inducing a haemorrhagic state. This approach may be applicable to other groups of patients.

# 12

# Primary and secondary vasospastic disorders (Raynaud's phenomenon) and vasculitis

Jill J.F. Belch

## Introduction

There are many inflammatory and vasospastic disorders that can present with ischaemia and thus come to the attention of the vascular clinician. These include Raynaud's phenomenon (RP) plus any associated connective tissue disorder, and the group of conditions known as 'vasculitis' (the vasculitides). Because of the systemic nature of these diseases, medical practitioners of all disciplines will be involved in their management at some stage in their career. Unfortunately, there is considerable overlap in the presenting features of these conditions and this can make diagnosis difficult. However, recent advances in immunopathological testing now allow the majority of disorders to be classified. On the other hand, the discovery of new autoantibodies makes the study of these disorders more difficult for the non-specialist. The aim of this chapter is to provide the vascular clinician with a grounding of knowledge in these disorders so that the initial diagnosis can be made. It describes the most common manifestations of these diseases, outlines their investigation (with particular emphasis on diagnostic autoantibody tests) and briefly delineates their treatment, with emphasis on recent advances.

## Vasospasm

Vasospasm is the key feature of RP. Maurice Raynaud's original description was of episodic digital ischaemia induced by cold and emotion.[1] The classical manifestation of pallor preceding cyanosis and rubor reflects the initial vasospasm (**Fig. 12.1**), followed by deoxygenation of the static venous blood (cyanosis) and then reactive hyperaemia (rubor) with the return of blood flow. The full triphasic colour change is not essential for the diagnosis of RP, and a history of cold-induced blanching with subsequent reactive hyperaemia can still reflect significant vasospasm. In addition, other stimuli can provoke an attack, for example chemicals (including drugs and those in tobacco smoke[2]), trauma and hormones. In addition to the digits, the vasospasm may involve the nose, tongue, ear lobes and nipples. A decrease in lung,[3] oesophageal[4] and myocardial[5] perfusion has been shown after cold challenge, which suggests systemic vasospasm, and these patients have a higher incidence of migraine, irritable bowel syndrome and angina.[6]

RP is nine times more common in women, with an overall population prevalence of about 10%. In the Framingham Offspring Study, the prevalence of RP was 9.6% in women and 5.8% in men. However, it may affect 20–30% of young women.[7] There also appears to be a familial predisposition, which is more marked if the age of onset of RP is under 30 years.[8]

### Nomenclature: phenomenon, syndrome or disease

Inconsistent terminology is a major problem for clinicians managing RP. Europeans use RP as a blanket term for all cold-related vasospasm, with secondary Raynaud's syndrome (RS) being associated with another disease, and primary Raynaud's disease (RD) where it occurs in isolation. However,

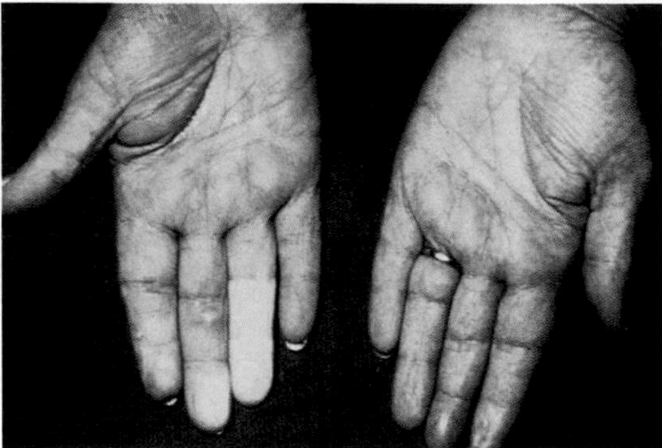

**Figure 12.1** • Digital pallor due to vasospasm.

American and Australasian researchers use the syndrome and phenomenon interchangeably,[9] and differentiate the types of RP by indicating whether primary RP or secondary RP. The former classification has been used in this chapter.

Many patients with mild disease never present to their general practitioners but of those who do, most will have primary RD. Patients with more severe disease are likely to be referred to a hospital specialist, and an early marker for secondary RS is the severity of vasospastic attacks,[10] although the RP may precede associated systemic disease by more than 20 years.[11] Hospital practitioners are therefore more likely to see a higher proportion of RS, and the important challenge is to differentiate between the primary and secondary conditions in order to facilitate early management of the underlying associated disorder.

The secondary associations of RS are shown in Box 12.1. Of the connective tissue diseases (CTDs), systemic sclerosis is the most frequent association. In the hyperviscosity syndromes, such as myeloma, the prevalence is similar to the normal population but the symptomatology tends to be more severe.

Occupational RS is also well recognised and a relatively common form is hand–arm vibration syndrome (HAVS; previously known as vibration white finger). As the name suggests, it occurs in workers exposed to vibrating instruments such as chainsaws, pneumatic road drills and buffing machines. An estimated 1.5 million workers in the USA use vibratory tools.[12] Before these tools were regulated, 90% of exposed workers developed symptoms of HAVS. Among American shipyard workers, 71% of full-time pneumatic grinders complained of white fingers[13] and in Japan 9.6% of forest workers had symptoms of this syndrome.[14]

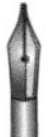

However, by using lighter chainsaws and reduced vibration, the frequency of clinical problems in Finnish forest workers was reduced from 40% to 5%.[15]

**Box 12.1** • Conditions associated with Raynaud's phenomenon

**Connective tissue diseases**

Systemic sclerosis
Systemic lupus erythematosus
Rheumatoid arthritis
Mixed connective tissue diseases
Sjögren's syndrome
Dermatomyositis/polymyositis

**Obstructive**

Atherosclerosis (especially thromboangiitis obliterans)
Microemboli
Thoracic outlet syndrome (especially cervical ribs)

**Drug therapy**

Beta-blockers
Cytotoxics, e.g. bleomycin
Ciclosporin
Ergotamine and other antimigraine therapies
Sulfasalazine

**Occupational**

Vibration white finger disease
Vinyl chloride disease
Ammunition workers (outside work)
Frozen food packers

**Miscellaneous**

Hypothyroidism
Cryoglobulinaemia
Reflex sympathetic dystrophy
Malignancy

The duration of exposure is important, with a latent period of often less than 5 years of full-time work. The severity of symptoms correlates with the length of exposure.[15] Vasospasm is not limited to the hands and has also been described in the toes.[16] It is likely that vibration-induced damage of the endothelium underlies this condition.[17] In approximately one-quarter of cases, the symptoms may resolve if a job change is effected early in the course of the disease.[18]

In the UK, HAVS has been a proscribed industrial disease since 1985. Patients may be eligible for industrial injuries disablement benefits if they fulfil certain criteria.[19] Specific daily time limits for different machines have been proposed and are being implemented opportunistically, often by use of a points system.

Other occupation-related causes of RP include vinyl chloride disease, which is estimated to occur in 3% of workers exposed to this chemical. Ammunition workers also develop RP outside their work environment when the vasodilatory effects of nitrates are removed.

Atherosclerotic obstructive arterial disease is a common cause of RP in those over 60 years of age, particularly in men, and screening and treatment of known risk factors, such as hyperlipidaemia are recommended. Various drugs may precipitate or exacerbate RP (e.g. beta-blockers for angina) and alternative drug therapies may be more appropriate (e.g. calcium channel blockers such as nifedipine). Vasospasm is also a feature of reflex sympathetic dystrophy and thoracic outlet syndrome, particularly occurring in the presence of a cervical rib (see Chapter 11).

## Pathophysiology

The precise mechanism that causes Raynaud's is unknown but four aetiological factors are considered to be important: (i) neurogenic; (ii) interactions between blood cells and the blood vessel wall; (iii) inflammatory and immunological responses; and (iv) genetic factors. It is likely that these mechanisms are interdependent and interact closely to produce the symptoms.

### Neurogenic

Most studies have focused on the peripheral nervous system. In patients with RP, α-adrenergic receptor sensitivity and density are increased[20] and the responsiveness of β-adrenergic presynaptic receptors in the peripheral vessels is also increased.[2] The role of the central sympathetic nervous system is not clear.[20–22]

### Interactions between blood and blood vessel walls

Microcirculatory flow depends on a functioning endothelium, plasma factors and the cellular elements of blood. Activated platelets aggregate and form clumps that can obstruct flow. They may also release vasoconstrictors such as thromboxane $A_2$ and serotonin, causing further platelet aggregation. Red blood cells (RBCs) appear less deformable in RP and cold temperatures further increase RBC stiffness.[23] Rigid RBCs and white blood cells (WBCs) may impede the microcirculation, and activated WBCs aggregate and adhere within the microcirculation and can narrow the vascular lumen. Additionally, WBC activation increases the formation of free radicals, which may be prothrombotic.[24] Elevated fibrinogen and globulin levels increase plasma viscosity and reduce blood flow. Increased platelet aggregation, rigid RBCs and activated WBCs have all been reported in patients with RS, together with raised plasma viscosity and reduced fibrinolysis.[25]

The intact endothelium is a functioning organ that produces many substances important in maintaining blood flow. Damage to it may impair blood flow in RP. Factor VIII von Willebrand factor (VWF) antigen is released following vascular damage and is increased in patients with RP.[26] VWF is active in the clotting cascade and platelet activation and may contribute to reduced blood flow. Tissue plasminogen activator is active in fibrinolysis and levels are reduced in RP, with a subsequent reduction in fibrinolysis.[25]

Endothelial vasoconstrictor/vasodilator production may also be impaired.[27–34] Most of these abnormalities are seen in patients with RS except for the increase in VWF, which occurs in the primary disease also. It is possible therefore that these are a consequence rather than the cause of the disorder. Nevertheless, they may still augment the impairment of blood flow and their correction by drug therapy may produce clinical benefit.

### Inflammatory and immunological mechanisms

Most cases of severe RS occur when associated with CTD, and disordered immunology and inflammation are found in these patients. Interestingly, however, abnormal WBC behaviour also occurs in HAVS,[25] which has no clear immunological/inflammatory basis. The interested reader is referred to the scientific literature.[35–37]

### Genetic factors

The link of genetic factors to RP has been suggested and primary RP has been found in monozygotic twins.[33] The concordance rate for RP in monozygotic twins is unknown, but significant familial aggregation of primary RD is well described. However, investigation of large series of twins and multicase families is needed to explore the role of genetics in the pathogenesis of RP.

## Clinical features

The initial features of demarcated blanching of extremities produced in response to cold, temperature change and emotion are episodic. Digital artery spasm is the cause of this pallor, although many people may complain of cold hands with some mild poorly delineated colour changes. They do not necessarily have RP but probably cold-induced closure of the arteriovenous shunts in the skin, which decreases cutaneous blood flow and limits body heat loss. Patients with RP subsequently experience the cyanotic phase and/or the redness of the reactive hyperaemia phase. This last phase may be associated with rewarming paraesthesia and pain. RP is therefore characterised by being biphasic or triphasic, and usually affects the fingers and toes though finger symptoms tend to be more prominent. This may be asymmetrical in that, for example, only one or two digits may be affected on each hand, although all digits may be equally affected.

As documented earlier, other extremities such as the ears, tongue and nose may also be affected, but a bluish discoloration in isolation is due to acrocyanosis and not RP. The occurrence of other skin-related problems (e.g. digital ulcers and recurrent chilblains), an onset in children under 10 years of age, an older adult onset (>30 years) and perennial attacks suggest secondary RP.

## Investigations

These should be directed at confirming the diagnosis of RP, if appropriate, and differentiating between the primary and secondary disease with elucidation of the underlying cause. In the majority of patients, the diagnosis of RP is made clinically from the history and examination if they present during a Raynaud's attack. Objective measures of blood flow are not usually required unless the clinical findings are vague. There are a variety of techniques available, many involving cold challenge, but there is no gold standard because of practical difficulties and interindividual differences.

The test we use most involves the measurement of digital systolic blood pressure changes before and after local cooling at 15°C. A pressure drop of >30 mmHg is considered to be significant, but precautions are required to avoid false-negative results. Ideally, patients should not be tested if they have had a Raynaud's attack earlier in the day as they may still be in the reactive hyperaemia stage and relatively protected from further vasospasm. In practice, the test may be carried out 2–3 hours after an attack if there is good clinical recovery. All vasoactive medication should be stopped for 24 hours before testing and testing should be avoided during mid-cycle in premenopausal women as poor flow can occur during ovulation.[38] Patients should be warm and not vasoconstricted prior to baseline measurements and this is best done by resting in a temperature-controlled laboratory for 30 minutes prior to testing. In warmer weather, additional total body cooling may be required as a warm body may protect a patient from the vasospastic effects of localised digital cooling.

Strain gauge plethysmography is the usual method of measuring digital systolic blood pressure. Considerable operator skill is required and flow cannot be measured. Photoplethysmography with more sophisticated Doppler ultrasound equipment allows the measurement of the pressure at which blood flow returns.

Computerised thermography uses skin temperature as an indicator of finger blood flow. This technique allows dynamic measurement of all phases of the attack but results must be interpreted with care as skin temperature is also dependent on venous and arterial blood temperature.

Associated diseases should be sought by carrying out screening blood tests. A full blood count, urea and electrolytes and urinalysis should detect anaemia of chronic disease and renal disease, and thyroid function tests detect hypothyroidism. Erythrocyte sedimentation rate (ESR) or plasma viscosity and rheumatoid antibody and antinuclear antibody tests help to detect associated CTD. Other tests, for example for cryoglobulins, may be carried out if appropriate. A chest radiograph will show basal fibrosis associated with CTD and a bony cervical rib.

Nail-fold capillaroscopy can be performed using an ophthalmoscope at high power. Normal vessels are not visualised (**Fig. 12.2**) but abnormally enlarged vessels, for example as seen in systemic sclerosis, will be seen quite easily (**Fig. 12.3**). These may also be examined by formal high-power microscopy but it should be noted that nail-fold changes also occur with trauma and in diabetes mellitus. The combination of abnormal nail-fold vessels and an abnormal immunological test has a 90% prediction value for later CTD.[9] Using structured classification systems, nail-fold patterns may be useful in assessing progression of the CTD.[39]

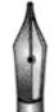

The diagnostic value of nail-fold capillaroscopy is now fully recognised with a clear diagnostic pattern seen for associated CTD: dilatation and tortuosity of the capillary with patches of so-called 'drop-out' where the vessel has been obliterated by the CTD process.[40]

Other tests, such as laser Doppler flowmetry, are used as research tools but are not helpful in making the diagnosis.[41]

## Management

A proportion of patients with mild disease will not require drug treatment. Associated disorders such as hypothyroidism should be treated and causative drug therapy (e.g. beta-blockers for hypertension) changed. Good symptomatic relief can be achieved in many patients despite the current lack of cure. A suggested management plan is shown in **Fig. 12.4**.

### General measures

Explanation of the disorder and reassurance is important in these patients who are often

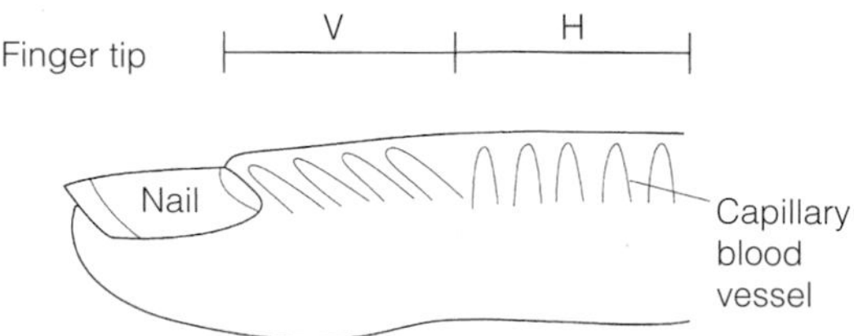


**Figure 12.2** • Diagram of nail-fold vessels. H, vessels perpendicular, not visible; V, vessels becoming parallel, visible if enlarged.

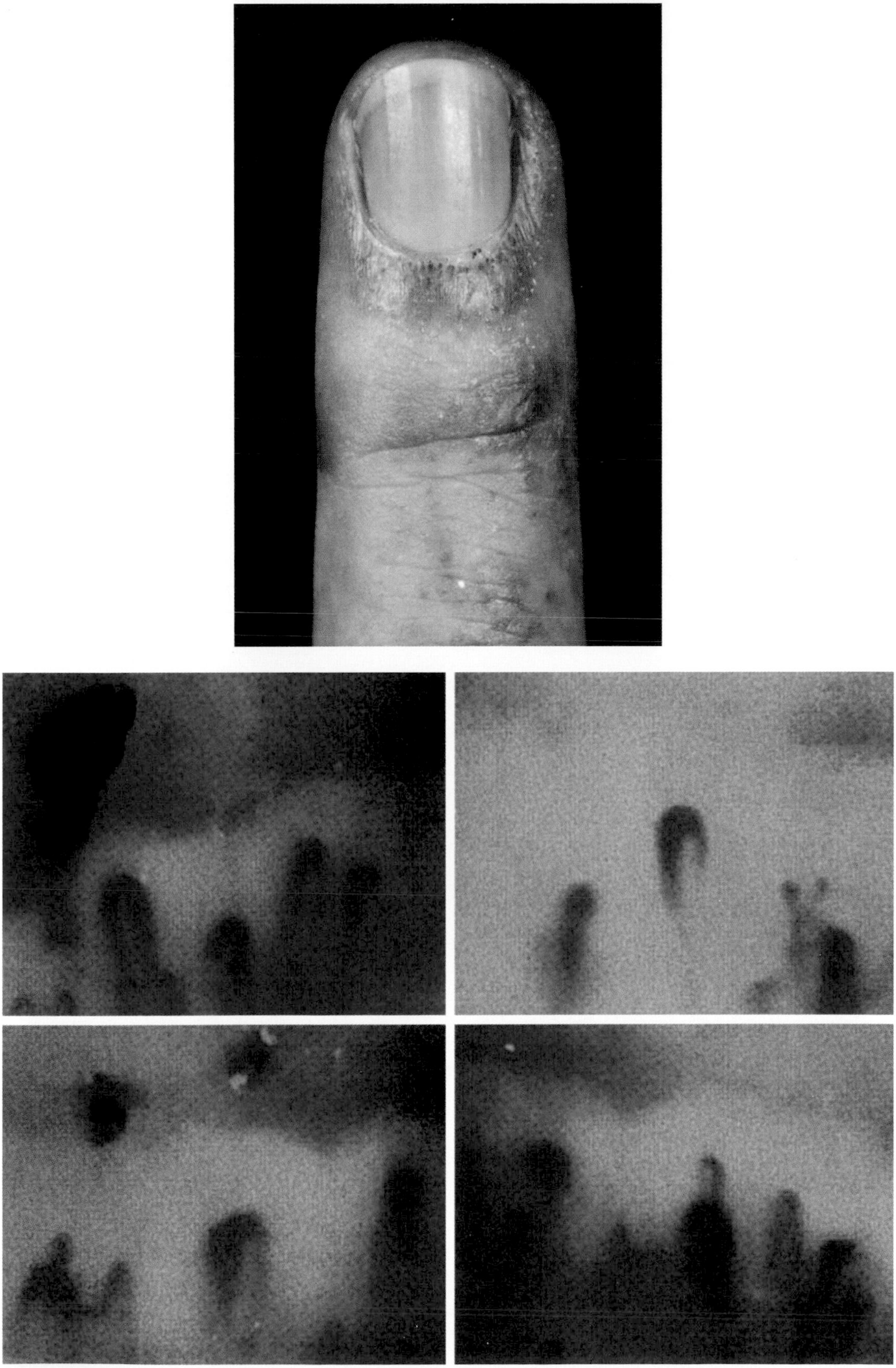

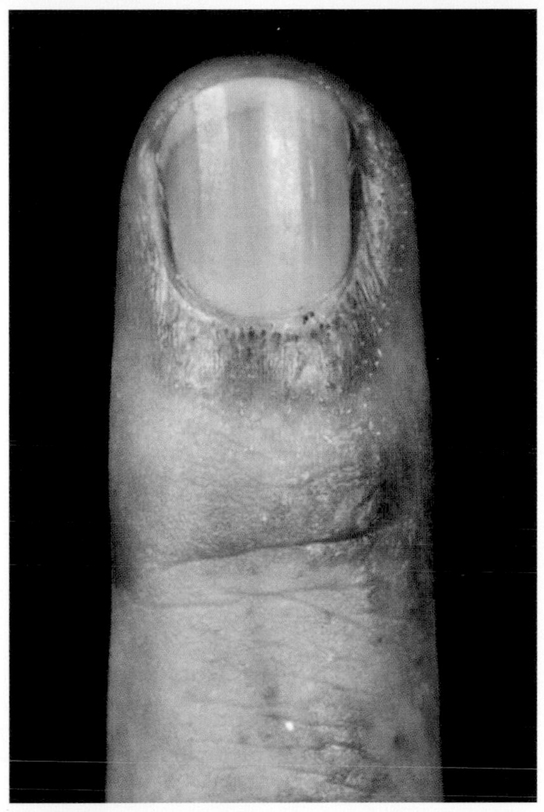

**Figure 12.3** • Enlarged nail-fold capillaries in a patient with systemic sclerosis.

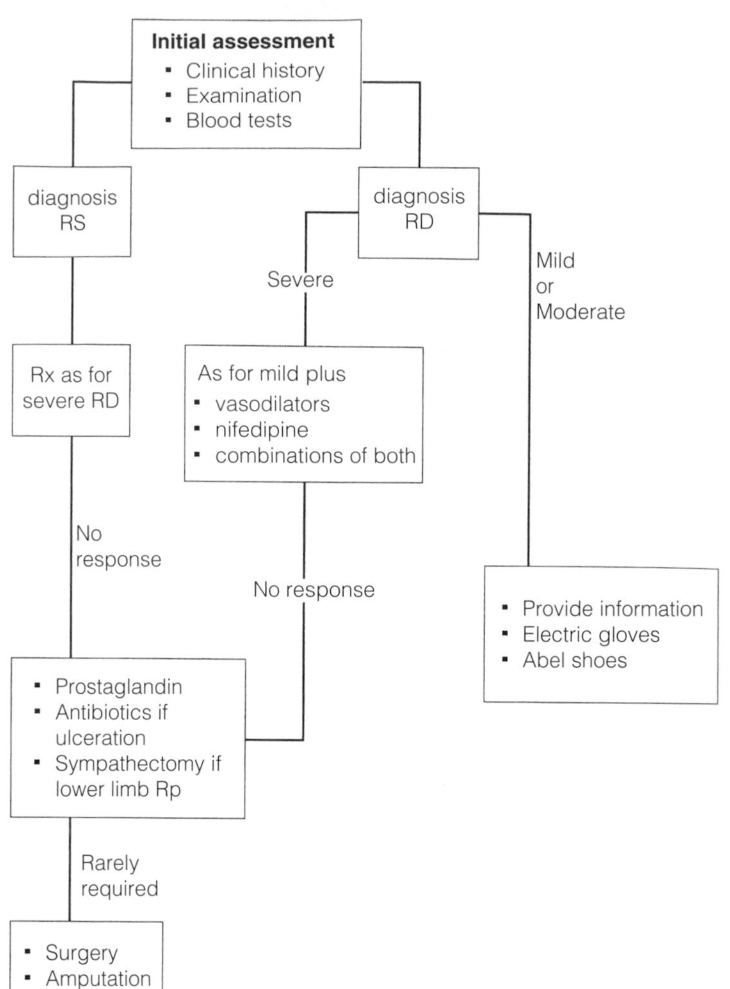


**Figure 12.4** • Flow chart for the management of Raynaud's phenomenon.

apprehensive about their condition. The Raynaud's and Scleroderma Association in the UK issues free information booklets, and local self-help groups can be invaluable for support.

Smokers should stop cigarette smoking. Pocket-sized thermochemical warming agents are available and convenient to use. Electrically heated gloves and socks are ideal for some and provide warmth for up to 3 hours. However, they require heavy batteries to be worn around the waist and are cumbersome, which means elderly patients may not be able to carry the battery. Newer designs are becoming available with the batteries inserted in a pocket on the gloves or socks themselves and should be more acceptable for many patients. Nevertheless, patients should be warned that the heat may irritate existing skin ulcers. 'Abel' shoes, available from surgical appliance suppliers, are padded and broad fitting and therefore warm while relieving pressure around the toes. Good ulcer care with early and adequate treatment of infection is important. It should be noted that the usual signs of infection, i.e. warmth, erythema and pus formation, may be absent because of poor blood flow. A high index of suspicion is required.

## Drug therapy

This should be offered when symptoms are severe enough to interfere with work or lifestyle. Most patients with RS and some with RD will fall into this category. A selection of the drugs used in the treatment of RP is shown in Box 12.2.

### Calcium channel blockers

These drugs are vasodilatory. Nifedipine is the gold standard and the most frequently prescribed drug, and has additional antiplatelet[42] and anti-WBC activity. However, its use is limited by the vasodilatory effects of flushing, headache and ankle swelling. These will be attenuated by using the slow-release, or 'retard', preparations and starting with 10 mg once daily gradually increasing to a maximum of 20 mg t.d.s. if required. Apart from ankle swelling, the

Box 12.2 • Commonly used drugs in the treatment of Raynaud's phenomenon

**Nifedipine**

Slow-release or retard preparation preferred, 10 mg b.d. then t.d.s.

Change to 20 mg b.d. then t.d.s. if required

Capsule as 'rescue medication' crushed under tongue if chronic dosing not tolerated

Can be combined at low dose (e.g. 10 mg once daily) with vasodilator if higher dose not tolerated

**Naftidrofuryl**

Initially 100 mg t.d.s. then 200 mg t.d.s. if required

**Inositol nicotinate**

Start at 500 mg t.d.s. increasing to forte 750 mg b.d. if required

Maximum dose is 1 g q.i.d.

Administer for a 3-month trial

**Pentoxifylline**

400 mg b.d. increasing to t.d.s. if required

**Moxisylyte (thymoxamine)**

40 mg q.d.s. increasing to 80 mg q.d.s.

Discontinue if no response in 2 weeks

vasodilatory adverse effects often abate with continued use. Nifedipine has no licence for use in pregnancy and patients should be advised accordingly. Other potentially useful calcium blockers include amlodipine,[43] diltiazem[44] and isradipine.[45] These tend to have, fewer vasodilatory effects but at the expense of efficacy. Verapamil and ketanserin are ineffective.

### Other vasodilators

Naftidrofuryl oxalate (Praxilene) is a mild peripheral vasodilator with a serotonin receptor antagonist effect. An oral dose of 200 mg t.d.s. has been evaluated in many studies and mild improvement can be expected in terms of severity of pain and duration of attacks.

It is our experience that patients with primary RD respond better to vasodilators than those with RS, the limiting factor often being adverse effects at higher doses. Occasionally, we also find that a combination of a low-dose calcium blocker with a vasodilator such as naftidrofuryl can produce benefit while minimising the adverse effects seen with higher doses of either drug given in isolation.

### Prostaglandins

Prostaglandins such as $PGI_2$ and $PGE_1$ have potent vasodilatory and antiplatelet effects but are both very unstable and require intravenous administration. Iloprost is a stable prostacyclin analogue that is effective in RP.[46] It is given intravenously for 6 hours daily for 3–5 days per treatment. The dose is gradually increased during each 6-hour period to a maximum tolerated dose, which should never be greater than 2 ng/kg per min. It is often less than this, particularly in women, because of flushing, headache or rarely hypotension. The same maximum dose is used each day. It is probably equipotent with nifedipine but remains a second choice in Europe because of its parenteral mode of administration and lack of licence in some countries. Newer studies of oral iloprost[47] and oral limaprost[48] have been encouraging, and these may become available in the relatively near future. Oral beraprost seems to be ineffective.

### Other drugs

Case reports and pilot studies suggest interesting areas for future work. Sildenafil improved pulmonary hypertension and peripheral blood flow in a patient with scleroderma-associated lung fibrosis and RP,[49] while *Ginkgo biloba* extracts[50] may also be effective in some cases. Cilostazol, a synthetic phosphodiesterase III inhibitor that reversibly inhibits platelet aggregation, is used for the treatment of intermittent claudication, and was tested in a randomised controlled trial in RP patients. Treatment was associated with vasodilation of the brachial arteries and conduit vessels.[51] However, the drug had no effects on microvascular blood flow or on the frequency and severity of RP attacks in both primary and secondary RP.

## Sympathectomy

This involves the injection of phenol into the sympathetic chain. Lumbar sympathectomy has an important role in intractable RP of the feet and is often worth considering. Cervical sympathectomy has a poor response and a high relapse rate and is no longer indicated for upper limb RP. The more selective digital sympathectomy is popular in some specialised centres but long-term follow-up results have yet to be published.

# Conclusion

RP is a common condition affecting 10% of the female population. Differentiation between primary and secondary RP is important for the correct management strategy. Satisfactory symptomatic relief is possible with a combination of drug therapy and non-pharmacological aids despite the lack of a cure. Surgery may be appropriate in some cases with an obstructive, bony or fibrous cervical rib. Treatment of associated CTD is also important. Occupational RP can sometimes be improved by change of job or a change in work techniques and this should always be considered.

## Connective tissue disease

The commonest disease associations with RS are the CTDs. Table 12.1 lists these disorders and indicates the relevant incidence of RP. It is found in the majority of patients with systemic sclerosis and mixed CTD. At present, the frequency with which these secondary conditions are recognised varies widely in reported studies and may depend in part on the doctor's referral pattern and the thoroughness with which the screen for a CTD is undertaken.[11] One of the most challenging issue when evaluating patients with RP is the assessment of risk for transition to CTD. DeAngelis et al.[52] reported that, after an average follow-up of 3 years, 10% of their group developed systemic sclerosis. Ziegler et al.[53] reported a 9% transition in patents presenting with RP alone and 30% from 'possible' secondary RP after a 12.4-year mean follow-up. This study suggests that there is a continuum in transition to CTD and that clinicians should not confidently assure patients with what appears to be isolated primary RP of the benign nature of their symptoms. The early detection of patients destined to progress to CTD can be difficult but recently more clearly defined abnormalities have been documented in RP that have a strong link with disease progression. These include certain clinical features, the presence of abnormal nail-fold vessels as previously described, and abnormal tests of immunology. The value of positive antinuclear antibodies (ANAs) in predicting future development of CTD was examined by Myckatyn and Russell,[54] who described the outcome of such patients at the University of Alberta Hospital. After a mean follow-up of 5.4 years, 91% remained ANA-positive and 6% progressed to CTD. The study emphasised the long-term persistence of positive serology and the low rate of transition to CTD, so although a positive test should sound a warning bell, it is not conclusive in itself.

The American Rheumatism Association (ARA) criteria for CTDs have high specificity but low sensitivity for the diseases. Thus patients who do not fulfil the ARA criteria for a particular CTD but who have a single feature of the disease, for example sclerodactyly, digital pitting or photosensitivity, are likely with time to develop fully established CTD.[55] Thus isolated features of CTD occurring in association with RP should arouse clinical suspicion.

**Table 12.1** • Incidence of Raynaud's phenomenon in connective tissue disorders

| Disorder | Incidence |
|---|---|
| Systemic sclerosis | 95% |
| Systemic lupus erythematosus | 29–40% |
| Polymyositis/dermatomyositis | 40% |
| Sjögren's syndrome | 33% |
| Mixed connective tissue disease | 85% |
| Rheumatoid arthritis | 10% |

The age of onset of RP may also be important. As stated, RP is common among young women and most of these probably have primary RD. When RP develops in older subjects, the likelihood of an underlying CTD is increased. Kallenberg[56] reports a study in which the median age of onset of vasospastic symptoms in RD was 14 years, and 36 years in patients with definite CTD. About 80% of patients presenting with onset of RP at the age of 60 years or above also have an associated condition,[53] but the incidence of CTD is the same as in the general population. The larger numbers of secondary cases reflect a higher proportion of patients with atherosclerosis (29% vs. 5% in the total Raynaud's population), and to a lesser extent hyperviscosity syndromes secondary to malignancy. Conversely, RP occurring in very young children, though rare, is frequently due to an underlying CTD. It has been estimated in one childhood study that 70% had primary RP and 30% were associated with other diseases.[33] Other suspicious symptoms that should alert the clinician to the likelihood of secondary RS include the presence of digital ulceration. Digital ulceration does not occur in RD. The recurrence of chilblains in adults may also raise suspicions, as should the occurrence of severe attacks persisting throughout the summer.[57] Furthermore, asymmetrical colour change with fewer digits affected suggests RS rather than RD.[58]

The above clinical symptoms can act as a guide to the future development of CTD and suggest that close monitoring of the patient with repeated observations of nail-fold vessels and immunopathological testing may be of value.

RP is a frequent accompanying symptom of CTDs. In some of these the RP is reported as merely consisting of a biphasic or triphasic colour change with minimal discomfort. In other conditions RP is the most significant symptom, with the patients complaining of pain, ulcers and even gangrene. The most likely group of patients to be seen by the vascular clinician are those suffering from limited systemic sclerosis. This is because Raynaud's is severe in systemic sclerosis, thus meriting hospital referral. Furthermore, it often predates the other symptoms of CTD by many years. Thus a high index of suspicion for this particular disorder must be held by those seeing patients as a result of their vasospastic symptomatology.

## Vasculitis

Vasculitis is the term used to describe the group of conditions characterised by inflammation within the blood vessel wall and possibly damage to vessel integrity. The vasculitic process may involve only one or many blood vessels and therefore organ systems. In general, the clinical features result in ischaemia of the tissues supplied by the damaged vessel. These symptoms are often accompanied by the constitutional symptoms of fever, weight loss and anorexia that result from widespread inflammation. The vasculitic conditions may have a range of vessel involvement, from a mild obliterative disorder to necrotising vasculitis. Table 12.2 shows some of the common vasculitides, stratified by the size of the vessel most commonly involved. The classification of vasculitis is confusing as there is considerable clinical overlap between the different vasculitic syndromes and often the cause is unknown. Because the diagnosis of vasculitis still requires histological confirmation in most cases, the classification based on the size of the predominant vessel involved and the type of inflammatory change is most frequently used. Non-invasive imaging using whole-body contrast-enhanced magnetic resonance angiography (CE-MRA) and multislice computed tomography have made significant inroads into conventional angiography in assessing the distribution of many vasculitic conditions. Increasingly, [$^{18}$F]fluorodeoxy glucose positron emission tomography/computed tomography can be used to demonstrate the presence, distribution and activity of vasculitis as well as to monitor its response to treatment.

## Takayasu's arteritis

This is an inflammatory and obliterative arteritis that primarily affects the large elastic arteries. It affects all levels of the aorta, its branches and the pulmonary arteries. The disorder has a striking female predominance, affecting women five to nine times more frequently than men. It usually presents between 10 and 30 years of age, although case reports of older patients have been published. The disease symptomatology can be divided into two phases: the acute systemic phase (pre-pulseless) and the chronic obliterative (pulseless) phase. The acute symptoms are often non-specific and are those one would expect to see with a generalised inflammatory process, and include fatigue and malaise, weight loss and fever. Arthralgia and myalgia are common. The symptoms of the chronic phase are the result of the obliterative arterial lesion and depend on which vessels are affected. Possible findings include diminished or absent arterial pulses, vascular bruits, hypertension, inequality of blood pressure between arms and legs, and abnormalities on auscultation of the heart. Upper limb claudication can occur in association with the reduced or absent upper limb pulses.

Laboratory studies in Takayasu's arteritis reflect the inflammatory nature of the disorder. The ESR is elevated in the majority of patients during active disease. CE-MRA plays an important role in the diagnosis of this disease, with findings of vessel occlusions, stenoses (**Fig. 12.5**), aneurysm formation and the development of collaterals around occlusions. All levels of the aorta as well as its major branches may be involved and should be visualised. Pulmonary artery involvement has been seen in up to half of patients with this disorder. Of six diagnostic clinical and imaging criteria issued by the American College of Rheumatology, three are required to reach the diagnosis of Takayasu's arteritis.[59] Biopsy during the early phase shows granulomatous inflammation with patchy involvement of the vessel wall. Later, the changes are characterised by intimal proliferation and band fibrosis of the adventitia and media.

**Table 12.2** • Relationship between vasculitis classification and vessel size

| Type of vasculitis | Aorta and branches | Large and medium-sized arteries | Medium-sized muscular arteries | Small muscular arteries | Arterioles, capillaries and venules |
|---|---|---|---|---|---|
| Takayasu's arteritis | ✓ | | | | |
| Buerger's disease (thromboangiitis obliterans) | ✓ | ✓ | | | |
| Giant cell arteritis (temporal arteritis) | ✓ | ✓ | | | |
| Polyarteritis nodosa | | ✓ | ✓ | | |
| Wegener's granulomatosis | | | ✓ | ✓ | |
| Connective tissue disorders | | | | ✓ | ✓ |
| Rheumatoid vasculitis | | | | ✓ | ✓ |
| Cutaneous vasculitis (leucocytoclastic/allergic) | | | | | ✓ |

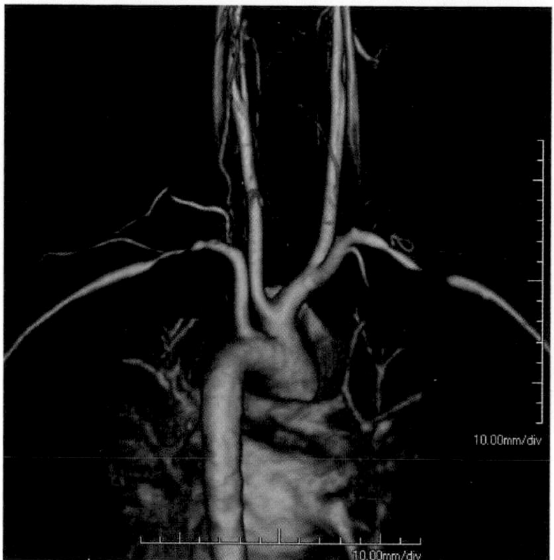


**Figure 12.5** • Posterior view of a 3D volume-rendered thoracic aorta magnetic resonance angiogram showing severe bilateral subclavian artery stenoses in a 35-year-old woman who presented with chest pain. In addition there were severe stenoses and occlusions of visceral and lower limb arteries. Image courtesy of Dr John Bottomley, Sheffield Vascular Institute, UK.

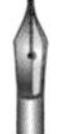

During the acute inflammatory phase immunosuppression with corticosteroids and/or cyclophosphamide has been found to be effective in halting the angiographic progression.[59]

Symptomatic management of the patient is also important and symptoms such as hypertension should be treated aggressively. Therapeutic response is best assessed by improvement in symptoms, a fall in ESR and improvement in serial angiographic studies. Surgery may be required to bypass stenosed or occluded segments of vessels that are producing significant ischaemia.[60]

## Buerger's disease (thromboangiitis obliterans)

Buerger's disease is the clinical syndrome characterised by segmental thrombotic occlusions of the small and medium-sized arteries usually of the distal lower limb but occasionally also involving the upper extremities. Buerger's disease usually occurs in young smokers and is frequently associated with both RP and superficial migratory thrombophlebitis. Although previously mainly described in young men, the increased incidence of smoking in women has caused an increase in Buerger's disease in this sex.[61] In a recent review the changing pattern of this disease was recorded, confirming the increased prevalence of Buerger's disease in women.[62] It also documented that older patients (>40 years of age) are being more frequently diagnosed.

In the acute lesion, the internal elastic lamina of the arteries is almost always intact. Thrombus fills the vessel lumen and is hypercellular with an infiltration of lymphocytes, fibroblasts and later giant cells. There is no vessel wall necrosis or vascular wall calcification and atheromatous plaques and aneurysms are both absent. The consistent presence of an acute hypercellular occlusive thrombus is the hallmark of this disease.

Altered haemorheological parameters have been detected in thromboangiitis obliterans, opening up some new therapeutic avenues.[63]

The symptoms of Buerger's disease are usually related to lower extremity ischaemia and include rest pain and tissue loss. Claudication is a rare symptom, but when present is usually confined to the foot. Femoral or popliteal pulses are usually present but the pedal pulses are absent.[64] The diagnosis of Buerger's disease depends to a great extent on the exclusion of other conditions, particularly early-onset atherosclerosis and immune disorders.

Investigation of the lower limb ischaemia reveals angiographically normal vessels proximal to the popliteal. The tibial and peroneal vessels are frequently normal to a point of sudden occlusion.

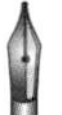

Tobacco abstinence is the cornerstone of management for Buerger's disease. In patients who do manage to stop smoking the appearance of new lesions and gangrene requiring amputation is unusual.[64]

However, persistent smoking leads to continued progression of the disease. Upper limb RP, finger ulceration and gangrene are treated as described earlier (Fig. 12.4). There have been a large number of medical treatments proposed for the treatment of Buerger's disease affecting the lower limb and the variety of the treatments proposed testifies to the fact that none are completely satisfactory and nearly all lack documentary efficacy. Corticosteroids,[65] antiplatelet therapy and iloprost infusions[66] are just a few of the treatments that have been used. The evidence for corticosteroid therapy is tenuous, whilst that for the use of iloprost and aspirin-like compounds is more convincing. Further research is required into the benefits of the various medical treatment regimens currently available.

## Giant cell arteritis

Giant cell arteritis, or temporal arteritis, is a systemic granulomatous vasculitis that predominantly affects large and medium-sized blood vessels. It usually involves the cranial branches of the aorta. It is most often seen in patients over 50 years of age and is an important preventable cause of blindness. However, it is recognised that temporal arteritis is a disease with many different manifestations and extracranial presentations are not uncommon. Among the vasculitic disorders, temporal arteritis is one of the more commonly occurring disorders, though it is still relatively rare. The estimated overall incidence rate in persons older than 50 years of age is approximately 17 per 100000 annually.[67] There is a three to five times higher incidence in women than in men. The risk of this disease occurring is increased in smokers and patients with already established atherosclerotic disease.[68]

Temporal arteritis may present acutely or insidiously. Although headaches and sudden blindness are the classical symptoms, constitutional symptoms such as fever, weight loss and fatigue may be the earliest manifestations.[69] Headaches are the usual complaint and these may be localised to the area overlying the superficial temporal arteries or may be generalised, resembling tension headaches. Scalp tenderness can also be a prominent feature and this can produce difficulty for the patients when combing their hair or sleeping at night on a pillow. This symptom is secondary to the involvement of the superficial temporal and occipital arteries. Jaw claudication occurs in approximately half of patients with this disease. This results from facial and maxillary artery involvement. Tongue claudication and dysphagia have also been reported and rarely glossitis and tongue necrosis are seen.[70] Sudden visual loss is a consequence of disease in the ophthalmic or posterior ciliary artery. Once blindness is established it is irreversible, but amaurosis fugax, a warning sign of impending blindness, is responsive to steroids. Pulmonary, renal and neurological symptomatology have also been reported as has synovitis, but cutaneous or limb vessel manifestations are rare. This disease is therefore unlikely to present to the vascular clinician.

The diagnosis of temporal arteritis is made by finding an elevated acute-phase response such as the ESR. However, it should be noted that the ESR is not necessarily always elevated in patients with this disorder. The diagnostic hallmark of temporal arteritis is a biopsy that shows granulomatous inflammation (**Fig. 12.6**). Because of the intermittent or skip pattern of the lesions, biopsy can be negative in 50% of cases. Thus a negative biopsy in the setting of a high suspicion for the disease does not rule out the disease and should not preclude steroid therapy.

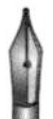

On occasions a trial of steroid therapy can in itself be used to make the diagnosis. Corticosteroids are the mainstay of treatment. This therapy is efficacious in preventing but not reversing blindness.[71]

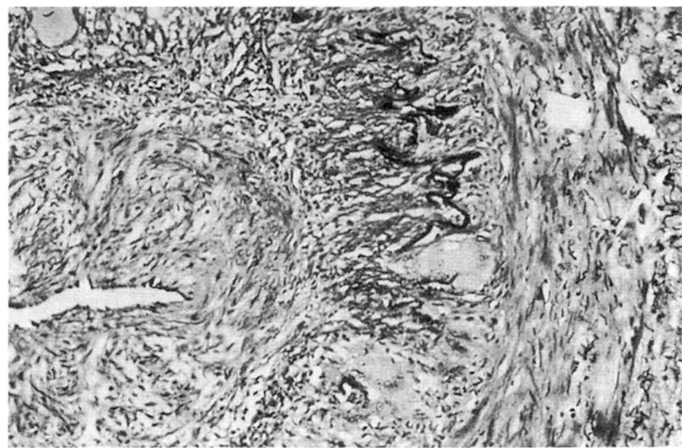

**Figure 12.6** • Temporal artery biopsy demonstrating granulomatous inflammation and disruption of the internal elastic lamina.

In studies of cytotoxic agents, methotrexate has been used as a corticosteroid-sparing drug in patients with polymyalgia rheumatica and giant cell arteritis, with conflicting results.[72,73] However, this drug may be tried in patients who are taking high doses of corticosteroids to control active disease and who have serious adverse effects from the steroids. Subjects with a raised platelet count are at higher risk of visual loss and should be treated effectively.[74] ESR/plasma viscosity and C-reactive protein (CRP) are generally used to monitor disease activity, but anticardiolipin antibodies if present may also be of benefit if there is confounding pathology that will increase ESR/CRP (e.g. infection).[75] Levels of interleukin (IL)-6 may be a sensitive indicator of active disease in polymyalgia rheumatica;[76] however, a recent paper suggests that in giant cell arteritis, subjects with a raised titre of IL-6 may in fact be at lower risk of ischaemic events.[77] Calcium and vitamin D supplementation should be given with corticosteroid therapy in all patients. In patients with reduced bone mineral density, bisphosphonates are recommended.[78]

## Polyarteritis nodosa

Polyarteritis nodosa (PAN) is a unique process characterised by a systemic necrotising vasculitis involving the small and medium-sized muscular arteries. The prevalence of PAN ranges between 5 and 77 per million population, with the higher incidence being reported in hepatitis B hyperendemic populations.[79] PAN is twice as common in men than women and the average age of diagnosis is between 40 and 60 years, although PAN has been seen in both children and the elderly.

The symptoms reported depend on the vessels affected. The presenting symptoms are often constitutional, such as malaise, abdominal pain, weight loss, fever and myalgia. Organ involvement can occur at the same time or may develop later in the disease process. Renal disease with proteinuria and progressive renal failure occurs in about 70% of patients.[80] Hypertension is a frequent finding. Gastrointestinal involvement is common and manifests as abdominal pain, nausea and vomiting. Acute events such as infarction of the bowel, perforation and haemorrhage are rare but produce the high mortality associated with this condition. Skin manifestations include nail-fold infarcts (**Fig. 12.7**), palpable purpura and livedo reticularis (**Fig. 12.8**). Damage to the blood vessel wall can result in aneurysm formation. Mononeuritis multiplex is common and other important sites of involvement include the retina and testes. Laboratory findings can be non-specific, making the diagnosis difficult, but include anaemia, elevated ESR and a positive test for antineutrophil cytoplasmic antibody (ANCA). Hepatitis B surface antigen and antibodies should be measured in all patients with PAN. Angiography may be diagnostic, showing the characteristic findings of saccular or fusiform aneurysms and arterial narrowing.[81] The diagnosis of PAN must be based on the demonstration of vasculitis by angiography or biopsy.

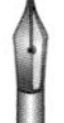

Corticosteroids are the cornerstone of treatment and cyclophosphamide can be added if the disease proves difficult to control.

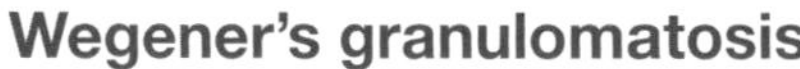

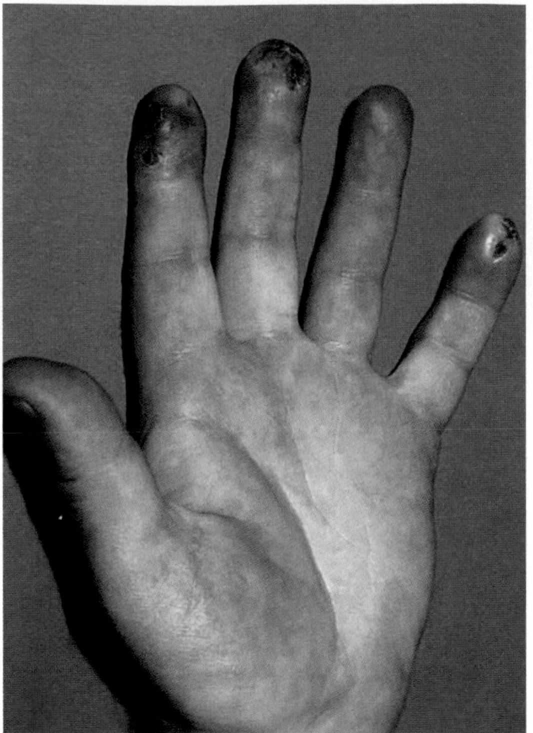

**Figure 12.7** • Digital infarct in polyarteritis nodosa.

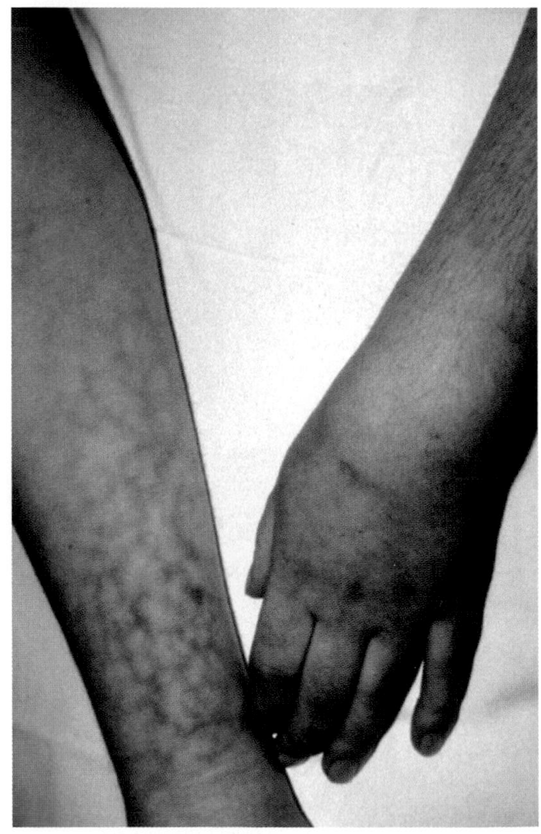

**Figure 12.8** • Livedo reticularis in polyarteritis nodosa.

## Wegener's granulomatosis

Wegener's granulomatosis is a form of vasculitis that involves mainly the medium and small arteries and veins of the upper and lower respiratory tract and kidneys. Although it is a systemic necrotising granulomatous vasculitis, it is classically associated with the triad of upper respiratory tract, lung and kidney involvement. The manifestations and severity of the disease at presentation are variable but cutaneous vascular symptoms tend to be less frequently seen.[82] These consist of cutaneous ulceration, subcutaneous nodules and palpable purpura.

Laboratory findings show an inflammatory response. Sinus radiographs or computed tomography may show evidence of mucosal thickening, sinus opacification or air–fluid levels. The chest X-ray may show mass lesions. Diagnosis is made through biopsy. The finding of elevated blood c-ANCA levels is strongly associated with Wegener's granulomatosis and these should be measured in cases of clinical suspicion.

Circulating endothelial cells may be a novel marker of active ANCA-associated small-vessel vasculitis. The clinical use of this tool and the pathogenic mechanisms leading to these findings require further investigation.[83] Treatment is with immunosuppressants.

**Box 12.3** • Clinical syndromes of cutaneous vasculitis

**Idiopathic cutaneous vasculitis**

**Necrotising vasculitis secondary to**

Drugs, e.g. antibiotics, diuretics, NSAIDs, anticonvulsants

Infection, e.g. upper respiratory tract virus, *Streptococcus*, hepatitis B, HIV

Immunological disorders, e.g. connective tissue diseases

**Cutaneous vasculitis as a manifestation of systemic disease**

Connective tissue disease

Mixed cryoglobulinaemia

Allergic granulomatosis (Churg–Strauss syndrome)

Behçet's disease

HIV, human immunodeficiency virus; NSAIDs, non-steroidal anti-inflammatory drugs.

## Cutaneous vasculitis/small-vessel vasculitis

The vessels primarily involved in small-vessel vasculitis are the postcapillary venules, although capillaries and arterioles may also be involved. When first described, small-vessel vasculitis was named hypersensitivity angiitis. At one time, small-vessel vasculitis was thought to be identical to the microscopic form of PAN. However, the latter affects mainly small arteries and arterioles rather than venules. Box 12.3 lists the clinical syndromes associated with cutaneous vasculitis.

### Idiopathic cutaneous vasculitis

This is the most common form of vasculitis in the skin.[8] It is usually manifest by palpable purpura most commonly occurring in the lower limb, often below the knee. The involvement of the lower limb tends to be symmetrical and is worsened by periods of sitting or standing. The lesions occur in crops, initially appearing as macular erythema and then progressing to purpura. Uncommonly, this type of vasculitis can present as urticaria and it can be distinguished from typical urticaria by the fact that the lesions persist for more than 24 hours. Biopsies of the lesion shows leucocytoclastic vasculitis with endothelial cell swelling, often necrosis as well as haemorrhage, fibrin deposition and infiltration with polymorphonuclear neutrophils.

### Necrotising vasculitis associated with infections, drugs or CTD

The aetiology of this form of vasculitis is presumed to be hypersensitivity to various factors, including infective agents and drugs, or underlying systemic disease. Nevertheless, in approximately half the cases no definitive precipitating agent can be found.[83] Infection is associated with cutaneous necrotising vasculitis in approximately 10% of cases. Most often these are viruses associated with the upper respiratory tract and cause vasculitis such as Henoch–Schönlein purpura, although bacterial organisms have also been found capable of inducing a hypersensitivity vasculitis. The most commonly implicated drugs are antibiotics, particularly penicillin and sulphonamides. Diuretics and non-steroidal anti-inflammatory drugs (NSAIDs) have also been linked to the condition. Leucocytoclastic vasculitis may also be associated with a number of immunological disorders with systemic manifestations; most commonly these are of the CTD type.

### Cutaneous vasculitis as a manifestation of systemic disease

Small-vessel vasculitis affecting the skin may be a manifestation of underlying systemic disease. The most common diseases in this category are the CTDs, particularly systemic lupus erythematosus but also mixed cryoglobulinaemia. The clinical and histological appearances of this type of vasculitis are often indistinguishable from those of the lesions of idiopathic cutaneous vasculitis. It is of crucial importance to examine any patient with skin vasculitis in a thorough fashion, focusing on the potential for the presence of CTD.

In Churg–Strauss vasculitis the most common type of skin manifestation appears mainly in the extremities and is maculopapular in appearance. It may be accompanied by vesicles and occasionally by bullae. Behçet's disease, which is characterised by oral and genital ulceration, may also present with a variety of non-specific skin changes including papules, vesicles, pyoderma and erythema nodosum-like lesions. Most patients with small-vessel vasculitis have disease limited to the skin.[83] Investigation of these patients should be aimed at confirming the diagnosis by biopsy and then elucidating potential aetiological agents or underlying systemic disorder.

Most patients with small-vessel vasculitis limited to the skin experience a single episode that is often short-lived and associated with minimal symptomatology. Therapy for these individuals may not be required or may be limited to the use of antihistamines or NSAIDs. However, for individuals with more severe or recurrent episodes, treatment with corticosteroids may have to be considered.

Human immunodeficiency virus (HIV) is becoming a rare but reported cause of vasculitis, and it is important for the clinican to be aware of these emerging data in this regard. A broad spectrum of vasculitis is reported in HIV-infected patients ranging from involvement of the small vessels, in hypersensitivity vasculitis secondary to drug treatment, to involvement of the aorta and branches. Corticosteroids or other immunosuppressive therapies such as intravenous immunoglobulin and cyclophosphamide are used to treat life-threatening vasculitic complications that involve the lungs, kidneys or central nervous system, in conjunction with effective antiretroviral therapy.

## Conclusion

Vasculitis will present to the vascular clinician as skin ischaemia. The predilection of a number of vasculitic disorders for the lower limb may mimic large-vessel disease or emboli. The cornerstone of diagnosis is the finding of an acute-phase response, e.g. elevated ESR, plasma viscosity and CRP levels. Screening for autoantibodies may be helpful, but diagnosis is often only made by analysis of biopsy material and this should be considered in all cases of vasculitis, unless the tissue is too ischaemic to sustain wound healing.

### Key points

- Raynaud's phenomenon should be classified appropriately into primary Raynaud's disease and secondary Raynaud's syndrome. Management includes general measures, drugs, sympathectomy and attention to any underlying disease.
- Vasculitis may present to the vascular clinician as skin ischaemia. Constitutional symptoms of fever, weight loss and fatigue are often clues to the diagnosis. Key investigations are ESR/plasma viscosity, CRP, autoantibodies and biopsy. Immunosuppression is the cornerstone of treatment of vasculitis.

## References


1. Raynaud MD. Asphyxre et de la gangrene symetriques des extremities. Paris, 1862. (Trans. Thomas Barlow, London, New Sydenham Society, 1988.)
2. Brotzu G, Falchi S, Mannu B et al. The importance of presynaptic beta receptors in Raynaud's disease. J Vasc Surg 1989; 9:767–71.
3. Baron M, Feiglin D, Hyland R et al. $^{67}$Gallium lung scans in progressive systemic sclerosis. Arth Rheum 1983; 26:969–74.
4. Belch JJ, Land D, Park RH et al. Decreased oesophageal blood flow in patients with Raynaud's phenomenon. Br J Rheumatol 1988; 27:426–30.
5. Kahan A, Devaux JY, Amor B et al. Nifedipine and thallium-201 myocardial perfusion in progressive systemic sclerosis. N Engl J Med 1986; 314:1397–402.
6. De Trafford JC, Lafferty K, Potter CE et al. An epidemiological survey of Raynaud's phenomenon. Eur J Vasc Surg 1988; 2:167–70.
7. Olsen N, Nielsen SL. Prevalence of primary Raynaud phenomena in young females. Scand J Clin Lab Invest 1978; 38:761–4.
8. Porter JM, Bardana EJ Jr, Baur GM et al. The clinical significance of Raynaud's syndrome. Surgery 1976; 80:756–64.
9. Porter JM, Rivers SP, Anderson CJ et al. Evaluation and management of patients with Raynaud's syndrome. Am J Surg 1981; 142:183–9.
10. Kallenberg CG, Wouda AA, The TH. Systemic involvement and immunologic findings in patients presenting with Raynaud's phenomenon. Am J Med 1980; 69:675–80.
11. Allen EV, Brown GE. Raynaud's disease: a critical review of minimal requisites for diagnosis. Am J Med Sci 1932; 183:187–200.
12. Taylor W. The hand–arm vibration syndrome: diagnosis, assessment and objective tests. A review. J R Soc Med 1993; 86:101–3.
13. Letz R, Cherniack MG, Gerr F et al. A cross sectional epidemiological survey of shipyard workers exposed to hand–arm vibration. Br J Ind Med 1992; 49:53–62.
14. Mirbod SM, Yoshida H, Nagata C et al. Hand–arm vibration syndrome and its prevalence in the present status of private forestry enterprises in Japan. Int Arch Occup Environ Health 1992; 64:93–9.
15. Koskimies K, Pyykko I, Starck J et al. Vibration syndrome among Finnish forest workers between 1972 and 1990. Int Arch Occup Environ Health 1992; 64:251–6.
16. Hedlund U. Raynaud's phenomenon of fingers and toes of miners exposed to local and whole-body vibration and cold. Int Arch Occup Environ Health 1989; 61:457–61.
17. Kennedy G, Khan F, McLaren M et al. Endothelial activation and response in patients with hand arm vibration syndrome. Eur J Clin Invest 1999; 29:577–81.
18. Taylor W, Pelmear PL. The hand–arm vibration syndrome: an update. Br J Ind Med 1990; 47:577–9.
19. Benefits Agency (Department of Social Security). If you have an industrial disease. NI 2August 1995; pp. 2–4.
20. Freedman RR, Sabharal SC, Desai N et al. Increased alpha-adrenergic responsiveness in idiopathic Raynaud's disease. Arth Rheum 1989; 32:61–5.
21. Olsen N, Petring OU. Vibration elicited vasoconstrictor reflex in Raynaud's phenomena. Br J Ind Med 1988; 45:415–19.
22. Carter SA, Dean E, Kroeger EA. Apparent finger systolic pressures during cooling in patients

with Raynaud's syndrome. Circulation 1988; 77:988–96.

23. Lau CS, O'Dowd A, Belch JJ. White blood cell activation in Raynaud's phenomenon of systemic sclerosis and vibration induced white finger syndrome. Ann Rheum Dis 1992; 51:249–52.
24. Lau CS, Bridges AB, Muir A et al. Further evidence of increased polymorphonuclear cell activity in patients with Raynaud's phenomenon. Br J Rheumatol 1992; 31:375–80.
25. Belch JJ, Drury J, McLaughlin K et al. Abnormal biochemical and cellular parameters in the blood of patients with Raynaud's phenomenon. Scott Med J 1987; 32:12–14.
26. Belch JJ, Zoma AA, Richards IM et al. Vascular damage and factor-VIII-related antigen in the rheumatic diseases. Rheumatol Int 1987; 7:107–11.
27. Belch JJ, McLaren M, Anderson J et al. Increased prostacyclin metabolites and decreased red cell deformability in patients with systemic sclerosis and Raynaud's syndrome. Prostaglandins Leukot Med 1985; 18:401–2.
28. Belch JJ, O'Dowd A, Forbes CD et al. Platelet sensitivity to a prostacyclin analogue in systemic sclerosis. Br J Rheumatol 1985; 24:346–50.
29. Zamora MR, O'Brien RF, Rutherford RB et al. Serum endothelin-1 concentrations and cold provocation in primary Raynaud's phenomenon. Lancet 1990; 336:1144–7.
30. Kahaleh B, Fan PS, Matucci-Cerinic M et al. Study of endothelial dependent relaxation in scleroderma (abstract). Am Coll Rheum 1993; B233:S180.
31. Khan F, Belch JJ. Skin blood flow in patients with systemic sclerosis and Raynaud's phenomenon: effects of oral l-arginine supplementation. J Rheumatol 1999; 26:2389–94.
32. Nakamura H, Matsuzaki I, Hatta K et al. Blood endothelin-1 and cold-induced vasodilation in patients with primary Raynaud's phenomenon and workers with vibration-induced white finger. Int Angiol 2003; 22:243–9.
33. Kahaleh MB. Raynaud phenomenon and the vascular diseases in scleroderma. Curr Opin Rheumatol 2004; 16(6):718–22.
34. Konttinen YT, Mackiewicz Z, Ruuttila P et al. Vascular damage and lack of angiogenesis in systemic sclerosis skin. Clin Rheumatol 2003; 22:196–202.
35. Kurozawa Y, Nasu Y. Circulating adhesion molecules in patients with vibration-induced white finger. Angiology 2000; 51:1003–6.
36. Lau CS. Haemostatic abnormalities in Raynaud's phenomenon and the potential for treatment with manipulation of the arachidonic acid pathway. MD thesis, University of Dundee, 1993.
37. Worda M, Sgonc R, Dietrich H et al. In vivo analysis of the apoptosis-inducing effect of anti-endothelial cell antibodies in systemic sclerosis by the chorionallantoic membrane assay. Arth Rheum 2003; 48:2605–14.
38. Lafferty K, De Trafford JC, Potter C et al. Reflex vascular responses in the finger to contralateral thermal stimuli during the normal menstrual cycle: a hormonal basis to Raynaud's phenomenon? Clin Sci 1985; 68:639–45.
39. Cutolo M, Sulli A, Pizzorni C et al. Nailfold videocapillaroscopy assessment of microvascular damage in systemic sclerosis. J Rheumatol 2000; 27:155–60.
40. Nagy Z, Czirjak L. Nailfold digital capillaroscopy in 447 patients with connective tissue disease and Raynaud's disease. J Eur Acad Dermatol Venereol 2004; 18:62–8.
41. Turner JB, Belch JJF, Khan F. Current concepts in assessment of microvascular function using laser Doppler imaging and iontophoresis. Trends Cardiovasc Med 2008; 18(4):109–16.
42. Maricq HR, Jennings JR, Valter I et al. Evaluation of treatment efficacy of Raynaud phenomenon by digital blood pressure response to cooling. Raynaud's Treatment Study Investigators. Vasc Med 2000; 5:135–40.
43. La Civita L, Pitaro N, Rossi M et al. Amlodipine in the treatment of Raynaud's phenomenon. Br J Rheumatol 1993; 32:524–5.
44. Rhedda A, McCans J, Willan AR et al. A double blind placebo controlled crossover randomized trial of diltiazem in Raynaud's phenomenon. J Rheumatol 1985; 12:724–7.
45. Leppert J, Jonasson T, Nilsson H et al. The effect of isradipine, a new calcium-channel antagonist, in patients with primary Raynaud's phenomenon: a single-blind dose–response study. Cardiovasc Drugs Ther 1989; 3:397–401.
46. Wigley F et al. Intravenous iloprost infusion in patients with Raynaud phenomenon secondary to systemic sclerosis: a multicenter, placebo-controlled, double-blind study. Ann Int Med 1994; 120:199–206.
47. Belch JJ, Capell HA, Cooke ED et al. Oral iloprost as a treatment for Raynaud's syndrome: a double blind multicentre placebo controlled study. Ann Rheum Dis 1995; 54:197–200.
48. Murai C, Sasaki T, Osaki H et al. Oral limaprost for Raynaud's phenomenon. Lancet 1989; ii:1218.
49. Rosenkranz S, Diet F, Karasch T et al. Sildenafil improved pulmonary hypertension and peripheral blood flow in a patient with scleroderma-associated lung fibrosis and the Raynaud phenomenon. Ann Intern Med 2003; 139:871–3.
50. Muir AH, Robb R, McLaren M et al. The use of Ginkgo biloba in Raynaud's disease: a double-blind placebo-controlled trial. Vasc Med 2002; 7:265–7.

51. Rajagopalan S, Pfenninger D, Somers E et al. Effects of cilostazol in patients with Raynaud's syndrome. Am J Cardiol 2003; 92(11):1310–15.
52. DeAngelis R, Del Medico R, Blasetti P et al. Raynaud's phenomenon: clinical spectrum of 118 patients. Clin Rheumatol 2003; 22:279–84.
53. Ziegler S, Brunner M, Eigenbauer E et al. Long-term outcome of primary Raynaud's phenomenon and its conversion to connective tissue disease: a 12-year retrospective patient analysis. Scand J Rheumatol 2003; 32:343–7.
54. Myckatyn SO, Russell AS. Outcome of positive antinuclear antibodies in individuals without connective tissue disease. J Rheumatol 2003; 30:736–9.
55. Belch JJ. Raynaud's phenomenon: its relevance to scleroderma. Ann Rheum Dis 1991; 50(Suppl 4): 839–45.
56. Kallenberg CG. Early detection of connective tissue disease in patients with Raynaud's phenomenon. Rheum Dis Clin North Am 1990; 16:11–30.
57. Franceschini F, Calzavara-Pinton P, Valsecchi L et al. Chilblain lupus erythematosus is associated with antibodies to SSA/Ro. Adv Exp Med Biol 1999; 455:167–71.
58. Cardelli MB, Kleinsmith DM. Raynaud's phenomenon and disease. Med Clin North Am 1989; 73:1127–41.
59. Arend WP, Michel BA, Bloch DA et al. The American College of Rheumatology 1990 criteria for the classification of Takayasu arteritis. Arth Rheum 1990; 33:1129–34.
60. Giordano JM. Surgical treatment of Takayasu's arteritis. Int J Cardiol 2000; 75(Suppl 1):S123–8.
61. Lie JT. The Canadian Rheumatism Association, 1991 Dunlop–Dottridge Lecture. Vasculitis, 1815 to 1991: classification and diagnostic specificity. J Rheumatol 1992; 19:83–9.
62. Stvrtinova V, Ambrozy E, Stvrtina S et al. 90 years of Buerger's disease: what has changed. Bratisl Lek Listy 1999; 100:123–8.
63. Bozkurt AK, Koksal C, Ercan M. The altered hemorheologic parameters in thromboangiitis obliterans: a new insight. Clin Appl Thromb Hemost 2004; 10:45–50.
64. Mills JL, Porter JM. Thromboangiitis obliterans (Buerger's disease). In: Churg A, Churg I (eds) Systemic vasculitides. Tokyo: Igaku-Shoin, 1991; pp. 229–39.
65. Cupps TR, Fauci AS. Thromboangiitis obliterans (Buerger's disease, endarteritis obliterans). In: The vasculitides. Philadelphia: WB Saunders, 1981; pp. 133–6.
66. Fiessinger JN, Schafer M. Trial of iloprost versus aspirin treatment for critical limb ischaemia of thromboangiitis obliterans. The TAO Study. Lancet 1990; 335:555–7.
67. Rao JK, Allen NB. Polymyalgia rheumatica and giant cell arteritis. In: Belch JJF, Zurier RB (eds) Connective tissue diseases. London: Chapman & Hall Medical, 1995; pp. 249–70.
68. Machado EB, Gabriel SE, Beard CM et al. A population-based case–control study of temporal arteritis: evidence for an association between temporal arteritis and degenerative vascular disease. Int J Epidemiol 1989; 18:836–41.
69. Goodman BW Jr. Temporal arteritis. Am J Med 1979; 67:839–52.
70. Sonnenblick M, Nesher G, Rosin A. Nonclassical organ involvement in temporal arteritis. Semin Arth Rheum 1989; 19:183–90.
71. Kyle V, Hazelman BL. Stopping steroids in polymyalgia rheumatica and giant cell arteritis. Br Med J 1990; 300:344–5.
72. Hoffman GS, Cid MC, Hellmann DB et al. A multicenter, randomized, double-blind, placebo-controlled trial of adjuvant methotrexate treatment for giant cell arteritis. Arth Rheum 2002; 46:1309–18.
73. Jover JA, Hernandez-Garcia C, Morado IC et al. Combined treatment of giant-cell arteritis with methotrexate and prednisone: a randomized, double-blind, placebo-controlled trial. Ann Intern Med 2001; 134:106–14.
74. Liozon E, Herrmann F, Ly K et al. Risk factors for visual loss in giant cell (temporal) arteritis: a prospective study of 174 patients. Am J Med 2001; 111:211–17.
75. Liozon E, Roblot P, Paire D et al. Anticardiolipin antibody levels predict flares and relapses in patients with giant-cell (temporal) arteritis. A longitudinal study of 58 biopsy-proven cases. Rheumatology (Oxford) 2000; 39:1089–94.
76. Weyand CM, Fulbright JW, Evans JM et al. Corticosteroid requirements in polymyalgia rheumatica. Arch Intern Med 1999; 159:577–84.
77. Hernandez-Rodriguez J, Segarra M, Vilardell C et al. Elevated production of interleukin-6 is associated with a lower incidence of disease-related ischemic events in patients with giant-cell arteritis: angiogeni1c activity of interleukin-6 as a potential protective mechanism. Circulation 2003; 107:2428–34.
78. American College of Rheumatology Ad Hoc Committee on Glucocorticoid-induced Osteoporosis. Recommendations for the prevention and treatment of glucocorticoid-induced osteoporosis: 2001 update. Arth Rheum 2001; 44:1496–503.
79. McMahon BJ, Heyward WL, Templin DW et al. Hepatitis B-associated polyarteritis nodosa in Alaskan Eskimos: clinical and epidemiologic features and long-term follow-up. Hepatology 1989; 9:97–101.
80. Conn DL. Polyarteritis. Rheum Dis Clin North Am 1990; 16:341–62.

81. Schirmer M, Duftner C, Seiler R et al. Abdominal aortic aneurysms: an underestimated type of immune-mediated large vessel arteritis? Cur Opin Rheumatol 2006; 18(1):48–53.

82. Langford CA, McCallum RM. Idiopathic vasculitis. In: Belch JJF, Zurier RB (eds) Connective tissue diseases. London: Chapman & Hall Medical, 1995; pp. 179–217.

83. Woywodt A, Streiber F, de Groot K et al. Circulating endothelial cells as markers for ANCA-associated small-vessel vasculitis. Lancet 2003; 361:206–10.

84. Sanchez NP, Van Hale HM, Su WP. Clinical and histopathologic spectrum of necrotizing vasculitis. Report of findings in 101 cases. Arch Dermatol 1985; 121:220–4.

# 13

# Peripheral and abdominal aortic aneurysms

Philip Davey
John Rose
Michael Wyatt

## Definition of an aneurysm

Derived from the Greek word *aneurysma* describing 'a widening', an arterial aneurysm is defined by an increased vessel diameter of 50% or more than that of the non-dilated adjacent vessel.[1]

## Prevalence of arterial aneurysms

Population screening studies indicate that the prevalence of abdominal aortic aneurysm (AAA) increases with age,[2,3] occurring in 7–8% in men over 65 years.[3,4] The disease prevalence is six times higher in men than in women,[5] with AAA rupture the seventh most common cause of male death in the UK.

There is considerably less information about the prevalence of peripheral aneurysms, although it is recognised that these frequently occur in association with AAA. Approximately 25% of patients with AAA have coexisting femoral or popliteal aneurysms.[6] It is likely therefore that peripheral aneurysms share a common aetiology with AAAs and that changes in their prevalence match those of aortic aneurysms.

## Pathogenesis of aortic aneurysms

Metabolic regulation of both elastin and collagen proteins in the aortic wall is under the control of several enzymatic agents. The most important group of these mediators appears to belong to the zinc- and calcium-requiring matrix-degrading metalloproteinases (MMPs) and there is compelling evidence that abnormal local MMP production and regulation is associated with the pathogenesis of aortic aneurysms. The elastolytic subtypes MMP-9 and MMP-2 appear to be the most influential in AAA pathogenesis.[7,8] A chronic inflammatory infiltrate composed of T cells, macrophages, B lymphocytes and plasma cells is a typical histological feature of AAA. Although the antecedent trigger for this cellular migration remains unclear, much of the subsequent vessel wall destruction appears to be mediated by the cytokines and chemokines released by the infiltrate with induction and activation of MMP species.[9]

Although certain phenotypes have been associated with increased frequency of disease progression, as yet no single genetic anomaly or polymorphism has been universally identified within all AAA patients. This approach to pathogenesis may eventually form the basis of genetic testing of specific increased-risk populations, allowing more focused surveillance and early intervention.[7]

In an effort to unify all aspects of this complex process, Ailawadi et al. have proposed a model of aortic aneurysm pathogenesis. They postulate that the initial trigger for AAA may be a combination of factors such as fragmented medial proteins, localised haemodynamic stress or a genetic predisposition that causes inflammatory cells to migrate into the aortic wall. This inflammatory infiltrate is rich in cytokines, chemokines and reactive oxygen species and attracts further cellular influx with expression and activation of proteases, in particular those of the MMP group. Subsequent unregulated connective tissue turnover results in medial degeneration of the aorta and aneurysmal dilatation. The proteolysis is exacerbated by the inherent increase in wall stress with progressive AAA expansion. If untreated, the sequence cascades with eventual aortic rupture.[9]

## Infrarenal abdominal aortic aneurysms

Most AAAs remain asymptomatic until rupture, with approximately 75% being symptom free at diagnosis. The majority of these cases are detected as an incidental finding during the course of investigation of unrelated cause. Aetiological factors include increasing age, male sex, ethnic origin, family history, smoking, hypercholesterolaemia, hypertension and prior vascular disease. Of these, male sex and smoking are the most important, increasing the chances of AAA development by 4.5 and 5.6 times respectively.[10]

### Symptomatic and ruptured AAAs

Rapid expansion (>1 cm/year) or the development of symptoms such as abdominal pain and tenderness and/or back pain is usually an indication for prompt surgical intervention, irrespective of size. This is because of a higher rupture rate.[11]

Rupture of an aortic aneurysm is a sudden catastrophic event with severe abdominal and/or back pain and circulatory collapse. Frequently, rupture occurs into the retroperitoneal space and bleeding may be arrested by a combination of hypotension and tamponade within this space. Although transient and unstable, this circumstance does provide an opportunity for emergency life-saving surgery. Free rupture into the peritoneal cavity is rapidly fatal. Approximately 75% of patients with ruptured AAAs die before reaching hospital.

### Inflammatory abdominal aortic aneurysms (IAAAs)

IAAAs account for 3–10% of all AAAs and were not classified per se until the early 1970s.[12] Classical defining features are the triad of a thickened aneurysmal wall, marked perianeurysmal/retroperitoneal fibrosis and dense neighbouring visceral adhesions. Abdominal or back pain, weight loss and an elevated erythrocyte sedimentation rate in a patient with known aortic aneurysm confers a diagnosis of IAAA until proven otherwise.[13]

### Population screening for AAAs

Given that (i) the majority of AAAs are asymptomatic, (ii) 75% of patients with rupture die without reaching hospital and (iii) elective surgical treatment of AAAs is effective, then population screening for AAAs is an attractive proposition.

B-mode ultrasound scanning using portable equipment has been shown to be effective in detecting AAAs and is inexpensive.[14] Furthermore, it has been estimated that a single ultrasound scan in males of 65 years of age would detect 90% of aneurysms at risk of rupture.[15]

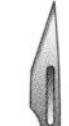

The Multicentre Aneurysm Screening Study (MASS) trial has provided good statistical evidence to show that the prevalence of aneurysm-related death is reduced significantly in a screened male population aged 65–74 years, with a 53% reduction in those who attended for screening.[2] Because other causes of death overshadow those due to ruptured AAAs, it has not been possible to demonstrate a statistically significant overall survival advantage for the screened population. Nevertheless, the case for extending population-based screening for AAAs is convincing.

Interestingly, the detection of aneurysms in a screened population does not appear to affect quality of life adversely.

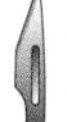

The MASS trial data show that over 4 years the mean incremental cost-effectiveness ratio for screening was £28 400 per life-year gained, equivalent to approximately £36 000 per quality-adjusted life-year. It was estimated that this would fall to approximately £8000 per life-year gained at 10 years.[16]

Compared with existing screening programmes, for example for breast and cervical cancer, screening for AAAs appears to be relatively cost-effective.

## Principles of AAA management

The fundamental principle underpinning AAA management strategy is the prevention of rupture. The role of medical therapy is important and includes blood pressure control, cholesterol reduction, antiplatelet therapy and smoking cessation. AAA size is still considered the most important factor in prediction of rupture. From a meta-analysis of 13 studies, Law et al. have quantified this annual risk for differing initial size[17] (Table 13.1).

The UK Small Aneurysm Trial and US Aneurysm Detection and Management (ADAM) trials were designed to provide guidelines as to when to offer elective surgery on the basis of aneurysm size.[11,18]

Table 13.1 • Annual AAA rupture risk in relation to size

| AAA size (cm) | Risk of rupture per year (%) |
|---|---|
| <3.0 | 0 |
| 3–3.9 | 0.4 |
| 4–4.9 | 1.1 |
| 5–5.9 | 3.3 |
| 6–6.9 | 9.4 |
| 7–7.9 | 24 |

Adapted from Law MR, Morris J, Wald NJ. Screening for abdominal aortic aneurysms. J Med Screening 1994; 1:110–15.[71] With permission from The Royal Society of Medicine Press Ltd.

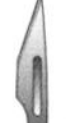

These two trials addressed the difficult dilemma of how to manage patients in whom the risks of surgery and rupture are similar. The Medical Research Council-sponsored UK Small Aneurysm Trial randomised 1090 patients with asymptomatic AAAs of 4.0–5.5 cm diameter to either initial ultrasound surveillance (527 patients) or surgery (563 patients). In the surveillance group, 321 patients eventually underwent surgery due to rapid expansion or growth to above the 5.5-cm threshold. In the early surgery group, the 30-day mortality rate was 5.8%. There was no difference in survival between the groups and concluded that early operative intervention for patients with AAAs of less than 5.5 cm diameter was not indicated. The rupture rate for untreated small aneurysms in this trial was less than 2% per annum. However, the rate was relatively higher in females and this suggests that elective surgery may be indicated for smaller aneurysms in this group of patients. However, at present the data are insufficiently robust to support this conclusion convincingly. The results of the ADAM trial and the conclusions drawn were similar.

## Surveillance of patients with small aneurysms

Since the publication of the small aneurysm trials, it has been recommended that patients with AAAs of less than 5.5 cm diameter should be managed conservatively with best medical therapy and regular surveillance by interval ultrasound scanning. The timing of such scans remains controversial, requiring a balance between cost/inconvenience and patient safety. It has recently been shown that an aorta with a diameter of <3 cm in a male aged 65 years of age or over is associated with minimal risk of eventual rupture, hence there is probably no justification for continued surveillance. For larger aneurysms, there is no robust evidence base upon which to base a surveillance programme. However, it is generally accepted that screening intervals of 1 year for aneurysms of 3.5–4.4 cm and 6 months for those of 4.5–5.4 cm would appear to be appropriate.

## AAA repair

Currently available evidence supports elective surgical intervention for the treatment of asymptomatic AAAs of 5.5 cm diameter or greater, subject to evaluation of the patient's general health and fitness for surgery.

### Investigation of the patient with known AAA

The aims of evaluation of patients diagnosed with an AAA are threefold:

1. to identify patients in whom the balance of risk favours operative intervention;
2. to reduce perioperative morbidity and mortality by identifying patients who may require further investigation or treatment of comorbidity prior to surgery;
3. to assess the anatomical suitability of the aneurysm for open or endovascular repair.

Accurate clinical assessment is imperative as it is recognised that perioperative mortality is related to the pre-existing physiological status of the patient.[18] The majority of early deaths following AAA repair are related to cardiac events and if pre-existing cardiac abnormalities are detected and treated prior to surgery, a substantial improvement in survival rates can potentially be achieved.[19] Respiratory complications are the most common form of morbidity after major abdominal surgery and occur after 25–50% of all such operations, including aortic aneurysm repair.[20] The risk of perioperative renal failure is increased in those with pre-existing renal disease, diabetes or coexisting cardiac disease, and in those aged over 60 years.

### Preprocedural imaging

Ultrasound is useful for the initial detection and outpatient surveillance of an AAA. Preoperatively, virtually all elective patients now undergo more detailed cross-sectional imaging with contrast-enhanced computed tomography (CT). With thin-slice acquisition of data, both spiral and multidetector row scanners provide excellent three-dimensional images from which to plan endovascular repair. Given the wide availability and high quality of multidetector CT angiography (MD-CTA), catheter angiography is rarely required preoperatively.

### Elective open AAA repair

General anaesthesia is preferred, and is frequently combined with epidural anaesthesia for postoperative pain control. Epidural anaesthesia may be employed as the sole method, particularly in those patients with severe respiratory disease. At induction, a broad-spectrum antibiotic should be administered as prophylaxis against graft infection. An intravenous bolus of heparin should be given prior to clamp application.

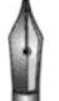

A trial conducted by the Joint Vascular Research Group of Great Britain and Ireland showed that while heparin does not have any influence on the risk of bleeding or thromboembolic complications, the incidence of perioperative myocardial infarction was reduced to 1.4% compared with 5.7% in patients who did not receive heparin.[21]

Although elective operative blood loss is usually minimal, excessive bleeding can occasionally be encountered either from back-bleeding lumbar arteries following opening of the sac or from the anastomotic suture lines. The routine use of a cell saver to preserve the patient's own red cells is a useful adjunct under these circumstances.[22]

The aorta is a longitudinal midline structure and most operations for aortic aneurysm repair involve proximal and distal anastomoses within the abdomen. Therefore, the preferred incision is longitudinal and midline and the approach transperitoneal. Alternatives include a transverse incision with a transperitoneal approach, and an oblique left-sided abdominal incision with an extraperitoneal approach, both of which may be advantageous in selected patients. With a transperitoneal approach, the intestines should be retained within the abdominal cavity, being packed to the right side and held in place with a suitable self-retaining retractor.

The aneurysm is exposed by incising the posterior parietal peritoneum and carefully mobilising the duodenum to the right. The renal vein marks the upper limit of dissection for an infrarenal aneurysm. Inferiorly, both common iliac arteries are dissected in preparation for clamping, care being taken to avoid damage to the hypogastric plexus of nerves in sexually active males. Minimal dissection is required to enable placement of clamps inserted from the front. Fabric grafts constructed from coated polyester (Dacron) or polytetrafluoroethylene may be used. Although ectatic dilatation of the common iliac arteries is commonly found in association with AAAs, true iliac aneurysms are comparatively infrequent. Therefore, 60–70% of AAAs can be repaired using a simple tube graft anastomosed to the infrarenal neck proximally and to the aortic bifurcation distally. In the remaining cases, it is necessary to use a bifurcated graft with anastomoses either to the common iliac bifurcation, or to the common femoral artery in the groin if the external iliac arteries are atheromatous or heavily calcified.

For repair of juxtarenal aneurysms, suprarenal clamping is essential. Under these circumstances, clamping of the supracoeliac aorta exposed through the lesser sac with separation of the fibres of the crura of the diaphragm may be preferable, since this allows more explicit exposure of the orifices of the renal arteries and less risk also of renal athero-embolisation than a clamp placed immediately above the renal arteries. A thoraco-abdominal approach with extraperitoneal exposure of the abdominal aorta is rarely necessary for juxtarenal aneurysms, but should be considered especially for obese patients in whom access is predicted to be problematical.

### Minimally invasive open AAA repair

The advent of endovascular techniques has stimulated interest in developing other less invasive alternatives to conventional open surgery. These include shorter (6-cm) incisions and totally laparoscopic techniques.[23] Custom-made retractors and other instrumentation have been developed for these procedures. It is claimed that surgical trauma is reduced significantly, with benefits in terms of lower operative mortality and morbidity rates and more rapid recovery of the patients. However, to date, reliable comparative data are lacking.

## Emergency open AAA repair

Successful emergency repair of ruptured AAAs relies on a precarious 'window of opportunity' when active bleeding is temporarily arrested by hypotension and tamponade of the haematoma by the posterior parietal peritoneum. In order to adequately conserve this clinical state, minimal resuscitation with permissive hypotension is desirable.

Survival following AAA rupture is poor in patients who have suffered a cardiac arrest, in the very elderly and in those who remain persistently unconscious. A decision not to offer surgical intervention to such patients is justified. Low or absent urinary output should not of itself be a contraindication to surgery, but its consideration within risk-scoring systems such as the Glasgow Aneurysm Score (see later) may help with appropriate patient selection for surgery.[24]

### Outcome following open surgical AAA repair

Elective open surgical repair of AAAs has been shown to be an effective procedure with good graft durability.

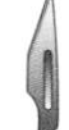

The Canadian Aneurysm Study demonstrated an in-hospital mortality rate of 4.7%, with a 5-year survival rate of 68%.[19] The UK Small Aneurysm Trial reported a 30-day mortality rate of 5.8% and the recent EVAR-1 trial a 30-day mortality rate of 4.7% in patients fit for surgery.[11,25]

Factors associated with a poorer outcome following open AAA repair include increased patient age, larger aneurysm size and the presence of preoperative renal failure.[26,27] In order to assist in the prediction of patients at high risk of perioperative mortality and morbidity after elective and ruptured AAA repair, the Glasgow Aneurysm Score (GAS) has been described.[24,28] In addition to the patient's age, differentially weighted patient-specific variables including the presence of cardiac, cerebrovascular and/or renal comorbidity with/without hypovolaemic shock are summed to yield a numerical value that can be extrapolated to a risk bracket (i.e. GAS = age ± cardiac disease (7 points) ± renal dysfunction (14 points) ± cerebrovascular disease (10 points) ± shock (17 points)). Naturally, the GAS alone should not dictate clinical practice, but it can serve as a useful adjunct for risk stratification in assessing a patient's suitability for AAA surgery.

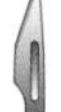

Another important determinant of patient outcome following AAA repair is the ability and experience of the operating surgeon. A recent meta-analysis demonstrated a significantly lower mortality following AAA repair with higher volume surgeons and suggested a minimum caseload of 13 open AAAs per annum for continued practice.[29] Naturally, this recommendation has significant implications for the provision of vascular services and would support the argument for fewer, larger, regional vascular centres linked directly to a nationwide targeted AAA screening programme.

Patients with AAAs have a markedly decreased life expectancy in comparison with age- and sex-matched control populations. The 5-year survival of patients postsurgery varies from 62% to 72% (compared with 83–90% in age- and sex-matched populations), with the majority of deaths due to coronary artery disease.[19,26] Quality-of-life studies have shown an improved perception of general health in the first 2 years after open repair in comparison with patients who are under surveillance.[30]

The UK Small Aneurysm Trial showed that only about 25% of patients with ruptured aneurysms make it to theatre for emergency repair.[11] A recent meta-analysis showed that there has been a gradual improvement in survival following surgery for ruptured AAAs over the last 40 years in the order of 3.5% per decade. However, this study also showed that the estimate of operative mortality rate remains high at approximately 41%.[31]

## Endovascular AAA repair (EVAR)

Since the first case of EVAR was reported by Parodi et al. in 1991,[32] this minimally invasive technique has become increasingly popular with both physicians and patients alike. The fundamental goal of EVAR is sustained aneurysm exclusion from the systemic circulation by means of a preoperatively sized stentgraft, preventing further aneurysm expansion and therefore eliminating rupture risk (**Fig. 13.1**).

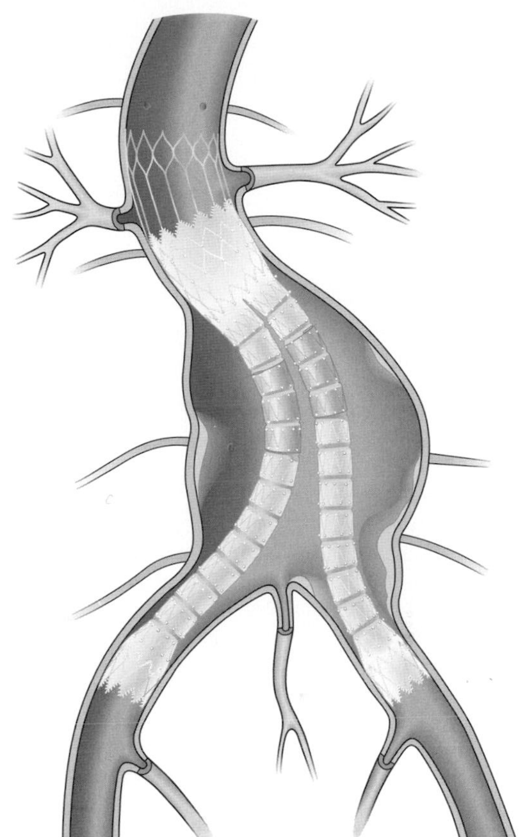

**Figure 13.1** • Model depicting the principle of AAA repair using an aortic stentgraft.

### Indications and eligibility for EVAR

Originally developed as a treatment option for those where existing comorbidity prohibited open surgical repair, the current indications for EVAR are less clear. The approach may well be preferable in cases of a hostile abdomen (e.g. peritoneal adhesions, intestinal stomas) and also where the risk of iatrogenic injury is significant (e.g. IAAA repair).[33] In the absence of such factors and in fitter patients the role of EVAR remains disputed.

Contrary to open AAA repair, EVAR suitability depends not only on patient fitness but also aneurysmal morphology. Limitations of contemporary endografts and their delivery platforms continue to preclude EVAR in many patients, with current elective eligibility rates quoted between 55% and 74%.[34,35] Features promoting EVAR suitability include a healthy proximal neck with limited angulation, at least 15 mm in length, no more then 30 mm in diameter and with smooth, parallel, endoluminal surfaces without significant mural thrombus. In addition the iliac arteries should be of sufficient calibre, at least 7 mm, to facilitate the passage of the delivery apparatus into the abdominal aorta. Short ectatic common iliac arteries represent relatively unfavourable anatomy for EVAR in view of the need for a reliable distal seal.[35,36]

### EVAR devices

Four distinct generic schemes are currently available for EVAR of infrarenal AAAs: straight aorto-aortic tube endografts, bifurcated systems, aorto-mono-iliac systems and combined bifurcated and iliac branched stentgrafts. All devices form their proximal seal within the infrarenal aortic segment but differences exist in the location of the distal 'landing site'. The pioneering aorto-aortic straight stentgraft resides entirely in the abdominal aorta but is only suitable for a very limited number of cases. The published early experience of EVAR showed that where aorto-aortic tube endografts were used for fusiform aortic aneurysms, an unacceptably high incidence of late device failure occurred due to extension of the pathological process into the distal neck and aorto-iliac segments.[37] There is still, however, a place for such tube grafts in localised saccular aneurysms, postoperative pseudoaneurysms and penetrating aortic ulcers.

Bifurcated systems offer the best solution by providing the potential for distal fixation beyond the vascular segments most likely to suffer further aneurysmal expansion in the long term, while maintaining normal anatomical relations. The currently available standard bifurcated devices may be appropriate for use in up to 50% of patients.[38] The remainder of EVAR-eligible aneurysms with more challenging anatomy (including those with aorto-iliac aneurysms) require the use of branched stentgrafts or the aorto-mono-iliac stentgraft.[39] Aorto-mono-iliac endografts require an extra-anatomical (femoro-femoral) crossover graft for maintenance of contralateral lower limb blood supply, following endoluminal plugging of the contralateral common iliac artery. Iliac branched stentgrafts are a relatively new and unproven development but provide an additional option for younger patients with bilateral aorto-iliac aneurysms.

### Patient assessment and EVAR technique

The patient should be formally assessed and prepared for EVAR as if for conventional open surgery. Detailed vascular imaging (preferably MD-CTA) should be obtained to enable calibration of the entire abdominal aorta and ilio-femoral segments in order to enable graft sizing and provide information regarding arterial access. Informed consent should include the routine morbidity and also the known EVAR-specific complications, including contrast nephropathy, endoleak (see later) and open surgical conversion. Ideally, the theatre should be designed for combined interventional/operative procedures and equipped with a C-arm or equivalent for intraoperative imaging.

After anaesthetic induction the patient is appropriately positioned, prepped and draped. The procedure usually commences by surgical cut-down to the femoral artery to gain access to the arterial circulation, although some advocate a percutaneous approach.[40] After femoral access is achieved, a soft wire and catheter are placed into the suprarenal aorta and a stiff guidewire is introduced through the catheter. Stiff guidewires are not intended to be 'working' wires and it is not sensible to try to negotiate tortuous iliac vessels with them. The stentgraft body is introduced over the stiff guidewire and the renal arteries are imaged. The image intensifier should be angled to optimise the view of the renal arteries and this typically requires a small amount of cranio-caudal and oblique tilt.

An imaging catheter is left alongside the graft body as the top stents are released in stages and short angiographic runs should be performed to ensure precise positioning relative to the renal arteries. Modular devices require cannulation in situ of the short leg or 'stump' of the main body of the device prior to introduction of the contralateral limb. This is generally performed by a retrograde approach from the contralateral femoral artery using angled catheters. Confirmation of successful cannulation is needed to avoid the error of inadvertently deploying the contralateral limb alongside rather than within the main graft. The iliac limbs are deployed close to the internal iliac origins, which are defined using oblique projections. Substantial overlap at the modular connections is essential to avoid late disconnections.

Completion angiography is performed to determine whether the aneurysm has been excluded and to ensure that there has been no encroachment by the fabric of the graft on the orifices of the visceral or internal iliac arteries (**Fig. 13.2**). Every effort must be made to resolve all primary type I endoleak before the patient is allowed to leave the operating room.

### EVAR-related complications and device failure

The physiological advantages of EVAR are reflected by the reduced requirement of postoperative critical care support and incidence of significant cardiac, pulmonary and renal complications. However, in addition to these routine causes of postoperative morbidity following AAA repair, EVAR unfortunately carries with it a distinct spectrum of its own specific complications.

*Endoleak.* Endoleak is defined as the persistence of blood flow outside the lumen of an endovascular graft but within an aneurysm sac or the adjacent vascular segment being treated by the stent.[41] The leak may be described as primary, originating at the time of EVAR, or secondary, referring to a leak not seen at completion angiography but demonstrated on

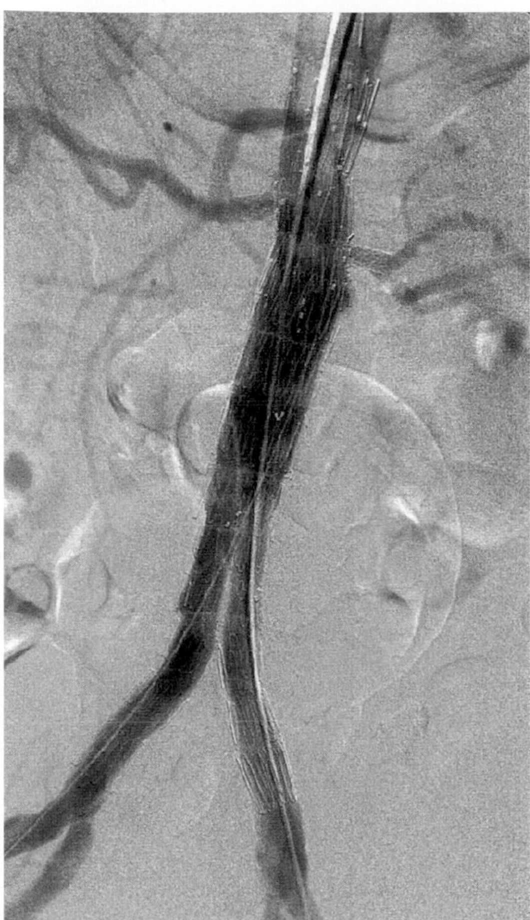

**Figure 13.2** • On-table angiogram showing satisfactory fenestrated EVAR placement with good filling of both renal arteries and no evidence of endoleak.

subsequent imaging. Endoleaks have been classified according to the source of aberrant blood flow, since this characterises the endoleak and hence the potential for deleterious sequelae (Table 13.2).[42]

Endoleaks are clinically important since they can be associated with aneurysm enlargement and eventual rupture. This is most often seen in type I (**Fig. 13.3a**) and III (Fig. 13.3c) leaks that communicate directly with the aortic lumen, and secondary intervention is almost always necessary in these patients.

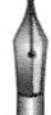

Of 4291 enrolled patients in the EUROSTAR registry in 2002, analysis of 34 patients with recorded rupture following EVAR showed that type I and III endoleaks and severe modes of structural disintegration of stentgrafts with or without migration were the most commonly documented findings at the time of rupture.[43]

Table 13.2 • Endoleak classification

| Endoleak type | | Source |
|---|---|---|
| I | A: Proximal<br>B: Distal<br>C: Iliac occluder | Graft attachment site |
| II | A: Simple (single vessel)<br>B: Complex (>2 vessels) | Collateral vessel |
| III | A: Junctional leak<br>B: Mid-graft hole<br>C: Other (e.g. suture hole) | Graft failure |
| IV | | Graft wall porosity |
| V | A: Without endoleak<br>B: With sealed endoleak<br>C: With type I or III leak<br>D: With type II leak | Endotension |

Type II (**Fig. 13.3b**) endoleaks denote continued blood flow into the aneurysmal sac from refilling collateral vessels, typically the lumbar and inferior mesenteric arteries. The clinical significance of type II endoleaks is contentious and there is no standard treatment protocol. Many consider these leaks self-limiting and recommend an expectant management course. Others advise early corrective intervention, arguing that any endoleak signifies systemic repressurisation of the aneurysmal sac with reintroduction of rupture risk.[44] Data from the EUROSTAR registry suggested that although they do not warrant urgent treatment, type II endoleaks are not harmless due to their observed association with aneurysm enlargement and reintervention.[45]

Transwall blood flow through an intact graft within 30 days of EVAR defines the type IV endoleak (**Fig. 13.3d**).[46] These leaks typically seal spontaneously and may be increasingly seen with the thinner and more porous later generation stents of today.

*Graft migration and dislocation.* Successful EVAR depends on the generation of a fluid-tight seal between stentgraft and healthy native vessel for AAA exclusion. Failure at any attachment site renders the endograft insecure and prone to abnormal movement (migration) that is facilitated by systemic arterial blood pressure. Significant device migration at the seal zones predisposes the patient to endoleak (type I), whereas unwanted mobility of modular systems may lead to component dislocation and potential type III endoleak (**Fig. 13.3c**).

Device migration most likely results from the combined effect of patient and device-related factors with a proximal attachment site failure most often described[47] (**Fig. 13.4**). In view of the significant risk of type I endoleak associated with distal migration of

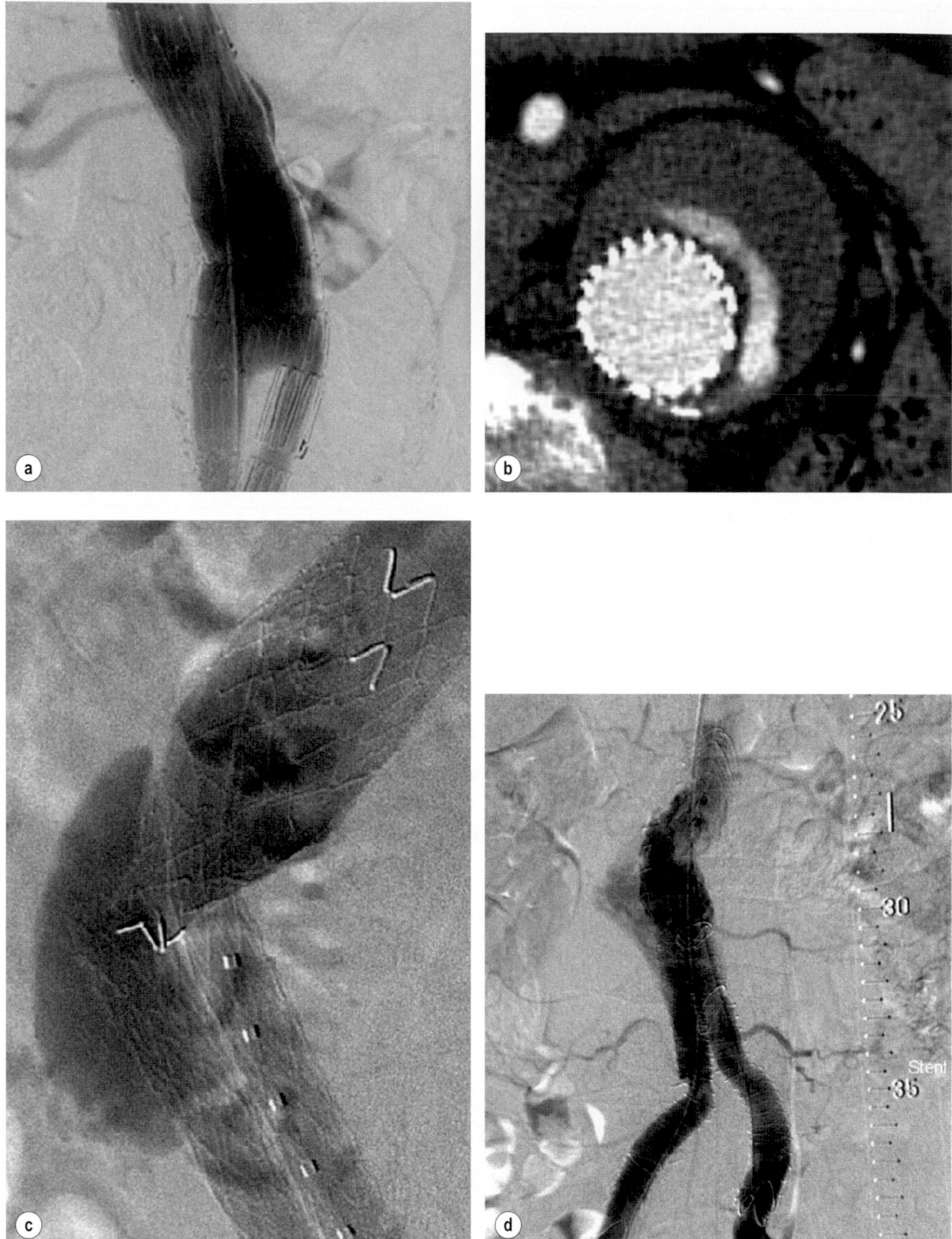


**Figure 13.3** • Images showing type I–IV endoleaks post-EVAR. **(a)** Completion angiogram showing a type I endoleak (proximal seal failure). **(b)** Post-EVAR contrast-enhanced CT scan showing a type II endoleak. **(c)** Delayed angiogram showing a type III endoleak (junctional graft failure). **(d)** Completion angiogram showing a type IV endoleak (graft porosity).

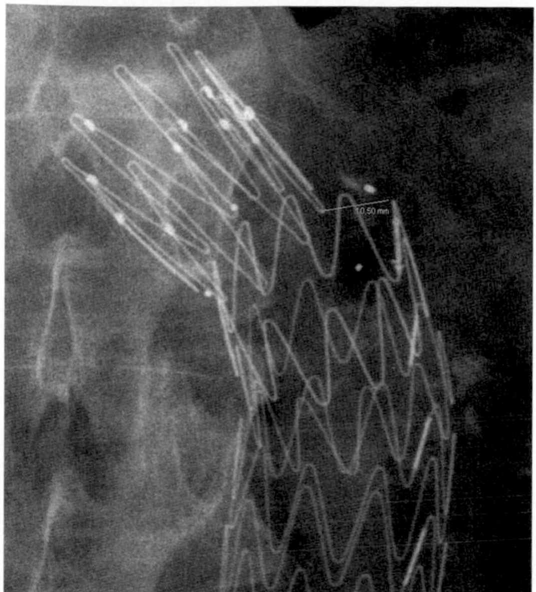

**Figure 13.4** • Post-EVAR imaging showing proximal stentgraft migration and impending endograft disruption.

the proximal stent, remedial intervention is almost always indicated. This can usually be achieved with aortic cuff deployment to repair the proximal seal, but occasionally stent revision is required.

*Kinking and occlusion.* Any distortion ('kinking') of the prosthetic conduit used in EVAR may result in stent stenosis, thrombosis and ultimately device (or limb) occlusion (see **Fig. 13.5**). In a review of 4613 EVAR cases submitted to the EUROSTAR registry over an 8-year period, postoperative graft kinking was described in 3.7% of cases.[48] Patent, symptomatic kinked stents can usually be treated by an endovascular approach (angioplasty or stenting) whereas occluded limbs typically require surgery.

*Other EVAR-related complications.* Stent manipulation within the aneurysmal sac during positioning and device deployment carries the risk of distal microembolisation of debris with potential for organ infarcts and limb ischaemia.[49–51] Introduction of guidewires, large-bore catheters and the endograft itself risks vessel injury such as rupture or dissection. Delayed presentations of iatrogenic arterial injury may occur with pseudo-aneurysm formation requiring prompt repair.

### Surveillance after EVAR

The modes of failure after endovascular grafting are well documented. It is mandatory that all patients are recruited onto a programme of systematic postoperative surveillance with the aim of detecting

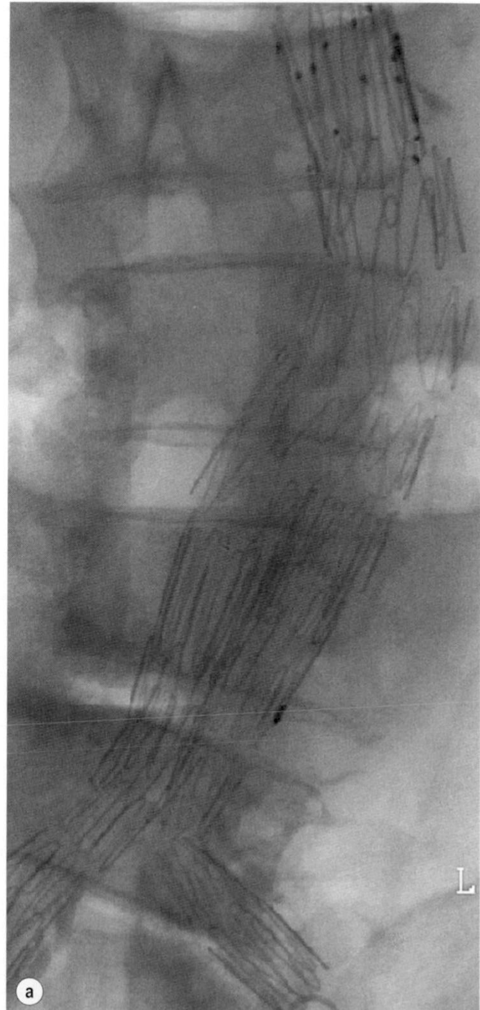


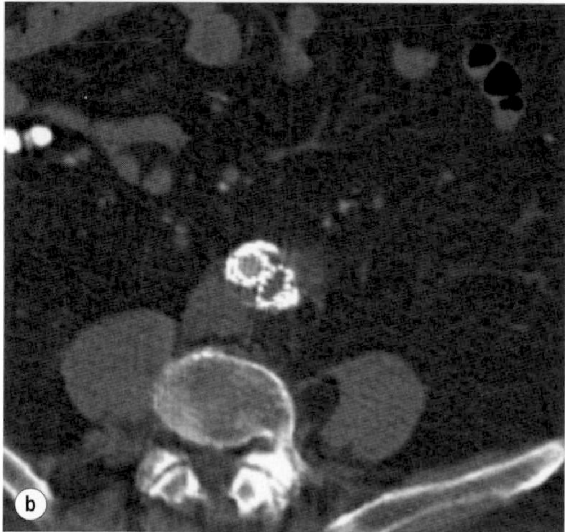


**Figure 13.5** • Post-EVAR imaging showing graft kinking and occlusion in the same patient. **(a)** Plain film showing left iliac limb kinking. **(b)** Contrast-enhanced CT scan showing consequent intraluminal occlusion.

causes of late rupture. The principal concerns are graft-related endoleak, aneurysm enlargement and migration of stents at the aortic or iliac landing zones or at the modular connections. Options for the method of surveillance include ultrasound, CT, magnetic resonance imaging (MRI) and plain radiography.

It has been shown that ultrasound can be used to detect graft-related (type I) endoleaks reliably.[52] Ultrasound is less effective for the detection of type II endoleaks, but since it is known that type II endoleaks without increased sac diameter are not associated with a significant risk of adverse clinical events, this may be regarded as an acceptable limitation. Plain radiography using a standardised protocol is an effective method for the detection of device migration.[53] Stent fractures and separation of modular components are also relatively easy to identify. It is comparatively inexpensive and usefully complements ultrasound scanning. Used in combination these two methods represent a potentially acceptable alternative to CT for surveillance.

It is generally accepted that surveillance after EVAR should be lifelong. The surveillance intervals vary but typically include baseline imaging with CT and plain radiography at 1 month after EVAR. Most protocols include more frequent surveillance intervals during the first 2 years, with annual surveillance thereafter.

### Outcomes after EVAR

Publication of two large multicentre European randomised controlled trials has finally provided some of the level I evidence required to support the continued use of EVAR in the normal AAA population.

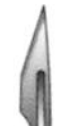

The UK EVAR-1 trial enrolled 1082 patients with suitable aneurysms (mean diameter 65 mm) that were considered fit enough for elective open AAA surgery and randomised them to either EVAR or conventional open repair (OR). Early outcome analysis revealed significantly lower 30-day mortality for the EVAR group (1.7%) compared to open surgical controls (4.7%).[25] Longer-term study follow-up reported EVAR to be as effective as surgery in protecting from late aneurysm-related death, although there was a significantly higher rate of graft-related complications following EVAR (35% vs. 8%).[54] In a smaller but similarly designed study, the Dutch DREAM trial compared outcome following EVAR and OR in 345 fit patients. A significantly lower operative mortality rate post-EVAR was confirmed (1.2% vs. 4.6%) with reduced incidence of early severe postoperative complications.[55] At 2-year follow-up, however, there was no observed survival advantage after EVAR or OR.[56] A recent meta-analysis of 42 trials involving 21 178 patients comparing open AAA repair with EVAR has reinforced these favourable EVAR findings.[57]

Renal failure after EVAR is associated with an increased rate of mortality and its aetiology is probably multifactorial. Implicated factors include radiological contrast-associated nephropathy, renal artery trauma, stent-induced stenosis and aortic neck thromboembolism following vessel instrumentation and manipulation.[58] It is rare for the renal ostia to be inadvertently covered by graft fabric, and careful planning and deployment decrease the risk of this occurring. There was concern that the introduction of suprarenal bare-stent fixation would lead to increased rates of renal failure, especially in patients with pre-existing renal impairment; however, studies have failed to demonstrate this.[58,59]

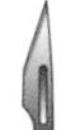

The UK EVAR-2 trial randomised 338 medically unfit patients who were anatomical candidates for endovascular AAA repair (>55 mm) to either EVAR or best medical therapy. The early mortality in the EVAR limb was 9% and at a mean follow-up of 3.3 years there was no difference in either the all-cause or aneurysm-related mortality between the groups.[60] Many clinicians have adopted these findings as justification not to offer EVAR in the higher-risk population. Caution is advised against this approach to management as closer scrutiny of the EVAR-2 results reveals some complicating issues. Firstly, there appeared to be an unacceptable delay from randomisation to treatment in the EVAR limb, so that nearly half (9 of 20) of the aneurysm-related mortality was explained by rupture prior to planned AAA repair. Operative (EVAR) mortality was surprisingly high (9%) and the rupture rate in the medically treated group (9 per 100 person-years) was significantly lower than expected, raising concern about disparate medical management between the two groups. Clearly though, EVAR-2 demonstrates the poor long-term prognosis of the unfit AAA patient irrespective of treatment, with only 62–66% alive at 4 years.

### The future of EVAR

There is little doubt that the principles of EVAR are particularly attractive in the case of AAA rupture, with several groups advocating its role. Avoidance of laparotomy confers a marked physiological advantage over open repair in an already dire situation.[61] However, the urgency associated with ruptured AAA repair results in little or no time being available to gather the required morphological information prior to EVAR. This is of particular importance since these aneurysms tend to have shorter and wider necks and are therefore more challenging for EVAR with current devices.[62] Furthermore, the requirement of a permanently available on-call endovascular team with access to the appropriate facilities for EVAR is a significant obstacle in most centres.[63]

The anatomical requirements for conventional endoluminal grafts exclude many patients from elective repair, primarily because of an unsuitable infrarenal aortic neck. The transrenal and juxtarenal aorta can be used to create a neck if holes or fenestrations are custom-manufactured in the graft to precise preoperative plans. The early data on the use of these devices are promising.[64,65] Fenestrations may be one of three types: scalloped, large or small. Scalloped grafts have a U-shaped defect in the leading edge of the endografts for preserved patency of the most proximal visceral arteries (**Fig. 13.6**). Both of the other types of fenestration reside in the body of the device fabric (**Fig. 13.7**). Large fenestrations are traversed by the bare metal scaffold, whereas small fenestrations lie between stent struts and require secondary stenting to prevent occlusion.[66]

Branched endografts have been used to preserve flow in hypogastric arteries and in the treatment of aortic arch and thoraco-abdominal aneurysms. Available evidence of efficacy is currently restricted to case reports and small case series.[67,68] Concerns about these devices include uncertainty regarding the long-term patency of stents in normal branch vessels, the increased number of modular connections and the possibility that the branches may kink if the aneurysm shrinks.

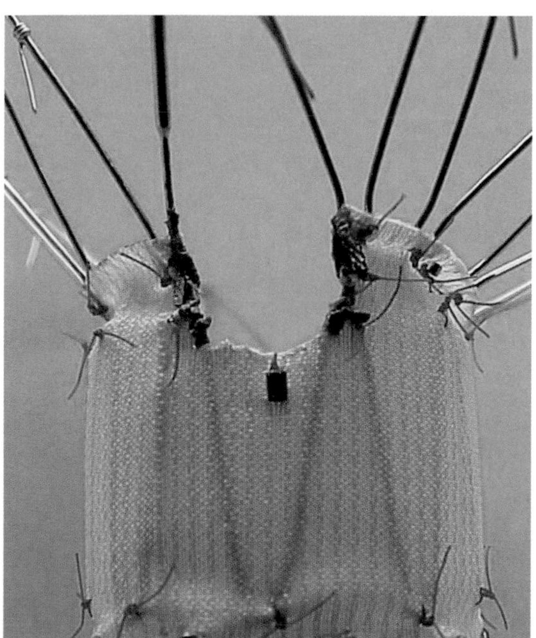

**Figure 13.6** • Scalloped stentgraft used for the endovascular treatment of AAA with short proximal necks.

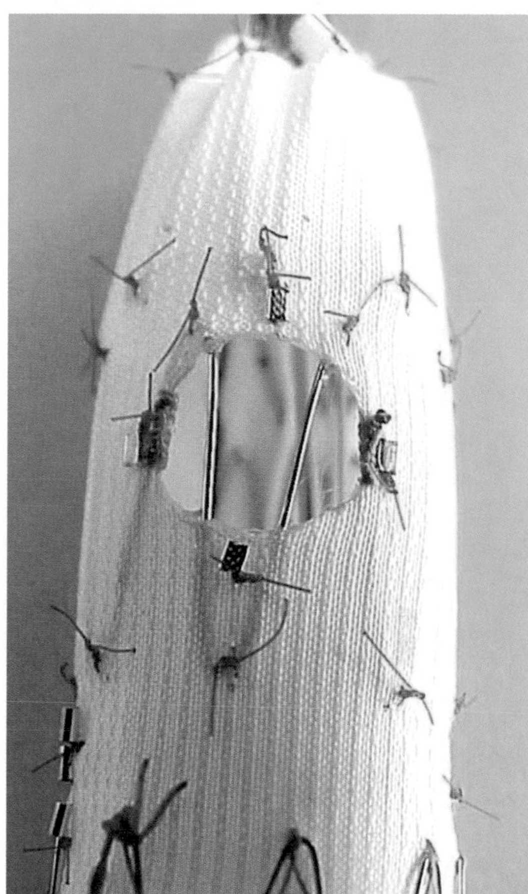

**Figure 13.7** • Fenestrated stentgraft used for the treatment of perirenal aortic aneurysms. Image courtesy of Cook Medical.

## Infected aneurysms

Although much less common than degenerative pathology, infected aneurysms remain an important subgroup of the disease. Since the introduction of antibiotic therapy and concomitant decline of endocarditis, true mycotic aneurysms are now rarely seen. Conversely, with increasingly invasive medical investigation and intravenous drug addiction (IVDA), post-traumatic infected false femoral aneurysms are now the major clinical problem to confront the vascular specialist. These are discussed in more detail in the section on femoral aneurysms.

### True mycotic aneurysms

True mycotic aneurysms result when septic emboli of cardiac source (endocarditis) lodge in the vasa vasorum or lumen of an artery. The patients tend to be middle-aged (30–50 years) and may have multiple aneurysms at differing sites. Both normal and abnormal vessels can be affected and although the pathology has a predilection for the aorta, intracranial, visceral and femoral arteries, any vessel can be affected. The usual infecting agents are Gram-positive cocci, in particular *Streptococcus* spp. and *Staphylococcus aureus*.[69]

## Microbial aneurysmal arteritis

With the ageing population and increasing incidence of atherosclerosis, microbial arteritis with aneurysm formation is now more frequently seen than the true mycotic aneurysm. The pathological process involves blood-borne bacteria 'seeding' into diseased arterial intima with subsequent suppuration, localised perforation and pseudo-aneurysm formation (**Fig. 13.8**). Contrary to mycotic aneurysms, healthy native vessels are not affected, atherosclerosis being the prime predisposing factor. Aortic involvement is typical, pathology in this location being three times more common than in the peripheral circulation. The classical infecting microorganisms are the *Salmonella* spp., but others have been reported, including *Escherichia coli, Staphylococcus* spp. and *Klebsiella pneumoniae*.[70]

## Clinical features and management principles of infected aneurysms

The clinical presentation of an infected aneurysm depends both on the site of involvement and underlying infective process. Usually, the patient presents with pyrexia of unknown origin and little else, therefore a high index of suspicion is required. Supporting features include positive blood cultures, leucocytosis, uncalcified aneurysms, vertebral erosion and a first presentation of aneurysm following an episode of bacterial sepsis. Classical radiological appearances on angiography may or may not be present: saccular aneurysm, multilobulated and/or eccentric pathology with a narrow neck.

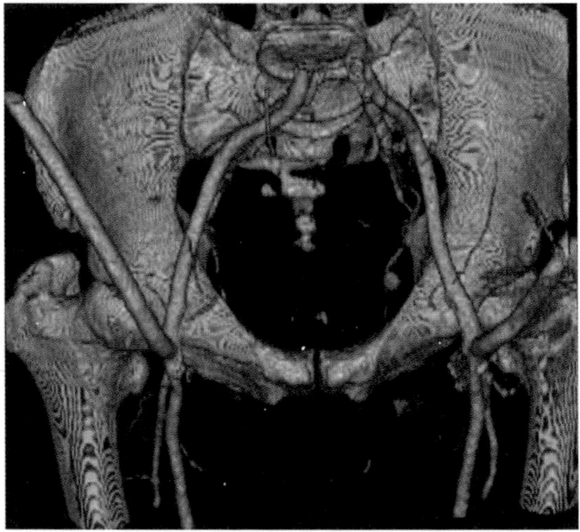

**Figure 13.8** • CT reconstruction of a peripheral seeded mycotic aneurysm of the left internal pudendal artery in a patient with an infected aortic stentgraft.

Following diagnosis, all patients should be commenced on appropriate antibiotic therapy. Unless the patient's general fitness is prohibitive, the definitive management plan is surgical. The principles of surgery for an infected aneurysm are generic, irrespective of site, and include: haemorrhage control; sepsis control (aneurysm resection, wide debridement, irrigation and drainage); confirmation of diagnosis (specimen cultures and sensitivity); and arterial reconstruction with autologous conduit if essential, e.g. superficial femoral vein harvest for aortic disease. Postoperatively, the patient should be prescribed a prolonged course of antibiotics that may be lifelong in some cases.[69]

Despite recent improvements in diagnosis, surgical techniques and pharmacology, the early outcome for patients with infected aortic aneurysms remains poor, with a mortality rate of 23%. Infected post-traumatic peripheral false aneurysms are associated with better survival (5% mortality), but the lower limb amputation rate can be up to 25–33% if the femoral artery is involved.

# Peripheral aneurysms

## Iliac aneurysms

Iliac aneurysms usually occur in association with aortic aneurysms. Isolated iliac aneurysms are comparatively unusual, the prevalence having been estimated to be less than 2% of that of aorto-iliac aneurysms. They tend to be large (4–8 cm) and typically involve either the common or internal iliac arteries. Aneurysmal disease of the external iliac artery is extremely rare.

Generally accepted guidance is that elective open or endovascular intervention is indicated for asymptomatic iliac aneurysms greater than 3–4 cm in diameter. Symptomatic and ruptured aneurysms require immediate surgical intervention.

## Common femoral aneurysms

Femoral arterial aneurysms can be divided simply into true or false (pseudo) aneurysms. True aneurysms relate to a distinct pathological process involving all three layers of the femoral arterial wall. False aneurysms are so-called due to their clinical mimicry of true disease but are, in actual fact, a vessel-associated contained blood collection and typically result from trauma.

Both disease processes may be symptomatic or asymptomatic. Symptomatic femoral aneurysms can present as a pulsatile groin mass which may or may not be painful, leg swelling (due to femoral vein compression and deep vein thrombosis) or features associated with chronic ischaemia attributable to aneurysm thrombosis/embolisation. Rupture can occur but is rare. Asymptomatic pathology is usually discovered incidentally on clinical examination of a patient with an aneurysm elsewhere or with chronic limb ischaemia.

### True femoral aneurysms

True femoral aneurysms are the second commonest peripheral aneurysm after the popliteal artery. They occur in between 2% and 3% of patients with aortic aneurysms and tend to be a disease of elderly men (male to female ratio 30:1). The condition is frequently bilateral and a coexistent generalised aneurysmal process may be manifest in other anatomical sites such as the aorto-iliac or popliteal arteries.

Small, asymptomatic true femoral artery aneurysms can be managed expectantly with clinical assessment at intervals. Surgical treatment is indicated for symptoms and probably for most aneurysms of 3 cm or more in size. Usually, a short interposition or inlay tube graft anastomosed proximally at the level of the inguinal ligament and distal to the common femoral bifurcation is required. This is a relatively small operation with durable results.

### False femoral aneurysms

Due to its ease of access and the trend for more invasive medical investigation and treatment (e.g. angiography, cardiac catheterisation, EVAR, intra-aortic balloon pumps, etc.), iatrogenic injury leading to false aneurysm is a relatively common occurrence that complicates approximately 1% of transfemoral interventions. The diagnosis should be suspected in any patient with a pulsatile mass at the site of a recent arterial cannulation. Initially, a duplex scan should be obtained to both confirm the diagnosis and characterise the false aneurysm. If the pathology is small and associated with minimal symptoms, simple observation with re-scanning may be justified as most of these pseudo-aneurysms will thrombose spontaneously within 2–4 weeks. Other options include compression therapy (direct pressure and/or ultrasound guided) in an effort to seal the feeding arterial jet. Thrombin injection is an effective treatment in this respect, with a reported success rate of over 95%. If these measures fail or in cases of tense swelling, threatened skin viability or neurology, open surgical repair is indicated. Unlike non-invasive methods, surgery has the advantage of combining both the arterial repair and field decompression. The former is usually a primary repair of the vessel with a prolene suture, although formal graft reconstruction is sometimes required.[71]

Infected femoral pseudo-aneurysms are now the most common type of infected aneurysm observed in clinical practice, largely explained by increased intravenous drug abuse in recent years. Although the usual microorganism cultured is a *Staphylococcus* species, the infection may be polymicrobial and close liaison with the microbiology team is required for appropriate antibiotic therapy. The surgical strategy for infected femoral false aneurysms depends largely on its cause. For non-IVDA patients, arterial excision and reconstruction with autologous conduit (e.g. long saphenous vein and obturator bypass) following the operative principles for infected aneurysms outlined earlier is preferred. In the IVDA patient, arterial excision with ligation alone (i.e. no reconstruction) is advised due to the unacceptable risk of subsequent graft infection with continued drug abuse. Ligation of the femoral artery does not necessarily mandate amputation if only one femoral segment is involved. If the femoral bifurcation is excised, however, the risk of limb loss is significant and reconstructive surgery may need to be considered, although this is contentious.[69]

## Popliteal artery aneurysms

Popliteal aneurysms are the most commonly encountered peripheral aneurysm, accounting for more than 80% of all peripheral aneurysms. The ratio of popliteal aneurysms to AAAs is approximately 1:15. Half are bilateral, a third asymptomatic and 40% are associated with AAAs.

Although rupture is rare, 50% of cases present with peripheral limb-threatening ischaemia. In common with aneurysms at all other sites, laminated thrombus develops within popliteal aneurysms. However, the fact that the popliteal artery is continually subjected to flexion and extension greatly increases the risk of disintegration and embolisation of this thrombus. In many patients, microembolisation of the peripheral circulation occurs silently prior to main vessel occlusion or thrombosis of the popliteal aneurysm itself. For this reason, the viability of the limb may be seriously threatened. Furthermore, compromise of the run-off circulation can impact adversely on the outcome from emergency bypass surgery. The bigger the aneurysm, the more likely there is to be thrombus. The presence of intraluminal thrombus is therefore a more important indication for elective surgical intervention than the size of the aneurysm. Any thrombus detected by ultrasound, CT or MRI constitutes an indication for elective treatment. In the absence of laminated thrombus, it is generally accepted that aneurysms with a diameter of 2 cm or greater warrant consideration for elective surgical repair.

Traditionally, popliteal aneurysms are treated by proximal and distal ligation and bypass using autologous vein undertaken via a medial approach. However, recent studies have identified persistent flow within the popliteal aneurysm in 30% of patients treated in this way.[72] Furthermore, there is a significant risk of continued expansion and even rupture due to pressurisation of the sac resulting from backflow through geniculate branches. Therefore, a posterior approach and insertion of an inlay graft is to be preferred.

An acutely thrombosed popliteal aneurysm is a clinical emergency. Preoperative or on-table thrombolysis has been used to open up the run-off vessels and thereby facilitate bypass surgery. There is some low-level evidence to suggest that this approach may improve the chances of successful limb salvage.[73] With the evolution of flexible endografts, endovascular repair is now a viable alternative to open surgery for the treatment of some popliteal aneurysms.[74]

Aneurysms of the upper limb, carotid and visceral arteries are discussed in their respective chapters.

## Key points

- The prevalence of AAAs has increased dramatically over the last four decades and this trend appears to be continuing.
- The clinical and financial cases for the introduction of a targeted population-based screening for AAAs are convincing.
- The Small Aneurysm Trial did not support a policy of early operative intervention for patients with AAAs of less than 5.5 cm diameter.
- Surgeons working in large-volume hospitals have lower mortality rates.
- The UK EVAR-1 trial reported a significant difference in the 30-day mortality, with 1.7% mortality in the EVAR group compared with 4.7% in those allocated to open repair.
- Both the EVAR-1 and DREAM trials confirm EVAR to be at least as effective as open repair in the prevention of aneurysm-related death in the longer term.
- EVAR requires annual surveillance and has an annual reintervention rate of 10%.
- EVAR should be used with caution in patients who are unfit for open surgery as 50% will die within 5 years, mostly from their comorbidity rather than rupture.
- Infected true aneurysms are associated with a poor prognosis but their incidence is declining.
- Post-traumatic false aneurysms are the most common infected aneurysms in clinical practice today and reflect both more invasive medical practice and intravenous drug abuse.

## References


1. Johnston KW, Rutherford RB, Tilson MD et al. Suggested standards for reporting on arterial aneurysms. Subcommittee on Reporting Standards for Arterial Aneurysms, Ad Hoc Committee on Reporting Standards, Society for Vascular Surgery and North American Chapter, International Society for Cardiovascular Surgery. J Vasc Surg 1991; 13:452–8.
2. Ashton HA, Buxton MJ, Day NE et al. The Multicentre Aneurysm Screening Study (MASS) into the effect of abdominal aortic aneurysm screening on mortality in men: a randomised controlled trial. Lancet 2002; 360:1531–9.

   **A UK multicentre population-based screening study of 67 800 men, aged 65–74 years, who were randomly allocated to be invited to attend for ultrasound assessment or not. The primary outcome measure was aneurysm-related death and there was a 42% risk reduction in the invited group.**
3. Lucarotti M, Shaw E, Poskitt K et al. The Gloucestershire Aneurysm Screening Programme: the first 2 years' experience. Eur J Vasc Surg 1993; 7:397–401.
4. Norman PE, Jamrozik K, Lawrence-Brown M et al. Population based randomised controlled trial on impact of screening on mortality from abdominal aortic aneurysm. Br Med J 2004; 329:1259–62.
5. Vardulaki KA, Walker NM, Day NE et al. Quantifying the risks of hypertension, age, sex and smoking in patients with abdominal aortic aneurysm. Br J Surg 2000; 87:195–200.
6. Cutler BS, Darling RC. Surgical management of arteriosclerotic femoral aneurysms. Surgery 1973; 74:764–73.
7. Wassef M, Baxter T, Chisholm RL et al. Pathogenesis of abdominal aortic aneurysms: a multidisciplinary research program supported by the National Heart, Lung and Blood Institute. J Vasc Surg 2001; 34:730–8.

8. Ailawadi G, Eliason JL, Upchurch GR. Current concepts in the pathogenesis of abdominal aortic aneurysm. J Vasc Surg 2003; 38:584–8.
9. Longo GM, Xiong W, Greiner TC et al. Matrix metalloproteinases 2 and 9 work in concert to produce aortic aneurysms. J Clin Invest 2002; 110:625–32.
10. Lederle FA, Johnson GR, Wilson SE et al. Prevalence and associations of abdominal aortic aneurysm detected through screening. Aneurysm Detection and Management (ADAM) Veterans Affairs Cooperative Study Group. Ann Intern Med 1997; 126:441–9.
11. The UK Small Aneurysm Trial Participants. Mortality results for randomised controlled trial of early elective surgery or ultrasound surveillance for small abdominal aortic aneurysms. Lancet 1998; 352(9141):1649–55.

    **A multicentre randomised controlled trial of 1090 patients with asymptomatic aneurysms of diameter 4.0–5.5 cm were randomly allocated to early elective surgery or ultrasound surveillance. There was no significant survival advantage at 6 years for those undergoing surgical repair.**
12. Walker DI, Bloor K, Williams G et al. Inflammatory aneurysms of the abdominal aorta. Br J Surg 1972; 59:609–14.
13. Rasmussen TE, Hallett JW. Inflammatory aortic aneurysms: a clinical review with new perspectives in pathogenesis. Ann Surg 1997; 225:155–64.
14. Lindholt JS, Vammen S, Juul S et al. The validity of ultrasonographic scanning as screening method for abdominal aortic aneurysm. Eur J Vasc Endovasc Surg 1999; 17:472–5.
15. Emerton ME, Shaw E, Poskitt K et al. Screening for abdominal aortic aneurysm: a single scan is enough. Br J Surg 1994; 81:1112–13.
16. Multicentre Aneurysm Screening Study Group. Multicentre aneurysm screening study MASS: cost effectiveness analysis of screening for abdominal aortic aneurysms based on four year results from randomised controlled trial. Br Med J 2002; 325:1135.

    **See also Ref. 2. Cost-effectiveness analysis at 4 years showed that the cost per quality-adjusted life-year was £36 000. It is projected that this value will fall to £8000 per quality-adjusted life-year at 10 years, which is well below the funding threshold in the UK health service.**
17. Law MR, Morris J, Wald NJ. Screening for abdominal aortic aneurysms. J Med Screening 1994; 1:110–15.
18. Katz DJ, Stanley JC, Zelenock GB. Operative mortality rates for intact and ruptured abdominal aortic aneurysms in Michigan: an eleven-year statewide experience. J Vasc Surg 1994; 19:804–15.
19. Johnston KW. Non-ruptured abdominal aortic aneurysm: six-year follow-up results from the multicenter prospective Canadian aneurysm study. Canadian Society for Vascular Surgery Aneurysm Study Group. J Vasc Surg 1994; 20:163–70.

    **A prospective analysis of 680 patients undergoing elective aneurysm surgery showed that cardiac-related death is the major perioperative risk and cardiac and cerebrovascular events are the major causes of death at 6 years.**
20. Zibrak JD, O'Donnell CR, Marton K. Indications for pulmonary function testing. Ann Intern Med 1990; 112:763–71.
21. Thompson JF, Mullee MA, Bell PR et al. Intraoperative heparinisation, blood loss and myocardial infarction during aortic aneurysm surgery: a Joint Vascular Research Group study. Eur J Vasc Endovasc Surg 1996; 12:86–90.
22. Goodnough LT, Monk TG, Sicard G et al. Intraoperative salvage in patients undergoing elective abdominal aortic aneurysm repair: an analysis of cost and benefit. J Vasc Surg 1996; 24: 213–18.
23. Kolvenbach R, Schwierz E, Wasilljew S et al. Total laparoscopically and robotically assisted aortic aneurysm surgery: a critical evaluation. J Vasc Surg 2004; 39:771–6.
24. Samy AK, Murray G, MacBain G. Glasgow Aneurysm Score. Cardiovasc Surg 1994; 2:41–4.
25. Greenhalgh RM, Brown LC, Kwong GP et al. Comparison of endovascular aneurysm repair with open repair in patients with abdominal aortic aneurysm (EVAR trial 1), 30-day operative mortality results: randomised controlled trial. Lancet 2004; 364:843–8.

    **A multicentre randomised controlled trial comparing open and endovascular repair in patients anatomically suitable for either. The 30-day mortality results show an initial survival advantage for patients treated with EVAR. See also Ref. 50.**
26. Batt M, Staccini P, Pittaluga P et al. Late survival after abdominal aortic aneurysm repair. Eur J Vasc Endovasc Surg 1999; 17:338–42.
27 Sahal M, Prusa AM, Wibmer A et al. Elective abdominal aortic aneurysm repair: does the aneurysm diameter influence long-term survival? Eur J Vasc Endovasc Surg 2008; 35:288–94.
28. Korhonen SJ, Ylonen K, Biancari F et al. Glasgow aneurysm score as a predictor of immediate outcome after surgery for ruptured abdominal aortic aneurysm. Br J Surg 2004; 91:1449–52.
29. Young EL, Holt PJE, Poloniecki JD et al. Meta-analysis and systematic review of the relationship between surgeon annual caseload and mortality for elective open abdominal aortic aneurysm repairs. J Vasc Surg 2007; 46:1287–94.

    **A meta-analysis involving 115 273 elective open AAA repairs demonstrating significantly lower mortality with higher caseload surgeons. The study suggested a critical case volume threshold of 13 open AAA repairs per annum.**

30. Lederle FA, Johnson GR, Wilson SE et al. Quality of life, impotence, and activity level in a randomized trial of immediate repair versus surveillance of small abdominal aortic aneurysm. J Vasc Surg 2003; 38:745–52.
31. Bown MJ, Sutton AJ, Bell PR et al. A meta-analysis of 50 years of ruptured abdominal aortic aneurysm repair. Br J Surg 2002; 89:714–30.
32. Parodi JC, Palmaz JC, Barone HD. Transfemoral intraluminal graft implantation for abdominal aortic aneurysms. Ann Vasc Surg 1991; 5:491–99.
33. Hinchliffe RJ, Macierewicz JA, Hopkinson BR. Endovascular repair of inflammatory abdominal aortic aneurysms. J Endovasc Ther 2002; 9:277–81.
34. Wolf YG, Fogarty TJ, Olcott CIV et al. Endovascular repair of abdominal aortic aneurysms: eligibility rate and impact on the rate of open repair. J Vasc Surg 2000; 32:519–523.
35. Arko FR, Filis KA, Seidel SA et al. How many patients with infrarenal aneurysms are candidates for endovascular repair? The Northern California experience. J Endovasc Ther 2004; 11:33–40.
36. Dillavou ED, Muluk SC, Rhee RY et al. Does hostile neck anatomy preclude successful endovascular aortic aneurysm repair? J Vasc Surg 2003; 38:657–63.
37. Faries PL, Briggs VL, Rhee JY et al. Failure of endovascular aortoaortic tube grafts: a plea for preferential use of bifurcated grafts. J Vasc Surg 2002; 35:868–73.
38. Simons P, van Overhagen H, Nawijn A et al. Endovascular aneurysm repair with a bifurcated endovascular graft at a primary referral center: influence of experience, age, gender, and aneurysm size on suitability. J Vasc Surg 2003; 38:758–61.
39. Moore WS, Brewster DC, Bernhard VM. Aorto-uni-iliac endograft for complex aortoiliac aneurysms compared with tube/bifurcation endografts: results of the EVT/Guidant trials. J Vasc Surg 2001; 33:S11–20.
40. Morasch MD, Kibbe MR, Evans ME et al. Percutaneous repair of abdominal aortic aneurysm. J Vasc Surg 2004; 40:12–16.
41. White GH, Yu W, May J. Endoleak: a proposed new terminology to describe incomplete aneurysm exclusion by an endoluminal graft. J Endovasc Surg 1996; 3:124–5.
42. Veith FJ, Baum RA, Ohki T et al. Nature and significance of endoleaks and endotension: summary of opinions expressed at an international conference. J Vasc Surg 2002; 35:1029–35.
43. Fransen GA, Vallabhaneni SR Sr, van Marrewijk CJ et al. Rupture of infra-renal aortic aneurysm after endovascular repair: a series from EUROSTAR registry. Eur J Vasc Endovasc Surg 2003; 26: 487–93.
44. Choke E, Thompson MM. Endoleak after endovascular aneurysm repair: current concepts. J Cardiovasc Surg 2004; 45:349–66.
45. van Marrewijk CJ, Fransen G, Laheij RJF et al. Is a type II endoleak after EVAR a harbinger of risk? Causes and outcome of open conversion and aneurysm rupture during follow-up. Eur J Vasc Endovasc Surg 2004; 27:128–37.
46. Chaikof E, Blankensteijn J, Harris P et al. Reporting standards for endovascular aortic aneurysm repair. J Vasc Surg 2002; 35:1048–60.
47. Lee JT, Lee J, Aziz I et al. Stent-graft migration following endovascular repair of aneurysms with large proximal necks: anatomical risk factors and long-term sequelae. J Endovasc Ther 2002; 9: 652–64.
48. Fransen GAJ, Desgranges P, Laheij RJF et al. Frequency, predictive factors, and consequences of stent-graft kink following endovascular AAA repair. J Endovasc Ther 2003; 10:913–18.
49. Zhang WW, Kulaylat MN, Anain PM et al. Embolization as cause of bowel ischemia after endovascular abdominal aortic aneurysm repair. J Vasc Surg 2004; 40:867–872.
50. Kramer SC, Seifarth H, Pamler H et al. Renal infarction following endovascular aortic aneurysm repair: incidence and clinical consequences. J Endovasc Ther 2002; 9:98–102.
51. Aljabri B, Obrand DI, Montreuil B et al. Early vascular complications after endovascular repair of aortoiliac aneurysms. Ann Vasc Surg 2001; 15:608–14.
52. McWilliams RG, Martin J, White D et al. Use of contrast-enhanced ultrasound in follow-up after endovascular aortic aneurysm repair. J Vasc Intervent Radiol 1999; 10:1107–14.
53. Murphy M, Hodgson R, Harris PI et al. Plain radiographic surveillance of abdominal aortic stent-grafts: the Liverpool/Perth protocol. J Endovasc Ther 2003; 10:911–12.
54. The EVAR Trial Participants. Comparison of endovascular aneurysm repair with open repair in patients with abdominal aortic aneurysm (EVAR trial 1): randomized controlled trial. Lancet 2005; 365:2179–86.
55. Prinssen M, Verhoeven EL, Buth J et al. A randomized trial comparing conventional and endovascular repair of abdominal aortic aneurysms. N Engl J Med 2004; 351:1607–18.

**A multicentre randomised trial comparing open surgical and endovascular repair in 345 patients with 5 cm or larger AAAs; 30-day mortality was 4.6% in the open repair group and 1.2% in the endovascular group.**

56. Blankensteijn JD, De Jong S, Prinssen M et al. Two year outcomes after conventional or endovascular repair of abdominal aortic aneurysms. N Engl J Med 2005; 352: 2398–405.

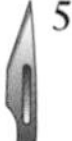

57. Lovegrove RE, Javid M, Magee TR et al. A meta-analysis of 21178 patients undergoing open or endovascular repair of abdominal aortic aneurysm Br J Surg 2008; 95:677–84.

    A meta-analysis of 42 studies comparing outcomes following open and endovascular AAA repair. EVAR was associated with significantly lower early 30-day mortality, postoperative morbidity and late aneurysm-related mortality.

58. Davey P, Peaston R, Rose J et al. Impact on renal function after endovascular aneurysm repair with uncovered supra-renal fixation (SR-EVR) assessed by serum cystatin C. Eur J Vasc Endovasc Surg 2008; 35:439–45.
59. Mehta M, Cayne N, Veith FJ et al. Relationship of proximal fixation to renal dysfunction in patients undergoing endovascular aneurysm repair. J Cardiovasc Surg 2004; 45:367–74.

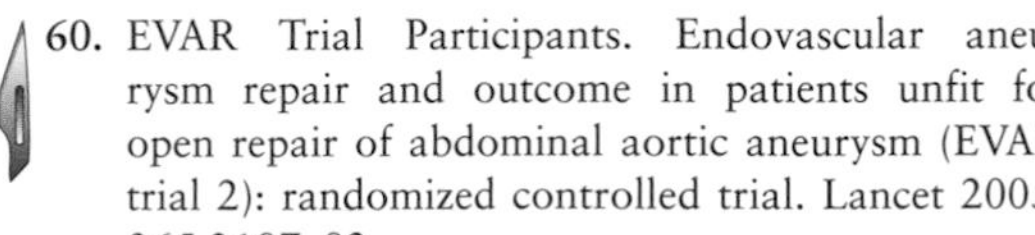

60. EVAR Trial Participants. Endovascular aneurysm repair and outcome in patients unfit for open repair of abdominal aortic aneurysm (EVAR trial 2): randomized controlled trial. Lancet 2005; 365:2187–92.

    A multicentre randomised trial comparing EVAR and best medical therapy in 338 unfit patients with morphologically suitable AAAs; 30-day mortality was 9% in the EVAR group and at a mean follow-up of 3.3 years there was no difference in either the all-cause or aneurysm-related mortality between groups.

61. Hinchliffe RJ, Hopkinson BR. Ruptured abdominal aortic aneurysm: time for a new approach. J Cardiovasc Surg 2002; 43:345–7.
62. Veith FJ, Ohki T. Endovascular approaches to ruptured infrarenal aortoiliac aneurysms. J Cardiovasc Surg 2002; 43:369–78.
63. Hinchliffe RJ, Yusuf SW, Macierewicz JA et al. Endovascular repair of ruptured abdominal aortic aneurysm – a challenge to open repair? Results of a single centre experience in 20 patients. Eur J Vasc Endovasc Surg 2001; 22:528–34.
64. Greenberg RK, Haulon S, O'Neill S et al. Primary endovascular repair of juxtarenal aneurysms with fenestrated endovascular grafting. Eur J Vasc Endovasc Surg 2004; 27:484–91.
65. Verhoeven EL, Prins TR, Tielliu IF et al. Treatment of short-necked infrarenal aortic aneurysms with fenestrated stent-grafts: short-term results. Eur J Vasc Endovasc Surg 2004; 27:477–83.
66. Parkinson TJ, Rose JD, Wyatt MG. Endovascular aneurysm repair: state of the art 2006. In: Earnshaw JJ, Murie JA (eds) The evidence for vascular surgery, 2nd edn. Shrewsbury: Tfm Publishers, 2007; pp. 153–64.
67. Abraham CZ, Reilly LM, Schneider DB et al. A modular multi-branched system for endovascular repair of bilateral common iliac artery aneurysms. J Endovasc Ther 2003; 10:203–7.
68. Chuter TA, Gordon RL, Reilly LM et al. Multi-branched stent-graft for type III thoracoabdominal aortic aneurysm. J Vasc Intervent Radiol 2001; 12:391–2.
69. Reddy DJ, Weaver MR. Infected aneurysms. In: Rutherford RB (ed) Vascular surgery, 6th edn. Philadelphia: Elsevier Saunders, 2005; pp. 1581–96.
70. Reddy DJ, Shepard AD, Evans JR et al. Management of infected aorto-iliac aneurysms. Arch Surg 1991; 126:873.
71. Knight CG, Healy DA, Thomas RL. Femoral artery pseudoaneurysms: risk factors, prevalence and treatment options. Ann Vasc Surg 2003; 17:503–8.
72. Kirkpatrick UJ, McWilliams RG, Martin J et al. Late complications after ligation and bypass for popliteal aneurysm. Br J Surg 2004; 91:174–7.
73. Marty B, Wicky S, Ris HB et al. Success of thrombolysis as a predictor of outcome in acute thrombosis of popliteal aneurysms. J Vasc Surg 2002; 35:487–93.
74. Gerasimidis T, Sfyroeras G, Papazoglou K et al. Endovascular treatment of popliteal artery aneurysms. Eur J Vasc Endovasc Surg 2003; 26:506–11.

# 14

# Thoracic and thoraco-abdominal aortic disease

Matt Thompson
Rob Morgan

## Introduction

There are few conditions in vascular surgery that have undergone such a significant paradigm shift in the last few years than the management of the thoracic aorta. The evolution of endovascular techniques has revolutionised the treatment of thoracic aneurysms and type B aortic dissections. Once the province of cardiologists and cardiothoracic surgeons, these conditions should now be familiar to clinicians dealing with peripheral vascular disease, as they form a potentially important part of vascular practice.

Endovascular repair (EVR) of the thoracic aorta has become an established treatment modality despite a relatively poor evidence base. There are good explanations for the lack of randomised data when the clinical outcomes for pathologies with established indications for treatment are compared between endovascular procedures and open thoracic surgery. Case series and registry data would appear to show that the endovascular procedures offer significantly lower mortality, morbidity and paraplegia rates when compared to open thoracic repair of thoracic aneurysms or acute dissections.[1,2] The lack of randomised trials does, however, pose a problem for endovascular techniques as much of the evidence base is composed of small retrospective series and registries, which do not offer sufficient detail to facilitate the subgroup analysis that is mandatory to refine indications for treatment.

Despite the change in practice that has encompassed treatment of thoracic aneurysms and dissections, the treatment of thoraco-abdominal aneurysms continues to pose a fundamental clinical challenge, with significant mortality rates attesting to the pathophysiological derangements that accompany open surgical repair. This chapter reviews the contemporary treatment of thoracic and thoraco-abdominal aortic disease that would be of relevance to the vascular clinician. Readers are referred to more specialised texts for a detailed description of conditions that would still be within the province of cardiothoracic surgery, e.g. ascending aortic aneurysms, type A aortic dissection.

## Imaging of the thoracic aorta

The main imaging method used for the assessment of patients with thoracic aortic pathology is computed tomography (CT). Assessment should involve scrutiny of axial and multiplanar images. In general, the axial images are more useful images for assessment of aortic diameters and the multiplanar reconstructions are used for assessment of aortic length. Although not as popular as CT, many operators prefer magnetic resonance imaging and magnetic resonance (MR) angiography because of the avoidance of ionising radiation and iodinated contrast. Recent reports of nephrogenic fibrosis related to the use of gadolinium[3] only have impact for those patients with renal failure. MR is particularly useful for the follow-up of those patients with thoracic aortic disease.

Conventional angiography may be required for assessment prior to endografting in some patients with lesions close to or involving the aortic arch for improved depiction of the relation of the lesion to the origins of the supra-aortic vessels. Conventional angiography may also be used to image access vessels if they are considered to be suboptimal for passage of the stentgraft delivery system on the CT images.

Transoesophageal echocardiography has a significant role in the classification and diagnosis of thoracic aortic dissection.

# Thoracic aortic aneurysms (TAAs)

## Classification

The descending thoracic aorta is the commonest location for aneurysms. Descending thoracic aneurysms are classified on the basis of whether they involve the upper half, the lower half or the entire descending aorta with the thorax divided at the sixth intercostal space (types A, B and C).[4]

The vast majority of thoracic aneurysms are non-specific or degenerative in aetiology, although specific aneurysms are caused by Marfan syndrome, Ehler–Danlos syndrome, syphilis and connective tissue disorders, e.g. ankylosing spondylitis, rheumatoid arthritis, Reiter's disease and systemic lupus erythematosis. Approximately one-quarter of thoracic aneurysms are caused by chronic thoracic aortic dissections. Some common variants of thoracic aneurysms would include mycotic aneurysms,[5] false aneurysms following trauma or lesions complicating a previous coarctation repair. Aneurysms of the descending aorta may extend into the abdomen and are referred to as thoraco-abdominal aortic aneurysms.

The majority of aneurysms are fusiform in morphology. Saccular aneurysms are less common and are usually the result of infection or previous trauma. Thoracic aneurysms have a strong association with coronary artery disease and abdominal aortic aneurysm.

## Incidence and clinical presentation

Aneurysms of the descending thoracic aorta are a disease of increasing age and the male to female ratio is 3:1. TAAs are estimated to occur in 10 per 100 000 patient-years.[6] Thoracic aneurysms are usually discovered incidentally on routine chest radiography. Clinical presentations include substernal, back or shoulder pain, superior vena cava syndrome, dysphagia, dyspnoea, stridor and hoarseness (due to laryngeal nerve compression) and rupture. The survival of patients with untreated TAAs is bleak and is estimated to be 13–39% at 5 years.[7] Eighty percent of thoracic aneurysms detected at autopsy have ruptured. The risk of rupture increases with the size of the aneurysm, but data regarding estimated annual rupture rates and aortic diameter are sparse and less robust than for the abdominal aorta. Some data suggest that the rupture rate of thoracic aneurysms is 2.7 per 100 000 patient-years as compared to 9.2 per 100 000 patient-years for abdominal aneurysms.

## Indications for treatment

The main indications for intervention are symptoms and size. There is controversy regarding the size criteria for treatment of TAAs. Juvonen et al. reported that the 2-year rupture rate for TAAs was 23% in aneurysms less than 7 cm,[8] whereas Elefteriades observed a 30% 5-year rupture rate when the aorta exceeded 6 cm.[9] Practically, most clinicians regard 6 cm as an indication for possible repair in an asymptomatic patient, the threshold obviously being balanced by the surgical risk.

## Technique of surgical repair

The mainstay of traditional surgical repair of TAAs includes a left thoracotomy for access, aortic clamping and inlay grafting, with intercostal reimplantation. The procedures are technically challenging due to the need to maintain visceral and spinal cord perfusion during the procedure. Several surgical adjuncts are available to achieve these aims, including the use of a Gott shunt, left heart bypass and distal aortic perfusion, selective intercostal shunting and routine cerebrospinal fluid (CSF) drainage.

## Endovascular repair of thoracic aneurysms

Detailed preoperative imaging is required to assess the proximal and distal landing zones for the endograft and to plan an access route. A segment of normal aorta above and below the lesion to be treated is required (landing zone), so that a seal can be achieved between the endograft and the normal aortic wall. The landing zone length should be at least 15 mm, although 20 mm is optimal. With respect to the aortic arch, the landing zone length should be measured on the inner curve of the aortic arch and not the outer curve. If the landing zone is considered to be of inadequate length, surgical bypass may be performed to debranch the aortic arch or abdominal aorta so that an effective sealing zone is created. This is often referred to as a hybrid endovascular procedure and examples of surgical bypasses would include ascending aorta to innominate and left common carotid (**Fig. 14.1**), left to right carotid bypass (**Fig. 14.2**) and left carotid–subclavian bypass.

The diameter thresholds are dictated by the available device sizes. A degree of oversizing is required

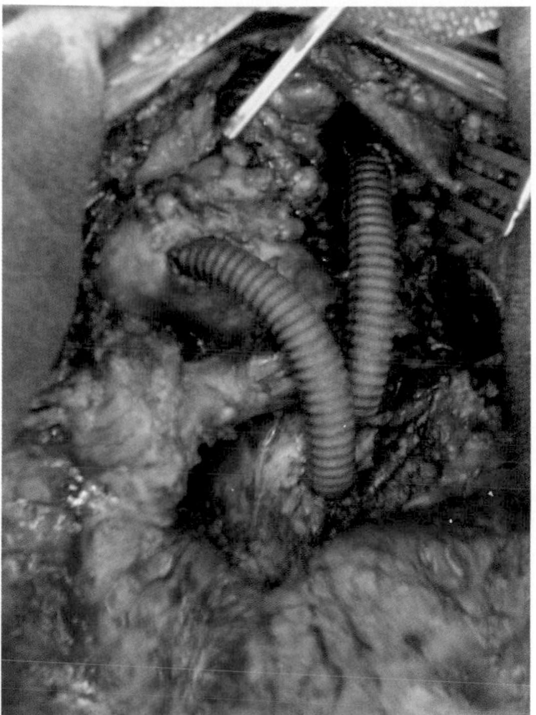

**Figure 14.1 •** Operative photograph of ascending aorta to innominate and left common carotid. Surgery performed to create an adequate landing zone in a patient with a very proximal thoracic aneurysm.

with respect to the aortic diameter during device selection. In general, for the treatment of aneurysms, devices are oversized by 15–20%. The maximum and minimum diameters of the available stent grafts are 46 and 22 mm. Therefore, the upper and lower limits of landing zone diameter are 18 and 40–42 mm respectively. If it is necessary to place more than one device because of the long length of aorta to be treated, the operator should also take into account the overlap required between adjacent devices, which is usually around 5 cm. Clearly, as with all endovascular aortic procedures, adequate access is required given the relatively large (25F) sizes of the endograft introducer sheaths.

The procedure is usually performed under general or regional anaesthesia, although stents can also be inserted using local anaesthesia alone. A diagnostic angiographic catheter is placed in the ascending aorta via the left brachial artery or the contralateral femoral artery. A femoral arteriotomy is usually required (although percutaneous procedures are feasible), and an exchange length extra-stiff guidewire (e.g. Lunderquist guidewire, Cook, UK) is advanced so that the tip is placed in the low ascending aorta. The systolic blood pressure should be reduced to below 100 mmHg peak systolic pressure to prevent the windsock effect of the cardiac output displacing the endograft.

The endograft delivery system is advanced over the guidewire to the desired deployment site. Accurate positioning is achieved by serial aortography. When the correct position is achieved, the stentgraft is released (Fig. 14.2). Further endografts are placed as necessary with at least 4–5 cm of overlap between endografts. After deployment, balloon dilation is performed to mould the endograft or endografts, and to eliminate any folds.

## Management of the spinal cord during endovascular thoracic procedures

Placement of an endograft in the thoracic aorta causes coverage of many intercostal vessels, with the risk of spinal cord ischaemia. Some centres advocate prophylactic CSF drainage whilst others adopt an expectant policy. Clearly if there is any sign of spinal cord ischaemia, the cord perfusion pressure

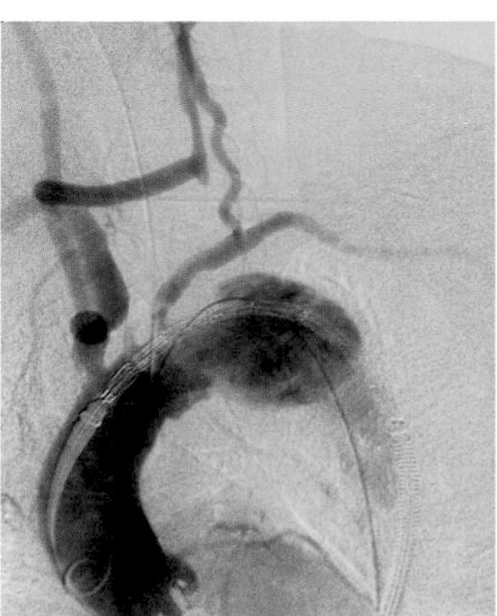

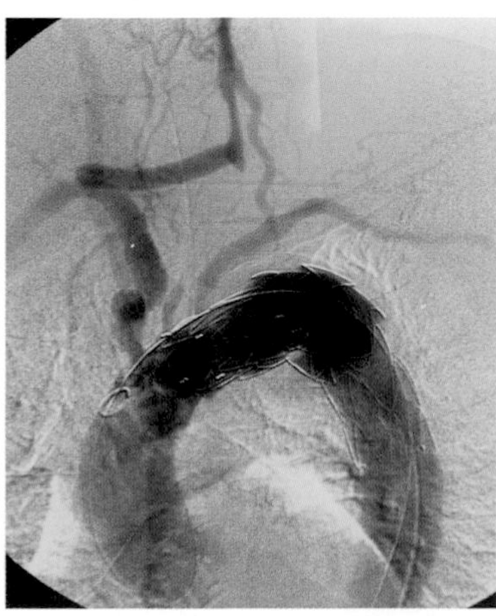

**Figure 14.2 •** Angiogram demonstrating a large thoracic aneurysm with the landing zone involving the left common carotid artery. To enable endovascular aneurysm repair a right to left common carotid bypass has been performed with ligation of the proximal left carotid artery (arrow).

must be increased by reducing CSF pressure and increasing mean arterial pressure.

Controversy has surrounded the management of the left subclavian artery during thoracic endografting. Early experience suggested that it was reasonably safe to cover the origin of the subclavian artery with respect to upper limb perfusion. However, more recent evidence has demonstrated that paraplegia rates are lower when subclavian perfusion is preserved, presumably due to the contribution of the vertebral artery to the anterior spinal artery.[10,11] Routine revascularisation of the left subclavian artery (via left carotid–subclavian bypass) is recommended in the authors' practice for all cases where coverage of the left subclavian origin is planned.

## Outcome of treatment

Results of open repair in centres of excellence are good, with 3-day mortality rates for all types of thoracic aneurysm below 12% and paraplegia rates below 4%.[12] Community results which incorporate several centres are more realistic of patient-centred outcomes and demonstrate 30-day mortality rates approaching 20%.[13] Mortality is predicted by renal insufficiency, age and emergency presentation.[14]

Outcome data for EVR of thoracic aneurysms are available from several sources. Leurs et al., on behalf of the EUROSTAR collaborators, reported data in 249 patients with 30-day mortality for elective total endovascular repair (TEVR) of 5.3% and paraplegia of 4%.[1] A cohort of patients with TAAs who underwent endografting with the Gore TAG device was compared retrospectively with the results of a cohort of 94 patients who underwent open surgical repair. The perioperative mortality (2.1% vs. 11.7%), paraplegia (3% vs. 14%) and freedom from major adverse event (48% vs. 20%) rates were all better in the endovascular group.[15]

Similarly, the European Talent Registry reported technical success of 98%, in-hospital mortality in 5% (4.1% and 7.9% for elective and emergency procedures respectively), paraplegia in 1.7% and stroke in 3.7%.[16] Similar outcomes have been reported for the newest generation of endografts, despite the fact the patients in these later data series had more challenging anatomy compared with earlier series.[10]

Endovascular thoracic aneurysm repair has a spectrum of complications unique to the procedure. The most common is endoleak. There seems little doubt that the most common endoleak is an attachment site (or type 1) endoleak. These may occur immediately or during follow-up and should be treated with additional devices. Type 3 leaks (between adjacent devices or through disrupted grafts) may occur and should also be treated with additional devices.

## Recommendations for practice

The advent of EVR for thoracic aneurysms has changed practice. In the authors' opinion, endovascular procedures should be used as first-line therapy for most thoracic aneurysms. Exclusions to this policy would be patients with unfavourable anatomy, poor long-term durability and possibly patients with documented connective tissue disease, in whom the results of endografting are not well defined.

The management of patients with Marfan syndrome have been the subject of much debate since the advent of endovascular therapy. Patients with Marfan's develop both thoracic aneurysms and dissections. However, the patients are usually younger and fitter than patients with non-specific aneurysms, have excellent outcomes from conventional surgery[17] and equivocal outcomes from EVR.[18] At present, there is no body of evidence to support the routine use of EVR in patients with Marfan syndrome.

# Thoraco-abdominal aortic aneurysms (TAAAs)

Aneurysms that involve the suprarenal portion of the abdominal aorta are traditionally described as thoraco-abdominal aneurysms and are classified according to the extent of the aneurysmal disease. The aetiology of thoraco-abdominal aneurysms differs from infrarenal aneurysms, with medial degenerative disease and chronic dissection particularly prevalent.[19] In contrast to infrarenal disease, the majority of patients with thoraco-abdominal aneurysms are symptomatic, the presence of back pain is particularly common, and this symptom may precede aortic rupture or intramural dissection.[20]

The rationale for treatment of thoraco-abdominal aneurysms largely derives from a natural history study from Crawford and DeNatale, who reported a series of 94 patients unsuitable for surgery.[21] After 24 months follow-up, only 24% of these patients were alive, which contrasted with the 59% 5-year survival of a concurrent cohort of patients who underwent operative repair. On the basis of these results, it was concluded that patients with significant thoraco-abdominal aneurysms should have an operative repair unless precluded by coexistent medical conditions.

## Surgical management

As with all complex aortic diseases, detailed imaging and careful assessment of comorbid risk factors is essential. Due to the high mortality rates associated with repair of TAAAs, consideration must be given to the balance between predicted surgical risk and aneurysm diameter. Preoperative cardiac revascularisation may be appropriate.

A left thoracotomy is usually required, although some type IV aneurysms may utilise an abdominal approach. The abdominal aorta is usually exposed by left medial visceral rotation. The diaphragm is partially divided with a circumferential incision preferred to preserve nerve supply. After the dissection has been completed the aneurysm is clamped at its proximal and distal extents, and an arteriotomy made in the lateral aneurysm wall. It is important that the arteriotomy is sited away from the visceral origins in the abdominal portion of the aneurysm. The proximal anastomosis is performed with a completely transected aorta to prevent aorto-oesophageal fistula. If possible, the proximal anastomosis is fashioned to include adjacent intercostal or visceral arteries, whilst any remaining intercostals are directly reimplanted into the graft or revascularised by separate jump grafts. The visceral arteries are then directly anastomosed into elliptical openings in the graft, utilising an inclusion technique. If possible, the coeliac, superior mesenteric and right renal arteries are taken on one patch; anastomosing the distal graft to the aortic bifurcation or iliac arteries completes the reconstruction (**Figs 14.3** and **14.4**).

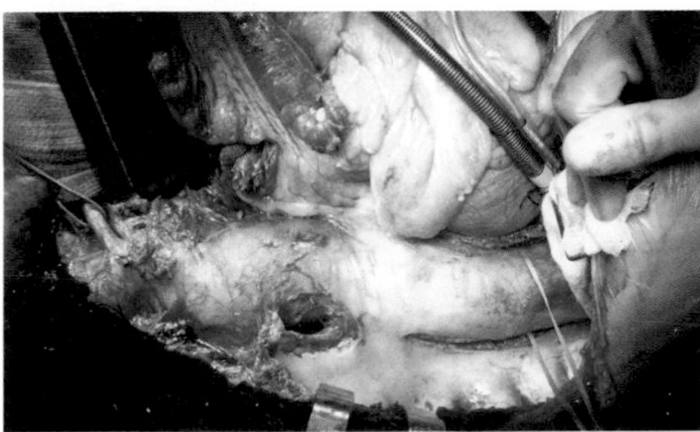

**Figure 14.3** • Operative picture demonstrating exposure of a type III TAAA using a left thoracolaparotomy. The diaphragm has been completely divided in this case. The left renal artery is controlled.

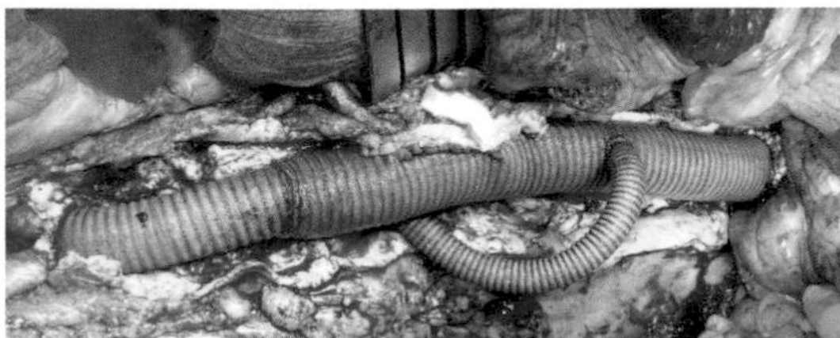

**Figure 14.4** • Operative picture of completed reconstruction of a TAAA. The visceral patch has been reinforced with Teflon pledgets. A separate graft has been anastomosed to a large intercostal.

## Adjunctive surgical techniques

During thoraco-abdominal aneurysm repair, prolonged visceral ischaemia is the main cause of postoperative renal dysfunction and can also contribute to multiple organ failure. To reduce the severity of organ hypoperfusion, partial left heart bypass with a centrifugal pump may be utilised to drain blood from the left atrium or upper pulmonary vein, and return it via the femoral artery or aorta. This facilitates renal and visceral perfusion whilst the proximal anastomosis is fashioned as long as the distal aortic clamp remains proximal to the visceral vessels.[22] During the abdominal part of the aneurysm repair, the coeliac trunk, superior mesenteric artery and both renal arteries can be selectively perfused with catheters which are connected to the left heart bypass.[23]

Paraplegia may complicate thoraco-abdominal aneurysm repair in up to 20% of cases and is increased in more proximal aneurysms, with lengthy clamp time, renal impairment, advanced age and emergency presentations. Paraplegia results from damage to the spinal cord due to a combination of division of spinal cord arteries, prolonged spinal cord ischaemia, reperfusion injury and postoperative hypotension. Maintenance of spinal cord blood supply may be achieved by reimplantation of patent intercostal arteries, and by distal aortic perfusion. CSF pressure increases during aortic clamping, and CSF drainage has been advocated to reduce paraplegia.[24,25]

A functional approach to the problem of neurological deficit aims at intraoperative monitoring of the spinal cord function. Somatosensory evoked potentials are widely used to detect spinal cord ischaemia during aortic cross-clamping and to identify vessels critical to spinal cord blood supply, which may then be perfused and reimplanted. An alternative approach is to use motor evoked potentials, which have been reported to improve paraplegia rates.[26–28]

## Results of surgical repair of thoraco-abdominal aneurysms

The mortality and morbidity rates following conventional repair of TAAAs are still significant, with specialised centres reporting mortality rates of 5–16% with paraplegia rates of 4–11%.[12,29–31] However, these excellent results are not representative of outcomes outside of these centres, with national/community mortality rates exceeding 20% at 30 days and 30% at 1 year.[13,32,33] Identifiable patient risk factors predicting adverse outcomes include emergent presentation, previous aortic replacement, diabetes, smoking history, renal and cardiorespiratory impairment, age beyond 80 years, acute dissection and the extent of TAAA.

## Hybrid visceral revascularisation and endovascular repair of thoraco-abdominal aortic aneurysms

The application of combining surgical and endovascular strategies in the management of complex aortic disease has been suggested to reduce the surgical insult, by obviating the need for thoracotomy and aortic cross-clamping whilst also reducing the duration of visceral and renal ischaemia. The exclusion of TAAAs by means of an endoluminal stent-graft delivered via a remote arteriotomy or conduit requires sufficient length of proximal and distal landing zones in non-diseased or replaced aorta and in addition needs to safeguard perfusion of the gut and kidneys. A hybrid repair may be defined as a combined surgical and endovascular approach in which transperitoneal retrograde visceral revascularisation is used to create an adequate distal landing zone for endovascular thoraco-abdominal aneurysm endograft exclusion. The retrograde visceral bypass maintains perfusion to the visceral and renal arteries. This approach may be combined with great vessel transposition or bypass to create an adequate proximal attachment site for the thoraco-abdominal endograft (**Fig. 14.5**).

At present, there are only a few case series reporting the results of this technique (Table 14.1).[34–40] Superficially, the results do not appear to show a significant advantage for the hybrid technique over conventional surgery, but in general patients have more comorbidity, are older, and have a higher proportion of type II and III aneurysms than comparable open series.

## Total endovascular repair of thoraco-abdominal aortic aneurysms

Recent technological advances in stentgraft design (**Fig. 14.6**) have realised the possibility of deploying

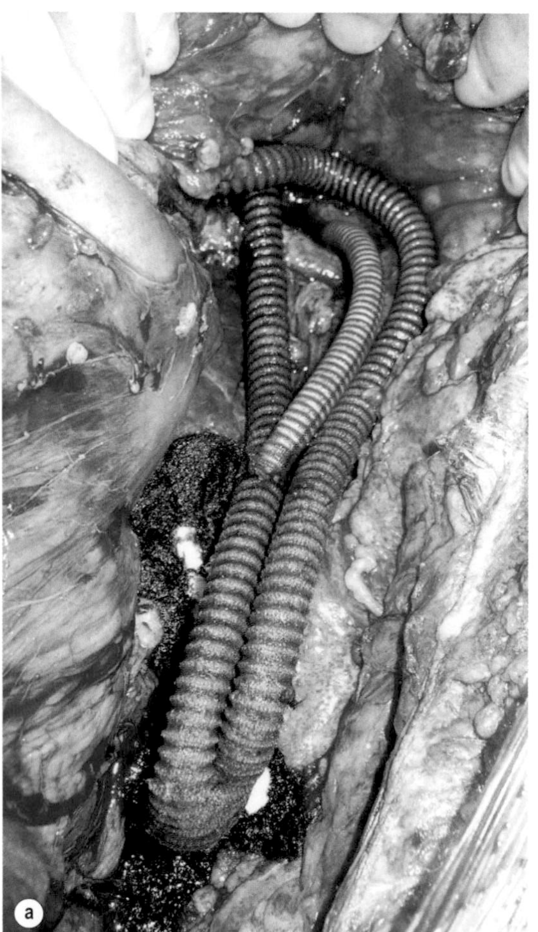


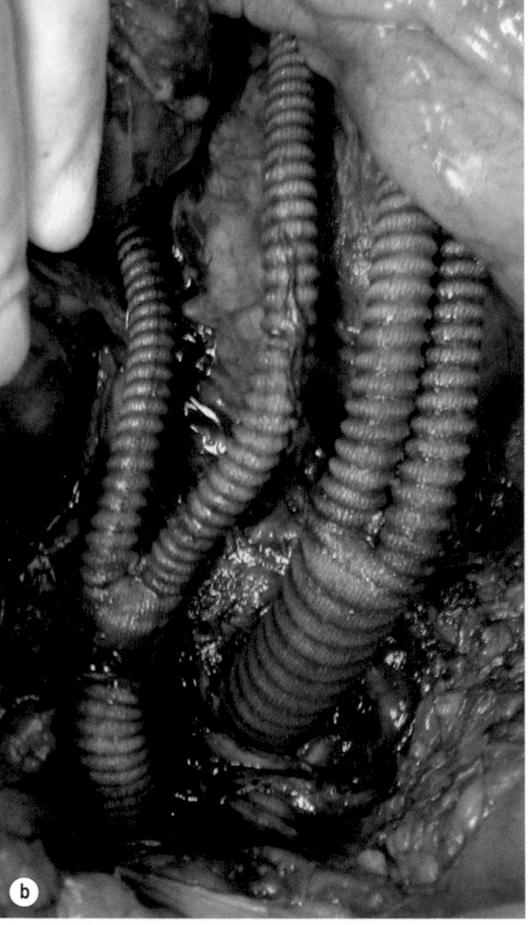


**Figure 14.5** • Operative pictures of two patients undergoing retrograde visceral revascularisation. Many different graft configurations are possible with varying numbers of vessels requiring revascularisation.

Table 14.1 • Summary of published series of combined surgical and endovascular repair of TAAAs ($n$ >10)

| Authors | Institution Year of pub. | Number | Type II (%) | Type III (%) | Visceral vessels bypassed | Mortality (%) | Permanent paraplegia (%) |
|---|---|---|---|---|---|---|---|
| Resch et al.[34] | Cleveland 2006 | 13 | 38.5 | 15.4 | N/A | 23.1 | 30.7 |
| Zhou et al.[35] | Houston 2006 | 15 | 0 | 53.3 | 40 | 6.7 | 0 |
| Black et al.[36] | St Mary's London 2006 | 26 | 62 | 26.9 | 94 | 23 | 0 |
| Bockler et al.[37] | Heidelberg 2007 | 11 | 18.2 | 9.1 | N/A | 18 | 0 |
| Chiesa et al.[38] | Milan 2007 | 13 | 15.4 | 0 | 32 | 23.0 | 7.7 |
| Lee et al.[39] | Gainesville 2007 | 17 | 11.8 | 47.0 | 56 | 24.0 | 0 |
| Biasi[40] | St George's London 2008 | 18 | 44.4 | 38.9 | 48 | 17.6 | 5.6 |

customised endografts with fenestrations, allowing target vessel cannulation with additional covered stents to afford antegrade perfusion of the visceral vessels.[41] Similarly, branched endovascular grafts have also been successfully deployed to preserve end-organ perfusion in selected patients, and some TAAAs can now be treated with four-vessel branched grafts.[42,43] The need for accurate measurements and precise manufacturing results in a lag time of several weeks in most, and anatomical constraints with access and vessel tortuosity may not allow all TAAAs to be treated with a total endovascular solution. This

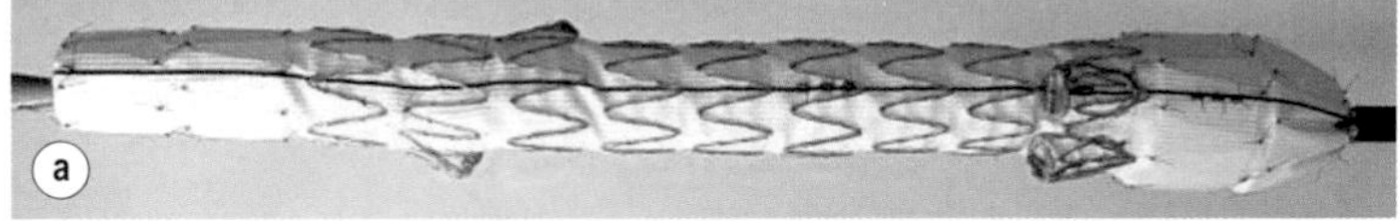

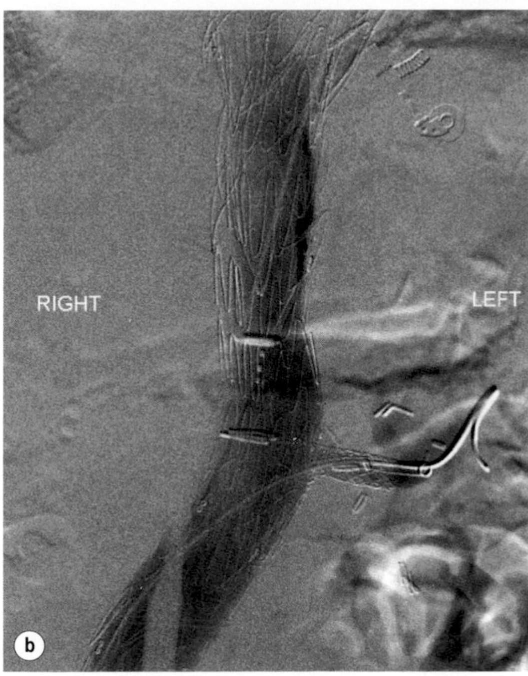


**Figure 14.6 • (a)** Picture of an endograft with four custom-made branches. **(b)** A procedural angiogram demonstrates completed reconstruction of a TAAA with a branched graft to the left renal artery. Part (a) courtesy of Cook, UK.

evolutionary technology shows significant promise in reducing the mortality and morbidity of TAAA repair, but at present case numbers are extremely small and highly selected. Further information will become available over the next few years to establish the place of this technology in complex aortic disease.

### Recommendations for practice

Open surgical repair remains the gold standard for the treatment of TAAAs. Endovascular techniques are evolving in this field but the complexities of maintaining visceral and renal perfusion make endovascular solutions technically complex. The hybrid approach is probably best seen as a bridge between traditional surgical techniques and the developing total endovascular solutions. At present, it would seem reasonable to reserve hybrid and endovascular solutions for those patients who have a high predicted mortality for open thoraco-abdominal replacement, whilst acknowledging that as endovascular experience develops, this technique is likely to play a more prominent role in the management of TAAAs.

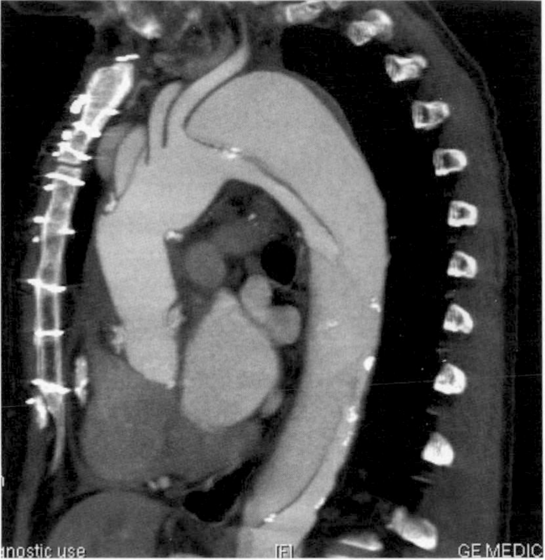

**Figure 14.7** • Sagittal reconstruction showing the classic appearance of a type B aortic dissection.

## Thoracic dissection and acute aortic syndrome

### Pathology and classification

The acute aortic syndrome may be described as a group of pathological conditions affecting the thoracic aorta that typically cause severe thoracic pain and may be misdiagnosed as acute coronary syndrome. The acute aortic syndrome encompasses classic aortic dissection (**Fig. 14.7**), intramural haematoma (IMH; **Fig. 14.8**) and penetrating aortic ulcers (PAUs; **Fig. 14.9**).[44] All three conditions may coexist and evolution from both IMH and penetrating ulcer to dissection has been described. To a large extent, the management of classic aortic dissection may be applied to both IMH and PAUs.

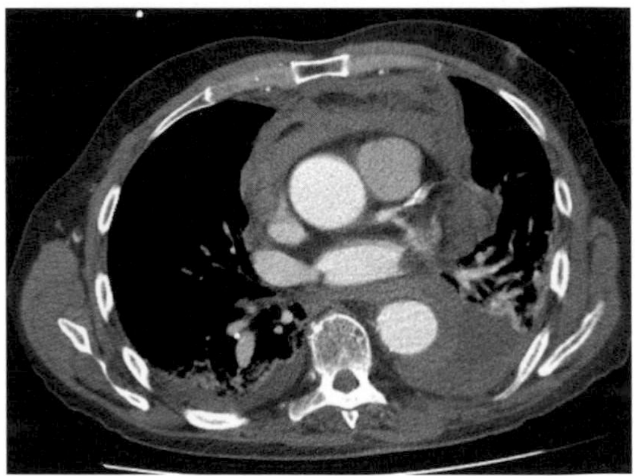

**Figure 14.8** • Axial CT appearance of intramural haematoma. There is a relatively high-density crescentic rim of fresh blood in the wall of the aorta (arrow).

Aortic dissections result from a tear in the aortic intima that allows blood to penetrate the aortic wall and propagate a cleavage plane between the intima and media. Two channels of flow result in the formation of true and false lumens. Common causes of dissection include hypertension, trauma and connective tissue disorders. Often, flow is preferentially directed into the false lumen due to the size of the entry tear. This may lead to compression of the true lumen, which can result in malperfusion or rupture of the false lumen. Malperfusion of the visceral, renal or lower limb arteries may complicate aortic dissection. This is usually due to branch vessel occlusion by an intimal flap and may be dynamic (due to true lumen compression) or static due to a blind-ending channel or significant thrombosis within the false lumen (**Fig. 14.10**).

IMH is defined by blood in the intramural space, without an obvious intimal tear. The condition may result from rupture of medial vasa vasora and is often regarded as a precursor to dissection. IMH accounts for up to 20% of acute aortic syndromes and has a prognosis similar to classic aortic dissection.[45] PAU results from focal ulceration of an atherosclerotic plaque, which may be associated with haematoma within the aortic wall. Penetrating ulcers have a poorer prognosis than classical dissection, with higher rates of aortic rupture.[46]

Aortic dissections are classified by site, chronicity and presentation. The most crucial classification

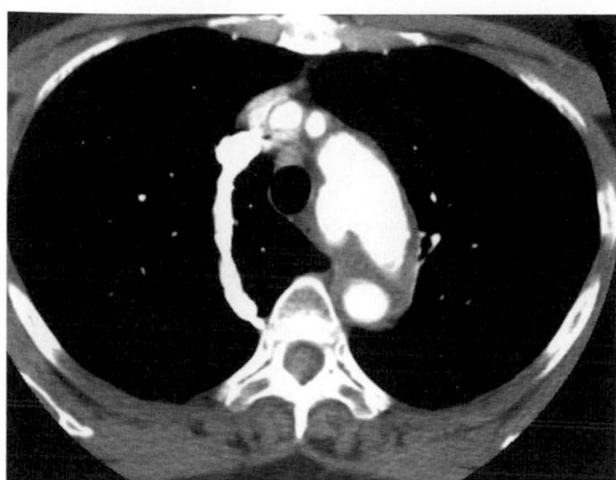

**Figure 14.9** • Axial CT appearance of penetrating aortic ulcer (arrow).

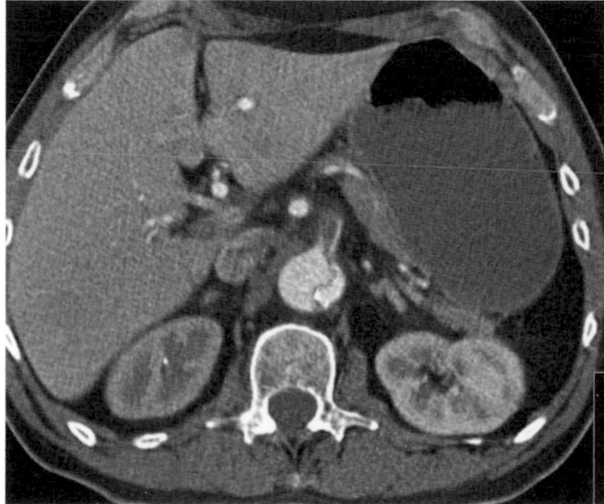

**Figure 14.10** • Axial CT demonstrating a patient with visceral ischaemia due to significant true lumen collapse (black arrows) and thrombosis of the false lumen in the SMA (white arrow).

involves the site of dissection. Under the commonly used Stanford classification, type A dissections involve the ascending aorta, whereas type B dissection does not. The DeBakey system is also used to classify site. Temporally, dissections are acute when less than 2 weeks after the onset of symptoms, and are termed chronic after this period. In addition dissections may be termed complicated or uncomplicated. Complications of aortic dissection would include rupture, malperfusion, impending rupture (persistent pain), refractory hypertension and false aneurysm formation.

## Conventional management of acute aortic dissection

Management of aortic dissection involves rapid pharmacological control of blood pressure and *dP/dt*. Type A dissection has a 1% mortality per hour from aortic rupture, aortic regurgitation, pericardial tamponade or coronary ischaemia and is treated by emergency surgical graft repair of the ascending aorta, with our without aortic valve replacement.[47] The management of type A aortic dissection will not be discussed further.

The management of type B dissections is principally medical, with intervention reserved for complications. Overall, medical management of patients with acute aortic dissection has a mortality rate of just over 10%; this includes a mixed group of patients with uncomplicated dissection and some patients with complicated dissection who would be considered unsuitable for surgical intervention. Surgical intervention in patients with complicated dissection has a mortality rate of approximately 30%.[48] Overall, the medical treatment of uncomplicated type B dissection appears appropriate, as in the acute phase uncomplicated type B dissections appear to have a relatively low mortality. In a series of 159 patients presenting with acute type B dissections, 47% of the patients had complicated dissections and had an overall, in-hospital mortality of 18%. In contrast, the 53% of patients with uncomplicated dissection had medical management, with mortality of just 1.2%.[49,50]

## Endovascular management of acute type B thoracic dissection

The advent of reliable endovascular therapy has revolutionised the treatment of complicated type B thoracic dissections. Endovascular therapy aims to cover the primary entry tear of type B dissections with an endovascular graft. This has the effect of depressurising the false lumen, allowing immediate true lumen expansion and movement of the intimal flap to facilitate aortic remodelling. Covering the primary entry tear will treat most complications of acute dissections by allowing thrombosis of the false lumen, minimising the effects of false lumen aortic rupture and by allowing true lumen expansion that will reverse many malperfusion syndromes (**Fig. 14.11**).

The technique of EVR is similar to that described above for thoracic aneurysms. An adequate sealing zone is required to effect coverage of the entry tear. Graft oversizing is limited to 10% so as not to traumatise the fragile proximal aorta, and balloon dilatation is contraindicated for the same reason. There is controversy as to the length of aorta that requires coverage in acute dissections. A short endograft will allow coverage of the primary tear but will rely on distal aortic remodelling to avoid false lumen perfusion in the lower thoracic aorta. A longer endograft will cause more false lumen thrombosis but will theoretically increase the risk

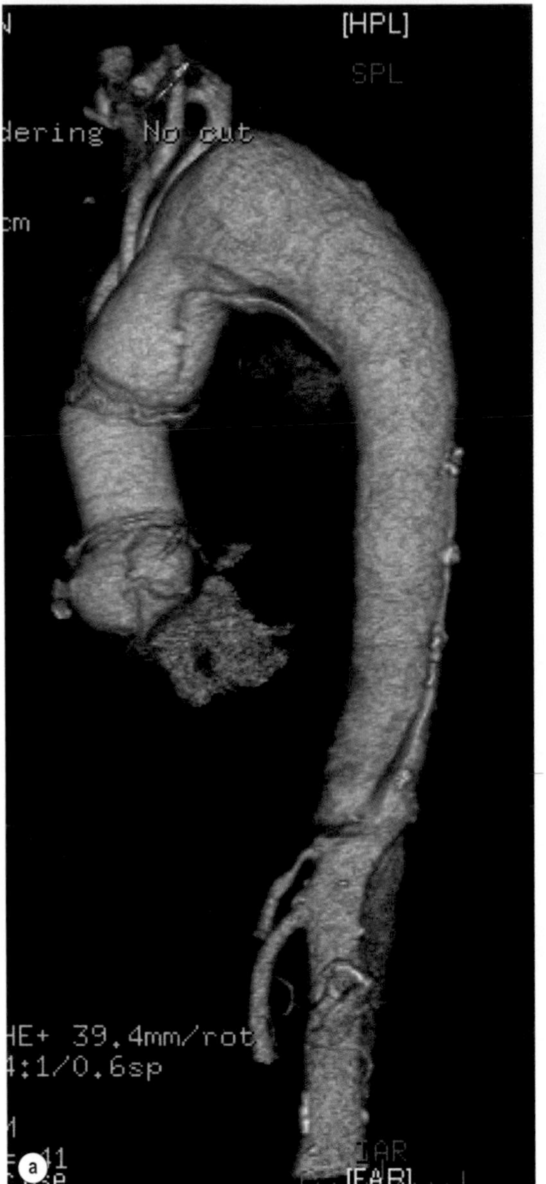


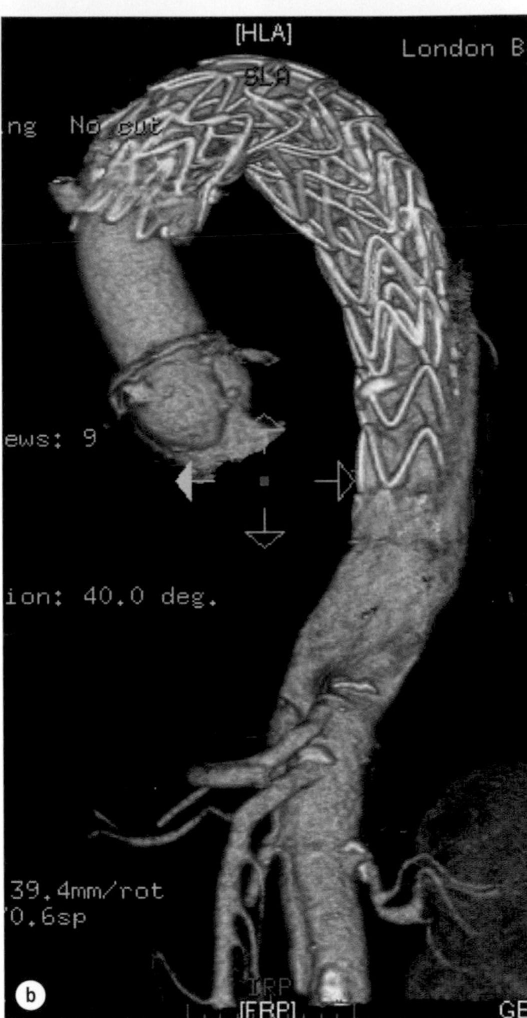


**Figure 14.11 • (a)** Patient with a residual dissection after a type A repair. **(b)** An endograft has been placed to cover the primary entry tear.

of paraplegia. One recent concept is to use a combination of a short covered endograft to cover the primary tear and an uncovered stent to facilitate remodelling.[51]

The early results of EVR of complicated type B dissections were vastly better than the open surgical alternative. Most series reported mortality rates below 10%, with paraplegia rates of less than 3%.[1,52–55] These findings stimulated a rapid change in management and most vascular centres would now regard endovascular therapy to be the first-line treatment for complicated type B dissections. EVR of thoracic aneurysms has its own set of perioperative complications, which include retrograde type A dissection, aortic rupture and continued perfusion of the false lumen.[10] In addition, other endovascular techniques including visceral stenting or fenestration[56] may be required to treat malperfusion.

In recent years several authors have suggested that asymptomatic acute type B dissections might benefit from EVR in preventing acute and long-term complications.[57] The rationale for this proposition revolves around the outcome for patients with asymptomatic dissection. Several historical studies have suggested that aortic-related death was high in this group of patients, and that mortality (from acute complications or late aortic rupture) might be reduced by EVR. It might be argued that newer data have revealed a low rate of complications in patients with stable, uncomplicated type B dissections[50,58] and that the key issue in this group of patients will be to define a subgroup that exhibits a high complication rate that might benefit from aortic repair in the acute phase.[59] Careful morphological studies and long-term follow-up will be required to define these groups, but some useful data have recently been published that identify a false lumen diameter exceeding 22 mm that predicts rapid aortic expansion.[59]

## Endovascular treatment of chronic dissections

Indications for repair of chronic dissections have usually been limited to the onset of complications, and an aortic diameter exceeding 5.5–6.0 cm. The literature surrounding the results of EVR for chronic dissections is particularly poor. In the series to date the mortality rates have been acceptable but the long-term success in preventing aortic expansion is unclear. There have been anecdotal reports that the false lumen below the stent may continue to expand after treatment and that the rate of repeated intervention is high.[10] This is an area that requires careful documentation to facilitate effective therapy. Again, procedural details require refinement as there is still uncertainty regarding the extent of aorta that should be covered, whether covering the entry tear is sufficient or if all re-entry tears should be treated, and whether aortic remodelling can be predicted by the morphology of the lesion.

### Recommendations for practice

EVR should now be considered the gold standard for complicated acute type B thoracic dissections. There appears no justification for repair of uncomplicated acute dissections. The indications and methodology for the treatment of chronic dissections remain undefined.

## Traumatic aortic injury (TAI)

TAI is the second commonest cause of death in patients after blunt injury: 15–30% of deaths from blunt trauma have aortic transaction at post-mortem. TAI is commonly associated with multiple injuries and a common occurrence after automobile accidents. The most common site of aortic injury is the isthmus, where the relatively mobile thoracic aorta joins the fixed arch. Aortic ruptures occur at this site in 80% of pathological series and in 90% of the clinical series.[60] There is a spectrum of degree of injury to the aorta ranging from intimal haemorrhage through to complete transection, periaortic haemorrhage and false aneurysm formation.[61]

The surgical approach to treatment has changed considerably in the last decade. Previously, it was thought that emergency repair was mandatory because of the belief that there was a high risk of early rupture (79% within 24 hours) in immediate survivors, although procedural mortality rates of this approach were in excess of 30%. Recent series suggest that the rupture risk in stable patients is only 10%. Therefore surgery can be delayed until the immediate threat to life from other injuries is controlled.[62]

In the last decade, due to its low complication rate, TEVR has in many centres superseded surgery for TAI. The procedural time is short and the operation confers very little in terms of additional morbidity to these severely ill patients. Due to the focal nature of the injury, only a short length of aorta requires covering with an endograft.

Although TEVR seems to have become the gold standard for TAI, there are relatively limited data on outcomes. Data from cohort series involve small numbers of patients. However, the procedural mortality is less than 10% throughout and the reported risk of paraplegia is negligible.[63–65]

The main disadvantage to TEVR for TAI is the relative unsuitability of the devices available for the patients who require TEVR. TAI occurs in a relatively young population with narrower aortas and more angulated aortic arches than older patients. None of the devices currently available conform very well to angulated arches. There are reports of endografts 'sitting up' in the arch, resulting in endograft collapse and pseudocoarctation.[66] The other problem is the lack of availability of small-calibre endografts. The smallest endograft is 22 mm, which limits the smallest size of aorta that can be stented to 18–19 mm. This may cause problems in young patients, and in some cases operators may resort to the use of smaller endografts not designed for use in the thoracic aorta, such as abdominal endograft limbs.

Nevertheless, at the very least endografting can act as a temporary measure to prevent rupture until the patient is well enough to undergo definitive surgical repair. In the future, we may expect to see the development of endografts specifically designed to treat aortic trauma.

## Key points

- There are a lack of randomised data to guide practice in diseases of the thoracic aorta. Most data derive from case series or registries. However, mortality differences, in some diseases, are so disparate between open surgical procedures and the endovascular equivalent that inferences can be drawn.
- Endovascular therapy may now be considered the first-line treatment for thoracic aneurysms and acute complicated dissections.
- There are no data, as yet, to support prophylactic endovascular repair of acute uncomplicated dissections.
- Thoraco-abdominal aneurysms remain a technical challenge with high mortality rates from all treatment modalities. Open surgery should still be considered as the first-line therapy for patients with low predicted mortality from open repair. Hybrid and total endovascular approaches might be considered appropriate for patients with high predicted mortality.
- The results of endovascular therapy in patients with Marfan syndrome are equivocal and open surgery should be considered preferable in this patient group.

# References


1. Leurs LJ, Bell R, Degrieck Y et al. Endovascular treatment of thoracic aortic diseases: combined experience from the EUROSTAR and United Kingdom Thoracic Endograft registries. J Vasc Surg 2004; 40(4):670–9; discussion 679–80.
2. Swee W, Dake MD. Endovascular management of thoracic dissections. Circulation 2008; 117(11):1460–73.
3. Bellin MF, Van Der Molen AJ. Extracellular gadolinium-based contrast media: an overview. Eur J Radiol 2008; 66(2):160–7.
4. Estrera AL, Miller CC 3rd, Porat E et al. Determinants of early and late outcome for reoperations of the proximal aorta. Ann Thorac Surg 2004; 78(3):837–45; discussion 845.
5. Sayed S, Choke E, Helme S et al. Endovascular stent graft repair of mycotic aneurysms of the thoracic aorta. J Cardiovasc Surg (Torino) 2005; 46(2):155–61.
6. Clouse WD, Hallett JW Jr, Schaff HV et al. Improved prognosis of thoracic aortic aneurysms: a population-based study. JAMA 1998; 280(22):1926–9.
7. Perko MJ, Norgaard M, Herzog TM et al. Unoperated aortic aneurysm: a survey of 170 patients. Ann Thorac Surg 1995; 59(5):1204–9.
8. Juvonen T, Ergin MA, Galla JD et al. Prospective study of the natural history of thoracic aortic aneurysms. Ann Thorac Surg 1997; 63(6):1533–45.
9. Elefteriades JA. Natural history of thoracic aortic aneurysms: indications for surgery, and surgical versus nonsurgical risks. Ann Thorac Surg 2002; 74(5):S1877–80; discussion S92–8.
10. Thompson M, Ivaz S, Cheshire N et al. Early results of endovascular treatment of the thoracic aorta using the Valiant endograft. Cardiovasc Interv Radiol 2007; 30(6):1130–8.
11. Buth J, Harris PL, Hobo R et al. Neurologic complications associated with endovascular repair of thoracic aortic pathology: incidence and risk factors. A study from the European Collaborators on Stent/Graft Techniques for Aortic Aneurysm Repair (EUROSTAR) registry. J Vasc Surg 2007; 46(6):1103–10; discussion 1110–11.
12. Estrera AL, Miller CC, Azizzadeh A et al. Thoracic aortic aneurysms. Acta Chir Belg 2006; 106(3):307–16.
13. Rigberg DA, McGory ML, Zingmond DS et al. Thirty-day mortality statistics underestimate the risk of repair of thoracoabdominal aortic aneurysms: a statewide experience. J Vasc Surg 2006; 43(2):217–22; discussion 223.
14. Safi HJ, Estrera AL, Miller CC et al. Evolution of risk for neurologic deficit after descending and thoracoabdominal aortic repair. Ann Thorac Surg 2005; 80(6):2173–9; discussion 2179.
15. Bavaria JE, Appoo JJ, Makaroun MS et al. Endovascular stent grafting versus open surgical repair of descending thoracic aortic aneurysms in low-risk patients: a multicenter comparative trial. J Thorac Cardiovasc Surg 2007; 133(2):369–77.
16. Fattori R, Nienaber CA, Rousseau H et al. Results of endovascular repair of the thoracic aorta with the Talent Thoracic stent graft: the Talent Thoracic Retrospective Registry. J Thorac Cardiovasc Surg 2006; 132(2):332–9.
17. Mommertz G, Sigala F, Langer S et al. Thoracoabdominal aortic aneurysm repair in patients with Marfan syndrome. Eur J Vasc Endovasc Surg 2008; 35(2):181–6.
18. Ince H, Rehders TC, Petzsch M et al. Stent-grafts in patients with Marfan syndrome. J Endovasc Ther 2005; 12(1):82–8.

19. Svensson LG, Crawford ES, Hess KR et al. Experience with 1509 patients undergoing thoracoabdominal aortic operations. J Vasc Surg 1993; 17(2):357–68; discussion 368–70.
20. Money SR, Hollier LH. The management of thoracoabdominal aneurysms. Adv Surg 1994; 27:285–94.
21. Crawford ES, DeNatale RW. Thoracoabdominal aortic aneurysm: observations regarding the natural course of the disease. J Vasc Surg 1986; 3(4): 578–82.
22. Safi HJ, Hess KR, Randel M et al. Cerebrospinal fluid drainage and distal aortic perfusion: reducing neurologic complications in repair of thoracoabdominal aortic aneurysm types I and II. J Vasc Surg 1996; 23(2):223–8; discussion 229.
23. Jacobs MJ, de Mol BA, Legemate DA et al. Retrograde aortic and selective organ perfusion during thoracoabdominal aortic aneurysm repair. Eur J Vasc Endovasc Surg 1997; 14(5):360–6.
24. Huynh TT, Miller CC 3rd, Estrera AL et al. Correlations of cerebrospinal fluid pressure with hemodynamic parameters during thoracoabdominal aortic aneurysm repair. Ann Vasc Surg 2005; 19(5):619–24.
25. Estrera AL, Miller CC 3rd, Huynh TT et al. Preoperative and operative predictors of delayed neurologic deficit following repair of thoracoabdominal aortic aneurysm. J Thorac Cardiovasc Surg 2003; 126(5):1288–94.
26. Jacobs MJ, Mommertz G, Koeppel TA et al. Surgical repair of thoracoabdominal aortic aneurysms. J Cardiovasc Surg (Torino) 2007; 48(1):49–58.
27. Jacobs MJ, Elenbaas TW, Schurink GW et al. Assessment of spinal cord integrity during thoracoabdominal aortic aneurysm repair. Ann Thorac Surg 2002; 74(5):S1864–6; discussion S92–8.
28. Shine TS, Harrison BA, De Ruyter ML et al. Motor and somatosensory evoked potentials: their role in predicting spinal cord ischemia in patients undergoing thoracoabdominal aortic aneurysm repair with regional lumbar epidural cooling. Anesthesiology 2008; 108(4):580–7.
29. Coselli JS, Bozinovski J, LeMaire SA. Open surgical repair of 2286 thoracoabdominal aortic aneurysms. Ann Thorac Surg 2007; 83(2):S862–4; discussion S90–2.
30. Conrad MF, Crawford RS, Davison JK et al. Thoracoabdominal aneurysm repair: a 20-year perspective. Ann Thorac Surg 2007; 83(2):S856–61; discussion S90–2.
31. Estrera AL, Miller CC 3rd, Huynh TT et al. Neurologic outcome after thoracic and thoracoabdominal aortic aneurysm repair. Ann Thorac Surg 2001; 72(4):1225–30; discussion 1230–1.
32. Cowan JA Jr, Dimick JB, Wainess RM et al. Ruptured thoracoabdominal aortic aneurysm treatment in the United States: 1988 to 1998. J Vasc Surg 2003; 38(2):319–22.
33. Derrow AE, Seeger JM, Dame DA et al. The outcome in the United States after thoracoabdominal aortic aneurysm repair, renal artery bypass, and mesenteric revascularization. J Vasc Surg 2001; 34(1):54–61.
34. Resch TA, Greenberg RK, Lyden SP et al. Combined staged procedures for the treatment of thoracoabdominal aneurysms. J Endovasc Ther 2006; 13(4):481–9.
35. Zhou W, Reardon M, Peden EK et al. Hybrid approach to complex thoracic aortic aneurysms in high-risk patients: surgical challenges and clinical outcomes. J Vasc Surg 2006; 44(4):688–93.
36. Black SA, Wolfe JH, Clark M et al. Complex thoracoabdominal aortic aneurysms: endovascular exclusion with visceral revascularization. J Vasc Surg 2006; 43(6):1081–9; discussion 1089.
37. Bockler D, Schumacher H, Klemm K et al. Hybrid procedures as a combined endovascular and open approach for pararenal and thoracoabdominal aortic pathologies. Langenbeck's Arch Surg 2007; 392(6):715–23.
38. Chiesa R, Tshomba Y, Melissano G et al. Hybrid approach to thoracoabdominal aortic aneurysms in patients with prior aortic surgery. J Vasc Surg 2007; 45(6):1128–35.
39. Lee WA, Brown MP, Martin TD et al. Early results after staged hybrid repair of thoracoabdominal aortic aneurysms. J Am Coll Surg 2007; 205(3):420–31.
40. Biasi L, Ali T, Lottus I. Hybrid repair of complex thoraco-abdominal aneurysms using applied endovascular strategies combined with visceral and renal revascularisation. J Thor Cardio Surg 2009 (In press).
41. Chuter TA. Fenestrated and branched stent-grafts for thoracoabdominal, pararenal and juxtarenal aortic aneurysm repair. Semin Vasc Surg 2007; 20(2):90–6.
42. Roselli EE, Greenberg RK, Pfaff K et al. Endovascular treatment of thoracoabdominal aortic aneurysms. J Thorac Cardiovasc Surg 2007; 133(6):1474–82.
43. Anderson JL, Adam DJ, Berce M et al. Repair of thoracoabdominal aortic aneurysms with fenestrated and branched endovascular stent grafts. J Vasc Surg 2005; 42(4):600–7.
44. Tsai TT, Nienaber CA, Eagle KA. Acute aortic syndromes. Circulation 2005; 112(24):3802–13.
45. Evangelista A, Mukherjee D, Mehta RH et al. Acute intramural hematoma of the aorta: a mystery in evolution. Circulation 2005; 111(8):1063–70.
46. Coady MA, Rizzo JA, Elefteriades JA. Pathologic variants of thoracic aortic dissections. Penetrating atherosclerotic ulcers and intramural hematomas. Cardiol Clin 1999; 17(4):637–57.
47. Mehta RH, Suzuki T, Hagan PG et al. Predicting death in patients with acute type A aortic dissection. Circulation 2002; 105(2):200–6.
48. Hagan PG, Nienaber CA, Isselbacher EM et al. The International Registry of Acute Aortic Dissection

(IRAD): new insights into an old disease. JAMA 2000; 283(7):897–903.

49. Estrera AL, Miller CC, Goodrick J et al. Update on outcomes of acute type B aortic dissection. Ann Thorac Surg 2007; 83(2):S842–5; discussion S846–50.

50. Estrera AL, Miller CC 3rd, Safi HJ et al. Outcomes of medical management of acute type B aortic dissection. Circulation 2006; 114(1, Suppl):I384–9.

51. Nienaber CA, Kische S, Zeller T et al. Provisional extension to induce complete attachment after stent-graft placement in type B aortic dissection: the PETTICOAT concept. J Endovasc Ther 2006; 13(6):738–46.

52. Eggebrecht H, Nienaber CA, Neuhauser M et al. Endovascular stent-graft placement in aortic dissection: a meta-analysis. Eur Heart J 2006; 27(4):489–98.

53. Bortone AS, De Cillis E, D'Agostino D et al. Endovascular treatment of thoracic aortic disease: four years of experience. Circulation 2004; 110(11, Suppl 1):II262–7.

54. Nathanson DR, Rodriguez-Lopez JA, Ramaiah VG et al. Endoluminal stent-graft stabilization for thoracic aortic dissection. J Endovasc Ther 2005; 12(3):354–9.

55. Chen S, Yei F, Zhou L et al. Endovascular stent-grafts treatment in acute aortic dissection (type B): clinical outcomes during early, late, or chronic phases. Catheter Cardiovasc Interv 2006; 68(2):319–25.

56. Beregi JP, Haulon S, Otal P et al. Endovascular treatment of acute complications associated with aortic dissection: midterm results from a multicenter study. J Endovasc Ther 2003; 10(3):486–93.

57. Nienaber CA, Zannetti S, Barbieri B et al. INvestigation of STEnt grafts in patients with type B Aortic Dissection: design of the INSTEAD trial – a prospective, multicenter, European randomized trial. Am Heart J 2005; 149(4):592–9.

58. Winnerkvist A, Lockowandt U, Rasmussen E et al. A prospective study of medically treated acute type B aortic dissection. Eur J Vasc Endovasc Surg 2006; 32(4):349–55.

59. Song JM, Kim SD, Kim JH et al. Long-term predictors of descending aorta aneurysmal change in patients with aortic dissection. J Am Coll Cardiol 2007; 50(8):799–804.

60. Shorr RM, Crittenden M, Indeck M et al. Blunt thoracic trauma. Analysis of 515 patients. Ann Surg 1987; 206(2):200–5.

61. Parmley LF, Mattingly TW, Manion WC. Penetrating wounds of the heart and aorta. Circulation 1958; 17(5):953–73.

62. Fabian TC, Davis KA, Gavant ML et al. Prospective study of blunt aortic injury: helical CT is diagnostic and antihypertensive therapy reduces rupture. Ann Surg 1998; 227(5):666–76; discussion 676–7.

63. Melnitchouk S, Pfammatter T, Kadner A et al. Emergency stent-graft placement for hemorrhage control in acute thoracic aortic rupture. Eur J Cardiothorac Surg 2004; 25(6):1032–8.

64. Waldenberger P, Fraedrich G, Mallouhi A et al. Emergency endovascular treatment of traumatic aortic arch rupture with multiple arch vessel involvement. J Endovasc Ther 2003; 10(4):728–32.

65. Fattori R, Napoli G, Lovato L et al. Descending thoracic aortic diseases: stent-graft repair. Radiology 2003; 229(1):176–83.

66. Hinchliffe RJ, Krasznai A, Schultzekool L et al. Observations on the failure of stent-grafts in the aortic arch. Eur J Vasc Endovasc Surg 2007; 34(4):451–6.

# 15

# Renal and intestinal vascular disease

Trevor Cleveland
Jonathan G. Moss
Philip Kalra
Michael Dialynas
Celia Riga
Nicholas Cheshire

## Renal artery disease

Renal artery stenosis is an anatomical description of a lesion that may represent a variety of pathophysiological disease processes or that may simply be silent throughout life. The pathological entity in the vast majority of patients in the Western world is atherosclerosis and the term 'atherosclerotic renovascular disease' has been coined. The remainder are mainly represented by fibromuscular dysplasia, which has little in common with its atherosclerotic counterpart, as well as by manifestations of systemic vasculitis.

### Fibromuscular dysplasia (FMD)

FMD is a non-inflammatory, non-atherosclerotic disorder that may be observed in almost any arterial bed and can lead to arterial stenosis. Five different types are recognised and usually affect younger patients with a female predominance, involving the distal main artery and/or the intrarenal branches. Rarely it may be complicated by a renal artery aneurysm. Patients may be asymptomatic but the most usual presentation is hypertension. Even though hypertension is commonly treated successfully with medication, and renal artery stenosis and renal dysfunction may progress in up to one-third of patients, this almost never leads to occlusion, and complete loss of renal function is exceptional. An abdominal bruit may be present. Magnetic resonance angiography (MRA) can detect fibromuscular disease in the proximal vessels, but is less sensitive for visualising the second- and third-order branches where fibromuscular disease can be located. The diagnosis will usually require conventional digital subtraction angiography. Selective angiographic views may be necessary to detect subtle branch lesions. When treating FMD, the results of percutaneous angioplasty (PTA) are good, with 10-year cumulative patency rates of 87% and up to 50% of patients cured of their hypertension, the remainder having a reduced drug burden and improved blood pressure control.[1] Stenting is usually reserved for suboptimal PTA or flow-limiting dissection.

### Arteritis

Involvement of the renal artery is not uncommon in systemic vasculitis. Polyarteritis nodosa, Wegener's granulomatosis, microscopic polyarteritis, Churg–Strauss syndrome as well as hypersensitivity vasculitides can affect the renal vessels. The diagnosis can be difficult and in the absence of other systemic symptoms may require a renal biopsy. Takayasu's arteritis is a non-specific inflammatory disease that mainly affects large arteries such as the aorta and its main branches including the renal artery, and is the most common cause of renovascular hypertension in India and China. The majority of patients can be managed medically on corticosteroids, with monitoring of disease activity using the erythrocyte sedimentation rate (ESR). In the chronic inactive stage, PTA can produce a reasonable blood pressure response.[2]

## Atherosclerotic renal vascular disease

### Definition and pathology

Atherosclerotic stenosis is the most common pathological condition of the renal arteries, affecting 1–5% of patients with hypertension.[3] Hypertension is common and by extrapolation there are 2–4 million individuals with renal artery stenosis (RAS) in the USA alone. Because occlusion of the renal artery is present in up to 50% of patients, the condition is best described as atherosclerotic renovascular disease (ARVD) rather than as RAS. Autopsy data demonstrate that the incidence of ARVD increases with age, affecting 18% of individuals between the ages 65 and 74 years and >40% of those over 75 years.[4] Medicare data from America indicate that ARVD has an incidence of 3.9 cases per 1000 of the population over 65 years.[5] Usually, ARVD is a manifestation of generalised atherosclerosis involving multiple vessels; however, in 15–20% of cases, ARVD is not associated with disease elsewhere.

Widespread atheroma is usually present in the aorta and typically compromises the proximal 1–2 cm of one or both renal arteries. If untreated, atherosclerotic stenosis progresses to renal artery occlusion in up to 50% of patients[6] and permanent loss of the renal parenchyma in 15–25% of patients, particularly in the elderly.[7] The exact level of angiographic stenosis that represents significant ARVD is controversial and varies between 50% and 75% in diameter loss. Large animal experiments have demonstrated a significant pressure gradient across a stenosis of 60%;[8] however, in humans a lesion even less than 50% can be associated with gradients of 15 mmHg.[9]

### Pathophysiology

#### Hypertension

The pathophysiology of hypertension differs in patients with unilateral and bilateral RAS. In both, a drop in renal perfusion pressure distal to the lesion induces an increase in the activity of the renin–angiotensin–aldosterone system (RAAS). Vasoconstriction as well as salt and water retention contribute to the initial rise in systemic blood pressure, which tends to increase perfusion pressure of the poststenotic kidney towards normal. In patients with unilateral disease, perfusion pressure also rises in the contralateral, non-stenotic kidney, inducing a pressure natriuresis response. Salt and water excretion increase in the non-stenotic kidney, promoting a return of extracellular volume towards normal. Initially, therefore, patients may experience marked reductions in blood pressure in response to RAAS blockade.

In patients with bilateral RAS, however, the increase in systemic pressure is never transmitted to a kidney, there is no pressure natriuresis, and salt and water retention can persist. Systemic hypertension and volume expansion return renal perfusion pressure toward normal, suppressing activity of the RAAS, and RAAS-blocking drugs may fail to reduce blood pressure effectively in these patients. Regardless of whether the disease is unilateral or bilateral, revascularisation may fail to cure hypertension, especially when the stenosis is long-standing.

#### Renal function

Existing consensus suggests that ARVD is an association, rather than the cause of the majority of cases of chronic and end-stage renal failure.[10] A haemodynamically significant RAS will lead to a reduction in renal artery perfusion pressure and a subsequent impairment of renal function simply due to a hydraulic effect in only a minority of patients. Most commonly, renin and angiotensin levels are increased in the poststenotic kidney, constricting the postglomerular efferent arteriole, which, in turn, helps to support glomerular capillary hydraulic pressure and filtration rate. This might explain why the use of RAAS-blocking agents such as angiotensin-converting enzyme (ACE) inhibitors is controversial in the management of ARVD. As glomerular perfusion in these patients is critically dependent upon angiotensin II, the risk of developing acute renal failure is significant, especially if the stenosis is bilateral or affects a solitary functioning kidney. Nonetheless, RAAS-blocking drugs are the only agents proven to slow progression to end-stage renal disease, and acute deterioration in renal function is usually immediately reversible on cessation of treatment without long-term adverse effects.

Cholesterol embolisation may cause acute renal failure in renovascular disease. Patients with severe aortic atheroma undergoing arterial surgical or angiographic procedures, thrombolysis or anticoagulation are at a significant risk of developing renal dysfunction secondary to cholesterol emboli. Associated clinical features include purpuric skin rash, proteinuria and eosinophilia. Proteinuria appears to be a key marker of renal histopathological damage in patients with ARVD and a recent prospective study has shown that it can be the main predictor of future deterioration in function.[11]

Studies in large cohorts of patients with ARVD have shown that there is often poor correlation between the degree of anatomic atheromatous stenosis, glomerular filtration rate (GFR) and overall renal function.[12,13] Patients with unilateral ARVD can have GFRs that range from normal to stage 5 kidney disease. Nuclear studies in patients with unilateral stenosis reveal that GFR is the same or even lower in the non-stenotic kidney as in the kidney distal to the stenosis. This lack of correlation between the severity of renal ischaemic injury and kidney function may explain why renal function often fails to improve significantly after revascularisation despite restoration of renal artery patency. Additional factors such as hypertensive damage, cholesterol atheroembolism, intrarenal vascular disease and focal segmental or global sclerosing glomerular lesions have been shown to contribute to renal parenchymal injury.

## ARVD and cardiovascular disease

There is an extremely high incidence of adverse cardiovascular events in patients with ARVD as compared with age-matched subjects with normal renal arteries. ARVD is present in 33–44% of patients with peripheral vascular disease and 38% of those found to have an abdominal aortic aneurysm.[14,15] In an autopsy series of 346 cases of brain infarcts, RAS was found in 10.4% and carotid artery stenosis in 33.6% of subjects.[16]

In a large group of patients in whom renal arteriography was performed at the time of cardiac catheterisation, 15% of patients were found to have significant RAS (>50% luminal narrowing) with a similar proportion having lesser degrees of RAS. Those with RAS had a much higher incidence of adverse cardiovascular events as compared with patients without ARVD. There was also a direct correlation between the degree of stenosis and overall survival rates. Patients with >95% narrowing had only an approximately 40% 4-year survival as compared with 80% in those with normal arteries. These findings were independent of whether or not the patients subsequently underwent revascularisation.[17,18]

Sudden-onset left heart failure in patients with no previous cardiac history and well-preserved overall cardiac function, also known as 'flash' pulmonary oedema, is a well-documented manifestation of ARVD. It affects over 10% of patients, especially those with evidence of bilateral RAS.[19]

A reasonable explanation for the increased risk of adverse cardiovascular events in ARVD is that the cardiovascular morbidity and mortality seen in this group of patients may be attributable to concomitant atherosclerosis found in other parts of the arterial tree, including the coronary and cerebral circulations.

## Diagnosis and presentation

The gold standard for diagnosing RAS is renal arteriography. Non-invasive tests are also used in the diagnosis of RAS, the choice of test based on local expertise and patient factors. MRA has been increasingly used in the evaluation of RAS. The use of contrast-enhanced MRA has improved the ability to visualise any accessory renal vessel. It is, however, important to note that for patients with moderate to severe renal disease the administration of some gadolinium contrast agents during MRA has been linked with the development of nephrogenic systemic fibrosis (NSF).

Assessing the clinical index of suspicion remains essential in determining an appropriate diagnostic and therapeutic strategy in ARVD. Specific clinical pointers include:

- hypertension;
- renal impairment;
- concominant cardiovascular disease;
- ACE-induced acute renal impairment;
- 'flash' pulmonary oedema;
- vascular bruits.

## Management options

Patients with ARVD will require both medical therapy and cosideration of revascularisation.

Definite indications for renal revascularisation are:

- recurrent flash pulmonary oedema;
- refractory hypertension;
- dialysis-dependent acute renal failure (in such patients there is little to be lost and much potentially to be gained by intervention).

Less certain indications are:

- those with ACE inhibitor-related uraemia who require ACE inhibitor treatment for cardiac disease;
- those with deteriorating renal function with bilateral RAS (or RAS in a solitary kidney);
- clinically stable patients with high-grade RAS.

### Medical therapy

Optimal medical management of patients with ARVD is not established; however, by analogy to patients with disease in other vascular beds, it should include tight blood pressure control, antiplatelet therapy, cholesterol management, adequate glycaemic control in diabetics, smoking cessation, diet and exercise (see Chapter 1). It should be noted that the addition of statin therapy to patients with RAS is associated with a reduced likelihood of the progression of the stenosis.[20]

*Antihypertensive therapy*

Although antihypertensive therapy is proven to be effective in preventing adverse events in patients with essential hypertension, there are no data on its effects on outcomes in patients with ARVD. Based on Joint National Committee on Prevention, Detection, Evaluation, and Treatment of High Blood Pressure VII recommendations, a target blood pressure of <140/90 mmHg is recommended for individuals without other comorbidities, whereas a lower goal of <130/80 mmHg is recommended for patients with hypertension and diabetes or renal disease with significant proteinuria. Most patients will require combinations of several antihypertensive agents to achieve optimal blood pressure control. Surprisingly, RAAS-blocking agents are the first-line antihypertensive choices in patients with ARVD, especially those with evidence of chronic parenchymal disease. Patients should be closely monitored for elevations in serum creatinine and potassium concentrations, particularly in the cases of bilateral RAS or in a solitary kidney.

### Endovascular therapy

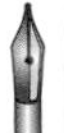

Stenting is now the first line of treatment in atherosclerotic RAS and has effectively replaced PTA in the vast majority of patients.

In patients at risk of contrast-induced nephropathy, alternative contrast agents such as carbon dioxide are available. In comparison to surgical techniques for revascularisation, renal stenting is a relatively simple procedure and less hazardous, although careful peri-interventional care is necessary.

*Work-up and postprocedure care*

As noted above, contrast-enhanced MRA had all but replaced other imaging techniques until the association with NSF was recognised. MRA provides the information required prior to renal artery stenting[21] (**Fig. 15.1**a,b). If a patient has an estimated GFR of <60 mL/min, then computed tomography angiography (CTA) should be considered, which carries the more benign risk of contrast-induced nephrotoxicity. If both MRA and CTA are contraindicated, then $CO_2$ angiography should be used. Determining the angle of origin of the renal arteries prior to the procedure allows optimal positioning of the fluoroscopic C arm and accurate placement of the renal stent (which should be placed to cover the renal ostium and protrude 1–3 mm into the aorta). Kidney size will also determine whether the patient will benefit from stenting. Kidneys less than 8 cm in length are generally unsuitable for revascularisation. Patients should be adequately hydrated at least 12 hours before and 12 hours following the procedure with intravenous fluids.[22] There is some evidence that administration of *N*-acetylcysteine reduces the incidence of contrast nephropathy and although the results of randomised controlled trials have been somewhat conflicting, many centres use it routinely.[23] Patients should receive antiplatelet therapy such as aspirin or clopidogrel for life, and be closely followed up for changes in renal function and blood pressure control.

*Procedure (Fig. 15.1c,d)*

Via a femoral approach (suitable for most cases), a 7Fr renal double-curve guiding catheter, or 5F similarly shaped sheath, is introduced into the abdominal aorta. The renal artery is cannulated directly from the guide catheter using a 0.014–0.018 inch wire. This allows for usage of low-profile systems for predilatation and stent placement. Vasospasm can be prevented with administration of vasodilators such as glyceryl trinitrate through the catheter. Balloon-expandable stents are now widely used as they are easier to position accurately to achieve full renal ostium coverage.

Cholesterol embolisation may occur at the time of renal artery stenting,[24] and some authors advocate the use of embolic protection devices.[25–27] None of the present devices are designed for renal intervention and may add to the complexity of the procedure.

*Complications*

For renal PTA/stenting the literature quotes complication rates ranging from 0% to 66%.[28] Major complications include:

- acute deterioration in renal function (usually secondary to contrast nephropathy);
- cholesterol embolisation (insidious onset, elevated ESR, eosinophilia, livedo reticularis rash);
- renal artery perforation (rare) – should this occur, it can usually be treated either by balloon tamponade or a stentgraft.

Most complications can be avoided by the use of low-profile systems, adequate hydration, closure devices, experienced operators and optimisation of patients prior to treatment.

*Results of angioplasty and stenting*

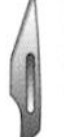

A recent meta-analysis[29] compared the results of PTA (10 articles, 644 patients) with stenting (14 articles, 678 patients). None were randomised controlled trials. Stent placement had a higher technical success rate and lower re-stenosis rate than PTA and the complication rate was similar for both techniques. The cure rate for

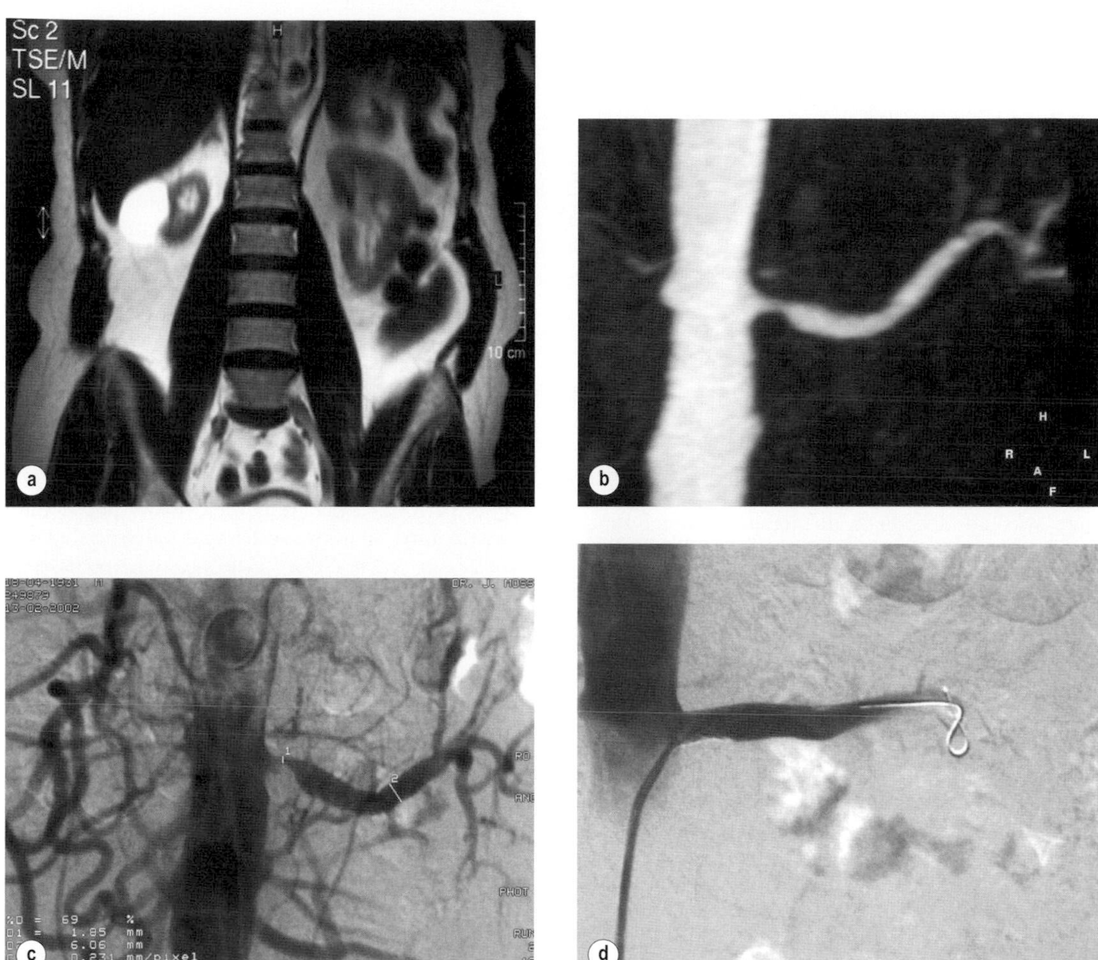


**Figure 15.1 • (a)** Magnetic resonance scan shows a small right kidney containing a cyst. **(b)** Magnetic resonance angiogram demonstrates an osteal stenosis of the left renal artery and an occluded right renal artery. **(c)** Conventional catheter angiogram at the time of treatment confirms these findings. **(d)** A stent has been placed at the ostium of the left renal artery.

hypertension was higher (20% vs. 10%) and the improvement rate for renal function was lower (30% vs. 38%) after stent placement compared with PTA.

At the present time there are only four published clinical trials that have tried to clarify the place of endovascular procedures in patients with ARVD, but all involved only relatively small patient numbers.

Van Jaarsveld et al.[30] randomised 106 patients with RAS of greater than 50% and significant hypertension (but only mild to moderate renal impairment; creatinine <200 μmol/L) to angioplasty or medical therapy. No differences were noted in the primary end-point of blood pressure control or in renal function. The other two trials incorporated a similar design but contained only 49 and 55 patients.[31,32] There are two published meta-analyses of the above trials.[33,34]

Both come to the same conclusion, namely that the effect of PTA on hypertension is at best modest and that none of these small trials were powered to detect changes in renal function. A moderate but clinically worthwhile benefit could not be excluded and further large-scale randomised trials are required. Two such trials (ASTRAL and STAR) are currently recruiting patients. Finally, a single randomised controlled trial has compared PTA with stenting in 85 patients with ostial lesions.[35] The technical success rate of stents was superior to PTA (88% vs. 55%) and the primary 6-month patency likewise superior (75% vs. 29%). The trial was stopped following an interim analysis of the data. The clinical outcomes in the two groups were similar, although the study was not powered to detect differences in blood pressure or renal function.

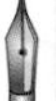

Very few radiologists would now use PTA alone for ostial atherosclerotic RAS.

(**Editor's note:** At the time of going to press the results of ASTRAL were starting to appear online. The trial randomised 806 patients in 56 centres to either best medical therapy or best medical therapy plus stenting for ARVD. Patients were randomised if they had at least one treatable renal artery and clinicians were in equipoise. The clinical status of the patients was heterogeneous and included hypertension and renal failure. At 1 year after treatment there was no difference in change in renal function, blood pressure control or rate of cardiovascular event, although at 4 years there was a trend towards better outcomes after RAS. Whilst the published outcomes are awaited, it will be interesting to witness how data from such a heterogeneous group of patients will, in time, affect the use of RAS.)

#### *Re-stenosis*

Re-stenosis is not such a major issue as in other vascular territories, presumably due to the relatively large-calibre (5–8 mm) vessel and high blood flow. Figures vary but a re-stenosis rate of 15% at 6 months seems realistic.[35] When re-stenosis does occur it is often clinically silent and requires no treatment. Consequently there is very little research on renal stent re-stenosis rates. The GREAT trial[36] compared sirolimus-eluting stents with bare metal stents in a small ($n$ = 106) non-randomised trial. Results showed a trend favouring sirolimus-eluting stents but none of the measures reached statistical significance, possibly due to underpowering.

### Surgical treatment

There are a range of surgical options available to treat renal artery disease (Box 15.1). Current guidelines recommend surgery in patients with ARVD who have indications for revascularisation and have multiple small renal arteries or require aortic reconstruction near the renal arteries for other indications (e.g. aneurysm, severe aortoiliac occlusive disease). The site of the lesion is also important, and if extra-anatomical bypass is considered, the condition of the donor visceral vessels must be optimal. In patients with renal artery occlusion, renal biopsy (performed either preoperatively or perioperatively) can indicate whether the kidney is viable and functionally salvageable on the basis of collateral vessels. The presence of extensive glomerular hyalinisation usually precludes revascularisation. However, this procedure is not without risk of bleeding and even the loss of a kidney.[37] Endarterectomy and bypass grafting are the two main surgical options for revascularisation.

Nephrectomy is the oldest surgical procedure used in the treatment of ARVD. In the presence of a normal contralateral kidney, it remains the option of choice if the affected kidney measures less than 8 cm. In this situation measurement of renal vein renin levels is of value, with nephrectomy being indicated when the ratio of renal vein renins is greater than 1.5.

In the presence of aortic aneurysmal disease affecting the renal ostium, aortic graft and renal bypass is indicated. This involves a 6–8 mm limb of Dacron and polytetrafluoroethylene (PTFE) sutured onto the aortic graft with an end-to-end renal anastomosis. Where bilateral RAS is present, an inverted bifurcated Dacron graft is preferred. Transaortic endarterectomy may be performed via a transverse or a trapdoor anterolateral aortic incision, and 5-year patencies in large centres can reach 90%.[38] The ostial lesion is then carefully endarterectomised and the procedure is completed with patch closure (**Fig. 15.2**).

Extra-anatomical bypass grafting is an attractive option for patients with unilateral RAS in the absence of significant aortic disease. Access is obtained via a simple subcostal incision, without the need for aortic cross-clamping or extensive dissection, and revascularisation is achieved using inflow from either the hepatic or splenic artery (**Fig. 15.3**a). An interposition saphenous vein graft may be used where there is insufficient arterial calibre and length for an end-to-end anastomosis (Fig. 15.3b). The inferior vena cava, the right renal vein and often the left renal vein must be fully mobilised. On the left side, the splenic artery is dissected from its midpoint from the pancreas. Splenectomy can be avoided as there is a rich collateral supply and perfusion via the short gastric arteries. The Cleveland clinic reports 175 extra-anatomical bypass procedures over a 12-year period,[39] with 2.9% operative mortality. Graft patency reached 96%, renal function improved in 40% and hypertension was improved or cured in three-quarters of the series.

Aortorenal bypass can be simply carried out using the long saphenous vein, PTFE, Dacron or rarely the internal iliac artery. The infrarenal aorta is preferred as an inflow site if it is relatively disease free. If not, then a 'rooftop' incision is necessary in order to expose the aorta above the coeliac axis. The thoracic aorta can

**Box 15.1** • Surgical revascularisation

Aortic graft and renal bypass
Aortorenal bypass
Aortorenal endarterectomy
Extra-anatomical bypass
Extracorporeal bench surgery

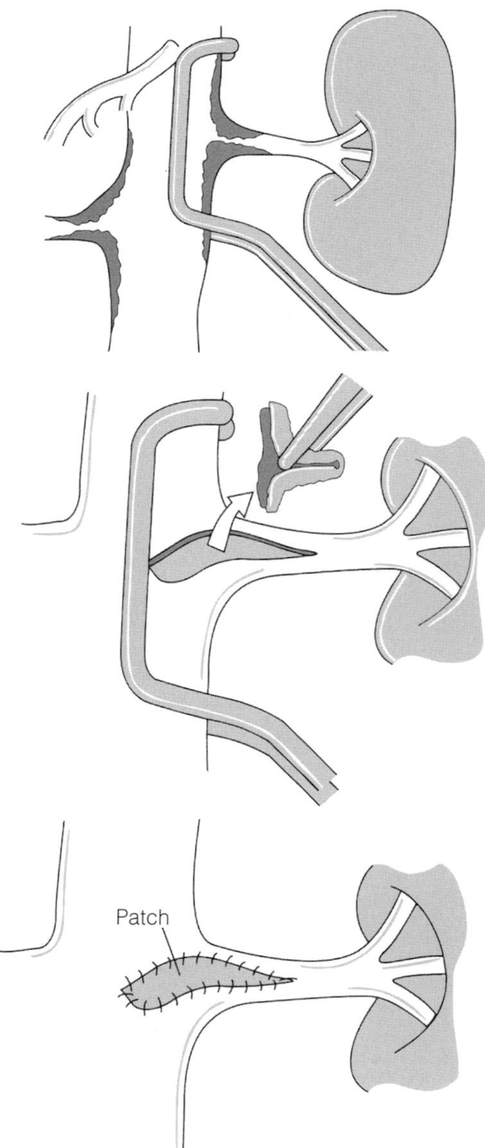


**Figure 15.2** • Transaortic renal endarterectomy with patch closure.

also be used as an inflow site. Where multiple small anastomoses are required, extracorporeal or bench surgery is performed for patients with disease affecting renal artery branches. Removal of the kidney, cooling and preservation as in renal transplantation surgery will allow multiple microvascular anastomoses to be performed before autotransplantation takes place. The internal iliac artery is commonly used for direct end-to-end anastomosis. Prefashioned branch saphenous vein grafts or the inferior epigastric artery can also be used. The Cleveland clinic again has the largest reported series of autotransplanation, with excellent long-term results.[37]

Surgical revascularisation is considered to be a high-risk option when compared to less invasive treatment methods. Reported results are shown in Table 15.1.[40–46] However, the quoted morbidity and mortality rates have set the standards against which other treatment modalities can be compared. There have been no large trials to date comparing the outcomes of stenting with surgical revascularisation in ARVD. In young, fit patients surgery may be preferred as it is cost-effective and the long-term re-stenosis rate is reported to be 3–4%. The management of ARVD can be complex and certainly requires a multidisciplinary approach to maximise the therapeutic potential for each individual patient.

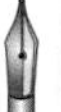
Stenting should be used as the primary mode of revascularisation as it is minimally invasive, reserving surgery for stent failure or more complex aortic and renal pathology.

# Intestinal vascular disease

Visceral arterial pathology, in common with any arterial disease, falls into two main categories: occlusive and aneurysmal disease. Intestinal ischaemia and visceral aneurysms are uncommon but potentially life-threatening conditions. Despite recent advances in therapeutic techniques and diagnostic tools, their management remains clinically challenging. Significant questions exist with regard to the optimal therapeutic choice and the predictors of clinical outcome. Surgery is the conventional treatment. The endovascular approach is an emerging option and the results have been constantly improving. Mesenteric venous thrombosis, non-occlusive mesenteric ischaemia and iatrogenic bowel ischaemia are all acute syndromes and will be discussed.

## Intestinal ischaemia

Mesenteric ischaemia results from hypoperfusion of the gut, most commonly due to occlusion, thrombosis or vasospasm. The clinical consequences depend upon the number of vessels affected, the adequacy of collateral circulation and the duration of the insult. Early diagnosis and treatment are imperative, otherwise outcomes can be catastrophic.

### Acute mesenteric ischaemia (AMI)

#### Aetiology and incidence

AMI can result from acute occlusion of the superior mesenteric artery (SMA; embolism, thrombosis or iatrogenic) or non-occlusive ischaemia secondary to inadequate mesenteric arterial blood flow and oxygenation. The commonest cause of AMI is embolic occlusion of the SMA (50% of all cases). Such emboli are usually cardiac in origin, but may arise

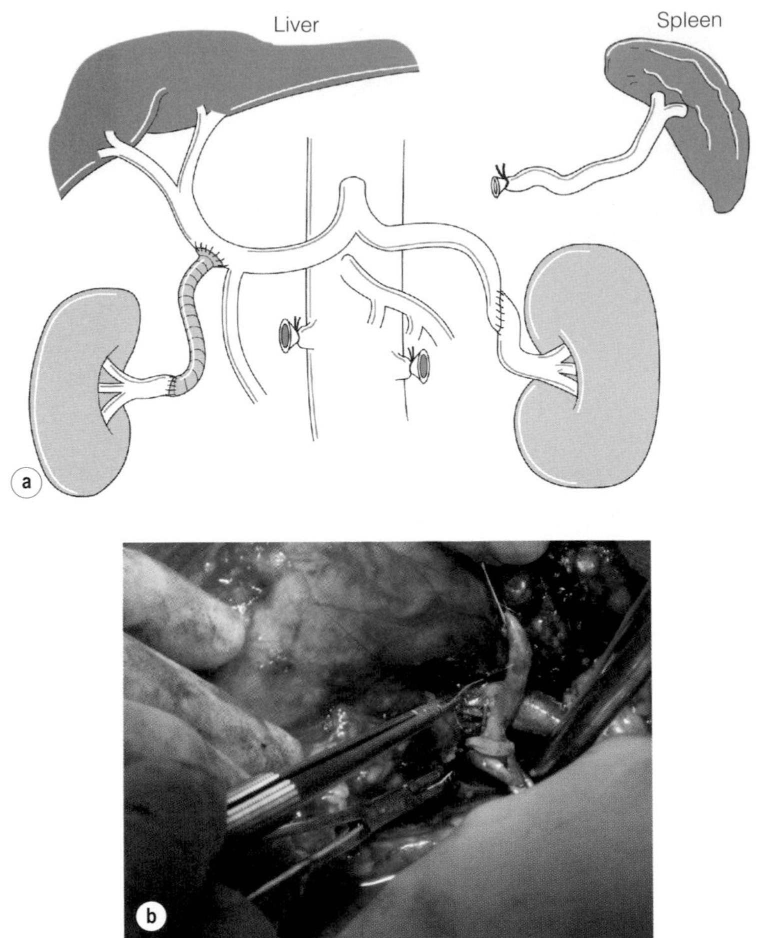


**Figure 15.3 • (a)** Extra-anatomical renal revascularisation from the hepatic or splenic arteries. **(b)** Hepatorenal bypass using the long saphenous vein.

**Table 15.1** • Reported results of surgical revascularisation

| | | |
|---|---|---|
| Benjamin et al. (1996)[40]<br>Dean (1997)[41] | Treatment of hypertension (cure or improvement) | 63–91% |
| Benjamin et al. (1996)[40]<br>Reilly et al. (1996)[42] | Treatment of renal failure (cure or improvement) | 33–91% |
| Steinbach et al. (1997)[43]<br>Darling et al. (1995)[44]<br>Novick et al. (1987)[45] | Primary patency rates | 93–97% |
| Darling et al. (1995)[44] | Morbidity | 6–43% |
| Reilly et al. (1996)[42]<br>Steinbach et al. (1997)[43]<br>Cambria et al. (1996)[46] | Mortality | 2–8% |

from atherosclerotic plaques or from arterial aneurysms. Acute disruption of the visceral arterial flow can occur during endovascular manipulation as a result of inadvertent plaque dislodgement and embolisation or accidental occlusion of the visceral artery origin with an endograft. Left colon ischaemia can also occur after aortic reconstruction.[47] The majority of emboli progress distally to the tapered segment of the SMA just past the origin of the middle colic artery. In 20% of cases, a pre-existing atherosclerotic lesion at the origin of the vessel will lead to visceral artery thrombosis. Most of these patients are female and have evidence of symptomatic vascular disease at other sites and have often previously undergone vascular interventions. Half of them have symptoms of chronic mesenteric ischaemia. Non-occlusive ischaemia caused during periods of low cardiac output and shock accounts for another 20% of cases.[48] A Swedish population-based study identified 997 cases of intestinal ischaemia using a clinical autopsy database. Fatal heart failure was the leading cause of intestinal hypoperfusion, although stenosis of the SMA and coeliac trunk, atrial fibrillation and recent surgery contributed significantly.[49] Other unusual arteriopathies, such as Takayasu's arteritis, fibromuscular dysplasia and polyarteritis nodosa, may first present with intestinal ischaemia. Isolated dissections of the SMA have also been reported, although more commonly it originates in the descending thoracic aorta and extends into the SMA.

### Pathophysiology

Intrinsic and extrinsic mechanisms are involved in the regulation of mesenteric blood flow. Intrinsic autoregulation of blood flow is most likely to involve direct arteriolar smooth muscle relaxation and metabolic response to adenosine and other metabolites of mucosal ischaemia. Extrinsic control is due to neural and humoral mechanisms. The intestine is able to compensate for a 75% acute reduction of blood flow for up to 12 hours without substantial injury. Extensive collateral circulation opens following occlusion of a major vessel. With prolonged ischaemic time, however, progressive vasoconstriction develops in the obstructed bed, increasing its pressure and reducing collateral flow. This vasoconstriction may persist even after restoration of flow, leading to continuing ischaemia. Ischaemia results in loss of mucosal barrier with translocation of bacteria, endotoxins and cytokines precipitating septicaemia and multiorgan failure. Ischaemic damage can also be caused by reperfusion injury, with the release of free radicals after successful reperfusion causing a pronounced inflammatory response.[50]

### Diagnosis and treatment

The classic presentation is with acute severe abdominal pain out of proportion to the physical signs. These patients are usually admitted with an acute abdomen. Left colon ischaemia following aortic reconstruction or aneurysm repair can present with watery diarrhoea (bloody or non-bloody) early in the postoperative period. These patients should all undergo urgent bedside colonoscopy. AMI can lead to sudden decompensation, and therefore a high index of suspicion and experience are required to avoid unnecessary delays in diagnosis and treatment. Mortality rates are high at 70–80%.[49] AMI is a true emergency, and confirmatory angiography should not delay treatment. Initial management includes volume resuscitation, correction of acidosis and intravenous antibiotics. Heparin anticoagulation should be started to prevent further propagation of thrombus. An emergency exploratory laparotomy is usually necessary.

Whilst reports exist of successful thrombolysis with percutaneous SMA angioplasty,[51] a laparotomy is still strongly advisable to assess bowel viability. The SMA is exposed and there often is a proximal SMA pulse if the cause is embolic. If the bowel is found to be viable, an embolectomy is performed via a transverse arteriotomy using a 3Fr Fogarty catheter. If a longitudinal arteriotomy is performed, it should be closed using a vein patch to prevent stenosis.

If the cause is thrombosis, no pulse is palpable in the SMA and surgical thromboembolectomy is unlikely to be successful or durable. A bypass graft distal to the occlusion is then required to restore arterial blood supply to the gut. This could be antegrade, taking inflow from the supracoeliac aorta, or retrograde from the infrarenal aorta or iliac arteries. Often the latter is chosen because the exposure is familiar and the risks associated with clamping and dissection are less.[52] If there is peritoneal contamination or extensive bowel gangrene, autologous vein as a conduit is preferable to a prosthetic graft. Caution, however, should be taken to avoid graft kinking and subsequent occlusion. Time should be allowed for reperfusion before assessing the bowel for viability. Necrotic bowel needs to be resected. Exteriorisation of the bowel with a planned second-look laparotomy and delayed bowel anastomosis is a safe option. Postoperatively, patients with emboli should be anticoagulated and those with evidence of atherosclerotic disease should receive optimal medical therapy and risk factor management.

Long-term patient outcomes depend on the cardiovascular status, underlying disease and extent of the bowel ischaemia. There have been no recent improvements in the diagnosis and treatment of AMI, and mortality rates remain high.

## Mesenteric venous thrombosis

This syndrome is rare and accounts for 5–15% of all cases of acute mesenteric ischaemia. It can be primary or secondary, following hypercoagulable states, portal venous stasis, intra-abdominal inflammation, infection, malignancy and oral contraceptive use (4–5% of all cases). Up to 75% of patients with mesenteric venous thrombosis have an inherited thrombotic disorder, the most common being factor V Leiden mutation. Conditions associated with acquired hypercoagulable states that are associated with mesenteric venous thrombosis are paroxysmal nocturnal haemoglobinuria and the myeloproliferative syndromes. Diagnosis is often delayed due to the absence of specific signs, symptoms and laboratory findings. Contrast-enhanced computed tomography (CT) can reveal the extent of thrombus, air in the mesenteric vein or portal system and the presence or absence of collateral flow. Unfortunately, the diagnosis is most commonly made at laparotomy or autopsy. Infarcted bowel should be resected and long-term anticoagulation should be established early as recurrence rates are high.

## Non-occlusive mesenteric thrombosis

This syndrome develops in severe systemic illness in association with cardiorespiratory shock and multiorgan failure. Typically, these are patients on the intensive care unit with congestive cardiac failure or severe cardiac dysfunction and the use of inotropic agents may further aggravate the situation. The administration of digoxin and α-adrenergic agonists as well as cocaine have also been implicated. The diagnosis is made with a high index of clinical suspicion and can be confirmed by angiography. This will show intestinal arterial vasospasm and exclude an intrinsic arterial lesion. Treatment depends on optimising cardiac output, treating underlying conditions such as sepsis and, where possible, removing adverse pharmacological agents such as the inotropes. In severe cases, intramesenteric arterial infusion of papaverine at a dose of 30–60 mg/hour is beneficial. Glucagon (2–4 mg/hour) will increase splanchnic blood flow and has the advantage of being given intravenously. However, mortality in this condition remains high at 70–80% despite these therapies.

## Chronic mesenteric ischaemia (CMI)

### Aetiology and incidence

CMI is the result of progressive atherosclerosis in more than 90% of cases. There is a significant gender difference, with females been affected in 76% of cases.[53] Half of the patients have significant coronary artery disease and/or peripheral arterial occlusive disease. Non-atherosclerotic causes of CMI are unusual and include thrombosis associated with thoracoabdominal aneurysms, aortic coarcation, aortic dissection, Takayasu's arteritis, systemic lupus erythematosus, polyarteritis nodosa, rheumatoid arthritis, fibromuscular hyperplasia, neurofibromatosis, radiation injury, cocaine abuse, Buerger's disease and extrinsic coeliac artery compression by the median arcuate ligament. Despite the frequency of visceral artery stenosis, symptomatic chronic intestinal ischaemia is rare because of the excellent collateral circulatory network between the main visceral arteries, namely the coeliac trunk, superior mesenteric and the inferior mesenteric arteries, and the systemic circulation (**Fig. 15.4**).

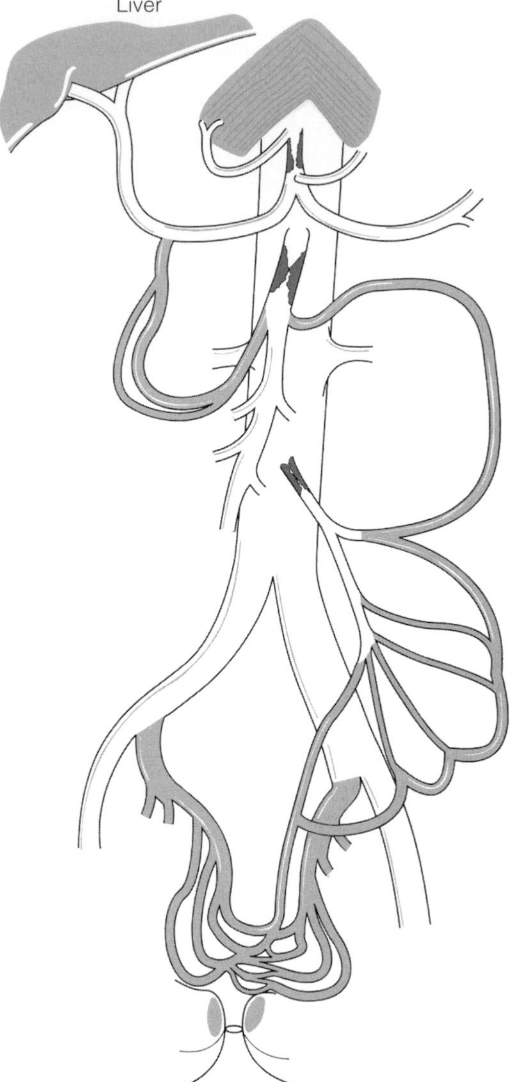


**Figure 15.4** • Collateral circulation of the intestine.

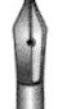

At least two of the three intestinal vessels must be stenotic or occluded for symptoms to occur,[53] and patients with single-vessel disease are rarely symptomatic.

### Diagnosis

Patients with visceral arterial insufficiency typically suffer from postprandial abdominal pain, which leads to food fear and progressive weight loss. This classical triad is only observed in half of the patients. The clinical picture can be quite non-specific and misdiagnosed for other conditions, such as gastritis, peptic ulcer disease, gastrointestinal malignancy and diverticular disease. Physical examination is also non-specific, although the manifestations of generalised atherosclerotis are very common and in up to 70% of the patients an abdominal bruit can be heard. The natural history is that of malnutrition, and progressive intestinal ischaemia may eventually lead to bowel infarction and death.

Until recently, catheter angiography was the only reliable method of assessing the splanchnic circulation in vivo. Newer techniques such as duplex ultrasound, gastrointestinal tonometry, CTA (**Fig. 15.5**) and magnetic resonance provide non-invasive or minimally invasive examination of the anatomy and function of the splanchnic circulation. As there is no effective medical treatment for CMI, its management is focused on restoration of blood flow.

### *Surgical intervention*

At present no information justifies visceral revascularisation for asymptomatic lesions except for patients with asymptomatic stenosis or occlusion of the SMA who need to undergo aortic surgery. Postoperative intestinal ischaemia can be prevented by grafting the SMA during the aortic procedure. Reconstruction of the inferior mesenteric artery should be strongly considered for those who have occlusion of all three major visceral trunks.

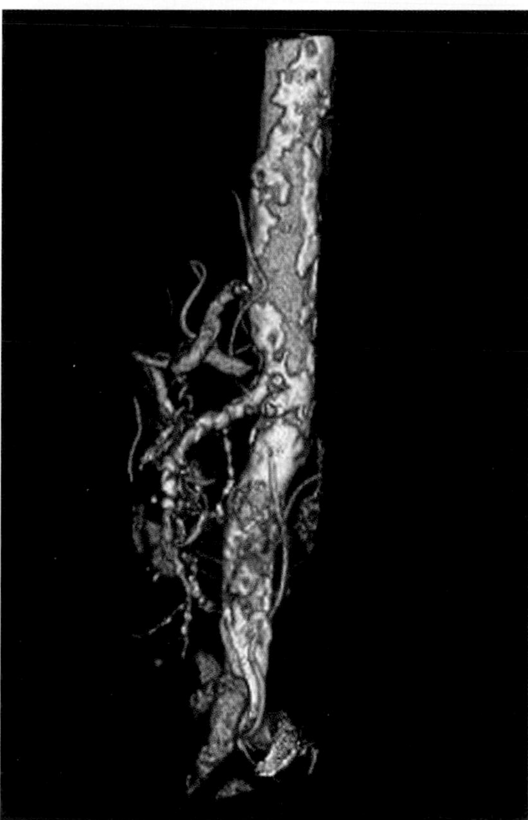

**Figure 15.5** • Reconstructed CT angiogram showing a tight coeliac artery stenosis and heavy aortic wall calcification, affecting the origins of the coeliac and superior mesenteric arteries.

Patients with symptomatic CMI benefit from surgical intervention but it is associated with greater risk of haemorrhage and death than other elective vascular procedures. The in-hospital mortality reaches 12.2%, with a postoperative complication rate of 54% including revascularisation syndrome.[54]

Current surgical techniques usually involve revascularisation of the stenotic or occluded mesenteric vessels using autologous or prosthetic grafts, although the precise configurations remain contraversial. Inflow may be from the supracoeliac aorta or distal thoracic aorta (antegrade reconstruction) or from the infrarenal aorta or the common iliac artery (retrograde reconstruction). Outflow may be either a single-vessel repair to only the coeliac or more commonly to the SMA, or as a multivessel repair. Hollier et al. showed that complete revascularisation in multivessel disease resulted in late recurrence of 11%, while revascularisation of one of the three stenotic vessels resulted in a 50% recurrence rate. They concluded that it is preferable to revascularise as many vessels as possible so that single-vessel thrombosis does not result in bowel infarction.[54] In contrast, Gentile et al. believe that retrograde isolated bypass grafts to the SMA provide comparable long-term prevention of recurrence.[55] Antegrade bypasses have the advantage that the bypass is placed in the direction of the normal blood flow, thus reducing the anastomotic turbulence. This design eliminates the possibility of kinking and thrombosis by compression or traction from the overlying intestinal mesentery which might be observed in retrograde grafts. Early experience with retrograde bypasses with vein as a conduit showed frequent graft kinking and occlusion. This is avoided by using a reinforced prosthetic graft in a lazy loop configuration. Foley et al. reported a 79% primary-assisted patency rate after 9 years. Most of these grafts were done in a retrograde fashion to the SMA only.[56] Taylor et al. prefer to perform a retrograde bypass graft starting from the infrarenal aorta because of its familiar exposure and reduced risks with clamping and dissection. They have a 5-year patency rate of 96% with an operative mortality rate of 7%.[57] Kansal et al. suggest that the retrograde bypass might be preferable to the antegrade bypass in a number of situations, including patients in whom previous surgery might prohibit a safe dissection of the supracoeliac aorta, medically high-risk patients in whom a shorter operative time might be preferable and the need for simultaneous infrarenal aortic and mesenteric revascularisation.[58]

Since graft occlusion may result in acute mesenteric ischaemia, graft stenoses are of concern. Kazmers found symptomatic assessment of patients insufficient amd therefore recommended graft surveillance using duplex every 4–6 months.[52]

The primary patency of surgical reconstruction has not been matched to date by endovascular techniques.[58–60] Non-randomised comparative studies of surgical revascularisation versus endovascular treatment show better primary and primary-assisted patency rates,[61–63] fewer reinterventions[63] and lower rates of symptom recurrence[64] in favour of surgical bypass. However, the major disadvantage of conventional surgery remains the high perioperative mortality and morbidity.

#### Endovascular options

The endovascular option for treating this condition is attractive as the open operations are a major undertaking in a group of patients who are almost exclusively elderly and in whom there is significant comorbidity. In addition, the nature of chronic mesenteric ischaemia dictates that such patients are chronically undernourished, dehydrated and lacking in metabolic reserves. In such circumstances subjecting these patients to a major surgical procedure, with its associated catabolic consequences, makes little sense.

The technique, although theoretically simple, may be technically challenging because of the difficult angles and heavily calcified, often fully occluded, lesions. Arterial access is obtained and heparin is routinely administered to ensure anticoagulation during catheter manipulation. The target lesion is identified following a flush aortogram (**Fig. 15.6**). A guide wire is then manipulated across the stenosis and the decision of primary angioplasty or stenting is made. When stenting has been performed, the literature mostly describes the use of short balloon-mounted stents, allowing as short a stent possible to cover the lesion (**Fig. 15.7**a,b).

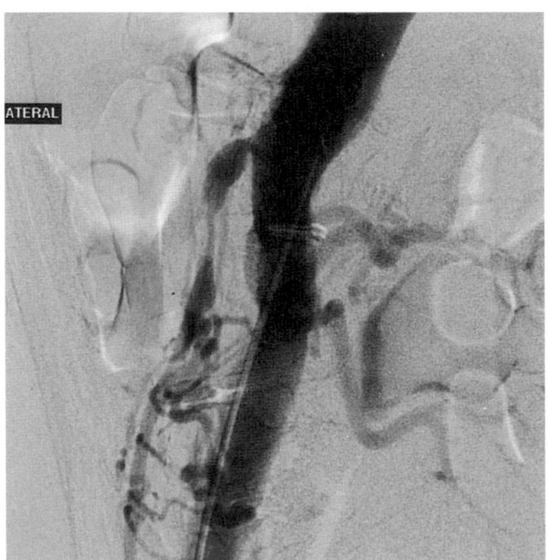


**Figure 15.6** • Catheter angiogram showing tandem tight superior mesenteric artery stenoses.

A recent series of 27 patients treated endovascularly showed a primary patency of 81% and a secondary patency of 100%.[65] Endovascular techniques are, however, limited by re-stenosis. The largest comparative series to date concluded that although the length of stay was reduced with endovascular treatment, stenting was associated with decreased primary patency, primary assisted patency and the need for earlier reintervention.[61] However, the reinterventions are generally of a less invasive nature than open procedures, and carry significantly reduced morbidity. In addition, patients treated endovascularly tend to be those with poorer overall prognosis, in whom long-term patency may be academic.

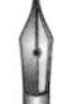

Vascular reconstruction may be more appropriate in younger and fitter patients, while endovascular treatment is preferable for the older, less fit, patients.

Most authors agree that the choice of treatment option should be selective.

#### Coeliac axis compression syndrome

External compression of the coeliac artery by the median arcuate ligament of the diaphragm may result in chronic mesenteric ischaemia and visceral artery aneurysm formation.[66] During inspiration, the aorta and coeliac axis move downward with the abdominal viscera. In expiration, the vessels move upwards and a maximal external compression on the coeliac artery occurs. Reilly et al. developed a group of positive and negative criteria to predict successful relief of symptoms with coeliac axis decompression: female gender, postprandial pain, age 40–60 years, profound weight loss, absence of a psychiatric or drug abuse history, arteriographic findings of coeliac artery decompression with post-stenotic dilatation or collateral flow.[67] The diagnosis remains one of exclusion. Surgical division of the arcuate ligament remains the only effective treatment.[68] This procedure can be performed laparoscopically and may be combined with coeliac artery stenting, which is a novel and attractive minimally invasive approach.[69] The debate regarding the clinical importance of this syndrome is compounded by the observation of recurrence after surgical treatment.[70]

## Visceral aneurysms

### Aetiology and incidence

Visceral artery aneurysms, whilst uncommon, are clinically important since 22% present as clinical emergencies, of which 8.5% result in death.[71] Although more than 3000 cases of visceral artery

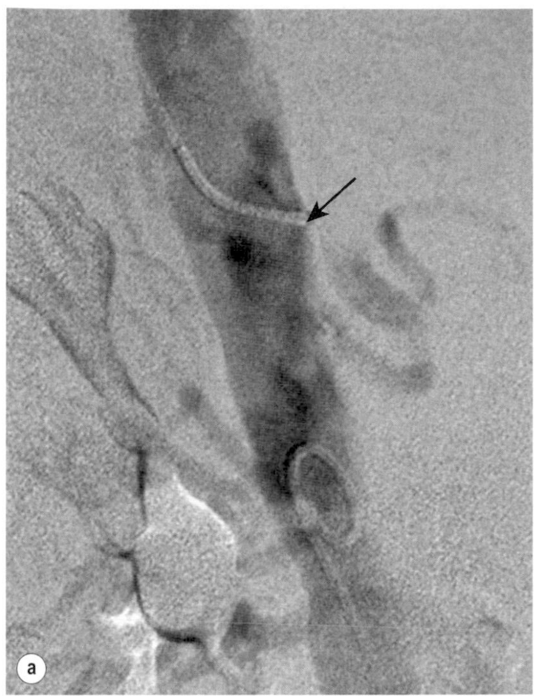

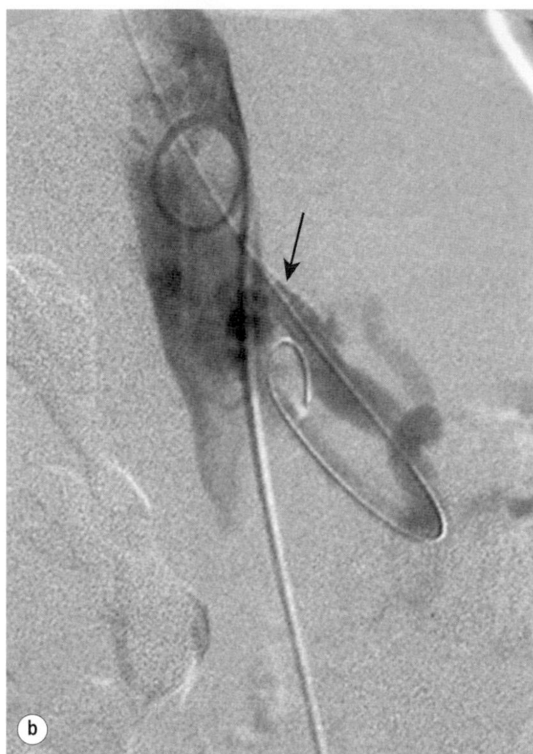

**Figure 15.7 • (a)** Angiogram showing a coeliac artery stenosis (arrow). **(b)** Angiogram after stenting of the stenosis (arrow).

aneurysms have been documented in the literature, their exact incidence is unknown. The natural history is one of expansion and eventual rupture. In the past, most visceral artery aneurysms were syphilitic or mycotic in origin, but today most true aneurysms are caused by atherosclerosis or medial degeneration, whereas false aneurysms are usually the result of trauma or inflammation (e.g. pancreatitis).[71] The clinical symptoms, natural history and mortality from visceral artery aneurysms vary depending on which vessels are involved.

Vessels affected, in descending order of involvement, include the splenic (60%), hepatic (20%), superior mesenteric (5.5%), coeliac (4%), gastric and gastroepiploic (4%), intestinal (3%), pancreaticoduodenal and pancreatic (2%), gastroduodenal (2%) and rarely inferior mesenteric arteries.[72] An example of a visceral aneurysm is shown in **Fig. 15.8.**

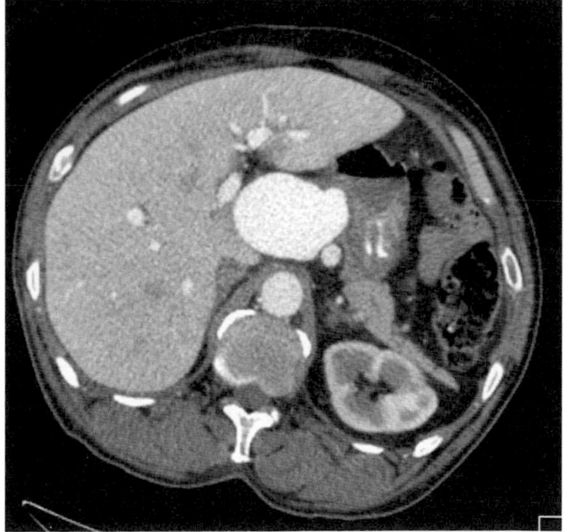

**Figure 15.8 •** CT angiogram showing a large gastric artery aneurysm.

## Diagnosis and treatment

Although in the past most visceral artery aneurysms were discovered at the time of rupture or at autopsy, many aneurysms are currently being recognised even in the asymptomatic state. This is mainly due to the greater availability of advanced imaging modalities.

Compared to other visceral aneurysms, SMA aneurysms are often symptomatic. This is due to their unique location near the origin of the pancreaticoduodenal and middle colic arteries. If dissection or occlusion of the aneurysm occurs, the distal mesenteric circulation will be isolated. Abdominal discomfort varies from mild to severe pain and in many is suggestive of intestinal angina. Gastrointestinal bleeding often associated with these lesions reflects their acute occlusion and bleeding from areas of intestinal infarction.[72]

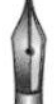

Modern treatment of splenic, hepatic and postinflammatory pseudoaneurysms is either by endoluminal embolisation or exclusion by placement of a stentgraft.[73,74]

Treatment is indicated to prevent catastrophic complications. Operative procedures include aneurysmorrhaphy or simple ligation.[70,72,75] Bypass reconstruction is seldom required using autologous vein or prosthetic graft.[76] Mortality associated with ruptured visceral artery aneurysms remain high, reaching 50%, whereas mortality from elective surgery is 5%.[76]

## Key points

**Renal disease**

- Angioplasty (PTA) is the procedure of choice for non-atheromatous lesions.
- The improvement of blood pressure control in non-atheromatous lesions is good to excellent following PTA.
- ARVD usually presents with hypertension, chronic renal failure, acute renal failure or pulmonary oedema. However, it is often asymptomatic and should not be forgotten in patients with extrarenal vascular disease.
- Stents have a higher technical success and patency rate compared with PTA in atheromatous ostial lesions.
- Surgery gives the lowest re-stenosis rates but should be reserved for stent failures or young fit patients.
- Improvement of blood pressure control in atheromatous lesions following stenting is marginal but may reduce the drug burden.
- Results in atheromatous patients with renal insufficiency following stenting are variable with no consensus.

**Intestinal ischaemia**

- Intestinal ischaemia is a rare condition that presents a major diagnostic and management challenge to the vascular specialist.
- Acute intestinal ischaemia remains a surgical emergency that should be treated by laparotomy, revascularisation and resection of dead bowel in most cases.
- Chronic intestinal ischaemia may be treated by surgical or endovascular methods. Endovascular techniques should be considered in poor-risk symptomatic patients and merit further objective assessment.

**Visceral aneurysms**

- Visceral artery aneurysms are uncommon but clinically important since 22% present as clinical emergencies, of which 8.5% result in death. Treatment is indicated to prevent catastrophic complications.

## References


1. de Fraissinette B, Garcier JM, Dieu V et al. Percutaneous transluminal angioplasty of dysplastic stenoses of the renal artery: results on 70 adults. Cardiovasc Intervent Radiol 2003; 26(1):46–51.
2. Tyagi S, Singh B, Kaul UA et al. Balloon angioplasty for renovascular hypertension in Takayasu's arteritis. Am Heart J 1993; 125:1386–93.
3. Rudnick KV, Sackett DL, Hirst S et al. Hypertension in a family practice. Can Med Assoc J 1997; 117(5):492–7.
4. Schwartz CJ, White TA. Stenosis of renal artery: an unselected necropsy study. Br Med J 1964; 2(5422):1415–21.
5. Kalra PA, Guo H, Kausz AT et al. Atherosclerotic renovascular disease in US medicare recipients aged 67 years or more: risk factors, revascularization and prognosis. Kidney Int 2005; 68(1):293–301.
6. Zierler RE, Bergelin RO, Isaacson JA et al. Natural history of atherosclerotic renal artery stenosis: a

prospective study with duplex ultrasonography. J Vasc Surg 1994; 19(2):250–7; discussion 257–8.

7. Herrera AH, Davidson RA. Renovascular disease in older adults. Clin Geriat Med 1998; 14(2):237–54.

8. Haimovici H, Zinicola N. Experimental renal-artery stenosis diagnostic significance of arterial hemodynamics. J Cardiovasc Surg 1962; 3:259–62.

9. Wasser MN, Westenberg J, van der Hulst VP et al. Hemodynamic significance of renal artery stenosis: digital subtraction angiography versus systolically gated three-dimensional phase-contrast MR angiography. Radiology 1997; 202(2):333–8.

10. Guo H, Kalra PA, Gilbertson DT et al. Atherosclerotic renovascular disease in older US patients starting dialysis, 1996 to 2001. Circulation 2007; 115(1):50–8.

11. Wright JR, Shurrab AE, Cheung C et al. A prospective study of the determinants of renal functional outcome and mortality in atherosclerotic renovascular disease. Am J Kidney Dis 2002; 39(6):1153–61.

12. Middleton JP. Ischemic disease of the kidney: how and why to consider revascularization. J Nephrol 1998; 11(3):123–36.

13. Textor SC. Revascularization in atherosclerotic renal artery disease. Kidney Int 1998; 53(3):799–811.

14. Missouris CG, Buckenham T, Cappuccio FP et al. Renal artery stenosis: a common and important problem in patients with peripheral vascular disease. Am J Med 1994; 96(1):10–14.

15. Olin JW, Melia M, Young JR et al. Prevalence of atherosclerotic renal artery stenosis in patients with atherosclerosis elsewhere. Am J Med 1990; 88(1N):46N–51N.

16. Kuroda S, Nishida N, Uzu T et al. Prevalence of renal artery stenosis in autopsy patients with stroke. Stroke 2000; 31(1):61–5.

17. Harding MB, Smith LR, Himmelstein SI et al. Renal artery stenosis: prevalence and associated risk factors in patients undergoing routine cardiac catheterization. J Am Soc Nephrol 1992; 2(11):1608–16.

18. Crowley JJ, Santos RM, Peter RH et al. Progression of renal artery stenosis in patients undergoing cardiac catheterization. Am Heart J 1998; 136(5):913–18.

19. MacDowall P, Kalra PA, O'Donoghue DJ et al. Risk of morbidity from renovascular disease in elderly patients with congestive cardiac failure. Lancet 1998; 352(9121):13–16.

20. Cheung CM, Patel A, Shaheen N et al. The effects of statins on the progression of atherosclerotic renovascular disease. Nephron Clin Pract 2007; 107(2):c35–42.

21. Tan KT, van Beek EJ, Brown PW et al. Magnetic resonance angiography for the diagnosis of renal artery stenosis: a meta-analysis. Clin Radiol 2002; 57(7):617–24.

22. Solomon R, Werner C, Mann D et al. Effects of saline, mannitol, and furosemide to prevent acute decreases in renal function induced by radiocontrast agents. New Engl J Med 1994; 331(21):1416–20.

23. Mainra R, Gallo K, Moist L. Effect of N-acetylcysteine on renal function in patients with chronic kidney disease. Nephrology 2007; 12(5):510–13.

24. Hiramoto J, Hansen KJ, Pan XM et al. Atheroemboli during renal artery angioplasty: an ex vivo study. J Vasc Surg 2005; 41:1026–30.

25. Holden A, Hill A, Jaff MR et al. Renal artery stent revascularization with embolic protection in patients with ischemic nephropathy. Kidney Int 2006; 70:948–55.

26. Henry M, Henry I, Klonaris C et al. Renal angioplasty and stenting under protection: the way for the future? Catheter Cardiovasc Intervent 2003; 60:299–312.

27. Hagspiel KD, Stone JR, Leung DA. Renal angioplasty and stent placement with distal protection: preliminary experience with the FilterWire EX. J Vasc Intervent Radiol 2005; 16:125–31.

28. Beek FJ, Kaatee R, Beutler JJ et al. Complications during renal artery stent placement for atherosclerotic ostial stenosis. Cardiovasc Intervent Radiol 1997; 20(3):184–90.

29. Leertouwer TC, Gussenhoven EJ, Bosch JL et al. Stent placement for renal arterial stenosis: where do we stand? A meta-analysis. Radiology 2000; 216:78–85.

Renal stenting is technically superior and clinically comparable to renal angioplasty alone.

30. Van Jaarsveld BC, Krijnen P, Pieterman H et al. The effects of balloon angioplasty on hypertension in atherosclerotic renal artery stenosis. N Engl J Med 2000; 342:1007–14.

The largest randomised controlled trial (106 patients). In patients with hypertension and atherosclerotic RAS, angioplasty has little advantage over drug therapy alone.

31. Plouin P-F, Chatellier G, Darne B et al. Blood pressure outcome of angioplasty in atherosclerotic renal artery stenosis. Hypertension 1998; 31:823–9.

In unilateral atherosclerotic RAS, angioplasty is a drug-sparing procedure that involves some morbidity. Previous uncontrolled studies have overestimated its effect on hypertension.

32. Webster J, Marshall F, Abdalla M et al. Randomised comparison of percutaneous angioplasty vs continued medical therapy for hypertensive patients with atheromatous renal artery stenosis. J Hum Hypertens 1998; 12:329–35.

Angioplasty results in a modest improvement in systolic blood pressure compared with drug therapy alone. This benefit was confined to bilateral disease. No patient was cured and renal function did not improve. Angioplasty was associated with significant morbidity.

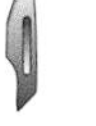

33. Ives N, Wheatley K, Stowe RL et al. Continuing uncertainty about the value of percutaneous revascularisation in atherosclerotic renovascular disease: a meta-analysis of randomised trials. Nephrol Dial Transplant 2003; 18:298–304.

Reported trials are too small to determine reliably the role of angioplasty in ARVD. Trials do exclude a large improvement in hypertension or renal function but are too small to exclude a clinically worthwhile benefit.

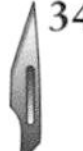

34. Nordmann AJ, Woo K, Parkes R et al. Balloon angioplasty or medical therapy for hypertensive patients with atherosclerotic renal artery stenosis? A meta-analysis of randomised controlled trials. Am J Med 2003; 114:44–50.

Angioplasty has a modest but significant effect on blood pressure and should be considered in poorly controlled hypertension in atherosclerotic patients. There is no evidence to support its use in improving or preserving renal function.

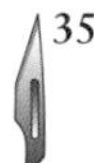

35. Van de Ven PJG, Kaatee R, Beutler JJ et al. Arterial stenting and balloon angioplasty in ostial atherosclerotic renovascular disease: a randomised trial. Lancet 1999; 353:282–6.

This trial showed convincing superiority of stenting over angioplasty regarding technical success and primary patency.

36. Zahringer M, Sapoval M, Pattynama PM et al. Sirolimus-eluting versus bare-metal low-profile stent for renal artery treatment (GREAT Trial): angiographic follow-up after 6 months and clinical outcome up to 2 years. J Endovasc Ther 2007; 14:460.
37. Novick AC. Extracorporeal microvascular reconstruction and autotransplantation for branch renal artery disease. In: Novick AC, Scoble J, Hamilton G (eds) Renal vascular disease. London: WB Saunders, 1996; pp. 497–511.
38. Bergentz SE, Weibull H, Novick AC. Long-term patency after reconstructive surgery and PTA for renal artery stenosis. In: Greenhalgh RM, Hollier L (eds) The maintenance of arterial reconstruction. London: WB Saunders, 1991; pp. 384–96.
39. Fergany A, Kolettis P, Novick AC. The contemporary role of extra-anatomical surgical renal revascularization in patients with atherosclerotic renal artery disease. J Urol 1995; 153(6):1798–801; discussion 1801–2.
40. Benjamin ME, Hansen KJ, Craven TE et al. Combined aortic and renal artery surgery. A contemporary experience. Ann Surg 1996; 223:555–65.
41. Dean RH. Surgical reconstruction of atherosclerotic renal artery disease. In: Branchereau A, Jacobs M (eds) Long term results of arterial interventions. Armonk, NY: Futura, 1997; pp. 205–16.
42. Reilly JM, Rubin BG, Thompson RW et al. Revascularization of the solitary kidney: a challenging problem in a high risk population. Surgery 1996; 120:732–6.
43. Steinbach F, Novick AC, Campbell S et al. Long-term survival after surgical revascularization for atherosclerotic renal artery disease. J Urol 1997; 158:38–41.
44. Darling RC III, Shah DM, Chang BB et al. Does concomitant aortic bypass and renal artery revascularization using the retroperitoneal approach increase perioperative risk? Cardiovasc Surg 1995; 3:421–3.
45. Novick AC, Ziegelbaum M, Vidt DG et al. Trends in surgical revascularization for renal artery disease. Ten years' experience. JAMA 1987; 257:498–501.
46. Cambria RP, Brewster DC, L'Italien G et al. Renal artery reconstruction for the preservation of renal function. J Vasc Surg 1996; 24:371–82.
47. Farkas JC, Calvo-Verjat N, Laurian C et al. Acute colorectal ischemia after aortic surgery: pathophysiology and prognostic criteria. Ann Vasc Surg 1992; 6(2):111–18.
48. Stoney RJ, Cunningham CG. Acute mesenteric ischemia. Surgery 1993; 114(3):489–90.
49. Acosta S, Ogren M, Sternby NH et al. Fatal nonocclusive mesenteric ischaemia: population-based incidence and risk factors. J Intern Med 2006; 259(3):305–13.
50. Granger DN, Hollwarth ME, Parks DA. Ischemia–reperfusion injury: role of oxygen-derived free radicals. Acta Physiol Scand Suppl 1986; 548:47–63.
51. Gartenschlaeger S, Bender S, Maeurer J et al. Successful percutaneous transluminal angioplasty and stenting in acute mesenteric ischemia. Cardiovasc Intervent Radiol 2008; 31(2):398–400.
52. Kazmers A. Operative management of acute mesenteric ischemia. Part 1. Ann Vasc Surg 1998; 12(2):187–97.
53. Hansen HJ, Christoffersen JK. Occlusive mesenteric infarction. A retrospective study of 83 cases. Acta Chir Scand Suppl 1976; 472:103–8.
54. Hollier LH, Bernatz PE, Pairolero PC et al. Surgical management of chronic intestinal ischemia: a reappraisal. Surgery 1981; 90(6):940–6.
55. Gentile AT, Moneta GL, Taylor LM Jr et al. Isolated bypass to the superior mesenteric artery for intestinal ischemia. Arch Surg 1994; 129(9):926–31; discussion 931–2.
56. Foley MI, Moneta GL, Abou-Zamzam AM Jr et al. Revascularization of the superior mesenteric artery alone for treatment of intestinal ischemia. J Vasc Surg 2000; 32(1):37–47.
57. Taylor L, Moneta G, Porter J. Treatment of chronic visceral ischemia. In: Rutherford RB (ed.) Vascular surgery. Philadelphia: WB Saunders, 2000; pp. 1532–41.
58. Kansal N, LoGerfo FW, Belfield AK et al. A comparison of antegrade and retrograde mesenteric bypass. Ann Vasc Surg 2002; 16(5):591–6.
59. Park WM, Cherry KJ Jr, Chua HK et al. Current results of open revascularization for chronic mesenteric ischemia: a standard for comparison. J Vasc Surg 2002; 35(5):853–9.

60. Kruger AJ, Walker PJ, Foster WJ et al. Open surgery for atherosclerotic chronic mesenteric ischemia. J Vasc Surg 2007; 46(5):941–5.

61. Atkins MD, Kwolek CJ, LaMuraglia GM et al. Surgical revascularization versus endovascular therapy for chronic mesenteric ischemia: a comparative experience. J Vasc Surg 2007; 45(6):1162–71.

62. Kasirajan K, O'Hara PJ, Gray BH et al. Chronic mesenteric ischemia: open surgery versus percutaneous angioplasty and stenting. J Vasc Surg 2001; 33(1):63–71.

63. Biebl L, Oldenburg W, Paz-Fumagalli R et al. Surgical and interventional visceral revascularization for the treatment of chronic mesenteric ischemia – when to prefer which? World J Surg 2007; 31(3):562–8.

64. Sivamurthy N, Rhodes JM, Lee D et al. Endovascular versus open mesenteric revascularization: immediate benefits do not equate with short-term functional outcomes. J Am Coll Surg 2006; 202(6):859–67.

65. van Wanroij JL, van Petersen AS, Huisman AB et al. Endovascular treatment of chronic splanchnic syndrome. Eur J Vasc Endovasc Surg 2004; 28(2):193–200.

66. Sugiyama K, Takehara Y. Analysis of five cases of splanchnic artery aneurysm associated with coeliac artery stenosis due to compression by the median arcuate ligament. Clin Radiol 2007; 62(7):688–93.

67. Reilly LM, Ammar AD, Stoney RJ et al. Late results following operative repair for celiac artery compression syndrome. J Vasc Surg 1985; 2(1):79–91.

68. Gloviczki P, Duncan AA. Treatment of celiac artery compression syndrome: does it really exist? Perspect Vasc Surg Endovasc Ther 2007; 19(3):259–63.

69. Carbonell AM, Kercher KW, Heniford BT et al. Multimedia article. Laparoscopic management of median arcuate ligament syndrome. Surg Endosc 2005; 19(5):729.

70. Geelkerken RH, van Bockel JH, de Roos WK et al. Surgical treatment of intestinal artery aneurysms. Eur J Vasc Surg 1990; 4(6):563–7.

71. Graham LM, Stanley JC, Whitehouse WM Jr et al. Celiac artery aneurysms: historic (1745–1949) versus contemporary (1950–1984) differences in etiology and clinical importance. J Vasc Surg 1985; 2(5):757–64.

72. Stanley JC, Thompson NW, Fry WJ. Splanchnic artery aneurysms. Arch Surg 1970; 101(6): 689–97.

73. Ishii A, Namimoto T, Morishita S et al. Embolization for ruptured superior mesenteric artery aneurysms. Br J Radiol 1996; 820(69):296–300.

74. Lorelli DR, Cambra RA, Seabrook GR et al. Diagnosis and management of aneurysms involving the superior mesenteric artery and its branches: a report of four cases. Vasc Endovasc Surg 2003; 37(1):59–66.

75. Jindal R, Pandey V, Natt R, Jenkins M. Ruptured mycotic aneurysm of a branch of the superior mesenteric artery and pulmonary tuberculosis. Eur J Vasc Endovasc Surg 2005; 30(1):107.

76. Huang YK, Hsieh HC, Tsai FC et al. Visceral artery aneurysm: risk factor analysis and therapeutic opinion. Eur J Vasc Endovasc Surg 2007; 33(3):293–301.

# 16

# Central venous and dialysis access

Peter W.G. Brown
Christopher P. Gibbons

## Introduction

Access to the venous circulation is an almost universal requirement in hospitalised patients for intravenous fluid administration or blood transfusion. This is most commonly achieved with an indwelling peripheral intravenous cannula but central venous access may be required for pressure monitoring, intravenous nutrition, haemodialysis, haemofiltration or the administration of cytotoxic drugs.

For acute haemodialysis, central venous catheters (CVCs) are the mainstay of access and provide high dialysis flows (>300 mL/min) but have high complication rates and are less suitable for chronic use. For long-term haemodialysis, an arteriovenous fistula (AVF) or graft (AVG) can provide a sufficiently high flow (>300 mL/min) to allow dialysis via two needles inserted into the efferent vein or the graft itself.

## Central venous access

### Indications

In addition to central venous pressure monitoring, CVCs can be used to infuse large volumes of irritating solutions, such as antibiotics, blood products, parenteral nutrition and chemotherapeutic agents, particularly if required over long periods. In an emergency, CVCs allow the rapid administration of large volumes of fluid if peripheral access cannot be achieved. Other indications include haemodialysis and plasmapheresis. Implantable injection ports, 'portacaths' (e.g. Bardport, Passport, Infuse-a-Port or Medi-Port), may be used for chemotherapy or long-term administration of other drugs.[1] One has also been developed for haemodialysis (Lifesite).[2]

### Methods

CVCs are generally inserted under local anaesthetic through the internal jugular, subclavian or femoral veins, preferably using ultrasound guidance, by the Seldinger technique.[3] If short-term access is required a multilumen catheter is inserted into the internal jugular vein so that the tip lies in the superior vena cava. For long-term access a catheter is used with a Dacron cuff in a subcutaneous tunnel (e.g. Hickman line) for fixation and to act as a barrier to infection.

Implantable access ports are usually inserted into the subclavian vein in the operating theatre and tunnelled so that the port lies over the anterior chest wall. They contain a diaphragm that may be accessed repeatedly using a special side-hole needle. Central vein access can also be achieved using a peripheral intravenous central catheter inserted in the antecubital or long saphenous vein. These are relatively small but widely used in neonates, as an alternative to umbilical vein catheters.

### Complications

Air embolus can be avoided by ensuring a head-down position during insertion, and accurate placement under ultrasound guidance will reduce the incidence of arterial puncture, haematoma, haemothorax and pneumothorax. The long-term complications of infection and thrombosis are dealt with below.

## Temporary dialysis access

Renal replacement therapy may be accomplished by renal transplantation or peritoneal dialysis but most patients require at least a period of haemodialysis. About 75% of patients are known to have deteriorating renal function at least 90 days before dialysis is required so that permanent haemodialysis access can be created in advance. Unfortunately, this opportunity is frequently missed in UK practice, with less than a third of patients starting haemodialysis with definitive access.[4] Dialysis is required for hyperkalaemia or when symptoms of weight loss, nausea, vomiting, anorexia or itching occur, usually at a serum creatinine level of 500–1500 µmol/L.

For patients presenting as an emergency with end-stage renal disease (ESRD) without prior access, haemodialysis can start using a double-lumen CVC whilst awaiting a permanent AVF. However, CVCs have a high risk of infection,[5] cause central venous stenosis or thrombosis[6] compromising further access in the upper limbs, and have a higher mortality than AVFs,[7] so should not be used long term except where other options have been exhausted.

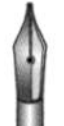

Temporary (non-tunnelled) catheters are used in patients who require short-term dialysis for transient renal failure, present acutely with ESRD or after failure of a permanent access, whilst awaiting maturation of a new AVF. Tunnelled catheters are preferred if dialysis is required for more than 2 weeks or for permanent access when the creation of an AVF or AVG is impossible.

The subcutaneous tunnel may reduce the rate of infection, but this has not been proven in a randomised trial.[8]

## Methods

Temporary femoral vein catheters are useful for acute dialysis but have a higher rate of infection than internal jugular CVCs[9] and should be replaced by a tunnelled (preferably jugular) venous catheter at the earliest opportunity. A median survival of 166 days has been reported for tunnelled femoral CVCs.[10]

The right internal jugular vein (IJV) is preferred as this provides the most direct route to the superior vena cava (SVC) and right atrium (RA). The left IJV has a greater complication rate because the catheter has to traverse two 90° bends to reach the RA. The subclavian route is discouraged because of the high incidence of subclavian vein stenosis and thrombosis that compromises future access in the ipsilateral arm. When other routes have been exhausted, tunnelled catheters can be placed in the femoral vein or even the inferior vena cava (IVC) via a transhepatic or translumbar approach.

The catheter tip is usually placed at the SVC/RA junction. Atrial placement minimises recirculation and reduces the risk of migration on standing,[12] but may cause arrhythmias.

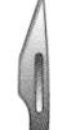

The preferred site for a CVC is the right IJV. CVCs should be inserted under fluoroscopic or ultrasound guidance, without which there is a malposition rate of 29%.[11]

## Complications of CVCs

### Insertion

The complications related to catheter insertion are the same as for other CVCs described above and can be reduced by ultrasound guidance and a micropuncture technique.

### Catheter dysfunction

Catheter dysfunction occurs when an adequate extracorporeal blood flow of 300 mL/min cannot be achieved. Early dysfunction is usually caused by malposition or kinking and is corrected by repositioning. Later dysfunction is primarily due to thrombosis or fibrin sheath formation. Rarely, tip migration demands repositioning with a snare or exchanging over a wire.

### Catheter lumen thrombosis

Catheter thrombosis is the most common cause of poor long-term function.[13] It may be cleared by instilling urokinase or tissue plasminogen activator (TPA). A urokinase infusion seems more effective than a urokinase lock.[14]

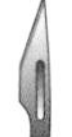

TPA may be superior to urokinase but this has not been proven in a randomised trial. Partial obstruction can be treated by infusing 2.5 mg of TPA over 3 hours.[15] A catheter lock between dialysis sessions is an alternative, which was better than placebo in a randomised trial.[16] Low-dose warfarin (1 mg/day) reduced thrombosis from 38% to 10% in CVCs used for chemotherapy, but there are no similar data in dialysis patients.[17]

### Central vein thrombosis

Mural thrombus is commonly seen in the SVC and RA with central venous catheters. If it compromises venous return, facial and arm oedema results. Central vein thrombus can be identified by magnetic resonance or conventional venography. Infusion of a fibrinolytic agent is usually successful, although organised thrombus may require angioplasty and stenting.

### Fibrin sheaths

Fibrin sheaths cause up to 43% of catheter dysfunction.[18] Contrast injection through the dialysis line may show a filling defect near the catheter tip or retrograde flow along the external surface of the catheter (**Fig. 16.1**). They may be treated by infusing a fibrinolytic agent over 6 hours, mechanical stripping using a snare from the femoral vein, or catheter exchange over a guide wire.

Stripping has a high technical success rate but the fibrin sheath frequently recurs. In a randomised trial there was no significant difference in additional patency between percutaneous stripping or urokinase.[19] In another randomised trial 4-month catheter patency was significantly better after catheter exchange than percutaneous stripping.[20]

If the catheter is exchanged over a guide wire, the sheath must be mechanically disrupted or the new catheter will be reinserted down the existing sheath. There are no controlled trials comparing all three techniques.

### Catheter-related infection

Catheter-related infection is a major cause of morbidity and mortality and is related to the duration of placement. Gram-positive bacteria are the usual cause[21] and resistant organisms such as methicillin-resistant *Staphylococcus aureus* (MRSA) are increasing. Catheter-associated sepsis can result in infective endocarditis, osteomyelitis, septic arthritis, epidural abscesses and death. Infection spreads either through the lumen of the catheter or along the outside from the exit site. An associated biofilm reduces the effectiveness of antibiotics.

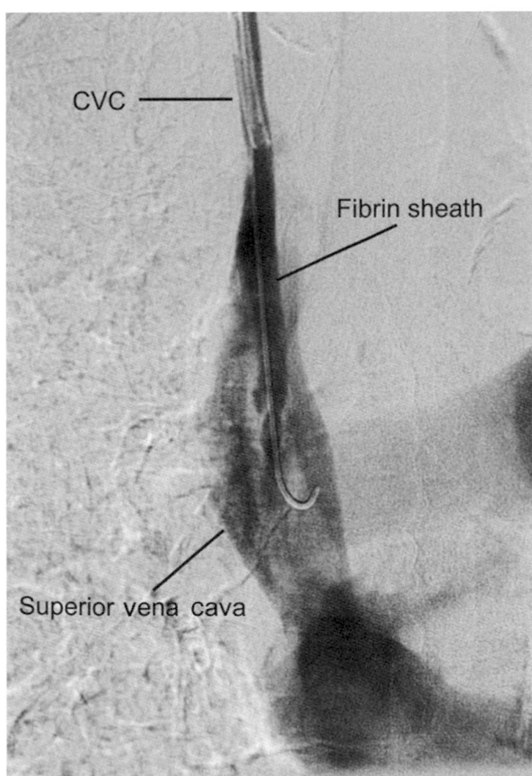


**Figure 16.1** • A venogram showing fibrin sheath around a partially withdrawn CVC.

Infections in non-tunnelled catheters should be treated by catheter removal and systemic antibiotics. In tunnelled catheters 90% of exit-site infections respond to oral antibiotics but intravenous antibiotics and catheter removal may be necessary for more serious tunnel infections. Systemic infections associated with tunnelled catheters can be treated initially with antibiotics but catheter removal is usually required. A new catheter should be inserted at a different site when the systemic sepsis has settled. Catheter exchange over a guide wire is controversial but there is some evidence that infection-free survival is similar to that after removal and delayed replacement.[22]

The cornerstone of prevention is scrupulous asepsis with regular exit-site inspection and dressing changes. Topical povidone–iodine reduces exit-site infections and bacteraemia in temporary dialysis catheters.[23] Mupirocin ointment is also effective,[24] but may increase colonisation by fungi and multiresistant organisms. Antibiotic-coated catheters reduce line sepsis in intensive care patients[25] and temporary dialysis catheters[26] but there is no evidence of benefit for long-term dialysis as the antibiotic is washed off over time. Antibiotic catheter locks have also been used. The antithrombotic antibacterial agent taurolidine citrate reduces bacteraemia but not exit-site infection in tunnelled catheters.[27]

## Permanent dialysis access

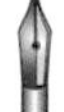

An AVF should be constructed 16–24 weeks before the anticipated need for dialysis, when the creatinine clearance falls to 25 mL/min or the serum creatinine level rises above 400 μmol/L (4 mg/dL) to allow time for maturation or redo surgery in the event of failure.[28–30]

Whereas CVCs are usually introduced on the ward or in the radiology department, peripheral arteriovenous (AV) access procedures require an operating theatre. However, most can be performed under local anaesthetic, often as day cases.

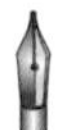

Dedicated operating lists organised by a dialysis access nurse are an enormous advantage and one such list is required per week for every 120 patients on dialysis to prevent unacceptable waiting times and prolonged CVC usage.[4]

## Access planning

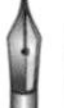

In patients with chronic renal failure it is essential that the cephalic and antecubital veins of both arms be reserved for dialysis access. Intravenous cannulas for other purposes should only be inserted into the back of the hand or the small veins on the anterior surface of the wrist, except in emergencies. A CVC, AVF or AVG should only be used for dialysis.[28–30]

An AVF should be created as distally as possible to preserve sites for future access. The non-dominant arm is preferred to allow greater freedom on dialysis or to facilitate self-cannulation for home dialysis patients. When upper limb access sites are exhausted the lower limbs may be used.[28–30]

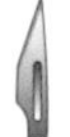

Autogenous AVFs are preferable to prosthetic AVGs as they have higher patency,[31] lower infection rates, require fewer revisions[32] and are associated with a slightly lower mortality, especially in diabetics.[7,33]

Whereas a side-to side radiocephalic AVF was originally described,[34] an end-to side configuration is now preferred as there is less risk of peripheral venous hypertension. Some advocate an end-to-end anastomosis for distal radiocephalic AVFs, provided there is a good ulnar pulse, to reduce the small incidence of steal.[35] Autogenous AVFs require a period of maturation to allow arterialisation of the venous outflow whereas AVGs can be needled directly as soon as the wounds have healed.

## Preoperative assessment

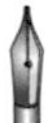

In many centres, patients proceed directly to primary AVF formation if there is a satisfactory radial pulse and suitable forearm veins. Opinion is divided on the need for preoperative imaging: the latest US National Kidney Foundation – Dialysis Outcomes Quality Initiative (NKF-KDOQI) clinical guidelines now recommend routine duplex imaging in all patients,[36] whereas the Vascular Access Society recommends a selective approach.[29]

However, there is an increasing trend for preoperative imaging to reduce primary failure, non-maturation and unnecessary surgery.[28–30,36]

Venography is advisable if central vein stenosis is suspected. In complex cases with unclear venous anatomy, particularly predialysis patients in whom iodinated contrast could exacerbate renal failure, duplex ultrasound or magnetic resonance imaging may be preferable in the first instance. Angiography or arterial duplex is recommended if arterial pulses are diminished.

### Duplex ultrasound

Preoperative duplex ultrasound is particularly useful for obese patients with impalpable superficial veins or following previous access failure, but cannot assess central vein patency. In studies from the USA, where AVGs are more frequently used than in Europe, routine preoperative ultrasound significantly increased the prevalence, reduced early failure rate and increased primary patency of autogenous AVFs compared with historical controls.[37–39] Prosthetic AV access reconstruction and access complications also decreased significantly. In another study duplex mapping changed the proposed procedure in a third of patients and almost doubled the proportion of AVFs constructed.[40] However, in a British study, duplex scanning rarely added any useful information except in those patients with poor vessels on clinical examination duplex, when the proposed procedure was altered in 50%. This suggests that patients with good pulses and clinically adequate veins may proceed to surgery without preoperative ultrasound mapping.[41]

A radial artery luminal diameter of less than 1.6 mm is associated with early fistula failure[42] and a minimum diameter of 2 mm is now usually advised.[29,30,36] Above this threshold there seems to be no correlation between arterial diameter or flow and fistula success.

Venous diameter is an important determinant of outcome. In prospective studies, mean cephalic vein diameters are significantly smaller in non-functioning AVFs. Minimum venous diameters (with a tourniquet) of 2–2.5 mm have been advised for AVFs and 3.5–4.0 mm for synthetic grafts.[29,30,36]

Venous distensibility is another important predictor of success. Veins were found to dilate 48% with a tourniquet in successful fistulas compared with only 12% in fistulas that subsequently failed.[43]

### Venography

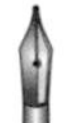

For many years, contrast venography was the gold standard and has the advantage of providing a venous map. It is mandatory in patients with prior ipsilateral central vein catheterisation, collateral vein development, oedema or arm swelling, indicating possible central vein obstruction.[29,30] Construction of a peripheral fistula in these patients can cause massive arm swelling.

Iodinated contrast may precipitate acute renal failure and is relatively contraindicated in predialysis patients. Duplex ultrasound is an alternative but is poor for assessing central vein stenosis. Contrast-enhanced magnetic resonance venography is promising, as the small volume of paramagnetic contrast agent used does not compromise renal function but requires further evaluation. Imaging is likely to improve significantly with new pulse sequences such as time-resolved magnetic resonance venography and the blood pool contrast agents.

Carbon dioxide venography is not nephrotoxic and is widely used in France but requires a costly injector, causes local pain during injection, overestimation of venous stenoses and occasionally acute right heart failure.

## Primary access

The snuffbox AVF is the most distal access possible and gives the longest length of vein for needling. It is possible in about 50% of patients and, in the event of failure, a wrist AVF can still be performed in half of the cases[44] (**Fig. 16.2**).

The wrist radiocephalic AVF (**Fig. 16.3**) was the first to be described[34] and remains the standard access in most units. It has a low complication rate and gives a good length of available vein. Patencies of 65% at 1 year are usual.[45] If a wrist AVF fails, further forearm radiocephalic fistulas can often be created more proximally. In obese patients the vein may remain difficult to needle so that it may be advisable to excise the subcutaneous fat overlying the vein through one or more transverse incisions.

The brachiocephalic AVF is the next option, which can be performed in a variety of configurations (**Fig. 16.4**), and gives excellent flows at the expense of a greater incidence of steal (see below). To avoid this, some authors advocate anastomosing the cephalic vein to the radial artery 2 cm beyond its origin instead of the brachial artery itself.[46]

The ulnobasilic AVF is often possible after a failed brachial fistula but is more difficult to needle and seems to have a poorer patency than other upper limb AVFs.[47]

When the options are limited by venous thrombosis or arterial disease an ulnocephalic or radiobasilic fistula may be possible in the forearm, but these require more extensive mobilisation and subcutaneous tunnelling of the vein across the forearm.[48]

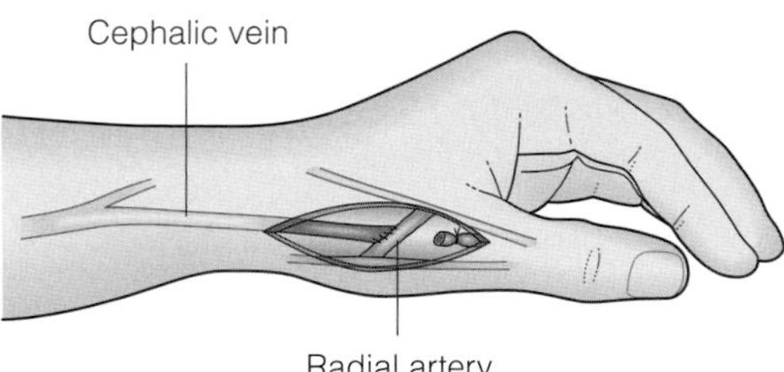


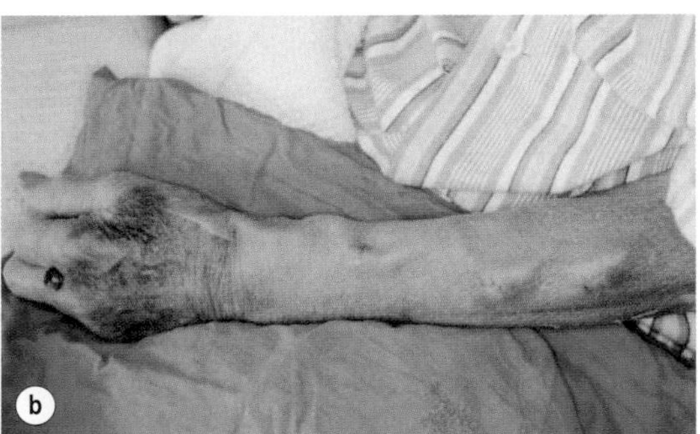


**Figure 16.2** • The snuffbox AVF. **(a)** Diagram showing position of anastomosis. **(b)** A mature snuffbox fistula showing the long length of available vein for needling.

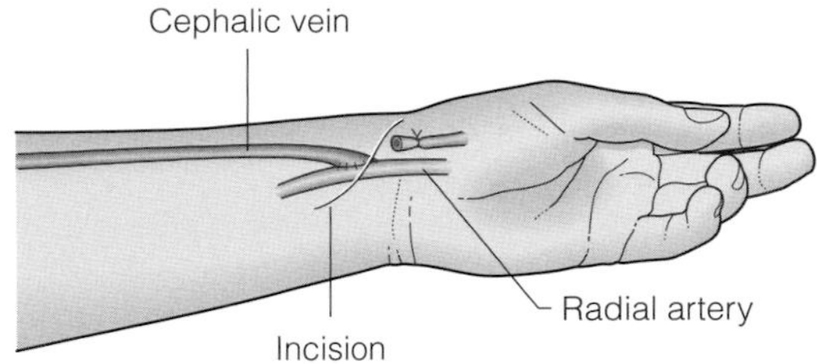


**Figure 16.3** • The radiocephalic AVF at the wrist.

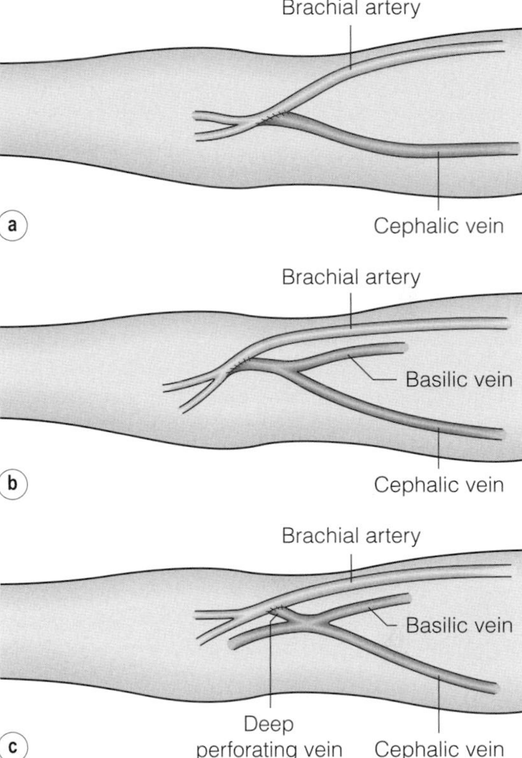


**Figure 16.4** • Configurations of the brachiocephalic AVF at the antecubital fossa. **(a)** Direct anastomosis between the cephalic vein and brachial artery. **(b)** Anastomosis including both median basilic and cephalic veins. **(c)** Gracz fistula between the deep perforating vein and the brachial artery.

## Secondary and tertiary access

When the cephalic vein is thrombosed, an antecubital brachiobasilic AVF may be possible but this leaves only a short length of vein for needling so the basilic vein is usually mobilised and rerouted superficially over the biceps muscle either in a single procedure or in a second stage after the vein has arterialised (the basilic vein transposition; **Fig. 16.5**).[49]

When an autogenous AVF cannot be performed, a prosthetic graft (AVG) can be used. A variety of graft materials are available, but polytetrafluoroethylene (PTFE) is the most popular. The graft itself is used for needling, which can be performed within 2–3 weeks, but has a higher rate of infection. There is also a high incidence of intimal hyperplasia, especially at or just beyond the venous anastomosis, which causes a higher rate of thrombosis and the need for more frequent revisions than autogenous fistulas. A wider graft,[50] a vein cuff[51] or an expansion of the venous end of the graft (Venoflo)[52] may reduce this and has better patency.

Biological grafts such as bovine mesenteric vein and bovine ureter are preferred in some units as they have greater resistance to infection, but they are prone to aneurysm formation.[53] Transposed long saphenous vein (LSV) is less popular as it is more difficult to needle but has fewer infective complications.[54] A forearm AVG either in a looped or straight configuration allows a basilic vein transposition to be performed if it fails, but has a poorer patency than the latter[55] so which should be performed first is a matter of dispute. A brachioaxillary AVG is the next option (**Fig. 16.6**).

Lower limb access is less popular but may be the only option when the SVC or both subclavian veins are occluded. An AVF at the ankle between the LSV and the posterior tibial artery is rarely possible because of underlying arterial disease. The LSV can be anastomosed to the popliteal artery above the knee or used as a subcutaneous loop from the femoral artery in the groin, but these are more difficult to needle. The superficial femoral vein can be used in the same configurations (or transposed to the forearm) and gives an excellent fistula at the expense of a high incidence of steal.

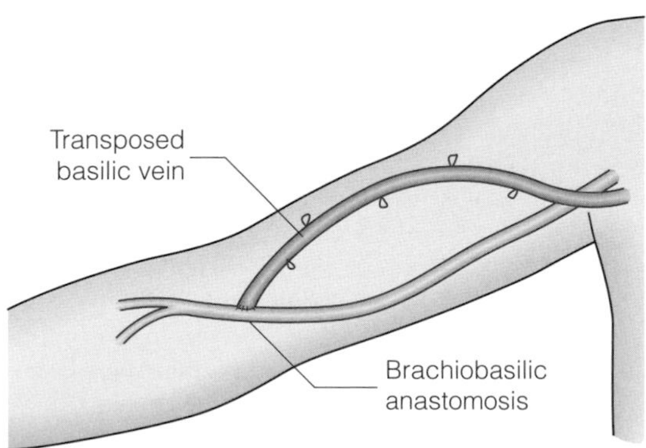


**Figure 16.5** • The basilic vein transposition AVF.

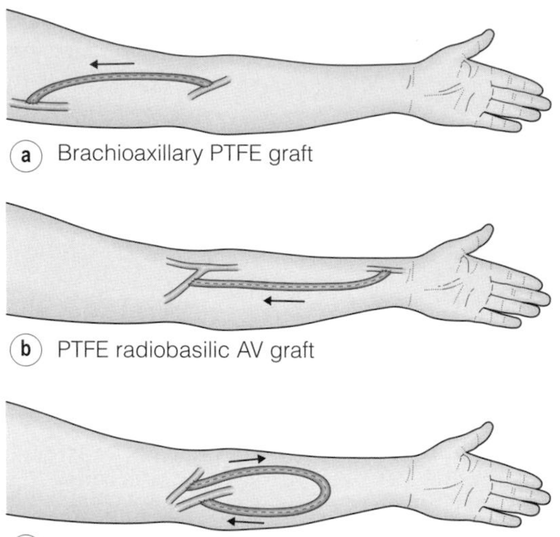


**Figure 16.6** • Popular configurations for upper limb AVGs: **(a)** straight **(b)** and looped brachioaxillary graft **(c)** forearm grafts.

In desperate cases, a variety of possibilities exist: axillo-femoral, axillo-axillary, ilio-iliac or even aorto-IVC AVGs can be used. Where there are no available veins the RA can be used as an outflow. Alternatively an arterio-arterial graft, usually in the axillary position, is possible but risks distal embolisation to the arm.[56]

## Factors affecting access patency

The following factors are known to affect access patency:

- **Vessel size.** Small arteries and veins have higher initial failure rates, more frequent failure to mature and poorer long-term patency.[42]
- **Fistula flow rate.** The flow rate the day after surgery correlates inversely with the risk of thrombosis, although intraoperative flow rates are less reliable.[42] The hyperaemic response of brachial artery blood flow is a strong predictor of access patency and maturation, presumably by detecting proximal arterial stenoses.[57]
- **Mode of presentation.** Patients presenting acutely with renal failure have poorer AVF

patency, which may be linked to the need for temporary access via a central venous catheter.[58]

- **Anastomotic method.** Non-penetrating vascular clips, which give an interrupted anastomosis with excellent endothelial apposition and less bleeding, are quicker and have improved patencies compared with sutured anastomoses in randomised trials.[59,60]
- **Access position.** More proximal AVFs have improved patency[61] but leave fewer options for access in the event of failure.
- **Gender.** Patency of AVFs is poorer in women than men.[44,58,61,62]
- **Diabetes.** There is conflicting evidence as to whether diabetes is an adverse factor, with some authors suggesting that AVF patency is poorer[61] whereas others have found no effect.[44,63,64]
- **Age.** In a meta-analysis, access patency was found to be worse in the elderly.[65]
- **Obesity.** Veins are more difficult to cannulate in obese patients, which may account for poorer patency reported by some authors.[66]
- **Smoking.** Smoking reduces AVF patency.[67]
- **Drugs.** Antiplatelet agents such as aspirin and dipyridamole prolong fistula survival and are used routinely.[68–70] A combination of aspirin and clopidogrel increased haemorrhagic complications without influencing patency in prosthetic AVGs in one study,[71] but clopidogrel alone significantly prolonged graft survival in another.[72] Warfarin reduces AVF thrombosis in patients with hypercoagulable states,[73] but routine use is best avoided because of the risk of haemorrhage. Surprisingly, warfarin was associated with poorer patency in the Dialysis Outcomes and Practice Patterns Study (DOPPS), but this may reflect its use in patients with a history of fistula thrombosis or known thrombotic disorders.[70] Calcium-channel blockers are associated with improved primary patency.[70] Angiotensin-converting enzyme inhibitors did not affect primary patency in one study[74] but were associated with improved secondary patency in DOPPS.[70] Fish oil reduced AVF thrombosis in one randomised trial.[75] Erythropoeitin does not reduce and may increase patency, at least in AVGs.[76,77]
- **Thrombotic tendencies and vasculitis.** Increased fibrinogen and vasculitis predispose to access thrombosis.[78]

## Access failure

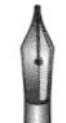

Percutaneous angioplasty of stenoses in AVFs and AVGs preserves veins and may prevent access thrombosis. Stenting is controversial but probably offers little extra advantage. Endovascular thrombolysis or thrombectomy of occluded AV accesses is effective provided that the underlying stenosis is dilated.[28–30]

### Failure to mature

About 10% of AVFs remain patent but never achieve an adequate flow for dialysis. A duplex scan may reveal a proximal arterial or a venous stenosis, treatable by angioplasty or surgery. Otherwise a more proximal fistula will be required.

### Stenosis and thrombosis

Early thrombosis may result from technical error, unrecognised pre-existing arterial stenoses or thrombophlebitis in the outflow vein, usually from previous intravenous cannulation. Late failure can result from hypotension, dehydration and hypercoagulable states, 'blowout' after traumatic needling or inappropriate use for intravenous infusions, but the most common cause is juxta-anastomostic venous intimal hyperplasia.

### Prevention of access failure

To prevent damage, careful needling and the avoidance of inappropriate use of AVFs are essential. Attempts to prevent intimal hyperplasia pharmacologically (e.g. with paclitaxel wraps) have yet to lead to routine clinical application.[79,80]

### Access surveillance

AVFs and AVGs may suddenly occlude without prior warning, resulting in hospitalisation and the need for a CVC. Most of these will have unrecognised stenoses due to intimal hyperplasia. Detection by routine surveillance and treatment of such stenoses could prevent thrombosis and allow continuous use of the access.

Impending failure may be indicated by the loss of a palpable thrill, needling difficulties or a reduction in dialysis efficiency (e.g. reduced Kt/V (the volume cleared of urea/distribution volume), a reduced urea reduction ratio at each dialysis, a rising predialysis serum potassium or evidence of recirculation through the dialysis machine). Such monitoring is useful but does not identify all failing fistulas.

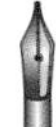

Access surveillance is controversial but there is increasing evidence that access flow monitoring can identify stenoses in AVFs and AVGs and allow endovascular treatment to prevent access failure.

A variety of surveillance methods using static (with the pump turned off) or dynamic (at a standard pump speed) venous pressure measurements during dialysis have been proposed but are unreliable because the direction of any pressure change depends on whether the venous needle is upstream or downstream of the stenosis. Flow measurements are usually performed by an indicator dilution technique (e.g. ultrasound dilution).[81,82] A low flow (<500 mL/min) is a strong predictor of impending thrombosis in AVGs and is better than dynamic venous pressure.[83–85] The change in graft flow over time is a better predictor than a single value[86] and a 25% drop has been proposed as the trigger for further imaging and intervention.

Detection of stenoses is worthwhile, as intervention-free survival is better for grafts after preemptive angioplasty than after thrombectomy and angioplasty,[87] and vascular access flow monitoring reduces access morbidity and costs.[88]

Surveillance using flow measurements also reduced thrombosis rates in AVFs in non-randomised[88,89] and randomised studies.[90] Others have failed to show improvement with surveillance but have been criticised on grounds of inadequate sensitivity[91] or inadequate angioplasty of detected stenoses.[92] Duplex surveillance also reduces thrombosis rates,[93] hospitalisation and CVC usage[94] in AVFs and AVGs.

## Access salvage

### AVF stenosis

In radiocephalic fistulas, most stenoses occur close to the AV anastomosis (**Fig. 16.7**), with the remainder more proximally in the vein. In upper arm AVFs they occur typically at the cephalic/subclavian vein junction. Intervention is indicated for stenoses greater than 50% associated with flow reduction, compromised dialysis or arm oedema. Fistulography is usually performed through the draining vein, reserving brachial artery puncture for inflow and anastomotic lesions. The venous run-off and central veins should also be demonstrated.

Primary angioplasty is indicated for upper forearm and upper arm significant stenoses, with technical success rates of over 90% and 1-year primary patency of 51% for forearm and 35% for upper arm fistulas.[95] Secondary patencies of over 80% can be achieved but more frequent interventions are needed in the upper arm. Stents offer no advantage.

Stenoses in the upper arm cephalic vein are a common cause of failure. Most respond well to angioplasty, but for those resistant to dilatation, stenting or surgical repair should be considered. Cutting and ultra-high-pressure balloons have given encouraging results but there are no randomised data.

If endovascular intervention fails, stenoses can be repaired surgically using a vein or prosthetic patch. Alternatively, inserting a short PTFE graft segment appears to be as good as an autogenous patch.[96] Stenoses adjacent to a distal AVF are best treated by creating a more proximal fistula, which may have better patency than angioplasty.[97]

### AVG stenosis

The most common cause for AVG dysfunction is a stenosis at or near the venous anastomosis. Indications for intervention are similar to those for AVFs, with similar high technical success rates. Restenosis is a greater problem and leads to poor primary patency rates of 23–44% at 1 year,[98] but 1-year secondary patencies of 92% can be achieved by repeated angioplasty.[95] Intragraft stenoses from excessive ingrowth of fibrous tissue through cannulation defects can be treated similarly, but may require surgical curettage or segmental replacement.

When angioplasty fails repeatedly, stents can be considered but their primary patency is generally no better than angioplasty. Stents are usually reserved for technical failure, rupture after angioplasty and central venous stenoses. However, in one randomised trial, adding a covered stent after AVG angioplasty increased the 6-month patency from 23% to 51%.[99]

Unassisted graft survival after thrombectomy and angioplasty is significantly worse than after elective angioplasty of patent grafts. Graft survival after thrombectomy and angioplasty may also be improved by stent implantation,[100] but there are no prospective controlled data.

There is no evidence favouring surgical revision over endovascular repair, but revisional surgery by segmental replacement or a jump graft to bypass a venous outflow stenosis may be required for recurrent stenoses.

### AVF and AVG thrombosis

Percutaneous declotting of AVGs is well established and effective, but AVFs are also being increasingly referred for radiological salvage. A thrombosed access should be declotted as soon as possible, preferably within 48 hours, and the underlying stenosis treated by angioplasty (with or without stenting). Available techniques include thrombolysis, thromboaspiration and mechanical thrombectomy. None seems superior but the expertise and experience of the operator are paramount.

Thrombus in an AVF causes phlebitis. The amount of thrombus can vary enormously. In some AVFs only a short segment of vein thromboses because a side-branch just proximal to a perianastomotic stenosis maintains patency. These can usually be treated by simple angioplasty. In others the large volume of thrombus in an aneurysmal draining vein has a risk of a significant pulmonary embolus unless it is aggressively aspirated or a mechanical clot-removing device is used.

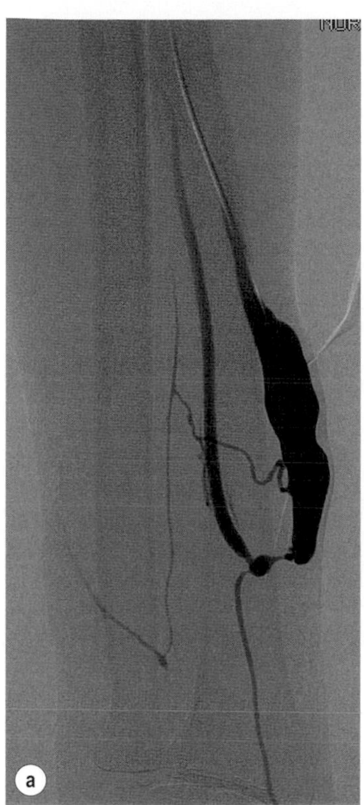


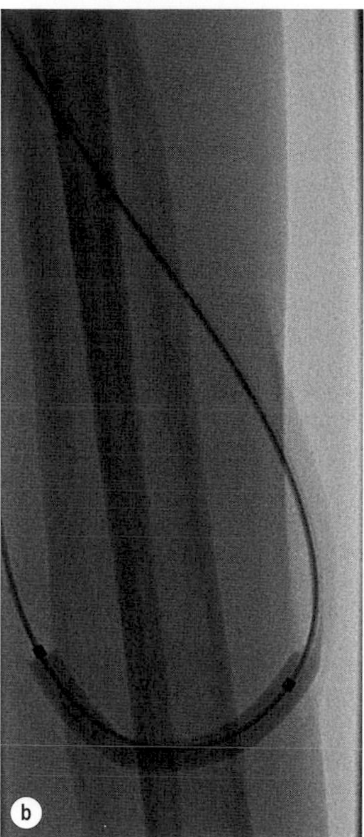


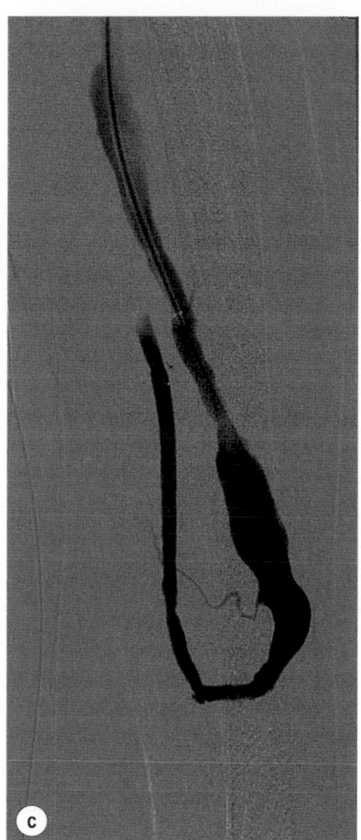


**Figure 16.7** • Fistulogram showing a stenosis adjacent to a radiocephalic AVF **(a)** successfully treated by angioplasty **(b, c).**

Technical success is reported as 73–90%, with widely differing 1-year primary and secondary patencies of 9–70% and 44–93% respectively.[101] Patencies are higher in the forearm than upper arm. There are no randomised trials of percutaneous intervention versus surgery for AVFs. Primary endovascular intervention has the advantage of preserving veins for needling, but surgical revision or a new AVF is often necessary.

AVGs thrombose more frequently than AVFs but are well suited to percutaneous intervention. Radiological declotting is less invasive than surgery and allows accurate treatment of the underlying cause, which is nearly always a venous outflow stenosis. No single device or declotting technique has been shown to be superior, and the success of treatment of the underlying stenosis seems to be the only predictive value for graft patency.[102] Thrombolysis or mechanical thrombectomy have clinical success rates of 74–94% but 6-month primary patencies are only 18–39%.[103] However, with repeated intervention secondary patency rates of up to 83% have been reported.[104] Whilst there has been no prospective randomised multicentre trial, a meta-analysis found surgical intervention to have higher primary patency than endovascular intervention.[105] In many centres endovascular declotting is preferred because of its low morbidity, reserving surgical revision for technical failures or repeated thromboses.[103]

The most common complication of endovascular declotting is distal arterial embolisation, which occurs in 1–9% of cases.[103] Others include vessel rupture (2–4%) and non-puncture site bleeding (2–3%). All methods of declotting, especially mechanical techniques, cause venous embolisation, but this is usually asymptomatic because of the small volume of thrombus displaced.

Surgical thrombectomy is usually easy if the access has failed recently. Any underlying stenosis must be corrected by bypass or patch angioplasty at the same time. If surgery is delayed for 10 days or more it may be best to abandon it and create a new access at another site.

## Other access complications

### Infection

Infection is the commonest cause of hospital admission and mortality in dialysis patients. It is most frequent in patients with CVCs and commoner in patients with AVGs than AVFs. The most frequent organism is *Staphylococcus aureus*. Bacteraemia or septicaemia may lead to endocarditis, mycotic aneurysms and septic arthritis.

Local needle-site infections may be controlled with antibiotics in the early stages but can lead to uncontrollable haemorrhage in autogenous fistulas, requiring emergency ligation or bypass of the infected area. AVGs with chronic needle-site infections or exposed segments (**Fig. 16.8**) may be salvaged by local excision and bypass of the area with appropriate antibiotic cover, but when the whole graft is infected it requires total excision. A further graft may be inserted once the wounds have healed.

## Haemorrhage

Traumatic cannulation leads to localised haematomas. Prosthetic grafts can be destroyed by repeated punctures in the same area that necessitate local graft replacement.

## Steal

An AVF tends to reduce digital arterial pressures[106] by lowering the peripheral resistance and may cause ischaemia (high-flow steal). The presence of a proximal arterial stenosis will amplify the reduction in finger pressures on AVF creation by limiting the increase in inflow (low-flow steal).

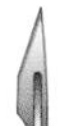

Mild steal symptoms, such as coldness, pain, cramps, diminished sensation or reduced grip strength, are common in patients with AVFs. At least one symptom is present in 80% of brachial AVFs, 50% of those with forearm AV loops and 40% of radiocephalic AVFs,[107] but clinically significant steal with rest pain or tissue loss occurs in only 1–8% of patients.

Four grades of steal are recognised (Table 16.1). Grades 1 and 2 can usually be managed conservatively, but grades 3 and 4 require surgical intervention.

**Table 16.1** • The stages of access steal syndrome

| Stage | Clinical features |
|---|---|
| I | Pale/cyanosed and/or cold hand without pain |
| II | Pain on exercise and/or dialysis |
| III | Rest pain |
| IV | Ulcer/necrosis/gangrene |

Predisposing factors include proximal AVF, diabetes mellitus, cardiac ischaemia, peripheral vascular disease[108] and low preoperative finger pressures.[106]

Steal is the most likely cause of unilateral hand or finger ischaemia occurring after AVF creation (**Fig. 16.9**). With proximal fistulas all fingers are ischaemic with a slow capillary return, whereas after a radiocephalic AVF only the thumb and index finger are affected. The radial pulse is absent but may return when the fistula is occluded. The diagnosis is confirmed by a digital pressure of 30 mmHg or less, increasing by at least 15 mmHg on AVF occlusion. A duplex scan will demonstrate any proximal stenosis, quantify AVF flow and show reversed flow in the artery distal to the AVF (although this is not diagnostic). Fistulography is rarely required.

Steal should be corrected expeditiously as ischaemic monomelic neuropathy may develop that persists after the successful treatment of the steal.

AVF ligation destroys the access but provides the most certain and may be wise in severe steal occurring immediately after AVF creation. Low-flow steal can usually be corrected by angioplasty or bypass of the inflow stenosis. There are a variety of treatment options for high-flow steal: arterial ligation distal to the fistula to prevent reversed flow is usually successful in radiocephalic AVFs with an intact ulnar artery and palmar arch.

Distal arterial ligation may also be sufficient in brachial AVFs but intraoperative monitoring with finger or needle pressures is essential as in most cases finger pressures rarely improve sufficiently.

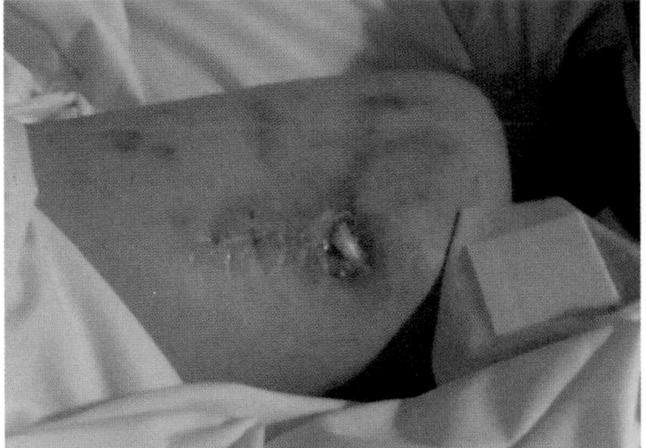

**Figure 16.8** • A PTFE thigh loop with an exposed segment.

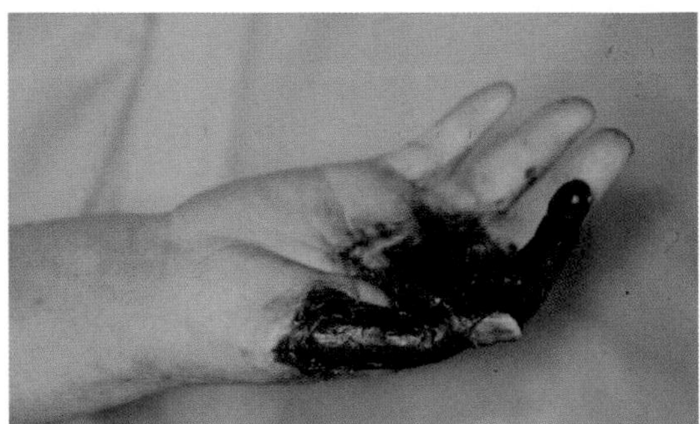

**Figure 16.9** • Severe steal with digital gangrene after a brachial AVF.

In these cases a bypass from the proximal brachial or the axillary artery to the brachial artery distal to the ligature increases the distal pressure enough to relieve symptoms in most cases. This is the so-called DRIL (distal revascularisation interval ligation) procedure[109] (**Fig. 16.10**).

Another technique to prevent distal reversed flow is 'proximalisation of the arterial inflow' in which a brachial AVF or AVG is taken down and a prosthetic graft is led from the axillary or proximal brachial artery and anastomosed to the outflow vein or the arterial end of the AVG[110] (**Fig. 16.11**). This preserves fistula flow but transfers the inflow to a larger, high-flow artery capable of adapting to the reduction in peripheral resistance without distal flow reversal. This may be useful in patients where a diseased run-off might compromise the distal revascularisation of a DRIL procedure.

Fistula flow can be reduced by narrowing the outflow vein ('banding'), but achieving the appropriate degree of stenosis is difficult so it frequently causes thrombosis or fails to relieve the steal. However, in a recent report the degree of stenosis was successfully controlled by tightening a polyester band in stages whilst monitoring the flow rate, digital pressures and subclavian venous oxygen saturation.[111] In another report banding was accomplished by a spindle-like suture and a PTFE strip during intraoperative flow monitoring.[112]

A further flow-reduction method is the 'extension procedure',[113] which is also known as the 'revision using distal inflow' (RUDI),[114] in which the cephalic vein or AVG is detached from its origin on the brachial artery and extended onto the radial artery 2–3 cm from its origin using a vein or prosthetic graft. This narrows the inflow and permits hand perfusion through the ulnar artery (**Fig. 16.12**). The choice of procedure depends on experience and personal preference, but the DRIL procedure is currently the most popular.

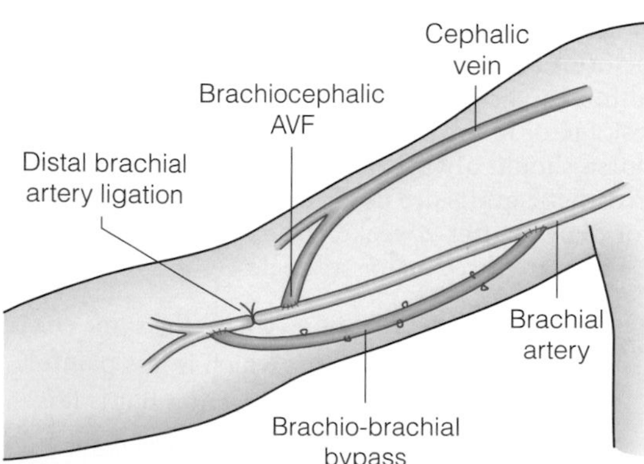


**Figure 16.10** • The DRIL procedure.

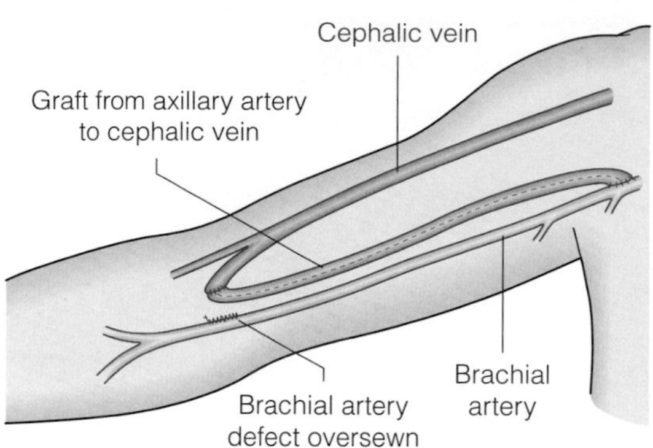


**Figure 16.11** • Proximalisation of the arterial inflow.

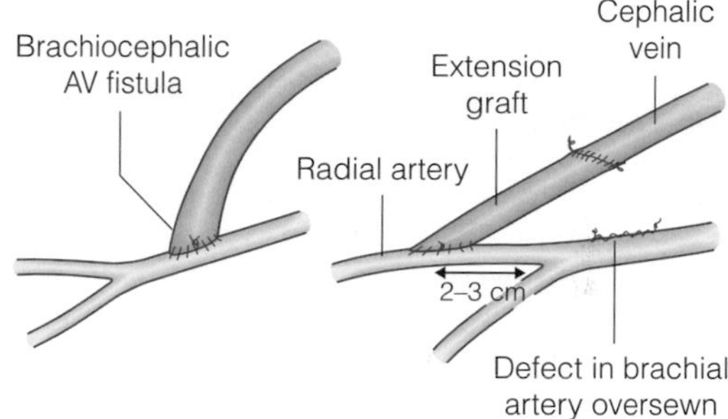


**Figure 16.12** • The extension procedure.

## Carpal tunnel syndrome

The incidence of carpal tunnel syndrome is increased by the presence of an AVF, possibly due to mild oedema due to venous hypertension.[115]

## Cardiac failure

High-output cardiac failure is a rare complication, occurring occasionally with proximal AVFs with fistula flows in excess of 1.5 litres per minute. Bramham's sign (slowing of the heart rate on AVF compression) confirms the diagnosis. Treatment is either by fistula ligation or flow reduction by the extension procedure or controlled banding.[111]

## Venous hypertension and central vein obstruction

Venous hypertension with oedema, venous collateral formation, or ulceration and tissue loss can occur with side-to-side AVFs but is more commonly associated with central venous obstruction (**Fig. 16.13**). If venous hypertension occurs with a side-to-side AVF, ligation of the distal vein draining the AVF is easy to perform and usually curative.

An AVF distal to a central obstruction is likely to exacerbate venous hypertension and may precipitate symptoms. Treatment of central vein obstruction by endovascular means or, as a last resort, surgical

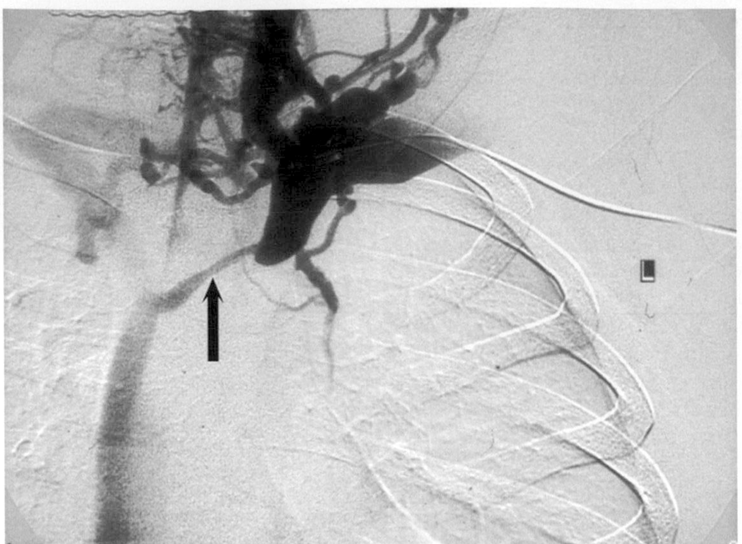

**Figure 16.13** • Venogram showing an innominate vein occlusion.

bypass will preserve the AVF, but sometimes the access must be ligated and created elsewhere, usually in the lower limb.

Subclavian stenosis or thrombosis is usually caused by a previous subclavian CVC. IJV catheters are now preferred but there is still a significant incidence of innominate and SVC stenosis (Fig. 16.13) or thrombosis. Endovascular treatment of these lesions is ideal, but simple angioplasty has a disappointing primary patency rate at 1 year of less than 40% in most studies.[6] Primary assisted or secondary patency rates are more encouraging at 35–97%.[116] Stents have a major role and can either be routinely placed at the initial intervention or reserved for early and frequent re-stenosis. There is no evidence at present advocating covered stents.

Surgical bypass had a similar primary patency rate (70–80%) at 1 year to primary angioplasty and stenting in one study,[117] but has significant morbidity and mortality. Isolated subclavian vein occlusions may be repaired surgically by direct patch angioplasty, an axillo-jugular venous bypass or the jugular turn-down operation. SVC obstruction usually requires a bypass, perhaps using a superficial femoral vein graft to the RA or a long subcutaneous graft from either the IJV or axillary vein to the femoral vein.[6]

### Aneurysm

The AVF outflow vein usually hypertrophies but sometimes reaches aneurysmal proportions (**Fig. 16.14**). In general, such aneurysms can be observed as rupture is rare, but occasionally the access must be ligated, the aneurysm bypassed or the vessel narrowed by a reefing suture if the skin overlying it becomes thin or haemorrhage occurs. The inflow artery may also become ectatic or aneurysmal but this rarely requires treatment.

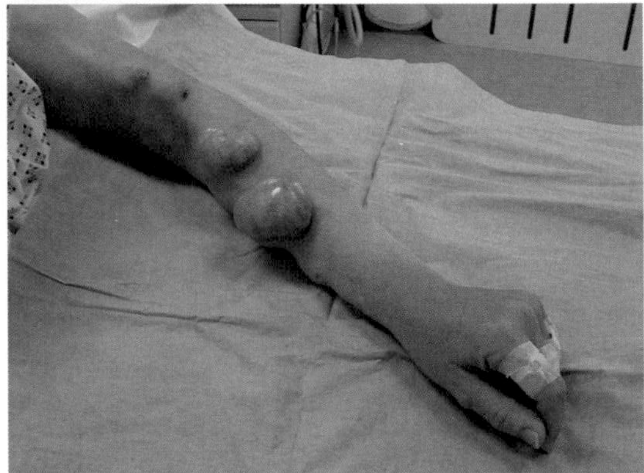

**Figure 16.14** • An aneurysmal wrist AVF.

## Cannulation

Cannulation of AVFs should be performed by adequately trained staff under strict aseptic conditions. A new autologous AVF is usually rested for 6 weeks before needling to allow the vein wall to thicken, although early cannulation did not appear to be a risk factor in the DOPPS.[118] An experienced dialysis nurse should always perform the first cannulation. Prosthetic grafts are needled directly and are usable for dialysis after 2 weeks.

There are three major strategies:

- The buttonhole technique, where the same site is needled at each dialysis, which is less painful and causes less aneurysm formation but is less suitable for grafts because it can cause local graft destruction.

- Area puncture, where the vein or graft is needled over a specific area for each of the withdrawal and reinfusion sites, results in venous dilatation over an area but can also cause stenoses between aneurysmal sections.
- The rope-ladder technique, where needles are inserted for each dialysis by moving along the vein or graft in a sequential pattern. This is probably most suitable for AVGs as the damage of repeated needling is distributed over a larger area and delays the need for revision.

## Access in children

The small calibre of the vessels has discouraged many surgeons from constructing AVFs in small children. Alternative methods such as CAPD are therefore preferred in many units, but when haemodialysis is unavoidable CVCs are commonly used. However, excellent results of radiocephalic or brachial AVFs constructed by microsurgery in small children have been reported from experienced units.[119]

### Key points

- The veins of the dorsum of the hand should be the preferred site for intravenous cannulation. The cephalic and antecubital veins should be reserved for dialysis access in patients with renal failure.
- The right IJV is the preferred site for central venous cannulation, which should be performed under ultrasound control.
- The use of CVCs for acute or short-term dialysis should be minimised because of the risks of septic complications, central venous thrombosis and a higher mortality than AVFs.
- Tunnelled CVCs should be used for dialysis if required for longer than 2 weeks but should only be used long term when an AVF or AVG cannot be constructed.
- Permanent vascular access should, wherever possible, be constructed 16–24 weeks before the anticipated need for dialysis.
- For permanent dialysis access an autogenous AVF should be constructed as distally as possible, preferably in the non-dominant arm.
- AVGs should only be used when the construction of an autogenous AVF is not possible.

## References


1. Sariego J, Bootorabi B, Matsumoto T et al. Major long-term complications in 1,422 permanent venous access devices. Am J Surg 1993; 165:249–51.
2. Rayan SS, Terramani, TT, Weiss VJ et al. The LifeSite hemodialysis access system in patients with limited access. J Vasc Surg 2003; 38:714–18.
3. Seldinger SI. Catheter replacement of the needle in percutaneous arteriography; a new technique. Acta Radiol 1953; 39:368–76.
4. Ansell D, Feest T, Williams AJ et al. (eds) UK Renal Registry Report 2005. Bristol: UK Renal Registry, Chapter 6. The National Dialysis Access Survey – preliminary results, 87–102. (http://www.renalreg.com/Report%202005/Cover_Frame2.htm)
5. Nasser GM, Ayus JC. Infectious complications of haemodialysis access. Kidney Int 2001; 60:1–13.
6. Mickley V. Central vein obstruction in vascular access. Eur J Vasc Endovasc Surg 2006; 32:439–44.
7. Dhingra RK, Young EW, Hulbert-Shearon TE et al. Type of vascular access and mortality in U.S. hemodialysis patients. Kidney Int 2001; 60:1443–51.
8. Tokars JI, Miller ER, Stein G. New national surveillance system for hemodialysis-associated infections: initial results. Am J Infect Control 2002; 30:288–95.
9. Merrer J, De Jonghe B, Golliot F et al. Complications of femoral and subclavian venous catheterisation in critically ill patients: a randomised controlled trial. JAMA 2001; 286:700–07.
10. Chow KM, Szeto CC, Leung CB et al. Cuffed tunneled femoral catheters for long-term hemodialysis. Int J Artif Organs 2001; 24:443–6.
11. Nazarian GK, Bjarnason H, Dietz CA et al. Changes in tunnelled catheter tip position when the patient is upright. J Vasc Intervent Radiol 1997; 8:437–41.
12. Mallory DL, Mcgee WT, Shawker TH et al. Ultrasound improves the success rate of internal jugular vein cannulation. A prospective, randomised trial. Chest 1990; 98:157–60.

In this prospective randomised trial ultrasound was shown to increase the success rate and reduce the complications of internal jugular cannulation.

13. Trerotola SO, Johnson MS, Harris VJ et al. Outcome of tunneled hemodialysis catheters placed via the right internal jugular vein by interventional radiologists. Radiology 1997; 203:489–95.
14. Twardowski ZJ. High-dose intradialytic urokinase to restore the patency of permanent central vein hemodialysis catheters. Am J Kidney Dis 1998; 31:841–7.
15. Savander SJ, Haikal LC, Ehrman KO et al. Hemodialysis catheter-associated fibrin sheaths: treatment with a low-dose rt-PA infusion. J Vasc Intervent Radiol 2000; 11:1131–6.
16. Ponec D, Irwin D, Haire WD et al. Recombinant tissue plasminogen activator (altepase) for restoration of flow in occluded central venous access devices. J Vasc Intervent Radiol 2001; 12:951–5.

    A randomised trial showing that a TPA lock is better than placebo in reopening occluded CVCs, clearing 74% of lines within 2 hours, increasing to 90% with a second treatment. Unfortunately dialysis catheters were excluded from this trial.
17. Bern MM, Lokich JJ, Wallach SR et al. Very low doses of warfarin can prevent thrombosis in central venous catheters. A randomised prospective trial. Ann Intern Med 1990; 112:423–8.
18. Suhocki PV, Conlon PJ, Knelson MH et al. Silastic cuffed catheters for hemodialyss vascular access: thrombotic and mechanical correction of malfunction. Am J Kidney Dis 1996; 28:379–86.
19. Gray RJ, Levitin A, Buck D et al. Percutaneous fibrin sheath stripping versus transcatheter urokinase for malfunctioning well-positioned central venous dialysis catheters: a prospective randomized trial. J Vasc Intervent Radiol 2000; 11:1121–9.
20. Merport M, Murphy TP, Egglin TK et al. Fibrin sheath stripping versus catheter exchange for the treatment of failed tunneled hemodialysis catheters: randomised clinical trial. J Vasc Intervent Radiol 2000; 11:1115–20.
21. Saad TF. Bacteraemia associated with tunnneled, cuffed hemodialysis catheters. Am J Kidney Dis 1999; 34:1114–24.
22. Tanriover B, Carlton D, Saddekni S et al. Bacteraemia associated with tunneled dialysis catheters: comparison of two treatment strategies. Kidney Int 2000; 57:2151–5.
23. Levin A, Mason AJ, Jindal KK et al. Prevention of hemodialysis subclavian vein catheter infections by topical povidone–iodine. Kidney Int 1991; 40:934–8.
24. Johnson DW, MacGinley R, Kay TD et al. A randomized, controlled trial of topical exit site mupirocin application in patients with tunnelled, cuffed haemodialysis catheters. Nephrol Dial Transplant 2002; 17:1802–7.
25. Kamal GD, Pfaller MA, Rempe LE et al. Reduced intravascular catheter infection by antibiotic bonding. JAMA 1991; 265:2364–8.
26. Chatzinikolaou I, Finkel K, Hanna H et al. Antibiotic-coated hemodialysis catheters for the prevention of vascular catheter-related infections: a prospective, randomised study. Am J Med 2003; 115:352–7.
27. Betjes MGH, van Agteren M. Prevention of dialysis catheter-related sepsis with a citrate–taurolidine-containing lock solution. Nephrol Dial Transplant 2004; 19:1546–51.
28. NKF-DOQI clinical practice guidelines for vascular access. National Kidney Foundation – Dialysis Outcomes Quality Initiative. Am J Kidney Dis 1997; 30 (4, Suppl 3):S150–91.

    The original US guidelines for vascular access that are widely recognised throughout the world.
29. Vascular Access Society Guidelines. http://www.vascularaccesssociety.com

    Online guidelines for vascular access produced by the Vascular Access Society – a predominantly European society for the promotion of vascular access for haemodialysis.
30. Winearls CG, Fluck R, Mitchell DC et al. The organization and delivery of the vascular access service for maintenance haemodialysis patients. Report of a joint working party, 2006; http://www.vascularsociety.org.uk/Docs/VASCULAR%20ACCESS%20JOINT%20WORKING%20PARTY%20REPORT.pdf

    Online guidelines and recommendations produced by a panel of UK nephrologists, vascular surgeons and interventional radiologists.
31. Huber TS, Carter JW, Carter RL et al. Patency of autogenous and polytetrafluoroethylene upper extremity arteriovenous hemodialysis accesses: a systematic review. J Vasc Surg 2003; 38:1005–11.

    A review and meta-analysis comparing 34 non-randomised studies of upper limb AV access showing a significantly better primary patency for autogenous AV fistulae at 6 months (72%) and 18 months (541%) than PTFE AV grafts (58% and 33% respectively).
32. Hodges TC, Fillinger MF, Zwolak RM et al. Longitudinal comparison of dialysis access methods: factors for failure. J Vasc Surg 1997; 26:1009–19.

    A large retrospective single centre study shwoing similar secondary patency for autogenous and prosthetic access but a much higher revision rate for AV grafts.
33. Astor BC, Eustace JA, Powe NR et al. Type of vascular access and survival among incident hemodialysis patients: the Choices for Healthy Outcomes in Caring for ESRD (CHOICE) Study. J Am Soc Nephrol 2005; 16:1449–55.

    A large non-randomised multicentre study on the outcome of different forms of AV access, showing a relative mortality for central venous catheters of 1.5 and prosthetic access 1.2 in comparison with autogenous AV fistulae.

34. Breschia MJ, Cimino JE, Appel K et al. Chronic hemodialysis using venepuncture and a surgically created arteriovenous fistula. N Engl J Med 1966; 275:1089–92.
35. Gelabert HA, Freischlag JA. Haemodialysis access. In: Rutherford RB (ed.) Vascular surgery, 5th edn. Philadelphia: Saunders, 2000; pp. 1466–77.
36. NKF-DOQI clinical practice guidelines for vascular access; www.kidney.org/professionals/kdoqi/guideline_upHD_PD_VA/index.htm

    The latest online US guidelines on vascular access.
37. Silva MB, Hobson RW, Pappas PJ et al. A strategy for increasing use of autogenous hemodialysis access procedures: impact of preoperative non invasive evaluation. J Vasc Surg 1998; 27:302–08.
38. Allon M, Lockhart ME, Lilly RZ et al. Effect of preoperative sonographic mapping on vascular access outcomes in hemodialysis patients. Kidney Int 2001; 60:2013–20.
39. Mihmanli I, Besirli K, Kurugoglu S et al. Cephalic vein and hemodialysis fistula. Surgeon's observation versus color Doppler utrasonographic findings. J Ultrasound Med 2001; 20:217–22.
40. Robbin M, Gallichio MH, Deierhoi MH et al. US vascular mapping before hemodialysis access placement. Radiology 2000; 217:83–8.
41. Wells AC, Fernando B, Butler A et al. Selective use of ultrasonographic vascular mapping in the assessment of patients before haemodialysis access surgery. Br J Surg 2005; 92:1439–43.
42. Wong V, Ward R, Taylor J et al. Factors associated with early failure of arteriovenous fistulae for haemodialysis access. Eur J Vasc Endovasc Surg 1996; 12:207–13.
43. Malovrh M. The role of sonography in the planning of arteriovenous fistulae for dialysis. Semin Dial 2003; 16:229–303.
44. Wolowczyk L, Williams AJ, Gibbons CP. The snuffbox arteriovenous fistula for vascular access. Eur J Vasc Endovasc Surg 2000; 19:70–6.
45. Rooijens PP, Tordoir JH, Stijnen T et al. Radiocephalic wrist arteriovenous fistula for hemodialysis: meta-analysis indicates a high primary failure rate. Eur J Vasc Endovasc Surg 2004; 28:583–9.
46. Ehsan O, Bhattacharya D, Darwish A et al. 'Extension technique': a modified technique for brachio-cephalic fistula to prevent dialysis access-associated steal syndrome. Eur J Vasc Endovasc Surg 2005; 29:324–7.
47. Salgado OJ, Chacon RE, Henriquez C. Ulnar–basilic fistula: indications, surgical aspects, puncture technique, and results. Artif Organs 2004; 28:634–8.
48. Tordoir JH, Keuter X, Planken N et al. Autogenous options in secondary and tertiary access for haemodialysis. Eur J Vasc Endovasc Surg 2006; 31:661–6.
49. Dix FP, Khan Y, Al-Khaffaf H. The brachial artery–basilic vein arterio-venous fistula in vascular access for haemodialysis – a review paper. Eur J Vasc Endovasc Surg 2006; 31:70–9.
50. Garcia-Pajares R, Polo JR, Flores A et al. Upper arm polytetrafluoroethylene grafts for dialysis access. Analysis of two different graft sizes: 6 mm and 6–8 mm. Vasc Endovasc Surg 2003; 37:335–43.
51. Lemson MS, Tordoir JH, van Det RJ et al. Effects of a venous cuff at the venous anastomosis of polytetrafluoroethylene grafts for hemodialysis vascular access. J Vasc Surg 2000; 32:1155–63.
52. Sorom AJ, Hughes CB, McCarthy JT et al. Prospective, randomized evaluation of a cuffed expanded polytetrafluoroethylene graft for hemodialysis vascular access. Surgery 2002; 132:135–40.
53. Berardinelli L. Grafts and graft materials as vascular substitutes for haemodialysis access construction. Eur J Vasc Endovasc Surg 2006; 32:203–11.
54. Bhandari Wilkinson A, Sellars L. Saphenous vein forearm grafts and gortex thigh grafts as alternative forms of vascular access. Clin Nephrol 1995; 44:325–8.
55. Keuter XH, De Smet AA, Kessels AG et al. A randomized multicenter study of the outcome of brachial–basilic arteriovenous fistula and prosthetic brachial–antecubital forearm loop as vascular access for haemodialysis. J Vasc Surg 2007 (Epub ahead of print).
56. Rudarakanchana N, Davies AH. Complex vascular access. In: Davies AH, Gibbons CP (eds) Vascular access simplified, 2nd edn. Shrewsbury, UK: tfm Publishing, 2007; Chap. 9, pp. 103–16.
57. Wall LP, Gasparis A, Callahan S et al. Impaired hyperemic response is predictive of early access failure. Ann Vasc Surg 2004; 18:167–71.
58. Rayner HC, Pisoni RL, Gillespie BW et al. Dialysis Outcomes and Practice Patterns Study. Creation, cannulation and survival of arteriovenous fistulae: data from the Dialysis Outcomes and Practice Patterns Study. Kidney Int 2003; 63:323–30.
59. Lin PH, Bush RL, Nelson JC et al. A prospective evaluation of interrupted nitinol surgical clips in arteriovenous fistula for hemodialysis. Am J Surg 2003; 186:625–30.
60. Shenoy S, Miller A, Petersen F et al. A multicentre study of permanent hemodialysis access patency: beneficial effect of clipped vascular anastomotic technique. J Vasc Surg 2003; 38:229–35.
61. Ernandez T, Saudan P, Berney T et al. Risk factors for early failure of native arteriovenous fistulae. Nephron Clin Pract 2005; 101:c39–4.
62. Rodriguez JA, Armadans L, Ferrer E et al. The function of permanent vascular access. Nephrol Dial Transplant 2000; 15:402–8.
63. Murphy GJ, Nicholson ML. Autogeneous elbow fistulae: the effect of diabetes mellitus on maturation, patency, and complication rates. Eur J Vasc Endovasc Surg 2002; 23:452–7.

64. Akoh JA, Sinha S, Dutta S et al. A 5-year audit of haemodialysis access. Int J Clin Pract 2005; 59:847–51.
65. Lazarides MK, Georgiadis GS, Antaniou GA et al. A meta-analysis of dialysis access outcome in elderly patients. J Vasc Surg 2007; 45:420–6.
66. Kats M, Hawxby AM, Barker J et al. Impact of obesity on arteriovenous fistula outcomes in dialysis patients. Kidney Int 2007; 71:39–3.
67. Weitzig GA, Gough IR, Furnival CM. One hundred cases of arteriovenous fistula for haemodialysis access: the effect of cigarette smoking on patency. Aust NZ J Surg 1985; 55:551–4.
68. Andrassy K, Malluche H, Bornfeld H et al. Prevention of PO clotting of AV. Cimino fistulae with acetylsalicyl acid: results of a prospective double blind study. Klin Wochenschr 1974; 52:348–9.
69. Sreedhara R, Himmelfarb J, Lazarus JM et al. Antiplatelet therapy in graft thrombosis: results of a prospective randomised double blind study. Kidney Int 1994; 45:1477–83.
70. Saran R, Dykstra DM, Wolfe RA et al. Dialysis Outcomes and Practice Patterns Study. Association between vascular access failure and the use of specific drugs: the Dialysis Outcomes and Practice Patterns Study (DOPPS). Am J Kidney Dis 2002; 40:1255–63.
71. Kaufman JS, O'Connor TZ, Zhang JH et al. Randomised controlled trial of clopidogrel plus aspirin to prevent hemodialysis access graft thrombosis. J Am Soc Nephrol 2003; 14:2313–21.
72. Trimarchi H, Young P, Forrester M et al. Clopidogrel diminishes hemodialysis access graft thrombosis. Nephron Clin Pract 2006; 102:c128–32.
73. LeSar CJ, Merrick HW, Smith MR. Thrombotic complications resulting from hypercoagulable states in chronic haemodialysis vascular access. J Am Coll Surg 1999; 189:73–9.
74. Heine GH, Ulrich C, Kohler H et al. Is AV fistula patency associated with angiotensin-converting enzyme (ACE) polymorphism and ACE inhibitor intake? Am J Nephrol 2004; 24:461–8.
75. Schmitz PG, McCloud LK, Reikes ST et al. Prophylaxis of hemodialysis graft thrombosis with fish oil: double-blind, randomized, prospective trial. J Am Soc Nephrol 2002; 13:184–90.
76. Fischer-Colbrie W, Clyne N, Jogenstrand T et al. The effect of erythropoietin treatment on arteriovenous haemodialysis fistula/graft: a prospective study with colour flow Doppler ultrasonography. Eur J Vasc Surg 1994; 8:346–50.
77. Martino MA, Vogel KM, O'Brien SP et al. Erythropoietin therapy improves graft patency with no increased incidence of thrombosis or thrombophlebitis. J Am Coll Surg 1998; 187:616–19.
78. Bumann M, Niebel W, Kribben A et al. Pimary failure of arteriovenous fistulae in auto-immune disease. Kidney Blood Press Res 2003; 26:362–7.
79. Kohler TR, Toleikis PM, Gravett DM et al. Inhibition of neointimal hyperplasia in a sheep model of dialysis access failure with the bioabsorbable Vascular Wrap paclitaxel-eluting mesh. J Vasc Surg 2007; 45:1029–37.
80. Kelly B, Melhem M, Zhang J et al. Perivascular paclitaxel wraps block arteriovenous graft stenosis in a pig model. Nephrol Dial Transplant 2006; 21:2425–31.
81. Krivitski NM. Access flow measurement during surveillance and percutaneous transluminal angioplasty intervention. Semin Dial 2003; 16:304–8.
82. Bosman PJ, Boereboom FT, Bakker CJ et al. Access flow measurements in hemodialysis patients: in vivo validation of an ultrasound dilution technique. J Am Soc Nephrol 1996; 7:966–9.
83. Bosman PJ, Boereboom FT, Smits HF et al. Pressure or flow recordings for the surveillance of hemodialysis grafts. Kidney Int 1997; 52:1084–8.
84. Bosman PJ, Boereboom FT, Eiklboom BC et al. Graft flow as a predictor in haemodialysis grafts. Kidney Int 1998; 54:1726–30.
85. May RE, Himmelfarb J, Yenicesu M et al. Predictive measures of vascular access thrombosis: a prospective study. Kidney Int 1997; 52:1656–62.
86. Neyra NR, Ikizler TA, May RE et al. Changes in access blood flow over time predicts vascular access thrombosis. Kidney Int 1998; 54:1714–19.
87. Lilly RZ, Carlton D, Barker J et al. Predictors of arteriovenous graft patency after radiological intervention in haemodialysis patients. Am J Kidney Dis 2001; 37:945–53.
88. McCarley P, Wingard RL, Shyr Y et al. Vascular access blood flow monitoring reduces access morbidity and costs. Kidney Int 2001; 60:1164–72.
89. Schwab SJ, Oliver MJ, Suhocki P et al. Hemodialysis arteriovenous access: detection of stenosis and response to treatment by vascular access blood flow. Kidney Int 2001; 59:358–62.
90. Tessitore N, Lipari G, Poli A et al. Can blood flow surveillance and pre-emptive repair of subclinical stenosis prolong the useful life of arteriovenous fistulae? A randomized controlled study. Nephrol Dial Transplant 2004; 19:2325–33.
91. Ram J, Nassar R, Sharaf et al. Thresholds for significant decrease in hemodialysis access blood flow. Semin Dial 2005; 18:558–64.
92. Krivitski N. Access flow surveillance – major criteria for success. Proc 5th Int Congress of the Vascular Access Society, Nice, 2007; L011.
93. Paulson WD. Access monitoring does not really improve outcomes. Blood Purif 2005; 23:50–6.
94. Dossabhoy NR, Ram SJ, Nassar R et al. Stenosis surveillance of hemodialysis grafts by duplex ultrasound reduces hospitalizations and cost of care. Semin Dial 2005; 18:550–7.

95. Turmel-Rodrigues L, Pengloan J, Baudin S et al. Treatment of stenoses and thrombosis in haemodialysis fistulae and grafts by interventional radiology. Nephrol Dial Transplant 2000; 15:2029–36.

96. Georgiadis GS, Lazarides MK, Lambidis CD et al. Use of short PTFE segments (<6 cm) compares favorably with pure autologous repair in failing or thrombosed native arteriovenous fistulae. J Vasc Surg 2005; 41:76–81.

97. Turmel-Rodrigues L, Pengloan J, Bourquelot P. Interventional radiology in hemodialysis fistulae and grafts: a multidisciplinary approach. Cardiovasc Intervent Radiol 2002; 25:3–16.

98. Gray RJ. AV shunt angioplasty – are patency results good enough? J Vasc Access 2007; 8:155–7.

99. Haskal ZJ, Schumann E, McClennan G et al. A prospective, multi-center randomised evaluation of an IMPRA/Bard ePTFE encapsulated carbon lined nitinol endoluminal device (ED) for AV access graft stenosis. J Vasc Iintervent Radiol 2005; 16:S49 (abstract).

100. Maya ID, Allon M. Outcomes of thrombosed arteriovenous grafts: comparison of stents vs angioplasty. Kidney Int 2006; 69:934–7.

101. Trerotola SO. AVF declotting: techniques and results. J Vasc Access 2007; 8:169–71.

102. Smits HFM, Smits JHM, Wust AF et al. Percutaneous thrombolysis of thrombosed haemodialysis access grafts: comparison of three mechanical devices. Nephrol Dial Transplant 2002; 17:467–73.

103. Aruny JE, Lewis CA, Cardella JF et al. Quality improvement guidelines for percutaneous management of thrombosed or dysfunctional dialysis access. J Vasc Intervent Radiol 2003; 14:S247–53.

104. Turmel-Rodrigues L, Pengloan J, Rodrique H et al. Treatment of failed native arteriovenous fistulae for hemodialysis by interventional radiology. Kidney Int 2000; 57:1124–40.

105. Green LD, Lee DS, Kucey DS. A metaanalysis comparing surgical thrombectomy, mechanical thrombectomy, and pharmacomechanical thrombolysis for thrombosed dialysis grafts. J Vasc Surg 2002; 36:939–45.

106. Valentine RJ, Bouch CW, Scott DJ et al. Do preoperative finger pressures predict early arterial steal in hemodialysis access patients? A prospective analysis. J Vasc Surg 2002; 36:351–6.

107. Van Hoek F, Scheltinga MR, Kouwenberg I et al. Steal in hemodialysis patients depends on type of vascular access. Eur J Vasc Endovasc Surg 2006; 32:710–17.

108. Yeager RA, Moneta GL, Edwards GL et al. Relationship of hemodialysis access to finger gangrene in patients with end-stage renal disease. J Vasc Surg 2002; 36:245–9.

109. Schanzer H, Schwartz M, Harrington W et al. Treatment of ischemia due to "steal" by arteriovenous fistula with distal artery ligation and revascularization. J Vasc Surg 1988; 7:770–3.

110. Zanow J, Kruger U, Scholz H. Proximalization of the arterial inflow: a new technique to treat access-related ischemia. J Vasc Surg 2006; 43:1216–21.

111. Van Hoek F, Scheltinga MR, Lurink M et al. Access flow, venous saturation, and digital pressures in hemodialysis. J Vasc Surg 2007; 45:968–3.

112. Zanow J, Petzold K, Petzold M et al. Flow reduction in high-flow arteriovenous access using intra-operative flow monitoring. J Vasc Surg 2006; 44:1273–8.

113. Ehsan O, Bhattacharya D, Darwish A et al. 'Extension technique': a modified technique for brachio-cephalic fistula to prevent dialysis access-associated steal syndrome. Eur J Vasc Endovasc Surg 2006; 29:324–7.

114. Minion DJ, Moore E, Endean E. Revision using distal inflow: a novel approach to dialysis-associated steal syndrome. Ann Vasc Surg 2005; 19:625–8.

115. Gousheh J, Iranpour A. Association between carpel tunnel syndrome and arteriovenous fistula in hemodialysis patients. Plast Reconstr Surg 2005; 116:508–13.

116. Peden EK. Central venous obstruction: When to treat? What to do? J Vasc Access 2007; 8:161–2.

117. Bhatia DS, Money SR, Ochsner JL et al. Comparison of surgical bypass and percutaneous balloon dilatation with primary stent placement in the treatment of central venous obstruction in the dilaysis patient: one year follow up. Ann Vasc Surg 1996; 10:452–5.

118. Saran R, Dykstra DM, Pisoni RL et al. Timing of first cannulation and vascular access failure in haemodialysis: an analysis of practice patterns at dialysis facilities in the DOPPS. Nephrol Dial Transplant 2004; 19:2334–40.

119. Bourquelot P. Vascular access in children: the importance of microsurgery for creation of autologous arteriovenous fistulae. Eur J Vasc Endovasc Surg 2006; 32:696–700.

# 17

# Varicose veins

Andrew W. Bradbury

## Introduction

In developed countries lower limb venous disease, including varicose veins (VVs) and their complications, affect up to half of the adult population, lead to significant reductions in health-related quality of life (HRQL) and account for 1–2% of total healthcare spending. Despite this, treatment of such disease is generally given a low priority, both clinically and in terms of research. VV surgery is a common cause of medico-legal claims and recurrence rates remain stubbornly high.[1] Successfully meeting the expectations of patients requires excellent communication skills, as well as thorough understanding of the anatomy, pathophysiology and available treatments.[2]

## Pathophysiology

VVs are nearly always due to superficial venous reflux (incompetence) which in the majority of patients is due to:

1. Primary valve failure – primary degenerative changes in the valve annulus and leaflets.
2. Secondary valve failure – developmental weakness in the vein wall leads to secondary widening of the valve commissures and incompetence.

It is likely that both mechanisms are involved, but to a variable extent in different patients.[3] In a small minority of patients, so-called secondary VVs develop following deep vein thrombosis (DVT).

The objective severity of VVs is largely determined by the severity of that reflux and the ability of the patient's calf muscle pump to overcome the haemodynamic consequences. In patients with VVs, during calf relaxation, large volumes of blood enter the (calf) muscle pump from the superficial varices. The muscle pump expels that blood from the leg only for it to re-enter the calf pump via the refluxing superficial veins and perforating veins (re-entry perforators). Mobile patients with mild to moderate superficial reflux and/or an efficient calf pump are able to compensate for this recirculation of venous blood, and to maintain (near) normal ambulatory venous pressures (AVPs), by increasing their calf muscle pump 'stroke volume'. However, those with immobility, severe reflux and/or a weak muscle pump develop sustained venous hypertension (high AVP) leading to the the skin changes of chronic venous insufficiency (CVI).[4] This accounts for two important clinical observations:

- CVI and ulceration can develop without primary deep venous pathology;
- in some patients with both VVs and deep (especially segmental) venous reflux, the latter disappears following eradication of superficial venous reflux.

## Epidemiology

The widespread adoption of the CEAP system to describe the severity and aetiology of lower venous disease has been a major advance (see Box 17.1).[5]

**Box 17.1** • CEAP classification of severity and aetiology of lower venous disease

**Clinical classification**

C0: no visible or palpable signs of venous disease
C1: telangiectasies or reticular veins
C2: varicose veins
C3: oedema
C4a: pigmentation or eczema
C4b: lipodermatosclerosis or atrophie blanche
C5: healed venous ulcer
C6: active venous ulcer
S: symptomatic, including ache, pain, tightness, skin irritation, heaviness and muscle cramps, and other complaints attributable to venous dysfunction
A: asymptomatic

**Aetiological classification**

Ec: congenital
Ep: primary
Es: secondary (post-thrombotic)
En: no venous cause identified

**Anatomical classification**

As: superficial veins
Ap: perforator veins
Ad: deep veins
An: no venous location identified

**Pathophysiological classification**

Pr: reflux
Po: obstruction
Pr,o: reflux and obstruction
Pn: no venous pathophysiology identifiable

A number of large studies has shown that of the adult populations of developed countries approximately 1% have a chronic venous ulcer (CVU); 5–10% have skin changes of CVI, 30–50% have trunk VVs and 80% have 'reticular' or 'hyphenweb' (spider) varices.[6] The prevalence of VVs increases sharply with age in both sexes. Although clinical series always contain an excess of women (usually about 3:1), age for age, lower limb venous disease probably affects men and women roughly equally. The effects of female sex hormones, increased blood volume and the gravid uterus on venous tone and function probably explain why so many female patients ascribe their VVs to pregnancy. A genetic element to the condition seems likely but is difficult to define. VVs are more commonly found in developed than in developing countries but it is difficult to know whether this is 'nature' or 'nurture'.[7] Obesity and a standing occupation (especially hairdressing) appear to aggravate the condition and make presentation to medical services more likely.[8]

## Types of varicose vein

### Primary trunk VVs

These are derived from the long (great) saphenous vein (LSV) and/or short (lesser) saphenous vein (SSV) and/or their major tributaries (**Fig. 17.1**). In slim patients, the superficial veins may be prominent but these 'athletic' veins are physiological and, unlike trunk VVs, are usually uniformly dilated and exhibit no tortuosity or elongation.

### Secondary trunk VVs

Dilated superficial trunk veins may be acting as collateral venous return in the presence of deep venous disease. The presence of the skin changes of CVI and an unusual distribution of varices should alert the clinician to this possibility. Although such veins are dilated, they may show little in the way of varicosity. They should not be removed unless testing confirms that they hinder the venous haemodynamics of the leg.

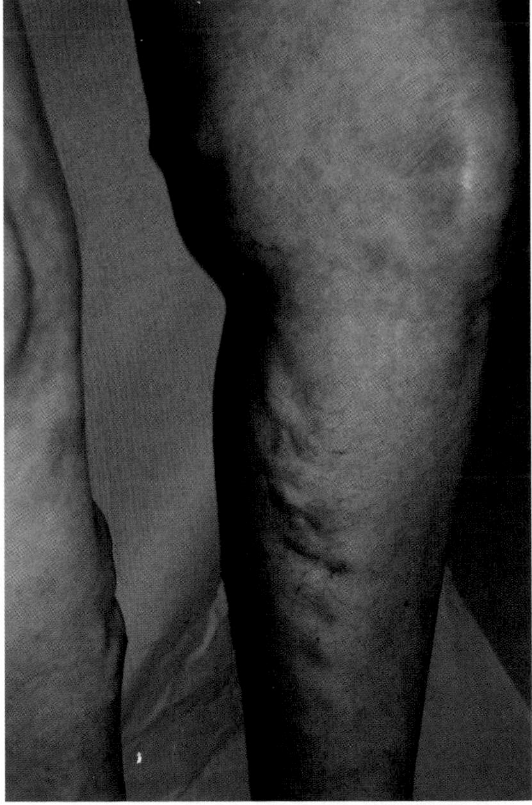

**Figure 17.1** • Typical long saphenous varicose veins affecting the medial calf.

## Reticular varices

These veins lie just beneath or in the deep layers of the skin and, even when normal, may form a highly visible 'reticular' pattern of dark blue veins, especially in those with thin pale skin (**Fig. 17.2**). The owners of such veins may find them unsightly and seek their ablation.

## Hyphenweb veins

These dilated intradermal venules (also called thread veins, spider veins, telangiectasia, venectasia, phlebectasia and venous 'flares') can be associated with trunk or reticular varices. They often appear on the legs of women after pregnancy and in those approaching menarche, and may be related to hormonal changes.

## Vascular malformations

The commonest venous malformation of the leg is Klippel–Trenaunay syndrome (KTS). KTS is characterised by a triad of port-wine stain, varicose veins, and bony and soft tissue hypertrophy, most patients having all three features (**Fig. 17.3**).[9] This is discussed in more detail in Chapter 20. In the author's experience surgery is best avoided. Recurrence of 'varicose veins' after surgery is inevitable and, as the deep venous system is often inadequate, removal of superficial veins may further impair the haemodynamic of the leg. The role of minimally invasive endovenous techniques has yet to be defined.

# Clinical presentation

Patients with VVs fall into two groups:

1. Uncomplicated group – patients in whom venous disease is confined to the superficial system and/or who have compensated mixed deep and superficial disease such that their AVP is (near) normal.

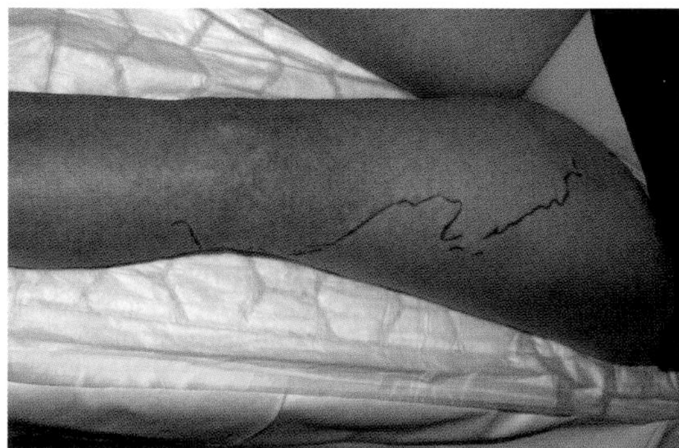

**Figure 17.2** • Typical reticular veins.

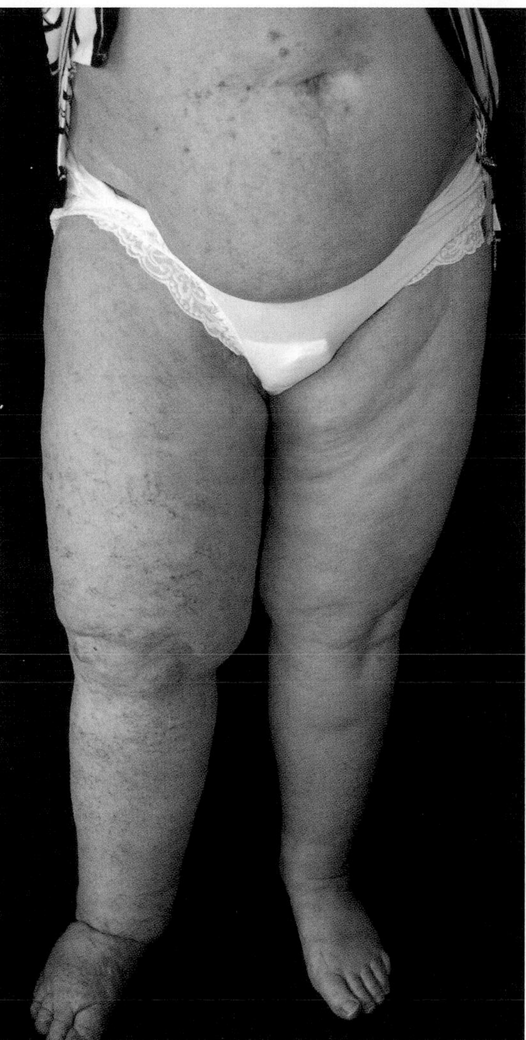

**Figure 17.3** • Klippel–Trenaunay syndrome of right leg also involving right pelvis and trunk.

2. Complicated group – patients who have combined superficial and deep venous disease and/or isolated superficial disease that has decompensated leading to high AVP and the risk of skin changes.

## Uncomplicated VVs

### Cosmesis

Many patients express dissatisfaction with the appearance of their legs and different factors determine whether this leads an individual to seek medical treatment. There is a general consensus that 'cosmetic' surgery should not normally be funded from the public purse. For this reason, some patients may attribute physical symptoms to their varices, fearing that they will not otherwise receive treatment.

## Symptoms

Many symptoms have been attributed to uncomplicated VVs. The Edinburgh Vein Study showed an inconsistent and gender-dependent relationship between a range of lower limb 'venous' symptoms (heaviness/tension, feeling of swelling, aching, restless leg, cramps, itching, tingling) and the presence and severity of trunk, reticular and hyphenweb varices. Clinical experience also suggests little concordance between symptoms and signs; some small varices are painful while many large varices are surprisingly asymptomatic. Some interpret these discrepancies as implying that uncomplicated VVs almost never cause lower limb symptoms and, as such, surgery is always 'cosmetic'. However, several studies have shown that VVs are associated with a reduced HRQL and that this can be improved by treatment.[10,11] This suggests that proper assessment and investigation does allow the genuinely symptomatic patients to be identified and that treatment directed at their VVs is beneficial.

## Reassurance

Many patients attending clinic have concerns about the future as well as their current symptoms; in particular, the subsequent risks of CVU and DVT.[12] The vast majority of patients with uncomplicated VVs never develop skin changes or CVU or DVT and can be confidently reassured. However, in older patients undergoing surgery or prolonged immobilisation, the presence of VVs (which in this age group may indicate previous DVT), together with other risk factors, must be taken into account when deciding upon thromboembolic prophylaxis.

## Superficial thrombophlebitis

This is a sterile inflammation of the vein wall and surrounding tissues secondary to thrombosis and is a common, painful and (rarely) life-threatening complication of VVs. Treatment includes analgesia and anti-inflammatory agents. Topical non-steroidal anti-inflammatory drug (NSAID) gels provide good relief (application under 'cling-film' aids absorption). Compression may prevent thrombus propagation, but the leg is often too tender for this, and early evacuation/aspiration of semiliquid haematoma may relieve symptoms. Duplex ultrasonography (DUS) should be performed to ensure that thrombus is not propagating into the deep system. If such thrombus is found, patients should be anticoagulated as for DVT and some surgeons recommend surgical removal of the thrombus and saphenofemoral ligation. Recurrence is common and the affected segments of vein should be removed once the inflammation has settled, although this can be difficult due to scarring. If thrombophlebitis is migratory, or occurs in the absence of VVs, then an underlying condition (e.g. malignancy, thrombophilia) should be suspected.[13]

# Complicated VVs

The complications of VVs include the following:

- **Corona phlebectatica.** This is also called malleolar flare and is one of the earliest skin manifestations of CVI. It comprises a leash of prominent, dilated, intradermal or subdermal veins at the medial malleolus (**Fig. 17.4**). The overlying skin is thin and fragile. Trauma can lead to haemorrhage and sometimes ulceration.
- **Lipodermatosclerosis.** Increased venous pressure can lead to extravasation of blood, with resulting inflammation and skin staining thought to be due to haemosiderin deposition (**Fig. 17.5**).[14] This may develop insidiously or can present acutely with acute pain and discoloration that mimics cellulitis.
- **Atrophie blanche.** Scar-like tissue that is thin and pale as a result of the reduction in papillary capillaries and collagen; it occurs at the site of previous ulceration.
- **Varicose eczema.** Itchy, scaly, dry skin over an area affected by CVI; scratch marks are often visible and often lead to ulceration (**Fig. 17.6**).
- **Oedema.** Other non-venous causes of oedema should be considered. A degree of lymphoedema may coexist with CVI.
- **Pain.** This may be described variably as aching affecting the whole leg or focal pain and tenderness related to particularly prominent varix.
- **Haemorrhage.** This is often alarming, even life-threatening, and frequently occurs following trauma. Direct pressure and elevation of the

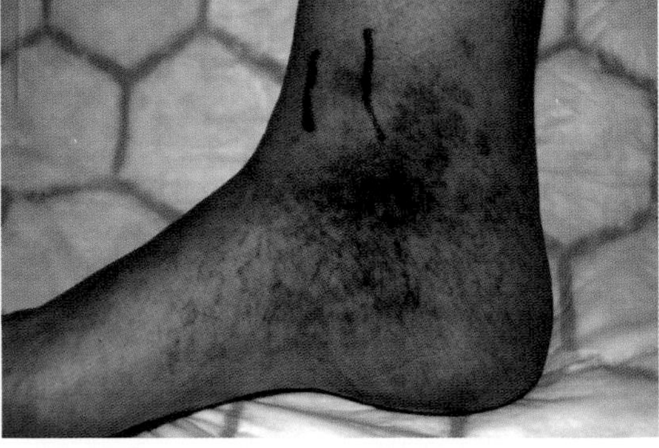

**Figure 17.4** • Corona phlebectatica (venous flare).

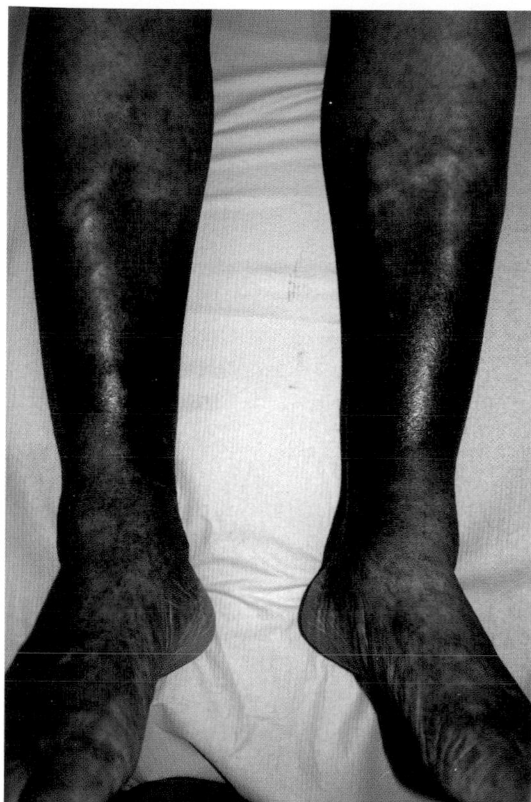

**Figure 17.5** • Bilateral lipodermatosclerosis.

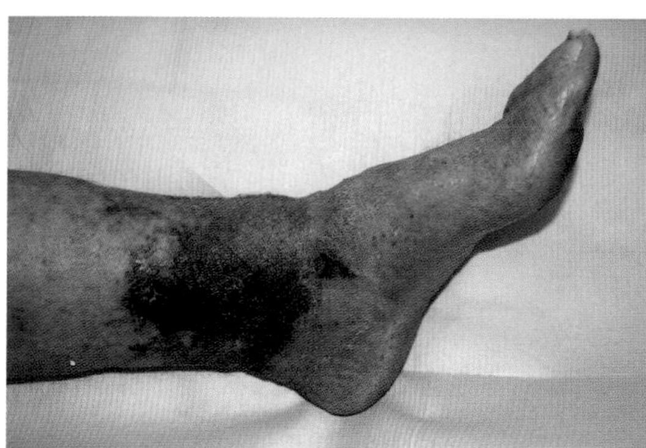

**Figure 17.6** • Varicose eczema (a prelude to ulceration).

limb will always arrest venous haemorrhage. Recurrent bleeding can be treated by underrunning the vein with an absorbable suture under local anaesthetic but inevitably further traumatises a vulnerable area of skin. The author has found foam sclerotherapy (see below) with compression to be an extremely effective and durable alternative.

## Clinical assessment and investigations

When assessing the patient with VVs, three important questions need to be answered:

- Are the symptoms due to venous disease?
- Is the presentation complicated or uncomplicated?
- Is there any other significant pathology, such as arterial disease?

### History

Orthopaedic, neurological and arterial causes of leg symptoms must be excluded. Particular attention must be paid to a history of previous DVT, leg trauma (fracture, joint replacement) and venous surgery. A family history of venous disease, particularly early-onset, recurrent or unusual thrombotic events, should be sought. It is has now been shown by several groups that many patients with CVI and CVU, even a significant proportion of those with simple VVs, have one or more underlying thrombophilias.[15]

### General examination

The patient should be examined in a warm room, standing with the hip and knee flexed to allow venous filling. The examiner must see the whole leg and lower abdominal wall to define the presence of scars and the pattern of varices.

In addition, the following should be recorded:

- oedema;
- skin changes of CVI;
- arterial pulses with or without ankle–brachial pressure index (ABPI).

Athletic veins and secondary varicose veins carry increased amounts of venous blood, *but in the correct physiological direction and without reflux*, and do not show varicosity. Reflux, leading to subvalvular turbulence, is necessary to produce varicosity, i.e. elongation, tortuosity and sacculation. A cough impulse and thrill are often palpable in the groin and over major varices.

Potentially misleadingly, many patients with advanced skin changes of CVI ± CVU, despite the presence of marked superficial reflux on DUS, have few visible VVs on inspection because of fibrosis of the vein wall and surrounding tissues. The presence of VVs can sometimes be inferred by the development of venous 'grooves' on elevating the leg.

### Hand-held Doppler examination

It is widely accepted that the clinical assessment of lower venous disease (inspection and tourniquet tests) is unreliable and so insufficient for the planning of treatment.[16] Proponents of hand-held (continuous wave) Doppler (HHD) argue that in the right hands it is accurate and allows DUS to be used selectively.[17,18] However, the advent of affordable, portable, 'user-friendly' DUS machines, and the move from surgical to non-surgical duplex-based treatment methods, means that an increasing number of vascular surgeons are choosing to undertake DUS (often themselves) on virtually all their patients.

### Duplex ultrasonography

It has been widely accepted for many years that patients with suspected deep venous disease, recurrent VVs and reflux in the politeal fossa should underdo DUS prior to intervention. However, there is growing evidence that a universal DUS policy improves outcomes. This is because:

1. Deep venous disease cannot be predicted and cannot be characterised without DUS.[19]
2. In patients with VVs on the back of the leg, only DUS can provide crucial information regarding (a) the relative contributions from tributaries of the LSV, the SSV, the vein of the popliteal fossa[20] and the Giacomini vein (GV),[21] and (b) the anatomy of the sapheno-popliteal junction (SPJ).
3. In patients with VVs on the front of the leg (of presumed LSV origin), only DUS can identify LSV duplication, reflux in the anterior accessory saphenous vein (AASV) and other major tributaries (all of which, if missed, are common causes of recurrence), segmental LSV hypoplasia (which can hinder conventional striping)[22] and locate incompetent perforating veins (IPVs).
4. In the context of an operation with a reputation for unacceptably high rates of recurrence and medico-legal interest, why risk 'getting it wrong'[23] for the sake of a harmless scan that with practice can be done as quickly as HHD (while continuing to take the history) and that allows one to demonstrate visually to the patient what is wrong?

There is also increasing evidence that DUS should be used postoperatively (at, say, 2–3 months) as a quality assurance tool and again (at, say, 12 months) to identify those patients who are likely to develop recurrent disease.[24]

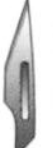
Routine preoperative duplex examination led to an improvement in results 2 years after surgery for patients with primary varicose veins.[18]

### Other investigations

In modern day-to-day practice there is almost no call for varicography or plethysmography, although the latter can be a useful tool for researchers when assessing global haemodynamic outcome following novel treatments and for health service providers wanting to 'ration' VV treatment.[25–27]

## Treatment

The perfect treatment for VVs would rapidly and permanently abolish all sources of superficial venous reflux, relieve all physical symptoms, significantly improve the appearance of the leg, be complication free, allow a fast (immediate) return to normal activities, be inexpensive, and be widely available and applicable to affected patients.[28] Such treatment does not and probably never will exist but, increasingly aware of the shortcomings of surgery, clinicians have devoted considerable energies into the development of minimally invasive alternatives such as radiofrequency ablation, endovenous laser ablation and ultrasound-guided foam sclerotherapy (also called endovenous chemical ablation, EVCA).[29]

### Compression therapy

Treatment during pregnancy should be conservative with compression hosiery, although for severe or recurrent thrombophlebitis sapheno-femoral junction (SFJ) ligation under local anaesthesia may be considered. Patients with uncomplicated VVs with concerns about future thrombosis, bleeding and/or ulceration can usually be reassured and discharged. Patients who request treatment purely for cosmetic reasons pose a potentially difficult problem in the present healthcare environment. In the absence of guidelines from the competent authority, surgeons have to make up their own minds on the merit of intervention in these cases.

Graduated compression hosiery may relieve symptoms, conceal veins and prevent deterioration of the skin changes associated with venous hypertension. However, stockings may be uncomfortable, their beneficial effect lasts only as long as they are worn and they must be replaced regularly. Class I compression may provide symptomatic relief for uncomplicated varicose veins but those with complications require class II or even class III (see Chapter 18). Although most patients require only a below-knee stocking, compliance remains a major problem. Compliance can be improved by providing patients with a stocking applicator and information about the wide range of stockings that are available.

There seems little doubt that compression stockings retard the progression of skin changes and prevent recurrent ulceration in patients with complicated VVs.

Such patients should be encouraged to wear their stockings for life. Stockings may be a useful diagnostic test when there is uncertainty about the extent to which leg symptoms are attributable to varices.

## Surgery

### General points

Not surprisingly, patients with VVs prefer, and get better outcomes from, surgery than they do compression only.

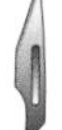

Surgical treatment provides symptomatic relief and significant improvements in quality of life in patients referred to secondary care with uncomplicated varicose veins.[30]

For patients with uncomplicated varicose veins and evidence of sapheno-femoral or sapheno-popliteal reflux, surgical treatment for varicose veins offers a modest health benefit for relatively little additional NHS cost relative to conservative treatment.[31]

Although VV surgery has a reputation for being associated with unacceptably high rates of recurrence and medico-legal claims, much can be done during preoperative assessment and the surgery itself to minimise these risks.

The patient should be warned about the common, almost inevitable, consequences of surgery as failure to do so may lead the patient to conclude that an unsatisfactory operation has been performed. These include bruising, areas of parasthesia[32] and the fact that it is sometimes impossible to remove all prominent veins with a stab avulsion technique. Any small residual veins can be dealt with by means of injection sclerotherapy, which should be viewed as an integral part of the overall treatment. The risk of recurrence, inevitable in a proportion of patients, should be discussed openly with the patient and documented in the case records. Information leaflets and specific consent forms may be useful but do not guarantee legal protection.

The operating surgeon must take personal responsibility for preoperative marking. Whether single lines or tramlines are used, incisions should not cut through markings to avoid tattooing. After marking, the patient should be asked if any varices have been missed. Some patients will point out prominent veins on the dorsum of the foot. Although these are usually physiological, many patients will express disappointment if these are still present when they return to the clinic. It is therefore worth discussing with the patient what should be done with these veins preoperatively, as their removal appears to carry no detriment to the patient (but beware tendons and nerves).

### Day-case surgery

An increasingly large proportion of VV operations are done as a day-case. The contraindications to day-case surgery include extensive varicose veins, advanced age, impaired fitness, obesity and lack of family support at home.

### Anaesthesia

Surgery for VVs can be performed under general, regional or local anaesthesia. The LSV can be stripped using a femoral nerve block but this inevitably leads to motor loss that prevents walking for several hours. Others inject along the course of the vein with a large volume of dilute local anaesthetic ('tumescent' anaesthesia) and stress the value of using adrenaline to reduce blood loss and bruising. When using local anaesthetic it is important not to exceed the toxic dose.

### Positioning

This is supine for LSV surgery with the legs spread apart on a board (especially if bilateral) and usually prone for SSV surgery. Some surgeons perform SSV surgery with the patient in the lateral position as this allows the anaesthetist to use a laryngeal mask rather than an armoured endotracheal tube. A head-down position reduces venous bleeding and the risk of air embolism but can lead to facial and laryngeal oedema and ventilatory problems.

### Sapheno-femoral ligation

- In a patient of normal build the SFJ usually lies directly beneath the groin crease; in the obese it lies above.
- Do not divide any vein until the SFJ has been unequivocally identified.
- The superficial external pudendal artery usually passes between the LSV and common femoral vein (CFV) but its course is variable and does not constitute a reliable landmark.
- Follow and divide all tributaries beyond secondary branch points.
- Ligate the LSV flush with the CFV using either a transfixion suture or double tie. Some authorities recommend the use of non-absorbable suture or other barrier method to reduce neovascularisation (see below).
- Divide the deep external pudendal vein as it comes off the CFV (optional if small).
- Directly ligate (and consider stripping) high posteromedial and anterolateral tributaries to reduce the risk of haematoma and thigh recurrence; look for (on preoperative duplex) and deal with a refluxing anterior accessory

saphenous vein (leaving this behind is a very common cause of recurrence).

- If the LSV cannot be stripped, then as much as possible should be removed to minimise recurrence.

## Neovascularisation

The controversy continues over whether neovascularisation exists and, if so, what it is, how it develops and the clinical consequences. There is no doubt that patients often develop new veins at the site of surgery, typically at the site of SFJ (or SPJ) dissection but also in stripper tunnels[33] and at the site of perforator ligation and even stab avulsions. The question is whether neovascularisation truly represents new blood vessel formation as a result of angiogenesis stimulated by factors released at the time of wound healing, or whether these veins have always been present and simply grown to a detectable size as a result of changes in haemodynamic forces. The author's view is that both mechanisms are involved to a varying degree. In practice, the development of significant recurrent VVs in the leg after previous SFJ (SPJ) ligation is nearly always associated with reflux in a non- or incompletely stripped LSV (SSV) or major tributary in the thigh. Numerous different methods of trying to prevent neovascularisation have been tried with varying success.[34]

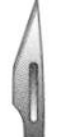

Insertion of a polytetrafluoroethylene (PTFE) patch following redo SFJ ligation and LSV stripping did not affect the rate of perioperative complications and it did not appear to contain neovascularisation.[35]

There is some evidence that using a non-absorbable suture to ligate and oversew the saphenous stump will reduce neovascularisation.

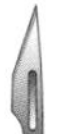

Recurrent reflux in the groin was reduced by oversewing the ligated SFJ in patients having varicose vein surgery.[36]

Many surgeons oversew the cribriform fascia and some oversew the LSV track after stripping to reduce the risk of haematoma formation. However, perhaps the only way to really avoid neovascularisation is to avoid surgery.[37] The best way to reduce the consequences of neovascularisation after surgery is to make sure it has nothing to connect to further down the leg by stripping the LSV (SSV) and major tributaries.

## Stripping

Several studies including randomised trials have clearly shown that LSV stripping improves HRQL by reducing the risk of recurrence, probably by (i) disconnecting the thigh perforators and saphenous tributaries and (ii) preventing any neovascularisation arising from the saphenous stump reconnecting with the LSV.[38]

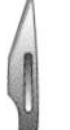

Stripping the LSV is recommended as part of routine varicose vein surgery as it reduced the risk of reoperation by 60% after 11 years, although it did not reduce the rate of visible recurrent veins.[39]

However, debate continues as to how the stripping should be undertaken.[40]

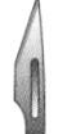

Flushing of the GSV tunnel with bupivacaine plus adrenaline significantly reduces postoperative pain and haematoma formation in patients undergoing GSV stripping for varicose veins.[41]

Cryosurgery has comparable postoperative results with conventional short stripping. Operation time is reduced with cryosurgery, but postoperative pain scores are higher. Patients favor cryosurgery because of better cosmetic results.[42]

It is widely recognised that LSV stripping is associated with a significant risk (up to about 20%) of (saphenous) nerve injury.[43] It is believed that those risks can be significantly reduced, although by no means eliminated by stripping from above downwards and only to the knee (as opposed to the ankle which was abandoned many years ago)[44] using an inversion stripping technique (as opposed to a stripper with an 'acorn'). This latter assertion has not been demonstrated in two randomised controlled trials. One drawback of stripping only to the knee is that reflux in the below-knee LSV, present either at the time of surgery or developing subsequently, is an important potential source of recurrence.[45] Sequential avulsion of the LSV is believed by some to be more complete and less likely to damage the saphenous nerve. However, it is less cosmetically acceptable and takes longer.

Properly counselled, most patients will not be unduly bothered by the usually uncomplicated sensory loss around their ankle despite the fact that is often quite persistent, even permanent. But a proportion will be and regret having had the operation, a big problem if they have not been told of the possibility. However, the biggest problem is that up to 1% of affected patients can develop saphenous neuralgia leading to chronic pain and dysaesthesia that is difficult to treat and may drive the patient to seek legal advice.

Whatever method is used, safe stripping requires that the groin anatomy is clearly displayed and that the stripper is passed from above downwards (minimising, it is believed, the danger of nerve injury and passage of the stripper through a perforator into the deep system) and is palpated subcutaneously throughout its course. Preoperative DUS mapping of the LSV allows the surgeon to know that the stripper is passing in the expected direction. Such DUS mapping will also show the site of major tributaries and perforators, allowing direct pressure to be applied to reduce haematoma; it will also identify LSV duplications, segmental LSV hypoplasia and the presence of an anterior accessory saphenous vein. This detailed anatomical knowledge is vital if the risks of leaving behind refluxing saphenous and non-saphenous superficial veins in the thigh, known to be the single greatest source of recurrence, are to be minimised.

Regrettably, the author has seen, in his capacity as an expert witness, patients who have had variously their deep veins and arteries stripped;[46] so, if in doubt, do not strip, re-evaluate the situation, ask for help and if you are still not happy leave the vein in situ!

## Sapheno-popliteal ligation

The practice of SSV surgery appears to vary widely,[47] but nearly everyone accepts that 'flush' SPJ ligation is much more difficult and less successful than surgeons would like it to be;[48] redo SSV surgery frightens most sensible surgeons. For these reasons, the author has virtually abandoned SSV surgery in favour of ultrasound-guided foam sclerotherapy; other surgeons have chosen other non-surgical inteventions.[49] A few points:

- Failure to mark preoperatively the SSV, the SPJ and the GV (if present) with DUS will lead to misplaced incisions, missed junctions, and an unacceptably high rate of collateral damage and recurrence; the author would suggest that nowadays such an omission is probably medico-legally indefensible.
- Traction on the SSV can tent up and damage the mobile and thin-walled popliteal vein. Palpation of the artery gives an indication of the depth of dissection.
- The common peroneal nerve runs adjacent to and then around the medial edge of biceps femoris and is at risk from lateral retraction or a careless stitch when closing the popliteal fascia.[50]
- Flush ligation of the SPJ, generally thought to reduce recurrence, can be difficult to achieve, especially in the obese. The anatomy may also be obscured by large gastrocnemius veins joining the SSV just before the junction. There is no consensus about whether to ligate these (the author does not). Therefore, in some patients, the possible benefits of a flush SPJ ligation (as opposed to one 1–2 cm distal to the junction) are outweighed by the risks of nerve and vascular injury.
- Stripping the SSV is widely believed to be associated with a significant risk of damage to the sural nerve, although practice is highly variable and the evidence base limited. In a recent prospective, non-randomised study (where the use of preoperatvie DUS was highly variable) 67 legs had SSV stripping (by a variety of techniques) and 116 had SPJ disconnection. The incidence of visible recurrent varicosities at 1 year was non-significantly lower after SSV stripping (18% vs. 24%). SSV stripping was not associated with an increase in numbness (both groups 28%) but was associated with significant reduction in SPJ incompetence (13% vs. 32%) at 1 year.[51] However, if you cause a sural nerve injury and you have not warned the patient of the risk then successful medico-legal action seems likely. Nowadays, there are non-surgical ways of 'stripping' the SSV that appear to carry no risk of nerve injury (see below).
- Failure to close the popliteal fascia as a definite layer will result in a rather unattractive 'bulge' at the back of the knee that is difficult to treat, although the author has had some success with mesh repair (of course, in patients operated elsewhere!).

## Tourniquets

Use of a tourniquet reduces blood loss but appears not be associated with any other benefits. The Boazul cuff is a sterile rubber exsanguinator/tourniquet that is rolled up the leg and held in place with a wedge (**Fig. 17.7**).

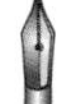

Use of a tourniquet appears to reduce blood loss during surgery. There were no reported differences between the use or non-use of a tourniquet in terms of complications and morbidity. However, the available trials were not of sufficient size to detect rarer complications such as nerve damage.[52]

The author is not a fan of tourniquets as he had found difficulty distinguishing vascular from non-vascular structures in a bloodless field (especially in the popliteal fossa); he is also aware of a number of patients who have suffered quite serious complications from tourniquet use leading to litigation.

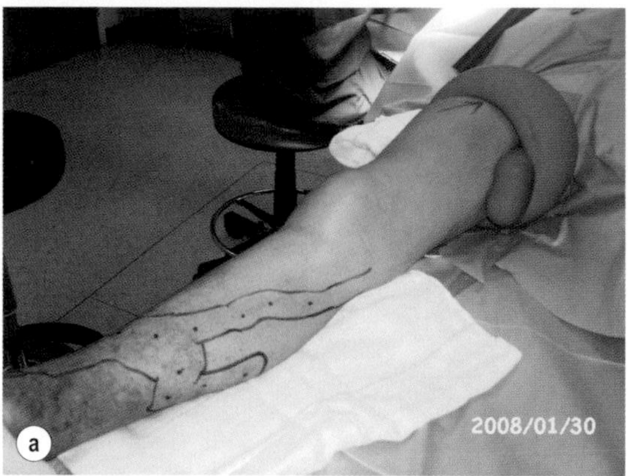


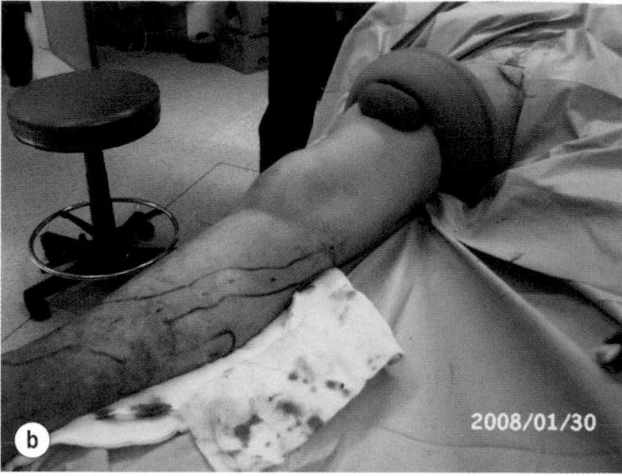


**Figure 17.7 •** **(a)** Boazul cuff in position. Note VVs marked with tramlines and phlebectomy hook. **(b)** Minimal blood loss after extensive phlebectomies.

## Avulsions

Some non-venous structures are at risk during avulsions: the lateral popliteal (common peroneal) nerve at the neck of fibula, the tibial nerves and vessels behind the medial malleolus, the sural nerve in the median line of the posterior calf or behind the lateral malleolus, and the saphenous nerve on the medial calf. Using a variety of hooks, veins can be removed through tiny stab incisions, requiring no suture. Stab incisions should normally be made vertically as these are closed naturally by the compression bandage. At the present time there is no evidence of benefit for powered phlebectomy.[53]

## Perforator ligation

Despite a lot of research into this topic, there is no clear evidence that interrupting IPVs by either open surgery or subfascial endoscopic perforator surgery (SEPS) is of clinical benefit in patients with VVs.[54]

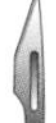

The addition of SEPS to standard LSV stripping reduced the number of IPVs but had no effect on recurrence rates or quality of life at 1 year.[55]

## Repeat groin dissection

The CFV and SFJ are approached through non-operated tissues, usually laterally. The CFV can then be skeletonised for 1–2 cm above and below the junction, which is then divided flush and repaired with non-absorbable suture. The LSV is often still present and its upper end can be difficult to locate, in which case it can be located at the knee, aided by preoperative duplex marking. The stripper is passed up to the groin and then stripped in the normal way. If the DUS shows large connections in the groin, then a formal groin redissection is performed. However, if the scan shows only neovascularisation with tiny channels, then groin dissection and its associated morbidity can be avoided; simply passing a stripper upwards from below removes the remaining LSV.

## Perioperative care

Although VV surgery should be 'clean', several studies have suggested that up to 10% of operated patients attend their GP in the postoperative period because of 'wound infection' and that many of these patients receive antibiotics. There is no evidence that using antibiotic prophylaxis at the time of VV surgery will reduce that occurrence but the author has taken to giving one dose of broad-spectrum antibiotic at induction. The risks of DVT following interventions for VVs, and what can be done to reduce them, are debated endlessly at venous meetings.

An extract from the author's patient information sheet is reproduced below:

- **Deep vein thrombosis** (DVT). Many patients are concerned and ask specifically about the risks of DVT after VV surgery and, indeed, there is continuing debate within the profession regarding magnitude of those risks and how to minimise them. The best study is of 377 patients scanned 2–4 weeks, 6 and 12 months after VV surgery.[56] DVT was detected in 20 patients (5.3%). Only eight patients had symptoms and no patient developed symptoms consistent with pulmonary embolus (PE). Eighteen of the 20 DVTs were confined to the calf veins. Half of the DVTs had resolved without any residual damage to the deep veins at 1 year. The authors of this paper concluded that incidence of DVT following varicose vein surgery was higher than previously thought, but these DVTs had minimal short- or long-term clinical significance.

- **Pulmonary embolus.** If a DVT develops after VV surgery then, as described above, there is a risk of clot travelling to the lung (PE) and causing problems (including potentially death). But this is very rare (probably much less than 1 in 10 000 risk).
- **Stopping the oral contraceptive pill (OCP) or hormone replacement therapy (HRT).** Both the OCP and HRT contain the female sex hormone estrogen and it is well recognised that this hormone increases the stickiness of the blood, and so the risks of blood clots including DVT and PE. Some surgeons ask their patients to stop their OCP/HRT 6 weeks before VV surgery and to recommence 6 weeks after their operation. The problem with that approach is that patients face a real risk of (presumably unwanted) pregnancy and a return of menopausal symptoms. In addition, there is no evidence that for the majority of patients this approach meaningfully reduces the risks of DVT/PE after VV surgery, which as discussed above are small. For these reasons I, along with many others surgeons, do not routinely recommend discontinuation of OCP/HRT.
- **Use of heparin to reduce the risk of DVT/PE.** Although there is no incontrovertible evidence that it reduces the risks of DVT/PE, I, along with many other surgeons, routinely prescribe one dose of low-molecular-weight heparin (a chemical that thins the blood) at the time of surgery.

When bandaging the leg, the surgeon should be aware of any arterial impairment and ensure the presence of good capillary return to the toes. There is no good evidence that any one bandaging system or postoperative schedule is superior and practice varies greatly.

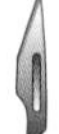

There was no benefit in wearing compression stockings for more than 1 week following uncomplicated high saphenous ligation with stripping of the great saphenous vein with respect to postoperative pain, number of complications, time to return to work or patient satisfaction for up to 12 weeks following surgery.[57]

Precise postoperative instructions and adequate analgesia should be given and the patient warned to return to hospital immediately if the operated leg becomes excessively painful.

## Endovenous laser ablation (EVLA)

EVLA involves using a percutaneously placed catheter to deliver laser light energy to create thermal damage of the vein wall. This results in destruction of the intima, collagen denaturation of the media and eventually fibrotic occlusion of the vein (**Fig. 17.8**).[58–61]

Potential patient advantages include:

- avoidance of general anaesthesia – it is usually performed as an outpatient procedure under local 'tumescent' anaesthetic (at the cannulation sites and around the vein to be treated) in a 'clean room' (as opposed to an operating theatre);
- less morbidity (pain and bruising) resulting in, potentially, an earlier return to normal acivities and work, although we know that outcome measure is affected by many factors other than the procedure;[62]
- no surgical wounds and so little or no risk of infection or scarring;
- reduced risk of nerve injury;
- avoidance of neovascularisation due to lack of wounds and, possibly, preservation of SFJ tributaries responsible for draining the perineum and anterior abdominal wall.

Although, as with any new technique, there is a learning curve in terms of patient selection and the procedure itself, once mastered it seems that EVLA can safely eradicate LSV, and with care (sural nerve) SSV, reflux in the short term (up to 2 years) in up to 95% of patients with a low rate of minor (bruising around the puncture site, transient paraesthesias, superficial phlebitis, pigmentation) and major (skin burns, DVT, PE) complications.

EVLA has not been around long enough to know what the 5- or 10-year results will be, but if we accept early duplex recurrence as a reliable surrogate for later symptomatic recurrence, then it seems unlikely that EVLA will be significantly worse than surgery. The potential downsides to EVLA are:

- Significant additional expense for equipment and consumables.
- Issues around the use of lasers (goggles, controlled environment, etc.).
- It does not treat the varices, only the trunk. Although it is argued that once trunkal reflux has been abolished, the varices shrink in a significant proportion of patients, one suspects that many patients require further treatment (e.g. stab avulsions, sclerotherapy).
- As with any catheter-based endovascular technique it can be difficult (impossible) to

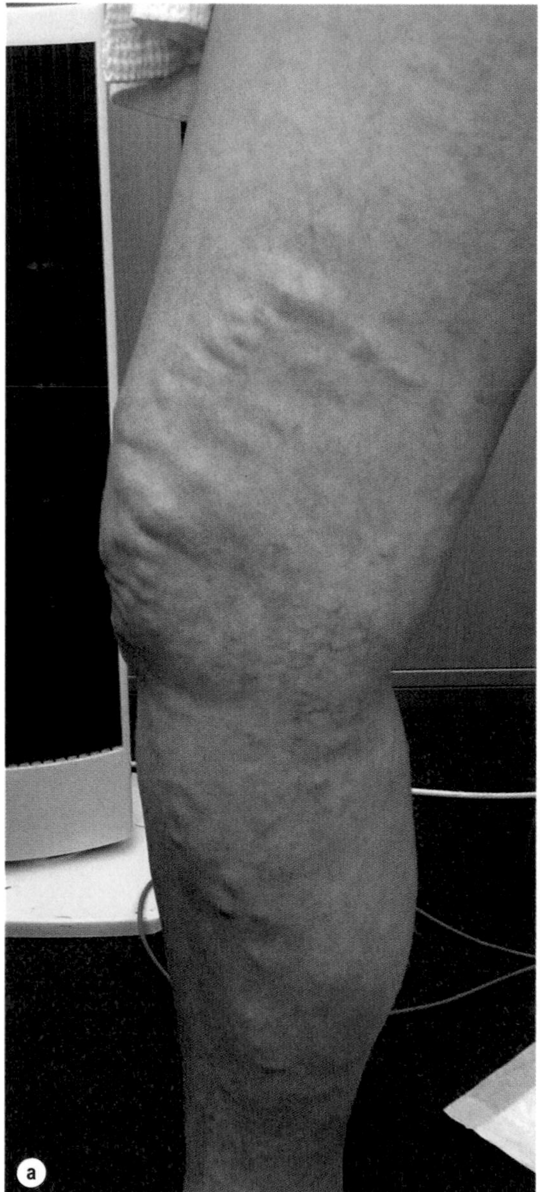
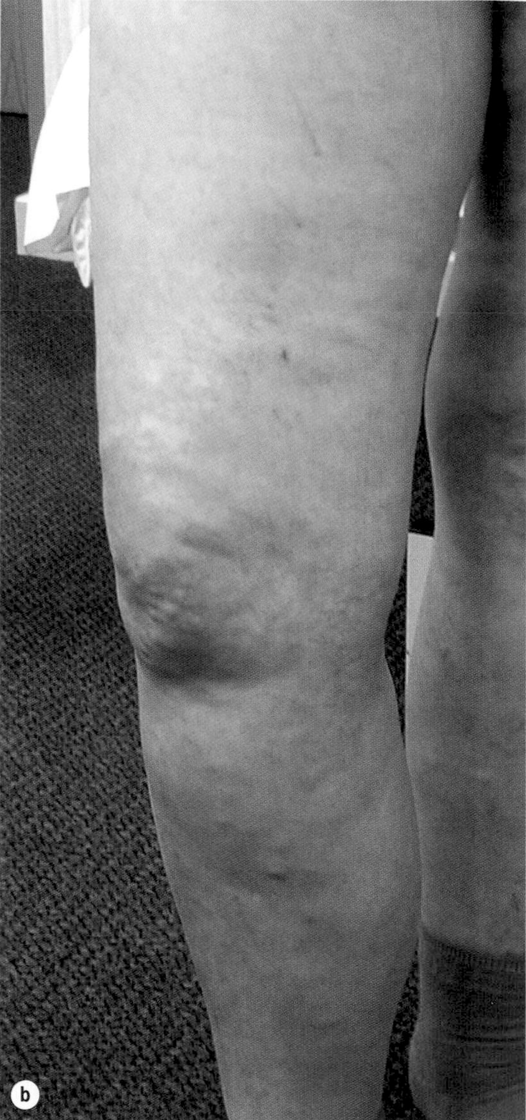

**Figure 17.8 • (a)** Right anterior accessory saphenous VVs affecting thigh and calf. **(b)** The same patient 6 weeks after EVLA. Courtesy of Mr Michael Gough.

negotiate tortuous, diseased (in this case alternately varicose and hypoplastic) vessels (veins). Thus, a variable (with experience) but nevertheless significant proportion of VV patients are not going to be suitable for EVLA.

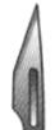

The short-term efficacy and safety of LSV EVLA (with mini-phlebectomies) is similar to high ligation and stripping (HL/S). Except for slightly increased postoperative pain and bruising in the HL/S group, no differences were found between the two treatment modalities, including time to return to normal activities and work. The treatments were equally safe and efficient in eliminating GSV reflux, alleviating symptoms and signs of LSV varicosities, and improving quality of life.[63]

Abolition of reflux and improvement in HRQL was comparable following both surgery and EVLA. The earlier return to work observed after EVLA may confer important socio-economic advantages.[64]

In summary, inexperienced EVLA of the main trunks plus (where necessary) mini-phlebectomies or sclerotherapy for the varices appears to be as effective as well-performed surgery but with less morbidity and 'down-time'.

## Radiofrequency ablation (RFA)

RFA involves using a percutaneous catheter to deliver radiofrequency energy to the vein. Thus, RFA is similar to EVLA in terms of principle and outcomes, and shares many of the potential advantages and disadvantages.[65–67]

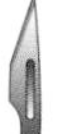

The 2-year clinical results of RFA are at least equal to those after HL/S of the GSV. Improved quality-of-life scores persisted through the 2-year observations in the radiofrequency obliteration group compared to the stripping and ligation group.[68]

RFA caused less pain and bruising and was performed more quickly than redo groin surgery. VNUS should be considered the treatment of choice for recurrent long saphenous varicose veins.[69]

RFA of the LSV is associated with somewhat poorer results at 3 years compared with the stripping operation.[70]

As with EVLA, although one can understand why patients might be attracted to, and surgeons might want to undertake, RFA the medium- and longer-term advantages over (well-performed) surgery are not overwhelming except, perhaps, in recurrent LSV disease, where RFA and EVLA allow redo groin dissection and stripping to be avoided.

## Sclerotherapy

The aim of sclerotherapy is to place a small volume of sclerosant in the lumen of a vein empty of blood, and then appose the walls of that vein with appropriate compression (class II) so that the vein undergoes occlusive fibrosis without the formation of clot.

Sclerosants fall into three categories:

- detergent, e.g. sodium tetradecyl sulphate (STS) and polidocanol (PD);
- osmotic, e.g. hypertonic saline (used in Europe and the USA);
- chemical irritant, e.g. chromated glycerine.

In the UK, most surgeons use STS and PD (the latter does not have a UK licence but is widely used 'off-licence' on a named-patient basis).

The appropriate strength of sclerosant depends upon:

- potency (STS is 2–3 times stronger than PD);
- the size of the vein being treated;
- whether (in respect of detergent sclerosants) it is being used as a liquid or as a foam (the latter is thought to have about twice the potency of the former).

Until recently, very few UK surgeons treated truncal (as opposed to small reticular and spider) VVs with sclerotherapy, largely because of randomised trials conducted in the 1970s showing poor long-term results compared with surgery. However, the advent of ultrasound-guided foam sclerotherapy (UGFS) has revolutionised the place of sclerotherapy in the treatment of VVs and is rapidly growing in popularity.[71]

The conversion of a detergent sclerosant (STS, PD) from its liquid phase to a foam by mixing it with air (Tessari method) has several beneficial consequences (**Fig. 17.9**):

- the potency of the sclerosant increases significantly, so allowing smaller volumes of sclerosant to be used;
- the foam 'pushes' the blood out of the vein, so preventing deactivation of the sclerosant by plasma proteins, thus increasing fibrosis while decreasing thrombosis.
- the sclerosant, because of the bubbles, becomes intensely echogenic, thus allowing it to be seen very clearly on ultrasound.

The result is that even very large trunk VVs, along with major tributaries and the varices themselves, can be reliably occluded with small volumes of sclerosant introduced through intravenous cannulae placed in the veins under duplex guidance (**Fig. 17.10**).

Although, as for the other endovenous techniques, randomised clinical trial (RCT) data are limited, several authors have published large series indicating that UGFS using STS or PD 'home-made foam' appears to be as effective, at least in the short term, as surgery, EVLA and RFA in the treatment of VVs.[72–77]

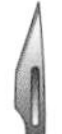

In an open-label, multicentre, prospective trial of 710 patients randomised to receive either Varisolve® (1% polidocanol microfoam) or alternative treatment (surgery or sclerotherapy), ultrasound-determined occlusion of trunk vein(s) and elimination of reflux were considered. Overall, Varisolve® was not inferior to alternative treatments, caused less pain and patients returned to normal more quickly.[78]

Ultrasound-guided sclerotherapy combined with sapheno-femoral ligation was less expensive, involved a shorter treatment time and resulted in more rapid recovery compared to sapheno-femoral ligation, saphenous stripping and phlebectomies.[79]

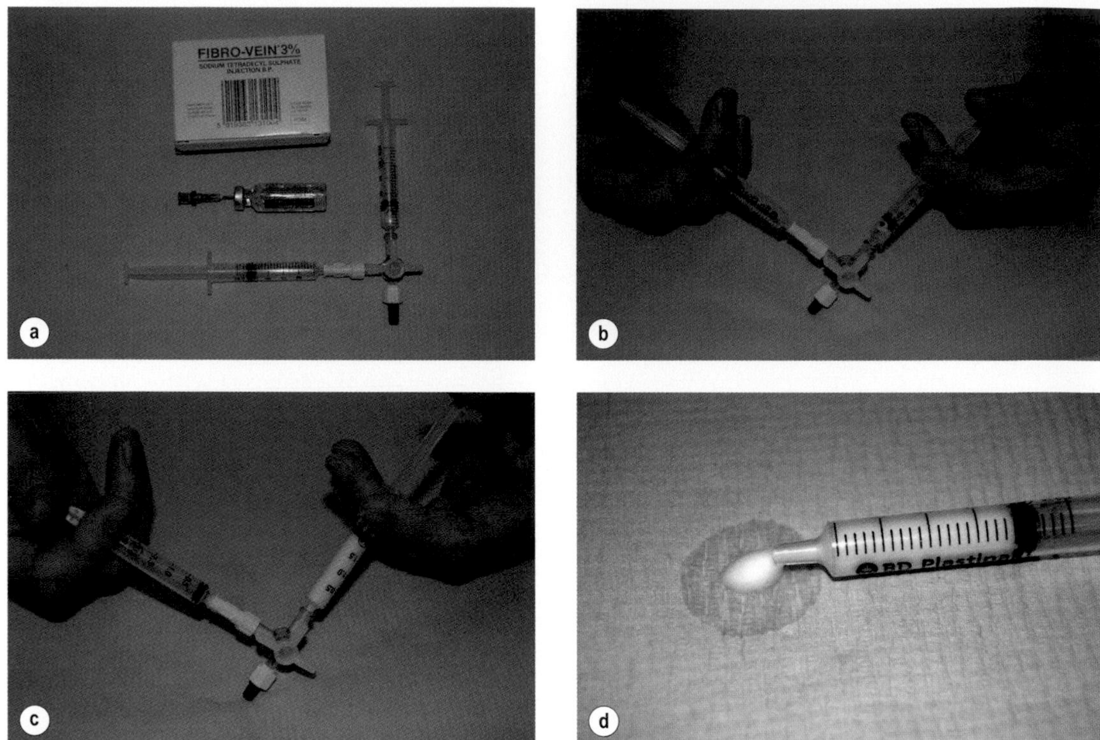


**Figure 17.9 •** Making foam using the Tessari method. **(a)** Two 2-mL syringes are connected via a three-way tap. **(b)** One syringe is filled with 0.5 mL of 3% STS and the other with 2 mL of air. **(c)** The STS is then 'squirted' back and forth through the three-way tap (typically 15 times). **(d)** This produces approximately 2.5 mL of microfoam.

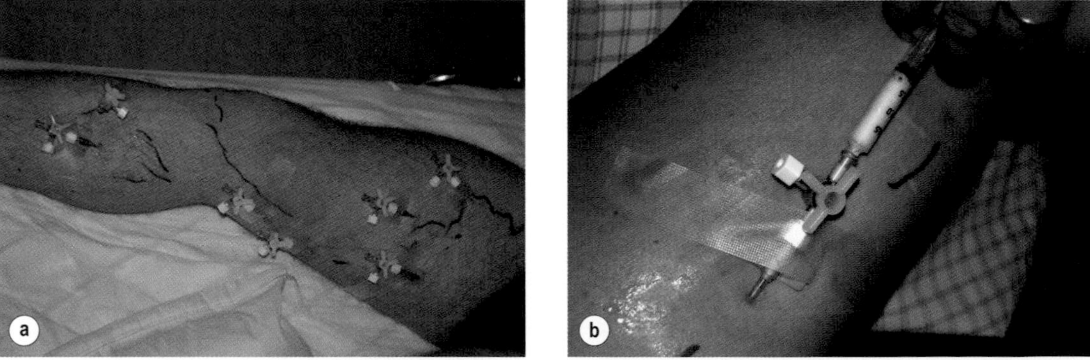


**Figure 17.10 • (a)** Multiple cannulae have been inserted under DUS guidance into the leg of a patient with extensive recurrent VVs. **(b)** Microfoam being injected. Notice that the leg is elevated to reduce 'dead space' within the veins.

Sclerotherapy is more of an art than a science and, as with the other endovenous techniques, there is a long learning curve to UGFS. The new practical skill that has to be mastered is the ability to reliably and accurately cannulate the VV (trunk, tributaries and varices) under DUS guidance; that, in turn, requires considerable facility with DUS. The author would strongly advise any surgeon wishing to embark upon UGFS (or any of the other minimally invasive endovenous techniques) to undergo some formal training in venous DUS. For although the principles of UGFS (EVLA, RFA) are simple, there are many pitfalls for the unwary and inadequately skilled.

Many of the complications of UGFS are the same as for 'standard' sclerotherapy and include skin pigmentation, lumpiness and superficial thrombophlebitis. Up to 20% of patients, especially those with fair skin and with large VVs near to the skin surface, can develop streaks of brown pigmentation over where the lumpy VVs used to be. This usually fades over a few months and in most patients is gone by 6–12 months; however, it can be permanent (**Fig. 17.11**). Superficial thrombophlebitis usually responds to topical NSAID gel, or aspiration of thrombus under local anaesthetic if severe. The risk of DVT is often a particular concern of surgeons thinking of embarking upon UGFS. Even with careful technique, some foam inevitable enters the deep venous system. This can be seen on DUS but can be cleared instantly by asking the patient to 'wiggle their ankle up and down'. The author has treated about 1000 patients with UGFS and has had two DVTs, giving a 0.2% risk; as discussed above, this appears significantly lower than with surgery. The big advantage of UGFS, as with the other endovenous techniques, is that the patient is fully mobile within a few minutes after completion of the procedure. The incidence of transient visual disturbance is reported to be 1% and is commoner in those who suffer from migraine; permanent visual loss has never been reported. The cause is probably a patent foramen ovale (also strongly associated with migraine), which allows the foam to bypass the filter of the lungs (a few patients develop a transient cough aftrer treatment) and enter the systemtic circulation. This is probably the mechanism underlying the other rare complications that have been reported, including transient confusion, fits and stroke (one reported case). With experience even very large VVs can be treated with small volumes of foam (often less than 10–12 mL), so minimising these already small risks. Some surgeons advocate the use of foam made with carbon dioxide (rather than air) but at this stage the advantages are not clear and it probably increases unnecessarily the complexity of the procedure.

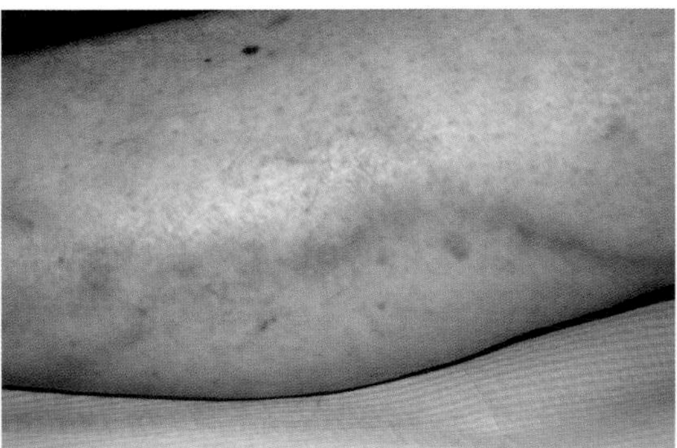

**Figure 17.11** • Pigmentation 6 months after UGFS.

## Which non-surgical treatment?

Although RCTs are few in number, those available suggest that (well-performed) surgical stripping, EVLA, RFA and UGFS are broadly similar in terms of their ability to eradicate reflux in LSV (SSV). There are pros and cons to each method but, having had experience of all three non-surgical alternatives, the author has chosen to concentrate exclusively on UGFS as the alternative surgery for a nunber of clinical and logistical reasons:

- UGFS can be used to treat the whole spectrum of venous disease from minor cosmetic varices to CVU to venous malformations.[80,81]
- There are very few VV patients who cannot be treated with UGFS but who could be treated by surgery, EVLA or RFA. Suggested contraindications to UGFS include: known allergy to sclerosant (very rare); arterial disease of a severity (ABPI <0.8) that prevents compression; severe immobility; severe obesity (difficult to cannulate, even harder to compress); severe postphlebitic deep venous disease. Most of these are also contraindications to all the other VV treatments.
- It is a complete treatment. In a patient with typical LSV and/or SSV VVs it is possible to treat the trunk, major and minor tributaries and the varices themselves in one session.
- No special equipment or facilities are required and the consumables are extremely inexpensive.
- It is very quick; once practised, treatment rarely takes more than 30 minutes (often much less), making it possible to treat 12 or more patients per day with ease.
- Recurrent VVs are just as easy to treat as primary VVs.
- There is no need to stop warfarin.

A recent review has suggested that conventional surgery should remain the treatment of choice, pending more evidence regarding these newer treatment modalities.[82]

However, the short-term advantages of the various endovenous alternatives over surgery are so obvious and attractive to patients, and to an ever increasing number of surgeons, that it is becoming increasingly difficult to persuade surgeons to randomise their patients and for their patients to be randomised.[64]

## Vulval and perineal varices

Vulval and perineal varices may arise in women as a complication of pregnancy or following pelvic

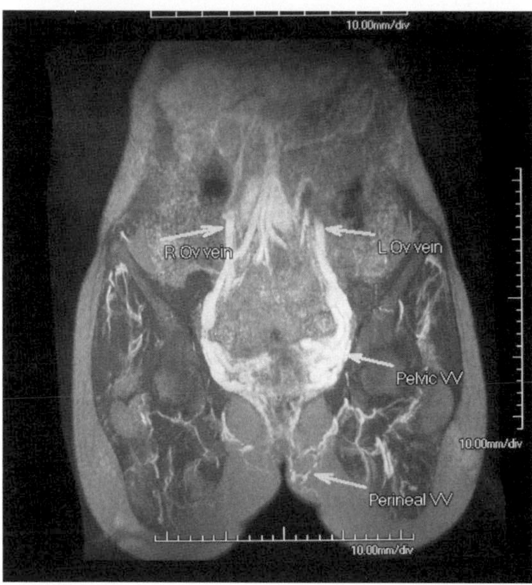


**Figure 17.12** • Magnetic resonance venogram showing reflux down the left ovarian vein communicating with perineal varices.

vein thrombosis (surgery, trauma or pelvic inflammatory disease), and are a consequence of ovarian and internal iliac venous valve incompetence.[83] They typically extend down the medial aspect of the thigh, and may join the saphenous system, which may also be incompetent.

The investigation of choice is magnetic resonance venography (**Fig. 17.12**). Treatment is carried out in two phases:

1. reflux in the ovarian vein is abolished;
2. the VVs themselves are dealt with locally by means of stab avulsions or sclerotherapy, with or without standard saphenous surgery.

Ovarian vein interruption was originally accomplished surgically through a loin incision and retroperitoneal approach. More recently, radiological ovarian vein embolisation has been successfully practised.[84] Ovarian vein reflux may be associated with the 'pelvic congestion syndrome', characterised by pelvic pain, backache, dysmenorrhoea, menorrhagia, dyspareunia and urological symptoms including dysuria.

## Key points

- Patients with asymptomatic uncomplicated VVs can generally be reassured as they are at low risk of developing complications.
- Interventions for symptomatic VVs clearly improve quality of life.
- Thorough pretreatment counselling and fully informed written consent are crucial.
- DUS is strongly recommended for all patients and certainly when there has been previous surgery, where there is suspicion of deep venous disease, and preoperatively in SSV surgery to mark the SPJ.
- Wherever possible, a refluxing LSV should be stripped (physically, thermally or chemically) to the knee to reduce the risk of recurrence.
- SSV surgery can be difficult, is often associated with suboptimal outcomes and is not for the inexperienced surgeon; modern endovenous techniques offer an attractive alteranative.
- Tourniquets reduce the amount of bleeding from VV surgery but appear to have no other advantages, as well as some disadvantages.
- Non-surgical alternatives such as EVLA, RFA and UGFS have the potential to offer considerable consumer and provider advantages, especially in patients with complex and recurrent disease.
- Each has its pros and cons but in experienced hands EVLA, RFA and UGFS are all probably at least as good as each other and as good as surgery, if not better.
- In an ideal world more randomised data would be forthcoming regarding the relative merits of surgery, EVLA, RFA and UGFS. However, for entirely understandable reasons, it is becoming increasingly difficult to persuade surgeons to randomise their patients and for their patients to be randomised.
- Proper training in the new endovenous techniques is mandatory if patients (and surgeons) are to be protected from the clinical and medico-legal consequences of adverse outcomes.

## References


1. Allegra C, Antignani PL, Carlizza A. Recurrent varicose veins following surgical treatment: our experience with five years follow-up. Eur J Vasc Endovasc Surg 2007; 33:751–6.
2. Dillon MF, Carr CJ, Feeley TM et al. Impact of the informed consent process on patients' understanding of varicose veins and their treatment. Irish J Med Sci 2005; 174:23–7.
3. Pascual G, Mendieta C, Mecham RP et al. Down-regulation of lysyl oxydase-like in aging and venous insufficiency. Histol Histopathol 2008; 23:179–86.
4. Bergan J. Molecular mechanisms in chronic venous insufficiency. Ann Vasc Surg 2007; 21:260–6.
5. Eklof B, Rutherford RB, Bergan JJ et al. American Venous Forum International Ad Hoc Committee for Revision of the CEAP Classification. Revision of the CEAP classification for chronic venous disorders: consensus statement. J Vasc Surg 2004; 40:1248–52.
6. Beebe-Dimmer JL, Pfeifer JR, Engle JS et al. The epidemiology of chronic venous insufficiency and varicose veins. Ann Epidemiol 2005; 15:175–84.
7. Sam RC, Hobbs SD, Darvall KA et al. Chronic venous disease in a cohort of healthy UK Asian men. Eur J Vasc Endovasc Surg 2007; 34:92–6.
8. Tuchsen F, Hannerz H, Burr H et al. Prolonged standing at work and hospitalisation due to varicose veins: a 12 year prospective study of the Danish population. Occup Environ Med 2005; 62:847–50.
9. Kihiczak GG, Meine JG, Schwartz RA et al. Klippel–Trenaunay syndrome: a multisystem disorder possibly resulting from a pathogenic gene for vascular and tissue overgrowth. Int J Dermatol 2006; 45:883–90.
10. Sam RC, Darvall KA, Adam DJ et al. A comparison of the changes in generic quality of life after superficial venous surgery with those after laparoscopic cholecystectomy. J Vasc Surg 2006; 44:606–10.
11. Ratcliffe J, Brazier J, Palfreyman S et al. A comparison of patient and population values for health states in varicose veins patients. Health Econ 2007; 16:395–405.
12. Campbell WB, Decaluwe H, Macintyre JB et al. Most patients with varicose veins have fears or concerns about the future, in addition to their presenting symptoms. Eur J Vasc Endovasc Surg 2006; 31:332–4.
13. Marchiori A, Mosena L, Prandoni P. Superficial vein thrombosis: risk factors, diagnosis, and treatment. Semin Thromb Hemostas 2006; 32:737–43.
14. Caggiati A, Rosi C, Franceschini M et al. The nature of skin pigmentations in chronic venous insufficiency: a preliminary report. Eur J Vasc Endovasc Surg 2008; 35:111–18.
15. Sam RC, Burns PJ, Hobbs SD et al. The prevalence of hyperhomocysteinemia, methylene tetrahydrofolate reductase C677T mutation, and vitamin B12 and folate deficiency in patients with chronic venous insufficiency. J Vasc Surg 2003; 38:904–8.
16. Bhasin N, Scott DJ. How should a candidate assess varicose veins in the MRCS clinical examination? A vascular viewpoint. Ann R Coll Surg Engl 2006; 88:309–12.
17. Campbell WB, Niblett PG, Peters AS et al. REACTIV (Randomised and Economic Analysis of Conservative Treatment or Interventions for Varicose veins) Study Participants. The clinical effectiveness of hand held Doppler examination for diagnosis of reflux in patients with varicose veins. Eur J Vasc Endovasc Surg 2005; 30:664–9.

   Selective use of HHD can avoid duplex imaging for many patients, with a low failure rate for detecting correctable venous reflux. Observed variations between individuals and units in results of HHD and duplex imaging have implications for the increasing use of duplex by clinicians.

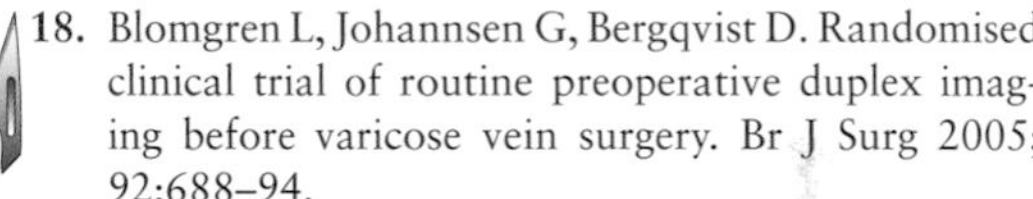

18. Blomgren L, Johannsen G, Bergqvist D. Randomised clinical trial of routine preoperative duplex imaging before varicose vein surgery. Br J Surg 2005; 92:688–94.

   Routine preoperative duplex examination led to an improvement in results 2 years after surgery for patients with primary varicose veins.

19. Ali SM, Callam MJ. Results and significance of colour duplex assessment of the deep venous system in recurrent varicose veins. Eur J Vasc Endovasc Surg 2007; 34:97–101.
20. Delis KT, Knaggs AL, Hobbs JT et al. The non-saphenous vein of the popliteal fossa: prevalence, patterns of reflux, hemodynamic quantification, and clinical significance. J Vasc Surg 2006; 44:611–19.
21. Bush RG, Hammond K. Treatment of incompetent vein of Giacomini (thigh extension branch). Ann Vasc Surg 2007; 21:245–8.
22. Caggiati A, Mendoza E. Segmental hypoplasia of the great saphenous vein and varicose disease. Eur J Vasc Endovasc Surg 2004; 28:257–61.
23. Makris SA, Karkos CD, Awad S et al. An "all-comers" venous duplex scan policy for patients with lower limb varicose veins attending a one-stop vascular clinic: is it justified? Eur J Vasc Endovasc Surg 2006; 32:718–24.
24. De Maeseneer MG, Vandenbroeck CP, Hendriks JM et al. Accuracy of duplex evaluation one year after varicose vein surgery to predict recurrence at the sapheno-femoral junction after five years. Eur J Vasc Endovasc Surg 2005; 29:308–12.
25. Harris MR, Davies RJ, Brown S et al. Surgical treatment of varicose veins: effect of rationing. Ann R Coll Surg Engl 2006; 88(1):37–9.
26. Sam RC, Darvall KA, Adam DJ et al. Digital venous photoplethysmography in the seated position is a reproducible noninvasive measure of lower limb venous function in patients with isolated superficial venous reflux. J Vasc Surg 2006; 43:335–41.
27. Beraldo S, Satpathy A, Dodds SR. A study of the routine use of venous photoplethysmography in a one-stop vascular surgery clinic. Ann R Coll Surg Engl 2007; 89:379–83.

28. Michaels JA, Campbell WB, Brazier JE et al. Randomised clinical trial, observational study and assessment of cost-effectiveness of the treatment of varicose veins (REACTIV trial). Health Technol Assess (Winchester, England) 2006; 10(13):1–196, iii–iv.

    **Standard surgical treatment of varicose veins by sapheno-femoral ligation, stripping and multiple phlebectomies is a clinically effective and cost-effective treatment for varicose veins, with an ICER well below the threshold normally considered appropriate for the funding of treatments within the NHS.**

29. Subramonia S, Lees TA. The treatment of varicose veins. Ann R Coll Surg Engl 2007; 89:96–100.

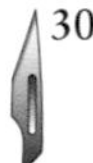

30. Michaels JA, Brazier JE, Campbell WB et al. Randomized clinical trial comparing surgery with conservative treatment for uncomplicated varicose veins. Br J Surg 2006; 93:175–81.

    **Surgical treatment provides symptomatic relief and significant improvements in quality of life in patients referred to secondary care with uncomplicated varicose veins.**

31. Ratcliffe J, Brazier JE, Campbell WB et al. Cost-effectiveness analysis of surgery versus conservative treatment for uncomplicated varicose veins in a randomized clinical trial. Br J Surg 2006; 93:182–6.
32. Subramonia S, Lees T. Sensory abnormalities and bruising after long saphenous vein stripping: impact on short-term quality of life. J Vasc Surg 2005; 42:510–14.
33. Munasinghe A, Smith C, Kianifard B et al. Strip-track revascularization after stripping of the great saphenous vein. Br J Surg 2007; 94:840–3.
34. De Maeseneer MG, Philipsen TE, Vandenbroeck CP et al. Closure of the cribriform fascia: an efficient anatomical barrier against postoperative neovascularisation at the saphenofemoral junction? A prospective study. Eur J Vasc Endovasc Surg 2007; 34:361–6.

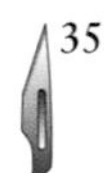

35. Winterborn RJ, Earnshaw JJ. Randomised trial of polytetrafluoroethylene patch insertion for recurrent great saphenous varicose veins. Eur J Vasc Endovasc Surg 2007; 34:367–73.

    **In this study, insertion of a PTFE patch did not affect the rate of perioperative complications and it did not appear to contain neovascularisation.**

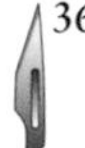

36. Frings N, Nelle A, Tran P et al. Reduction of neoreflux after correctly performed ligation of the saphenofemoral junction. A randomized trial. Eur J Vasc Endovasc Surg 2004; 28:246–52.

    **Recurrent reflux in the groin was reduced by oversewing the ligated SFJ in patients having varicose vein surgery. This adds weight to the theory of neovascularisation as a cause of recurrent veins and offers a means to reduce clinical recurrence rates.**

37. Kianifard B, Holdstock JM, Whiteley MS. Radiofrequency ablation (VNUS closure) does not cause neo-vascularisation at the groin at one year: results of a case controlled study. Surgeon –J R Coll Surg Edinb Ireland 2006; 4:71–4.

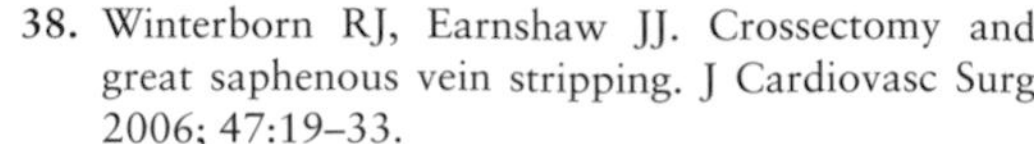

38. Winterborn RJ, Earnshaw JJ. Crossectomy and great saphenous vein stripping. J Cardiovasc Surg 2006; 47:19–33.

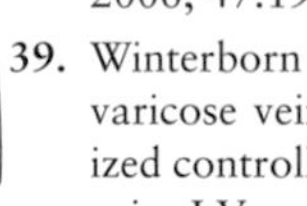

39. Winterborn RJ, Foy C, Earnshaw JJ. Causes of varicose vein recurrence: late results of a randomized controlled trial of stripping the long saphenous vein. J Vasc Surg 2004; 40:634–9.

    **Stripping the long saphenous vein is recommended as part of routine varicose vein surgery as it reduced the risk of reoperation by 60% after 11 years, although it did not reduce the rate of visible recurrent veins.**

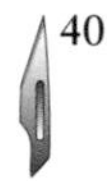

40. Lorenz D, Gabel W, Redtenbacher M et al. Randomized clinical trial comparing bipolar coagulating and standard great saphenous stripping for symptomatic varicose veins. Br J Surg 2007; 94:434–40.

    **A new bipolar coagulating electric vein stripper was safe and effective in avoiding painful haematomas following varicose vein surgery.**

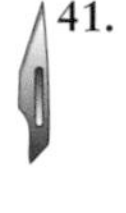

41. Nisar A, Shabbir J, Tubassam MA et al. Local anaesthetic flush reduces postoperative pain and haematoma formation after great saphenous vein stripping – a randomised controlled trial. Eur J Vasc Endovasc Surg 2006; 31:325–31.

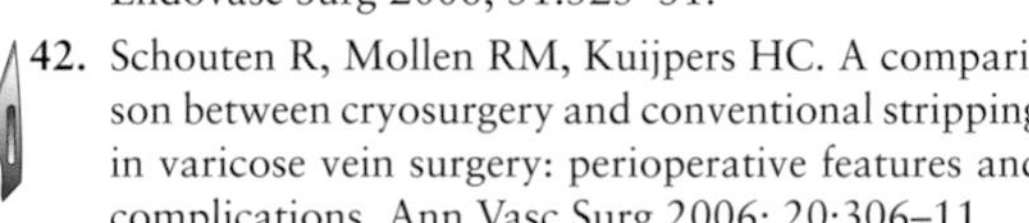

42. Schouten R, Mollen RM, Kuijpers HC. A comparison between cryosurgery and conventional stripping in varicose vein surgery: perioperative features and complications. Ann Vasc Surg 2006; 20:306–11.

    **Cryosurgery has comparable postoperative results with conventional short stripping. Operation time is reduced with cryosurgery, but postoperative pain scores are higher. Patients favour cryosurgery because of better cosmetic results.**

43. Sam RC, Silverman SH, Bradbury AW. Nerve injuries and varicose vein surgery. Eur J Vasc Endovasc Surg 2004; 27:113–20.
44. Wood JJ, Chant H, Laugharne M et al. A prospective study of cutaneous nerve injury following long saphenous vein surgery. Eur J Vasc Endovasc Surg 2005; 30:654–8.
45. van Neer P, Kessels A, de Haan E et al. Residual varicose veins below the knee after varicose vein surgery are not related to incompetent perforating veins. J Vasc Surg 2006; 44:1051–4.
46. Rudstrom H, Bjorck M, Bergqvist D. Iatrogenic vascular injuries in varicose vein surgery: a systematic review. World J Surg 2007; 31:228–33.
47. Winterborn RJ, Campbell WB, Heather BP et al. The management of short saphenous varicose veins: a survey of the members of the vascular surgical society of Great Britain and Ireland. Eur J Vasc Endovasc Surg 2004; 28:400–3.
48. Rashid HI, Ajeel A, Tyrrell MR. Persistent popliteal fossa reflux following saphenopopliteal disconnection. Br J Surg 2002; 89:748–51.
49. Theivacumar NS, Beale RJ, Mavor AI et al. Initial experience in endovenous laser ablation (EVLA) of varicose veins due to small saphenous vein reflux. Eur J Vasc Endovasc Surg 2007; 33:614–18.

50. Giannas J, Bayat A, Watson SJ. Common peroneal nerve injury during varicose vein operation. Eur J Vasc Endovasc Surg 2006; 31:443–5.

51. O'Hare JL, Vandenbroeck CP, Whitman B et al. on behalf of the Joint Vascular Research Group. A prospective evaluation of the outcome after small saphenous varicose vein surgery with one year follow-up. J Vasc Surg (in press).

52. Rigby KA, Palfreyman SJ, Beverley C et al. Surgery for varicose veins: use of tourniquet. Cochrane Database Syst Rev 2002; 4:CD001486.

Although there were significant quality issues with the available evidence, the use of a tourniquet would appear to reduce blood loss during surgery. There were no reported differences between the use or non-use of a tourniquet in terms of complications and morbidity. However, the available trials were not of sufficient size to detect rarer complications such as nerve damage.

53. Scavee V. Transilluminated powered phlebectomy: not enough advantages? Review of the literature. Eur J Vasc Endovasc Surg 2006; 31:316–19.

54. Recek C. Impact of the calf perforators on the venous hemodynamics in primary varicose veins. J Cardiovasc Surg 2006; 47:629–35.

55. Kianifard B, Holdstock J, Allen C et al. Randomized clinical trial of the effect of adding subfascial endoscopic perforator surgery to standard great saphenous vein stripping. Br J Surg 2007; 94:1075–80.

IPVs do not remain closed following standard varicose vein surgery. The addition of SEPS was not associated with significant morbidity but did reduce the number of IPVs. Up to 1 year this had no effect on recurrence rates or quality of life.

56. van Rij AM, Chai J, Hill GB et al. Incidence of deep vein thrombosis after varicose vein surgery. Br J Surg 2004; 91:1582–5.

57. Biswas S, Clark A, Shields DA. Randomised clinical trial of the duration of compression therapy after varicose vein surgery. Eur J Vasc Endovasc Surg 2007; 33:631–7.

There was no benefit in wearing compression stockings for more than 1 week following uncomplicated high saphenous ligation with stripping of the great saphenous vein with respect to postoperative pain, number of complications, time to return to work or patient satisfaction for up to 12 weeks following surgery.

58. Sharif MA, Soong CV, Lau LL et al. Endovenous laser treatment for long saphenous vein incompetence. Br J Surg 2006; 93:831–5.

59. Theivacumar NS, Dellagrammaticas D, Beale RJ et al. Fate and clinical significance of saphenofemoral junction tributaries following endovenous laser ablation of great saphenous vein. Br J Surg 2007; 94:722–5.

60. Theivacumar NS, Dellagrammaticas D, Beale RJ et al. Factors influencing the effectiveness of endovenous laser ablation (EVLA) in the treatment of great saphenous vein reflux. Eur J Vasc Endovasc Surg 2008; 35:119–23.

61. van den Bos RR, Kockaert MA, Neumann HA et al. Technical review of endovenous laser therapy for varicose veins. Eur J Vasc Endovasc Surg 2008; 35:88–95.

62. Wright AP, Berridge DC, Scott DJ. Return to work following varicose vein surgery: influence of type of operation, employment and social status. Eur J Vasc Endovasc Surg 2007; 31:553–7.

63. Rasmussen LH, Bjoern L, Lawaetz M et al. Randomized trial comparing endovenous laser ablation of the great saphenous vein with high ligation and stripping in patients with varicose veins: short-term results. J Vasc Surg 2007; 46:308–15.

The short-term efficacy and safety of LSV EVLA (with mini-phlebectomies) is similar to HL/S. Except for slightly increased postoperative pain and bruising in the HL/S group, no differences were found between the two treatment modalities, including time to return to normal activities and work. The treatments were equally safe and efficient in eliminating GSV reflux, alleviating symptoms and signs of LSV varicosities, and improving quality of life.

64. Darwood RJ, Theivacumar N, Dellagrammaticas D et al. Randomised clinical trial comparing laser ablation with surgery for the treatment of primary great saphenous varicose veins. Br J Surg 2008; 93:294–301.

Abolition of reflux and improvement in HRQL was comparable following both surgery and EVLA. The earlier return to work observed after EVLA may confer important socio-economic advantages.

65. Nicolini P. Closure Group. Treatment of primary varicose veins by endovenous obliteration with the VNUS closure system: results of a prospective multicentre study. Eur J Vasc Endovasc Surg 2005; 29:433–9.

66. Ravi R, Rodriguez-Lopez JA, Trayler EA et al. Endovenous ablation of incompetent saphenous veins: a large single-center experience. J Endovasc Ther 2006; 13:244–8.

67. Pannier F. Rabe E. Endovenous laser therapy and radiofrequency ablation of saphenous varicose veins. J Cardiovasc Surg 2006; 47:3–8.

68. Lurie F, Creton D, Eklof B et al. Prospective randomised study of endovenous radiofrequency obliteration (closure) versus ligation and vein stripping (EVOLVeS): two-year follow-up. Eur J Vasc Endovasc Surg 2005; 29:67–73.

The 2-year clinical results of radiofrequency obliteration (RFO) are at least equal to those after HL/S of the GSV. In the vast majority of RFO patients the GSV remained permanently closed and underwent progressive shrinkage to eventual sonographic disappearance. Recurrence and neovascularisation rates were similar in the two groups, although limited patient numbers prevent reliable statistical analysis. Improved quality-of-life scores persisted through the 2-year observations in the RFO group compared to the stripping and ligation group.

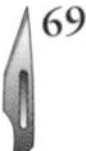
69. Hinchliffe RJ, Ubhi J, Beech A et al. A prospective randomised controlled trial of VNUS closure versus surgery for the treatment of recurrent long saphenous varicose veins. Eur J Vasc Endovasc Surg 2006; 31:212–18.

VNUS caused less pain and bruising and was performed more quickly than redo groin surgery. VNUS should be considered the treatment of choice for recurrent long saphenous varicose veins.

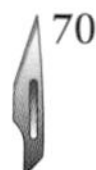
70. Perala J, Rautio T, Biancari F et al. Radiofrequency endovenous obliteration versus stripping of the long saphenous vein in the management of primary varicose veins: 3-year outcome of a randomized study. Ann Vasc Surg 2005; 19:669–72.

Radiofrequency endovenous obliteration of the LSV is associated with somewhat poorer short-term results compared with the stripping operation.

71. O'Hare JL, Earnshaw JJ. The use of foam sclerotherapy for varicose veins: a survey of the members of the Vascular Society of Great Britain and Ireland. Eur J Vasc Endovasc Surg 2007; 34:232–5.
72. Rabe E, Pannier-Fischer F, Gerlach H et al. German Society of Phlebology. Guidelines for sclerotherapy of varicose veins (ICD 10: I83.0, I83.1, I83.2, and I83.9). Dermatol Surg 2004; 30:687–93.
73. Darke SG, Baker SJ. Ultrasound-guided foam sclerotherapy for the treatment of varicose veins. Br J Surg 2006; 93:969–74.
74. Creton D, Uhl JF. Foam sclerotherapy combined with surgical treatment for recurrent varicose veins: short term results. Eur J Vasc Endovasc Surg 2007; 33:619–24.
75. Smith PC. Chronic venous disease treated by ultrasound guided foam sclerotherapy. Eur J Vasc Endovasc Surg 2006; 32:577–83.
76. Jia X, Mowatt G, Burr JM et al. Systematic review of foam sclerotherapy for varicose veins. Br J Surg 2007; 94:925–36.
77. Myers KA, Jolley D, Clough A et al. Outcome of ultrasound-guided sclerotherapy for varicose veins: medium-term results assessed by ultrasound surveillance. Eur J Vasc Endovasc Surg 2007; 33:116–21.

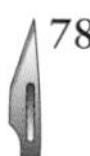
78. Wright D, Gobin JP, Bradbury AW et al. The Varisolve® European Phase III Investigators Group. Phlebology 2006; 21:180–90.

In an open-label, multicentre, prospective trial of 710 patients randomised to receive either Varisolve® (1% polidocanol microfoam) or alternative treatment (surgery or sclerotherapy), ultrasound-determined occlusion of trunk vein(s) and elimination of reflux were considered. Overall, Varisolve® was not inferior to alternative treatments, caused less pain and patients returned to normal more quickly.

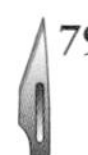
79. Bountouroglou DG, Azzam M, Kakkos SK et al. Ultrasound-guided foam sclerotherapy combined with sapheno-femoral ligation compared to surgical treatment of varicose veins: early results of a randomised controlled trial. Eur J Vasc Endovasc Surg 2006; 31:93–100.

Ultrasound-guided sclerotherapy combined with sapheno-femoral ligation was less expensive, involved a shorter treatment time and resulted in more rapid recovery compared to sapheno-femoral ligation, saphenous stripping and phlebectomies.

80. van Neer P, Veraart JC, Neumann H. Posterolateral thigh perforator varicosities in 12 patients: a normal deep venous system and successful treatment with ultrasound-guided sclerotherapy. Dermatol Surg 2006; 32:1346–52.
81. Nitecki S, Bass A. Ultrasound-guided foam sclerotherapy in patients with Klippel–Trenaunay syndrome. Isr Med Assoc J 2007; 9:72–5.
82. Campbell B. Varicose veins and their management. Br Med J 2006; 333:287–92.
83. Greiner M, Gilling-Smith GL. Leg varices originating from the pelvis: diagnosis and treatment. Vascular 2007; 15:70–8.
84. Creton D, Hennequin L, Kohler F et al. Embolisation of symptomatic pelvic veins in women presenting with non-saphenous varicose veins of pelvic origin – three-year follow-up. Eur J Vasc Endovasc Surg 2007; 34:112–17.

# 18

# Chronic leg swelling

Timothy A. Lees
Sherab G. Bhutia
Arun Balakrishnan
Nicholas F.W. Redwood

There are various conditions that cause chronic lower limb swelling (Box 18.1). The two most common are chronic venous insufficiency and lymphoedema.

## Chronic venous insufficiency (CVI)

CVI encompasses disease of the lower limb veins in which venous return is impaired, usually over a number of years, by reflux, obstruction or calf muscle pump failure. This leads to sustained venous hypertension and ultimately clinical complications including oedema, eczema, lipodermatosclerosis and ulceration.

### Clinical features

The clinical features of CVI include swelling, skin changes, ulceration, varicose veins and pain.

#### Swelling

Swelling is due to oedema fluid, which is initially pitting, but as the disease progresses subcutaneous fibrosis and induration occur. If there is any break in the skin, this leads to copious exudation of fluid.

#### Skin changes

Varicose eczema commences as dry, scaly and itchy skin. The skin becomes friable and may become infected following scratching. Pigmentation, due to the deposition of haemosiderin in the tissues, produces a brown discoloration characteristic of CVI, which together with fibrosis leads to the clinical picture of lipodermatosclerosis around the ankle (**Fig. 18.1**).

#### Ulceration

Ulceration is often precipitated by minor trauma and venous ulcers occur predominantly on the lower leg, more commonly on the medial aspect. These are usually surrounded by eczema or pigmentation and exude fluid that can cause maceration of the surrounding skin. In patients presenting with lower limb ulceration, approximately 80%[1,2] will have evidence of venous disease and 10–25%[3] of limbs will have Doppler-verified arterial disease. Approximately 12% will have coexisting diabetes or rheumatoid arthritis.[4] Although immobility is often a contributory cause, it can also cause stasis ulceration in isolation.

#### Varicose veins

It may be obvious that the patient has varicose veins, and a history of previous varicose vein treatment should be sought. However, the absence of visible varicose veins does not exclude the presence of significant superficial reflux.

#### Pain

The patient may complain of a general ache and heaviness in the leg after long periods of standing. This is worse towards the end of the day but improves with elevation or bed rest.

**Box 18.1** • Differential diagnosis of chronic leg swelling

**Venous disease**

Primary varicose veins
Primary deep venous incompetence
Post-thrombotic syndrome
Arteriovenous malformations

**Lymphoedema**

Primary
Secondary

**General disease**

Lipidema
Congestive cardiac failure
Pretibial myxoedema
Nephrotic syndrome
Hepatic failure

**Tumours**

Pelvic tumours causing extrinsic compression

**Drugs**

**Dependency**

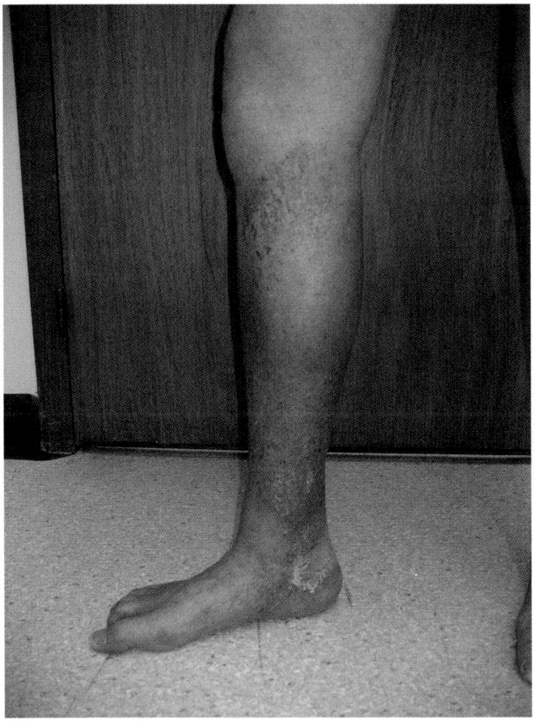

**Figure 18.1** • Bilateral chronic venous insufficiency with pigmentation and severe lipodermatosclerosis resulting in the typical 'inverted champagne bottle' shape.

A history of deep vein thrombosis (DVT) should be sought. Venous claudication is an uncommon symptom and is usually due to extensive iliofemoral vein occlusion. The symptoms differ from arterial claudication because the increase in arterial inflow during exercise combined with decreased outflow results in acute distension of the limb, giving rise to generalised pain in the leg and a severe bursting sensation. The pain does not stop immediately on cessation of exercise and often requires elevation for 10–20 minutes for relief.

## Epidemiology

The prevalence of chronic venous insufficiency in the adult population lies between 2% and 9%, and may be higher in males than females.[5,6] The most serious feature of chronic venous insufficiency is ulceration, which is a distressing and debilitating condition. Leg ulcers affect about 1% of the adult population in developed countries. It has been demonstrated that approximately 50% of ulcers have been present for more than 12 months and 72% are recurrent.[7] Within the UK, Australia, Sweden and Italy, overall rates for active ulceration range from 0.15% to 0.5%, and increase with age.[8–12] In the UK, the total cost to the NHS has been estimated to be £230–600 million a year.[13,14]

## Aetiology

To understand CVI, one must consider the changes that occur in both the larger veins (macrocirculation) and the capillary bed (microcirculation).

### Macrocirculation

During exercise in the normal individual, effective contraction of the calf muscles combined with vein patency and valvular competence aids venous return and reduces venous pressure in the lower leg from about 90 mmHg to 30 mmHg. Failure of any of these mechanisms may result in postambulatory venous hypertension, which is accepted as the underlying haemodynamic abnormality in CVI. The recognised causes are outlined in Box 18.2.

#### Deep and superficial reflux

Historically, most venous ulcers have been considered secondary to previous DVT. However, with the advent of duplex scanning it has become apparent that there is also a group with primary deep venous reflux. Isolated superficial venous incompetence without deep venous incompetence has been shown to occur in between 31%[15] and 57%[16] of patients with venous ulceration. Of the possible sites of reflux, the iliofemoral, long saphenous and popliteal veins have the greatest effect on haemodynamics and skin changes.[17]

Box 18.2 • Causes of venous hypertension

**Superficial venous reflux**

Long saphenous vein reflux
Short saphenous vein reflux

**Deep venous reflux and occlusion**

Primary (idiopathic)
Secondary to deep venous thrombosis or injury

**Perforating vein reflux**

**Abnormal calf pump**

Neurological
Musculoskeletal

**Combination of the above**

### Perforating vein reflux

The contribution of incompetent perforators to the development of CVI remains controversial. The studies which have looked at the patterns of reflux (discussed above) show that isolated perforator incompetence occurs in only 2–4% of limbs with skin changes, and perforator incompetence is usually associated with reflux in the superficial or deep systems. However, the prevalence of incompetent perforators increases linearly with the clinical severity of CVI.[18] Whereas ambulatory venous pressures normalise after correction of reflux in the superficial venous systems, no change is seen after perforator surgery and the pressures are very similar to those seen in deep venous reflux.[19] In those cases where superficial and perforator reflux coincide, treating only the former results in healing rates of 95%.[20]

## Microcirculation

The pathophysiology in CVI is still not fully understood and is best explained by the following two hypotheses:

1. **White cell trapping hypothesis.** White blood cells are larger and less deformable than red blood cells. The haemodynamic effect of this is that the white cell has a greater effect on blood flow through a narrow channel such as a capillary.[21] If the perfusion pressure across the capillary bed is reduced because of an increase in venous pressure, white cells plug the capillaries and red cells build up behind. On reaching the postcapillary venule, the white cells are forced to marginate by the red cells.[22] Adherence of white cells to the endothelium is then stimulated by (i) decreased shear force[23] and (ii) upregulation of adhesion molecules by the endothelium as a response to venous hypertension.[24] The trapped white cells release proteolytic enzymes and oxygen free radicals, causing endothelial and tissue damage. As a consequence there is a release of vascular endothelial growth factor. This increases microvascular permeability, which may explain the presence of a fibrin cuff, and also produces excessive amounts of nitric oxide. This in turn damages tissues.[25] White cell trapping also has the effect of generating local ischaemia by reducing perfusion,[26] which may be a trigger to white cell activation.
2. **Fibrin cuff hypothesis.** A rise in venous pressure is directly transmitted to the capillary bed, where there is capillary elongation[27] and widening of the pores between the endothelial cells.[28] This results in the passage of larger molecules out of the intravascular compartment into the tissues. Fibrinogen is one such molecule that is deposited in the presence of capillary hypertension and polymerises to form fibrin. Patients with CVI also appear to have a defective interstitial fibrinolytic system within the lower limb,[29] and therefore fibrin accumulates. This may act as a barrier to oxygen, resulting in local tissue ischaemia and cell death, producing ulceration.[30]

There is good evidence to support white cell-mediated damage, with the initiating event being endothelial derangement secondary to venous hypertension. However, neither hypothesis accounts for how lipodermatosclerosis becomes frank ulceration. A possible explanation lies with matrix metalloproteinases. These enzymes help remodel the extracellular matrix by protein degradation, and enhanced matrix metalloproteinase activity has been demonstrated in lipodermatosclerosis.[31] An imbalance in matrix turnover then exists, leading to unrestrained degradation and ulceration. Therefore it is not unreasonable to propose that matrix metalloproteinases finish what the white cells have started.

Other possible mechanisms for the development of ulceration include arteriovenous communications, the trap hypothesis (trapping of growth factors and other stimulatory substances by macromolecules leaking from the circulation), increased tissue pressure and cutaneous iron overload.

# Classification

CVI involves a variety of anatomical and physiological abnormalities and so a standardised system is required to allow uniformity of reporting.

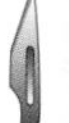

A classification was developed in 1994 by an international consensus conference under the auspices of the American Venous Forum and recommendations for change were made in 2004.[32]

This includes clinical signs (C), aetiology (E), anatomical distribution (A) and pathophysiological condition (P), and is therefore known by the acronym CEAP. Advanced CEAP is the same as the above basic CEAP but allows any of 18 named venous segments to be used as locators for venous pathology. Several definitions have been refined, C classes have been changed, a descriptor n (no venous abnormality identified) has been added, the date of classification has been introduced along with the level of investigation. The CEAP system is helpful in comparing limbs for the purposes of research, although it is rather unwieldy for everyday use (Box 18.3).

**Box 18.3 • CEAP classification**

**Clinical signs ($C_{0-6}$)**

Limbs are placed into one of seven clinical classes according to objective signs as follows:

Class 0: no visible or palpable signs of venous disease

Class 1: telangiectases, reticular veins, malleolar flare

Class 2: varicose veins

Class 3: oedema without skin changes

Class 4a: pigmentation or eczema class 4b, lipodermatosclerosis or atrophie blanche

Class 5: skin changes as above with healed ulceration

Class 6: skin changes as above with active ulceration

Each limb is further classified as asymptomatic (A) or symptomatic (S)

**Aetiology ($E_{C,P,S,N}$)**

This classification refers to congenital (C), primary (P; unknown cause but not congenital), secondary (S; acquired) and no aetiology identified (N). These groups are mutually exclusive

**Anatomical distribution ($A_{S,D,P,N}$)**

This refers to superficial (S), deep (D), perforating (P) veins and no venous location identified (N). More than one system may be involved

**Pathophysiological condition ($P_{R,O,N}$)**

This refers to reflux (R) or obstruction (O), or both may be present. $P_N$ implies no venous pathophysiology identified

## Investigation

Patients often present with mixed arterial and venous disease. The investigation of the venous disease is discussed below.

### Hand-held Doppler

Continuous-wave hand-held Doppler using an 8-MHz probe is a useful outpatient tool in screening for arterial and venous disease. Its limitations are that the exact vein being insonated is unknown, it is operator dependent and the significance of reflux of short duration may be uncertain.

### Duplex scanning

This combines a B-mode grey-scale ultrasound image with Doppler ultrasound, which allows the user to accurately select vessels for insonation and to determine the direction of flow. The Doppler flow information can also be incorporated onto the B-mode image as a colour, providing real-time images of blood flow within a vessel. This allows assessment of flow direction and is called colour flow imaging. Very low flow rates can be detected with power Doppler but this technique gives no information on the direction of flow.

Duplex is an important investigation of lower limb venous disease and is rapidly becoming the gold standard. Modern equipments allow easy identification of normal and abnormal venous anatomy, along with the presence of venous reflux. It is also extensively used for the diagnosis of DVT. A recent consensus document by UIP suggested duplex scan as an essential part of assessment of patients with CVI. The same document advocates use of duplex to predict the likely outcome after superficial venous surgery and to select patients requiring deep venous reconstruction.[33]

### Venography

Venography is invasive and to a large extent has been superseded by duplex scanning for the investigation of venous disease. Occasionally MR or VT Venography are required. Nevertheless, it can provide useful anatomical and functional information, particularly when the duplex findings are equivocal or duplex is limited, for example in the obese leg. Varicography, ascending and descending venography may be used in particular situations.

### Functional calf volume measurements

Various investigations may be used to examine the overall function of the venous system in the lower limb.

#### Ambulatory venous pressure measurement

This provides direct measurement of the superficial venous pressure at the ankle. This is achieved by cannulation of a vein on the dorsum of the foot connected to a pressure transducer, amplifier and a recorder. The pressure changes recorded in the long saphenous vein in the foot during and after 10 tiptoe exercises are shown in **Fig. 18.2**. This investigation is an indicator of overall lower limb venous function including calf muscle pump function.

### Plethysmography

There are many different types of plethysmography and these measure either alterations in calf volume directly or other parameters that indirectly reflect volume change. These include photoplethysmography, strain gauge plethysmography and air plethysmography.

## Treatment

The management of patients with CVI may be divided into either the prevention or the treatment of clinical complications such as lipodermatosclerosis and ulceration. Correcting the underlying cause will help to stop or reverse these complications. In addition, vigorous treatment of conditions known to lead to CVI, particularly acute DVT, may reduce the incidence of this problem in the long term. Management of patients with ulcers of mixed aetiology will require treatment aimed at each specific cause but this section deals predominantly with the treatment of isolated venous disease.

### General measures

These should include elevation of the legs at rest above the level of the heart. This helps to reduce oedema, decrease exudate from ulcers and accelerate regression of skin changes.[4] Immobility, occupation, obesity and coexisting disease may also influence the development of skin complications and should be addressed. Placing the patient in bed reduces the venous pressure at the ankle to about 12–15 mmHg and will therefore usually lead to ulcer healing. However, this is not a treatment enjoyed by most patients and may increase the risk of DVT. It is therefore generally reserved for ulcers that have failed to heal by all other methods.

### Graduated elastic compression

Compression therapy remains the primary treatment for CVI. It provides symptomatic relief, promotes ulcer healing and helps in preventing ulcer recurrence.

Applying a sustained graduated compressive force that is highest at the ankle and decreases proximally has been shown to reduce venous pressure at the ankle, increase femoral vein blood flow and increase venous refilling time. This improves venous function and can heal up to 93% of venous ulcers.[34] Graduated elastic compression may be applied using either bandages or stockings. It is important that these are applied by experienced staff as inexpertly applied compression can do more harm than good.

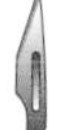

The Cochrane systematic review of compression treatment for venous leg ulcers provides a useful summary of the benefits of elastic stockings and bandaging systems.[35]

This concludes that in the healing of leg ulcers: (i) compression is more effective than no compression; (ii) elastic compression is more effective than non-elastic compression; (iii) multilayered high compression is more effective than single-layer compression; and (iv) there is no significant difference between four-layer bandaging and other high-compression multilayered systems.

In the prevention of ulcer recurrence, there are no randomised trials comparing compression with no compression.

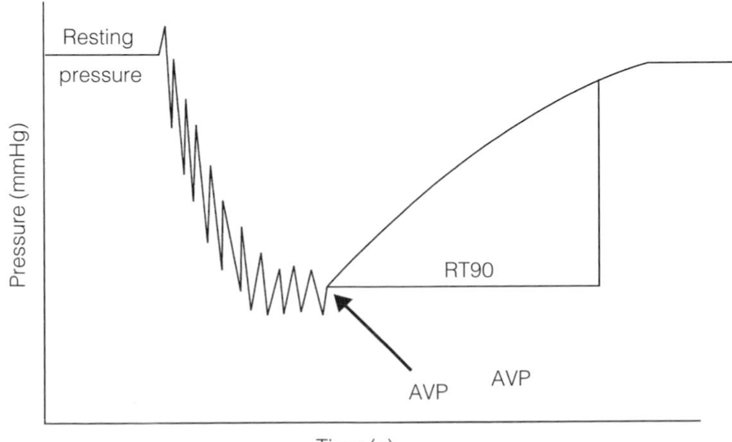


**Figure 18.2** • Venous pressure trace recorded from a superficial vein on the dorsum of the foot during 10 tiptoe exercises and return to the resting value after exercise. AVP, ambulatory venous pressure; RT90, time for 90% refilling.

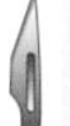

However, a review of trials comparing different grades of compression stocking concludes that higher grades of compression are associated with lower recurrence rates, but at a cost of lower patient compliance.[36] Approximately one-third of patients do not comply with the long-term use of compression hosiery.[37]

Stockings are classed according to the pressure they exert at the ankle and are designed to provide a linear graduated decrease in pressure above this, although in practice this may not always be the case. Pressures of up to 60 mmHg may be produced by elastic stockings and conventional pressure classes and indications are given in Table 18.1.

For the majority of patients with CVI or mild lymphoedema, a knee-length compression stocking designed to apply compression of 25–35 mmHg is ideal, but this will be influenced by how well they tolerate the stocking and their ability to apply them. Thigh-length stockings seem to confer little benefit over knee-length ones and as shorter stockings are easier to put on, compliance with these tends to be better. Stocking applicators may also aid patient compliance.

## Intermittent pneumatic compression

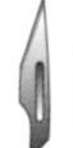

There is some evidence that intermittent pneumatic compression may provide accelerated ulcer healing when used either alone or in combination with elastic compression, although there is a need for further trials in this area.[38]

## Pharmacotherapy

### Dressings

For those patients with venous ulceration, there is a wide variety of topical dressings available. Trials to identify which of these produce the best healing rates have been difficult to construct because of many other treatment variables and therefore most of the dressings in everyday use have not been directly compared in the treatment of venous ulceration. Whatever dressing is chosen should be used in conjunction with treatment of the underlying venous insufficiency, usually by adequate graduated elastic compression. Simple non-adherent dressings are all that is required for many ulcers. Vacuum-assisted closure dressing systems are being increasingly used to treat troublesome venous ulcers. They help control the wound exudate, improve lymphatic and arterial flow and are known to accelerate wound healing in leg ulcers of various aetiologies.

### Emollients

These soothe, smooth and hydrate the skin and are indicated for all dry or scaling disorders. Therefore they may be of benefit in treating the skin changes associated with CVI, such as varicose eczema. Their effects are short-lived and frequent application is necessary. Preparations containing an antibacterial should be avoided unless infection is present.

### Oxpentifylline (pentoxifylline)

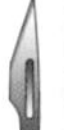

There have been several randomised controlled trials of oxpentifylline compared with placebo, with or without compression, in the healing of venous leg ulcers.[39] These have demonstrated that this drug is more effective than placebo in ulcer healing.

### Nutrition

Adequate nutrition is important for ulcer healing, and protein, vitamins A and C, zinc and other trace elements are all important. It may be appropriate to consider dietary supplements if these are deficient.

## Surgical intervention

### Superficial venous surgery

Superficial surgery may be of benefit in healing ulcers in situations of isolated superficial venous incompetence or combined superficial and deep venous incompetence. Surgery for isolated superficial venous incompetence may also reduce long-term recurrence rates.

**Table 18.1** • Conventional pressure classes of compression stockings

| Class | Pressure at ankle (mmHg) | Indications |
|---|---|---|
| I | <25 | Mild varicosis, venous thrombosis prophylaxis |
| II | 25–35 | Marked varicose veins, oedema, chronic venous insufficiency |
| III | 35–45 | Chronic venous insufficiency, lymphoedema, following venous ulceration to prevent recurrence |
| IV | 45–60 | Severe lymphoedema and chronic venous insufficiency |

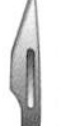

A recent randomised controlled trial comparing superficial venous surgery plus elastic compression with compression alone for venous ulceration has demonstrated no difference in initial healing rates but a reduction in recurrence rates at 12 months in the surgical group (12% vs. 28%). The authors concluded that most patients with chronic venous ulceration will benefit from addition of simple venous surgery.[40]

### Perforating vein surgery

There was renewed interest in medial calf-perforating vein incompetence with the advent of subfascial endoscopic perforating vein surgery. This new type of surgery is associated with less morbidity than open perforator surgery[41] and ulcer healing rates in the region of 90% at 1 year have been reported.[42] However, although there have been many studies on this new technique, it is usually carried out in combination with other reflux corrective surgery and the precise indications and benefit of perforator surgery remain unclear.

### Deep venous reconstruction

Worldwide experience of deep venous valvular reconstruction is limited as most patients with CVI can be managed very adequately with superficial venous surgery and the conservative measures described above. Therefore it is usually reserved for those patients with severe symptoms that prove resistant to conservative treatment.

The benefit of deep venous reconstructive surgery is unclear as many of the published series have included ancillary procedures such as high saphenous ligation and stripping, and in the few series where the influence of these procedures has been excluded the numbers involved tend to be small or the follow-up short. A number of different procedures have been described and these are shown in Box 18.4.

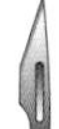

A recent Cochrane review has found only one randomised trial of deep venous reconstructive surgery.[43] This trial compared external valvuloplasty plus superficial venous ligation with superficial venous ligation only. There was a moderate improvement in clinical outcome in the valvuloplasty plus ligation group compared with mild clinical improvement in the ligation-only group.

### Venous bypass

Following DVT, recanalisation will occur in all affected venous segments in over 50% of limbs by 90 days.[44] However, the resultant destruction of the valves produces a functional obstruction. There may also be a failure in recanalisation that leaves a persistent mechanical venous outflow obstruction.

**Box 18.4** • Procedures for correction of deep venous valvular incompetence

**Valvular repair**

Valvuloplasty
Valve transposition
Valve transplantation

**External support of vein wall**

Dacron cuff
Vein wall plication

If severe, this gives rise to a swollen leg and ultimately skin changes associated with CVI, and may also cause venous claudication. Surgical bypass of an obstructed vein may be possible, but this should be reserved for those patients in whom there is measured evidence of outflow obstruction and in whom there are severe symptoms. As spontaneous improvement may occur due to the development of collaterals up to 4 years after DVT, surgery should not usually be considered before this time. Two principal surgical procedures have been described:

1. The femoro-femoral crossover graft for iliac obstruction (Palma operation; **Fig. 18.3**).[45] Only a small number of patients are suitable for this procedure, but in these patients long-term patency and relief of symptoms may be achieved in up to 70% of cases.[46] The long saphenous vein on the unaffected side is used as a crossover graft.

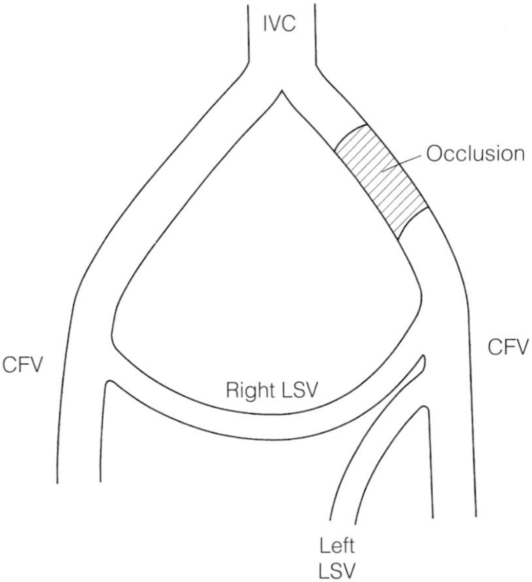


**Figure 18.3** • Femoro-femoral crossover graft using the long saphenous vein (LSV) to bypass unilateral iliac obstruction. CFV, common femoral vein; IVC, inferior vena cava.

2. Limbs with functional outflow obstruction due to stenosed or occluded deep thigh veins may be suitable for sapheno-popliteal bypass, which uses the long saphenous vein as a bypass channel. The theoretical difficulty with this procedure is that the long saphenous vein may already be acting as a collateral channel and to interfere with this may make matters worse should thrombosis occur. However, good long-term patency rates have been reported.[47]

### Skin grafting

Large ulcers may be usefully treated with a split-skin graft or pinch grafts which, if successful, will reduce the healing time. Before this is undertaken, it is important that the ulcer bed is clear from slough and not infected (particularly β-haemolytic streptococci, *Pseudomonas* and *Staphylococcus aureus*). However, unless the underlying venous abnormality is also treated, failure of the graft and subsequent recurrence is inevitable.

### Endovascular management of venous outflow obstruction

With the development of endovascular treatments in recent years it has become clear that iliac venous occlusions and stenoses may be treated by endoluminal stenting, although the long-term results have not been directly compared with surgery. Raju et al.[48] have reported treating a small series of long iliac venous occlusions, with primary and secondary patency rates at 2 years of 49% and 76% respectively. Further studies have reported patency rates in the region of 90% at 1 year for stenting of iliac venous stenoses (May–Thurner syndrome).[49,50] This refers to the chronic pulsatile compression of the proximal left common iliac vein by the overlying right common iliac artery or aortic bifurcation, resulting in an intraluminal venous spur, web or membrane. This common lesion (20% of the adult population) is an increasingly well-recognised cause of left iliac vein thrombo-occlusive disease, particularly in young patients. The clinical picture is of left leg venous hypertension or DVT and is likely to explain the preponderance for left-sided DVT in general.

## Preventing the post-thrombotic limb

CVI developing secondary to previous DVT is commonly referred to as post-thrombotic syndrome (PTS) or postphlebitic syndrome. The management of DVT has historically been directed at preventing thrombus extension and pulmonary embolus in the acute phase. There has been little focus on long-term treatment in order to prevent the development of PTS.

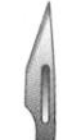

The risk of developing severe CVI with ulceration following DVT is of the order of 2–10% at 10 years.[51–53]

However, 30% or more will develop features of mild or moderate PTS.[53–55] This risk increases with more proximal DVT and recurrent episodes of thrombosis. Even with isolated calf vein thrombosis there is a risk of development of PTS, although this risk is lower than with popliteal or more proximal thromboses.

The causes of PTS related to previous DVT are either valvular incompetence or residual outflow obstruction with eventual calf muscle pump failure. Therefore treatment of the primary DVT should be aimed not only at preventing thrombus propagation and pulmonary embolism, but also at preventing venous damage and preserving or restoring venous function. This may include anticoagulation, limb elevation, elastic compression therapy and, in some cases, thrombolysis. Patients who have had DVT should be considered for long-term elastic compression hosiery, in particular those patients with residual reflux and who are on their feet all day or travel long journeys.[52] They should be encouraged to take regular exercise to stimulate the calf muscle pump. These simple measures may be required for life but are often all that is needed to prevent a lifetime of debility due to PTS.

### Summary

Investigation and treatment must be tailored to the individual patient but a simplified everyday management plan is shown in **Fig. 18.4**.

## Dependency and inactivity

Patients who sit for long periods are exposed to a raised venous pressure at the ankle for longer periods of time. Normal daily activity includes activation of the calf muscle pump by walking, thereby decreasing the venous pressure, but without this pressure reduction the effects on the lower limb are similar to those seen in venous reflux due to prolonged venous 'hypertension'. Therefore inactive patients, for example those confined to a wheelchair, can develop venous-type leg swelling in the absence on any true venous pathology.

## Lymphoedema

Lymphoedema is the progressive swelling of a limb that occurs when the lymphatic system fails to transport fluid via the lymphatic vessels and lymph nodes.

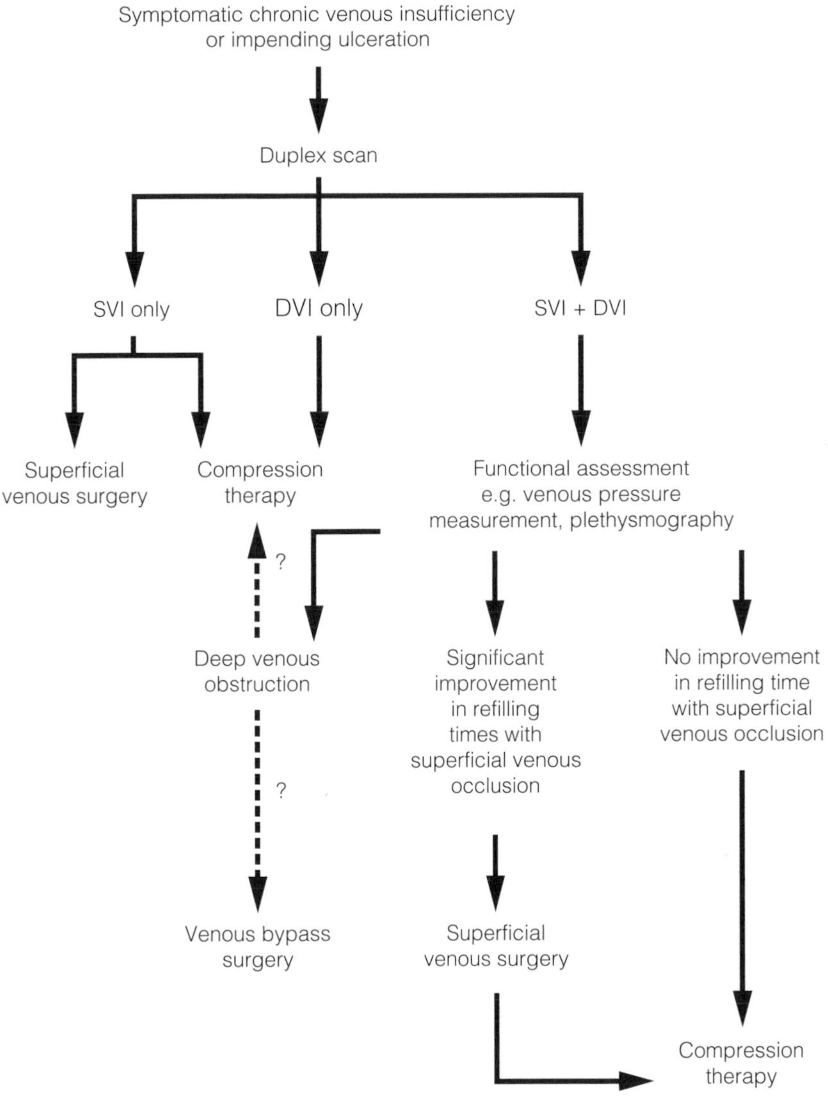


**Figure 18.4** • Flow diagram for the management of chronic venous insufficiency. DVI, deep venous incompetence; SVI, superficial venous incompetence.

## Aetiology

Lymphoedema can be primary or secondary.

### Primary

The traditional classification of primary lymphoedema is shown in Box 18.5. Congenital lymphoedema occurs at or soon after birth and in some rare cases it is autosomally inherited (Milroy's disease). Lymphoedema praecox presents up to the age of 35 years and is more common in women than men. Lymphoedema tarda presents over the age of 35 years. It is likely that these three groups represent different parts of the same spectrum of disease, which has been attributed to aplasia, hypoplasia or hyperplasia of the lymph vessels during development. However, a fibrotic obstruction in the lymph nodes has also been described.[56,57]

In addition to this, a functional classification more orientated to the treatment of these conditions may be used. This type of classification was first described by Browse.[58]

- Obliterative (80%): the distal lymphatics undergo progressive obliteration. This occurs predominantly in females and is often bilateral.
- Proximal obstruction (10%): proximal occlusion occurs in the abdominal, pelvic or inguinal lymph nodes. This is predominantly unilateral.

- Lymphatic valvular incompetence and hyperplasia (10%): development of the valve system is incomplete and lymphatic dilatation and hyperplasia occur. This is usually bilateral.

### Secondary

Secondary lymphoedema occurs when the lymphatic channels become occluded due to an acquired cause. The lymphatic channels distal to the obstruction become dilated and the valves secondarily incompetent. The commonest cause worldwide is filarial infestation but in Europe the commonest cause is neoplasia and its treatment, for example postmastectomy lymphoedema. The causes of secondary lymphoedema are also listed in Box 18.5.

## Presentation

Initial presentation is with peripheral oedema. History and examination will usually be able to differentiate lymphoedema from other causes of limb swelling and may distinguish between primary and secondary causes.

### History

The patient complains of a slowly progressive swelling of the limb and difficulties with footwear, and as the oedema progresses skin complications develop. Limb swelling usually commences distally and may progress during the day, particularly on standing. Although rarely painful, the leg may feel heavy and uncomfortable and there may be a history of recurrent lymphangitis. Primary lymphoedema occurs predominantly in females in their early teens, especially around puberty,[59] whereas patients with secondary lymphoedema will commonly have a history of previous surgery, neoplastic disease or radiotherapy.

### Examination

Examination reveals swelling of the limb, which may be unilateral or bilateral. Initially it will pit like other types of oedema, but with time the swelling becomes non-pitting due to hypertrophy of adipose tissue and increasing subcutaneous fibrosis. The swelling is uniform and as it progresses the leg becomes like a tree-trunk (**Fig. 18.5**). The skin develops a 'peau d'orange' appearance with hyperkeratosis of the toes and skin fissuring with secondary fungal infection. The skin gradually thickens, becoming less elastic until it is not possible to pick up a fold in the lower leg. This inelasticity produces a positive Stemmer sign (the inability to pinch the skin of the dorsum of the second toe between the thumb and forefinger). The dorsum of the foot is usually involved, producing the characteristic 'buffalo hump' appearance, and chylous vesicles may occur on the pretibial area.

**Box 18.5** • Causes of lymphoedema

**Primary**

- Congenital (age <1 year)
  - Familial (Milroy's disease)
  - Non-familial
- Praecox (age <35 years)
  - Familial
  - Non-familial
- Tarda (age >35 years)

**Secondary**

- Malignant disease
- Surgery
  - Radical mastectomy
  - Radical groin dissection
- Radiotherapy
- Infection
  - Parasitic (filariasis)
  - Pyogenic (β-haemolytic streptococci, *Staphylococcus aureus*)
  - Tuberculosis
- Impairment
  - Arterial surgery
  - Venous disease and venous surgery

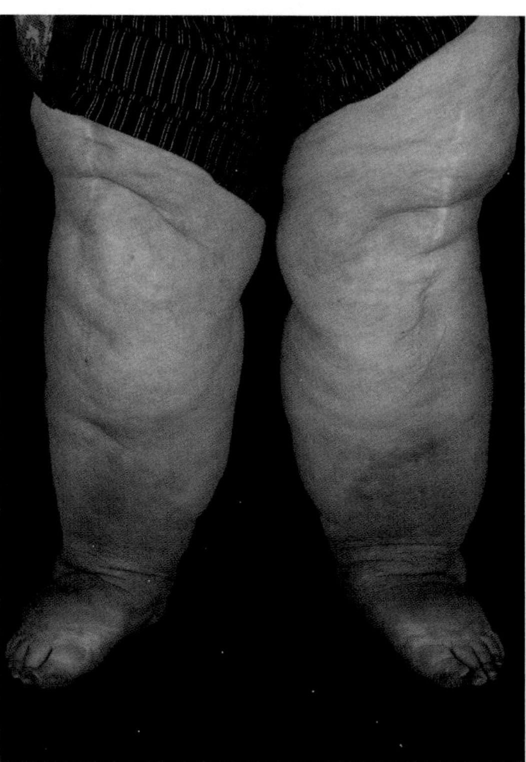

**Figure 18.5** • Chronic lymphoedema of the leg with tree-trunk appearance and 'buffalo hump' of the foot.

Ankle ulceration is not usually found with lymphoedema. It has been suggested that the reason for this is that the skin remains more elastic than in venous disease, allowing expansion to occur without increased tension.[60] The presence of surgical scars or skin telangiectasia following radiotherapy may indicate a cause of secondary lymphoedema.

## Clinical staging

Clinical staging is used to standardise reporting and to guide treatment. There is no consensus on a universal staging system that applies to all forms of lymphoedema. The consensus document of the International Society of Lymphology suggests the staging system given in Table 18.2.[61] Within each stage, severity based on volume difference can be assessed as minimal (<20% increase) in limb volume, moderate (20–40% increase) or severe (>40% increase).

## Investigation

The diagnosis of lymphoedema can usually be made clinically. Investigation is needed when the diagnosis is uncertain, to exclude sinister underlying causes or, if surgery is being considered, to confirm the diagnosis and plan treatment.

### Duplex ultrasonography

This is useful to exclude CVI. The B-mode image will also detect the changes in the dermis and subcutaneous layers and can therefore be used as a means of monitoring the disease.

### Lymphangioscintigraphy (isotope lymphography)

This is now one of the most frequently performed investigations as it provides an overall assessment of lymphatic drainage and in the majority of cases avoids the need for conventional lymphangiography (**Fig. 18.6**). Radiolabelled (usually technetium) colloid is injected into the interdigital space between the second and third toes on both sides and gamma-camera pictures are taken at 5-minute intervals to assess transit through the lymph channels. Scintigraphy has been demonstrated to have a sensitivity of 92% and a specificity of 100% for the diagnosis of lymphoedema.[62] A negative scintigram effectively excludes the diagnosis. Primary and secondary lymphoedemas are frequently associated with similar scintigraphic appearances, including delayed transit, the presence of collaterals, dermal backflow, and reduced uptake in one or more groups of lymph nodes. However, it can be used to distinguish between a venous and lymphatic cause of limb swelling and is a good method to assess treatment responses.

### Computed tomography

Computed tomography may show the presence of dilated lymphatic channels, thereby aiding the diagnosis of obstructive lymphoedema and lymphatic valvular incompetence. It will also provide evidence of lymphoedema by the presence of a honeycomb appearance of fluid in the subcutaneous tissues, and has been used to monitor the response to compression therapy by measuring the cross-sectional area of limb compartments.[63] Patients with a previous history of pelvic or abdominal malignancy should be scanned for recurrent disease in order to diagnose

**Table 18.2** • Clinical staging of lymphoedema

| | |
|---|---|
| Stage 0 | Latent or subclinical condition where swelling is not evident despite impaired lymph transport |
| Stage I | Early accumulation of fluid that subsides with limb elevation. Pitting may occur |
| Stage II | Limb elevation alone rarely reduces tissue swelling and pitting is manifest.<br>Late in stage II, the limb may or may not pit as tissue fibrosis supervenes |
| Stage III | Lymphostatic elephantiasis where pitting is absent and trophic skin changes such as acanthosis, fat deposits and warty overgrowths develop |

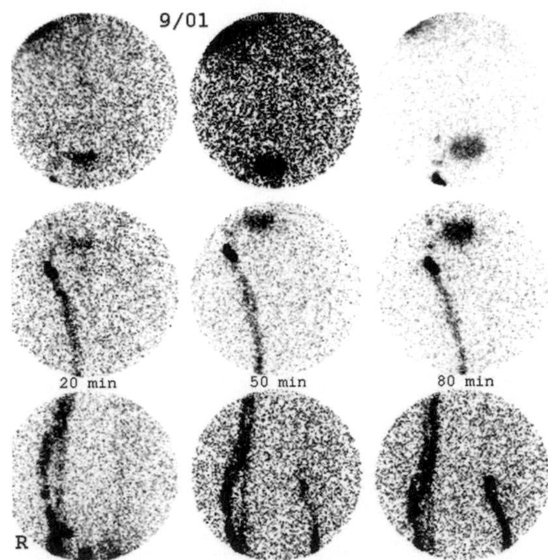


**Figure 18.6** • Lymphoscintigram confirming left-sided lymphoedema. On the right, the isotope is travelling up the lymphatics of the leg with concentration in the ilioinguinal nodes (normal). On the left the isotope has remained in the leg.

enlarged lymph nodes or pelvic masses that may be compressing the lymphatic channels.

### Magnetic resonance imaging (MRI)

In patients with chronic lymphoedema, MRI has been shown to demonstrate circumferential subcutaneous oedema, thickening of dermis and a honeycomb pattern of fibrosis between the muscle and subcutis.[64,65] Case et al.[66] found that MRI characteristically showed diffuse dermal and subcutaneous oedema, a non-oedematous occasionally hypertrophied skeletal muscle compartment, variability in regional lymph node size and appearance (depending on the underlying clinical disorder), serpiginous 'channels' or 'lakes' consistent with dermal collateral lymphangiectasis, and increased subcutaneous fat. They showed that, unlike scintigraphy, MRI can demonstrate anatomical definition of the lymphatics proximal to an obstruction and advocate its combined use with scintigraphy. It can distinguish between lymphatic and venous swelling, but is not good at separating primary and secondary causes of lymphoedema.

### Interstitial magnetic resonance lymphangiography

Interstitial magnetic resonance lymphography involves intracutaneous injection of a paramagnetic contrast agent for the visualisation of lymphatic vessels. Animal and human studies have demonstrated the feasibility and safety of this method.[67–69] Lohrmann et al. used intracuteous injections of gadodiamide mixed with mepivacaine into the interdigital webs. A 3-D spoiled gradient echo sequence revealed beaded appearance of lymphatic vessels in all cases. Lower leg lymphatics were best delineated after 35–45 minutes and the upper leg lymphatics and inguinal nodes after 55 minutes. Dilated lymphatic channels were the common finding among patients with lymphoedema. Collateral vessels along with dermal backflow indicated proximal obstruction.[70–72]

### Fluorescence microlymphangiography (FML)

FML involves visualisation of the superficial network of lymphatics with a fluorescence microscope following intracutaneous injection of fluorescein isothiocyanate–dextran 150 000 using microneedles. Emanating from the fluorescent spot, the surrounding network of microvessels is filled and becomes easily visible; documentation is performed by photography or video film. In Milroy's disease, a lack of microlymphatics (aplasia) is typical, while in other primary and secondary lymphoedema the network remains intact but the depicted area is enlarged. Lymphatic microangiopathy characterised by obliterations of capillary meshes or mesh segments develops in phleboedema with trophic skin changes, progressive systemic sclerosis and Fabry's disease. In lipoedema, lymphatic microaneurysms are seen. Microlymphatic pressure may also be measured using FML. Normal subjects produced significantly lower pressure (7.9 ± 3.4 mmHg) compared to patients with primary lymphoedema (15.0 ± 5.1 mmHg, $P < 0.001$). FML can confirm the clinical diagnosis of lymphoedema, distinguish among various forms of oedema and is useful in clinical research.[61,73]

### Contrast lymphangiography

This investigation is now used only rarely in the diagnosis of lymphoedema and has been largely replaced by scintigraphy. It is for patients being considered for microvascular lymphatic reconstruction.

### Volumetry

This is not a diagnostic test but is used as a reliable method of measuring upper or lower limb volume by water displacement, allowing an objective assessment of treatment.

## Treatment

The aim of treatment is to reduce limb swelling, reduce the risk of infection and improve function. If management begins early in the disease process when pitting oedema is present, conservative measures should be successful. Once achieved the improvement must be maintained. Surgical options are available in a few centres for resistant and severely symptomatic cases.

### General measures

Once the diagnosis is made, a clear explanation of the condition and its non-life-threatening nature is given to the patient. Information leaflets help to reassure the patient and encourage good compliance, which is needed for a lifetime of careful attention. Simple elevation of a lymphoedematous limb while resting and at night reduces oedema by increasing venous return and reducing the production of interstitial fluid. Exercise, such as on an exercise bicycle, encourages movement of lymph along non-contractile vessels and increased contractility of collecting lymph vessels.[74]

### Manual lymphatic drainage

This can be initiated by the physiotherapist. It involves manipulating the leg by squeezing just above the most proximal area of oedema and then working from proximal to distal. This enhances lymphatic flow.

### Graduated elastic compression

Compression stockings need to exert a pressure of approximately 50 mmHg or higher. The stockings can be used for maintenance of the limb after oedema reduction but compliance is low in the summer months, and the elderly and frail find them difficult to apply. Compression can also be achieved by multilayer bandaging.

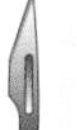

If graduated elastic compression is used initially followed by a stocking for maintenance, a greater and more sustained limb volume reduction is achieved than if stockings alone are used throughout.[75]

### Intermittent pneumatic compression (IPC)

IPC involves placement of the limb in a multicompartmental sleeve. Each compartment consists of air cells which are sequentially inflated to a pressure of about 80 mmHg and deflated from distal to proximal, thus massaging the lymph centrally. Patients use this for 4 hours a day and it can be done at home. If the lymphatic system is obliterated or obstructed more proximally, massaging the lymph centrally can precipitate collections elsewhere, such as the genitals, and high pressures may injure peripheral lymphatics. Reports combining IPC with stockings quote figures of 90% for immediate benefit and long-term maintenance.[76] The poor responders have usually had oedema for more than 10 years. In these chronic patients, compression using the hydrostatic pressure of mercury has had some effect.[77] The leg is placed in a cylinder and is covered by two membranes, which are filled and emptied with mercury in cycles. Pressures of up to 800 mmHg are generated at the foot and this linearly decreases towards normal atmospheric pressure at the surface. This is well tolerated and improvement is even seen in those with fibrosclerotic oedema. Despite its theoretical simplicity, the application and safety precautions are complex.

### Thermal treatment

Hyperthermia of the leg is produced by microwave heating or immersion in hot water. There is no change to the flow of lymph but it does reduce the local inflammatory infiltrate and extracellular protein matrix.[78] A reduction in limb volume follows, along with a decrease in the rate of recurrent infections.

### Complex decongestive physiotherapy (complex physical therapy)

Complex decongestive physiotherapy generally involves a two-stage treatment programme over 2–4 weeks. The first phase consists of skin care, light manual massage, range of motion exercise and compression typically applied with multilayered bandage wrapping. Phase 2 aims to conserve and optimise the results obtained in phase 1. It consists of compression by a low-stretch elastic stocking or sleeve, skin care, continued 'remedial' exercise, and repeated light massage as needed. With good compliance a 65–67% reduction in limb volume can be achieved, with 90% of the reduction being maintained at 9 months.[79,80] As an added benefit the incidence of infection almost halves. There is evidence to suggest that complex decongestive physiotherapy significantly improves quality of life.[81]

### Prevention of infection

The lymphatic system transports lymphocytes, enabling rapid response to foreign antigens. Stagnation of lymph prevents this and so increases the risk and severity of infection. The common pathogens are β-haemolytic streptococci and *Staphylococcus aureus*. With each attack of cellulitis or erysipelas the organisms further obliterate the lymph channels, making the oedema worse. Well-fitting comfortable shoes prevent small cracks in the skin that may act as a portal of entry. The affected limb should be washed daily with a mild soap and the feet must be dry before putting on shoes. The patient must keep a very careful eye on the foot and any early signs of infection must be treated aggressively with antibiotics. Recurrent infection can be managed by long-term, prophylactic, low-dose antibiotics such as amoxicillin, flucloxacillin or a cephalosporin.

### Drugs

Benzopyrones are thought to reduce oedema by reducing vascular permeability and thus the amount of fluid forming in the subcutaneous tissues. Advocates for this treatment method believe that the drugs have some beneficial effect on pain and discomfort in the swollen areas. Proponents also claim that these drugs increase macrophage activity, encouraging the lysis of protein, which in turn reduces the formation of fibrotic tissue in the lymphoedematous limb. A Cochrane review of available literature in 2004 concluded that there is not enough evidence from the research to show that benzopyrones are either beneficial or unhelpful in reducing lymphoedema.[82]

Diuretics may help for a short time in early oedema in combination with other modalities, but long-term therapy is of no value.

Underlying filarial infection should be treated with diethylcarbamazine.

Lymphangiogenesis is mediated through the vascular endothelial growth factor (VEGF)-3 receptor on lymphatic endothelia. Some early work on animal models has shown that stimulation of this receptor by VEGF-C will improve lymphatic function.[83,84]

## Surgical treatments

These can be divided into debulking operations and bypass procedures. Surgery is indicated if conservative measures have failed and there is disability, lymphorrhagia or recurrent lymphangitis. Obliterative causes are best treated by debulking procedures, whereas in lymphatic obstruction physiological bypass is recommended.

### Debulking operations

These procedures aim to excise variable amounts of the excess skin and subcutaneous tissue from the affected limb. The techniques range from removal of ellipses of tissue and primary closure (Homan's operation; **Fig. 18.7**) to the radical Charles operation, which excises all the skin and subcutaneous tissues of the calf down to and sometimes including the deep fascia. Primary skin grafting is then required. Good functional results have been obtained with this method but cosmesis is poor and it may be complicated by warts, resistant ulceration, lymph weeping and pantalooning of the thigh. Suction lipectomy, which has good results in the postmastectomy arm,[85] has been advocated in order to overcome these problems but only in the less severe situation,[86] because there is a tendency for greater fibrosis in the lower limb. Modern liposuction devices along with the use of tumescent solution and power-assisted cannula are thought to improve efficacy.[87]

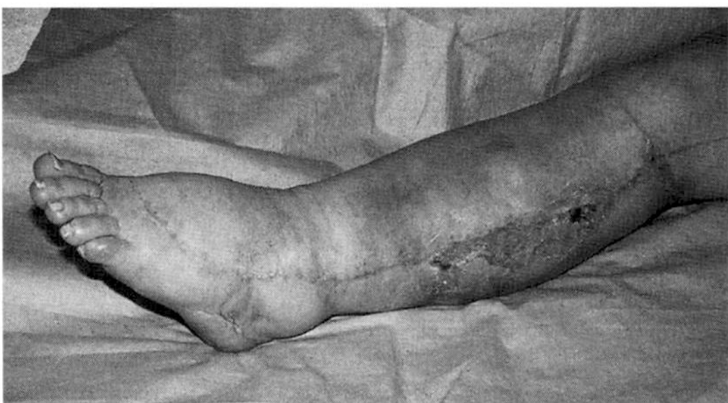

**Figure 18.7** • Homan's operation. A long ellipse of skin and subcutaneous tissue has been excised from the lateral side of the leg after a previous procedure on the medial side. Poor wound healing is common.

### Bypass procedures

These are reserved for regional blockage of the lymphatics, which could be due to either primary obstructive or secondary causes. If an iatrogenic secondary cause is suspected, a period of 6 months should elapse to allow any procedural swelling to subside before embarking on a lymphatic bypass. The bypass procedures are listed in Box 18.6.

Skin, muscle and omentum have been used to bypass regional obstructions but these tissues tend to have a paucity of lymphatics and as the technique relies on the development of new channels, high levels of success have not been reported. The technique of enteromesenteric bridging was designed to overcome this problem.[88] A 10-cm segment of ileum is resected on its mesentery and opened along its antimesenteric border. The mucosa is dissected off, leaving a submucosal area rich in lymphatics and blood vessels. The uppermost normal nodes are identified and bisected. The submucosal patch is then stitched in place over the top. Investigation has shown the early development of a lymphatic bridge and follow-up for 6 years has demonstrated a maintained improvement in 75% of legs, but the numbers are very small.[89]

Autologous lymphatic vessels harvested from the contralateral normal limb are used to perform lymphatico-lymphatic anastomoses and bypass obstruction. A suitable conduit is identified after the injection of patent blue dye into the interdigital spaces. The anastomoses are technically demanding. Limb volumetry reveals initial improvements in 66% of cases but this falls to about 50% at 1 year. Recent studies show that lower limb bypasses maintain improvement for 8 years and those in the upper limb for 10 years.[90,91]

Lymphatico-venous anastomosis is physiological if one considers the termination of the thoracic duct at the subclavian vein. Excellent long-term results have been published, with volume reductions on average of 67% lasting more than 7 years in the 85% of patients followed up along with an 87% reduction in the incidence of cellulitis.[92,93]

**Box 18.6** • Bypass procedures for lymphoedema

- Skin and muscle flaps
- Omental bridges
- Enteromesenteric bridges
- Lymphatico-lymphatic anastomosis
- Lymphatico-venous anastomosis

## Key points

- CVI is the commonest cause of leg swelling.
- The risk of mild to moderate chronic venous insufficiency after DVT is 30% at 10 years.
- The risk of severe CVI after DVT is 2–10% at 10 years.
- Superficial venous reflux alone may cause CVI.
- Graduated elastic compression is effective in healing ulcers and preventing recurrence.
- Superficial venous surgery may be of benefit in isolated superficial venous incompetence and combined superficial and deep venous incompetence.
- There is only limited evidence for the benefit of deep venous reconstructive surgery and endovascular therapy.
- Lymphoedema may be classified as primary or secondary.
- A further functional classification of obliterative, proximal obstruction, and valvular incompetence and hyperplasia may be used.
- The commonest cause of lymphoedema worldwide is filariasis but in Europe the commonest cause is malignancy and its treatment.
- Oedema is initially pitting, but becomes non-pitting due to subcutaneous fat deposition and fibrosis.
- Ulceration is rare in lymphoedema.
- Diagnosis is usually confirmed by isotope lymphangioscintigraphy.
- Satisfactory treatment can usually be achieved by conservative measures, including manual drainage, elastic compression, complex decongestive therapy and prevention of infection.

# References


1. Ruckley CV, Callam MJ, Dale JJ. Causes of chronic leg ulceration. Lancet 1982; ii:615–16.
2. Cornwall JV, Lewis JD. Leg ulcers: epidemiology and aetiology. Br J Surg 1986; 73:693–6.
3. Callam MJ, Harper DR, Dale JJ . Arterial disease in chronic leg ulceration: an underestimated hazard. Lothian and Forth Valley leg ulcer study. Br Med J 1987; 294:1389–91.
4. The Alexander House Group. Consensus paper venous leg ulcers. J Dermatol Surg Oncol 1992; 18:592–602.

   A condensed consensus report summarising the status of various aspects of epidemiology, diagnosis and treatment of venous ulcers. Various investigational and treatment approaches are summarised and recommendations given. Level II evidence.
5. Evans CJ, Fowkes FG, Ruckley CV et al. Prevalence of varicose veins and chronic venous insufficiency in men and women in the general population: Edinburgh Vein Study. J Epidemiol Community Health 1999; 53:149–53.
6. Van den Oever R, Hepp B, Bebbaut B et al. Socio-economic impact of chronic venous insufficiency. An underestimated public health problem. Int Angiol 1998; 17:161–7.
7. Nelzen O, Bergqvist D, Lindhagen A. Venous and non-venous leg ulcers: clinical history and appearance in a population study. Br J Surg 1994; 81:182–7.
8. Callam MJ, Ruckley CV, Harper DR et al. Chronic ulceration of the leg: extent of the problem and provision of care. Br Med J 1985; 290:1855–6.
9. Cornwall JV, Dore CJ, Lewis JD. Leg ulcers: epidemiology and aetiology. Br J Surg 1986; 73:693–9.
10. Baker SR, Stacey MC, Jopp-McKay AG et al. Epidemiology of chronic venous ulcers. Br J Surg 1991; 78:864–7.
11. Lees TA, Lambert D. Prevalence of lower limb ulceration in an urban health district. Br J Surg 1992; 79:1032–4.
12. Cesarone MR, Belcaro G, Nicolaides AN et al. 'Real' epidemiology of varicose veins and chronic venous disease: the San Valentino Vascular Screening Project. Angiology 2002; 53:119–30.
13. Harding K. Wound management in general practice. In: Royal College of General Practice members' reference book. London: Sabre-crown, 1991; pp. 313–16.
14. Bosanquet N. Costs of venous ulcers: from maintenance therapy to investment programmes. Phlebology 1992; 7:44–6.
15. Ruckley CV, Evans CJ, Allan PL et al. Chronic venous insufficiency: clinical and duplex correlations. The Edinburgh Vein Study of venous disorders in the general population. J Vasc Surg 2002; 36:520–5.
16. Lees TA, Lambert D. Patterns of venous reflux in limbs with skin changes associated with chronic venous insufficiency. Br J Surg 1993; 80:725–8.

17. Payne SPK, London NJM, Jagger C et al. Clinical significance of venous reflux detected by duplex scanning. Br J Surg 1994; 81:39–41.
18. Delis KT, Ibegbuna V, Nicolaides AN et al. Prevalence and distribution of incompetent perforating veins in chronic venous insufficiency. J Vasc Surg 1998; 28:815–25.
19. Burnand KG, O'Donnell TF, Lea Thomas M et al. The relative importance of incompetent communicating veins in the production of varicose veins and venous ulcers. Surgery 1977; 82:9–14.
20. Darke SG, Penfold C. Venous ulceration and saphenous ligation. Eur J Vasc Surg 1992; 6:4–9.
21. Chien S, Schmalzer EA, Lee MML et al. Role of white blood cells in filtration of blood cell suspension. Biorheology 1983; 20:11–27.
22. Schmid-Schonbein GW, Usami S, Skalak R et al. The interaction of leukocytes and erythrocytes in capillary and postcapillary vessels. Microvasc Res 1980; 19:45–70.
23. Lawrence MB, McIntire LV, Eskin SG. Effect of flow on polymorphonuclear leukocyte/endothelial cell adhesion. Blood 1987; 70:1284–90.
24. Sahary M, Shields DA, Georgiannos SN et al. Endothelial activation in patients with chronic venous disease. Eur J Vasc Endovasc Surg 1998; 15:342–9.
25. Shoab SS, Scurr JH, Coleridge Smith PD. Increased plasma vascular endothelial growth factor among patients with chronic venous disease. J Vasc Surg 1998; 28:535–40.
26. Coleridge Smith PD, Thomas P, Scurr JH et al. Causes of venous ulceration: a new hypothesis. Br Med J 1988; 296:1726–7.
27. Vanscheidt W, Laaf H, Weiss JM et al. Immunohistochemical investigation of dermal capillaries in chronic venous insufficiency. Acta Derm Venereol (Stockh) 1991; 71:17–19.
28. Wenner A, Leu HJ, Spycher M et al. Ultrastructural changes of capillaries in chronic venous insufficiency. Exp Cell Biol 1980; 48:1–14.
29. Gajraj H, Browse NL. Fibrinolytic activity of the arms and legs of patients with lower limb venous disease. Br J Surg 1991; 78:853–6.
30. Browse NL, Burnand KG. The cause of venous ulceration. Lancet 1982; ii:243–5.
31. Herouy Y, Nockowski P, Schopf E et al. Lipodermatosclerosis and the significance of proteolytic remodeling in the pathogenesis of venous ulceration. Int J Molec Med 1999; 3:511–15.
32. Eklof B, Rutherford RB, Bergan JJ et al. Revision of CEAP classification for chronic venous disorders: consensus statement. J Vasc Surg 2004; 40:1248–52.

    **This is an international consensus document produced under the auspice of the American Venous Forum that provides a classification for CVI.**
33. Coleridge-Smith P, Labropoulos N, Partsch H et al. Duplex ultrasound investigation of the veins in chronic venous disease of the lower limbs – UIP consensus document, part I. Basic principles. Eur J Vasc Endovasc Surg 2006; 31:83–92.
34. Mayberry JC, Moneta GL, Taylor LM Jr et al. Fifteen year results of ambulatory compression therapy for chronic venous ulcers. Surgery 1991; 109:575–81.
35. Cullum N, Nelson EA, Fletcher AW et al. Compression for venous leg ulcers (Cochrane review). In: The Cochrane Library, issue4. Chicester: John Wiley & Sons, 2003.

    **This is a meta-analysis of 22 trials comparing compression with no compression and various types of compression in the healing of venous leg ulcers. Six trials compared compression with no compression, five trials compared elastic with non-elastic compression, three trials compared four-layer bandaging with other multilayered systems, four trials compared healing rates between elastomeric multilayered systems, and four trials compared multilayered high compression with single-layer compression. Results are given in the text.**
36. Nelson EA, Bell-Syer SEM, Cullum NA. Compression for preventing recurrence of venous ulcers (Cochrane review). In: The Cochrane Library, issue 4. Chicester: John Wiley & Sons, 2003.

    **This is a review of two randomised controlled trials, one of which compared class III stockings with class II stockings and the other compared two different makes of class II stocking in the prevention of ulcer recurrence. Higher grades of compression are associated with lower recurrence rates. Also, not wearing stockings is strongly associated with ulcer recurrence.**
37. Ruckley CV. Treatment of venous ulceration: compression therapy. Phlebology 1992; 1(Suppl):22–6.
38. Mani R, Vowden K, Nelson EA. Intermittent pneumatic compression for treating venous leg ulcers (Cochrane review). In: The Cochrane Library, issue 4. Chicester: John Wiley & Sons, 2003.

    **This is a review of four randomised controlled trials; three compared IPC plus compression with compression alone. One of these found increased ulcer healing with IPC, while two found no evidence of benefit. One trial compared IPC without additional compression with compression alone and found no difference.**
39. Jull AB, Waters J, Arroo B. Pentoxifylline for treating venous leg ulcers (Cochrane review). In: The Cochrane Library, issue 4. Chicester: John Wiley & Sons, 2003.

    **This is a meta-analysis of nine trials, eight of which compared pentoxifylline (oxpentifylline) with placebo. Oxpentifylline is more effective than placebo in terms of complete ulcer healing or significant improvement. The relative risk of ulcer healing with oxpentifylline compared with placebo is 1.41.**
40. Barwell J, Davies C, Deacon J et al. Comparison of surgery and compression with compression alone

in chronic venous ulceration (ESCHAR study): randomized controlled trial. Lancet 2004; 363:1854.

This is a randomised controlled trial of 500 consecutive patients with chronic venous ulcers randomly assigned to compression alone or in combination with surgery to assess the role of superficial venous surgery in the healing and prevention of recurrence of leg ulcers. There was no difference in initial healing rates but a reduction in recurrence at 12 months in the surgical group (12% vs. 28%).

41. Stuart WP, Adam DJ, Bradbury AW et al. Subfascial endoscopic perforator surgery is associated with significantly less morbidity and shorter hospital stay than open operation. Br J Surg 1997; 84:1364–5.

42. Gloviczki P, Bergan JJ, Rhodes JM et al. Mid-term results of endoscopic perforator vein interruption for chronic venous insufficiency: lessons learned from the North American subfascial endoscopic perforator surgery registry. The North American Study Group. J Vasc Surg 1999; 29:489–502.

43. Abidia A, Hardy SC. Surgery for deep venous incompetence. In: The Cochrane Library, issue 4. Chicester: John Wiley & Sons, 2003.

This is a review of randomised trials of surgical treatment of patients with deep venous incompetence. Only one trial was found comparing superficial venous ligation and limited deep anterior valve plication with superficial ligation alone, with moderate improvement in clinical outcome in the former group compared with mild improvement in the latter group.

44. Killewich LA, Bedford GR, Beach KW et al. Spontaneous lysis of deep venous thrombi: rate and outcome. J Vasc Surg 1989; 9:89–97.

45. Palma EC, Esperon R. Vein transplants and grafts in the surgical treatment of the postphlebitic syndrome. J Cardiovasc Surg (Torino) 1960; 1:94–107.

46. Halliday P, Harris J, May J. Femoro-femoral crossover grafts (Palma operation), a long term follow up study. In: Bergan JF, Yao JST (eds.) Surgery of the veins. New York: Grune & Stratton, 1985; p. 241.

47. Husni EA. Venous reconstruction in postphlebitic disease. Circulation 1971; 43(Suppl 1):147–50.

48. Raju S, McAllister S, Neglen P. Recanalisation of totally occluded iliac and adjacent venous segments. J Vasc Surg 2002; 36:903–11.

49. O'Sullivan GJ, Semba CP, Bittner CA et al. Endovascular management of iliac vein compression (May–Thurner syndrome). J Vasc Intervent Radiol 2000; 11:823–36.

50. Raju S, Owen S Jr, Neglen P. The clinical impact of iliac venous stents in the management of chronic venous insufficiency. J Vasc Surg 2002; 35:8–15.

51. Leizorovicz A. Long-term consequences of deep venous thrombosis. Haemostasis 1998; 28(Suppl 3): 1–7.

52. McCollum C. Avoiding the consequences of deep venous thrombosis. Br Med J 1998; 517:696.

53. Janssen MC, Haenen JH, van Asten WN et al. Clinical and haemodynamic sequelae of deep venous thrombosis: retrospective evaluation after 7–13 years. Clin Sci 1997; 93:7–12.

In this study, 81 patients with venographically confirmed lower-extremity DVT were clinically and haemodynamically re-examined 7–13 years after DVT (mean 10 years) to assess PTS; 7–13 years after DVT 31% of the patients had moderate and 2% had severe clinical PTS, while 57% of the patients had abnormal haemodynamic findings. Level II evidence.

54. Franzeck UK, Schalch I, Bollinger A. On the relationship between changes in the deep veins evaluated by duplex sonography and the post-thrombotic syndrome 12 years after deep venous thrombosis. Thromb Haemost 1997; 77:1109–12.

55. Johnson BF, Manzo RA, Bergelin RO et al. Relationship between changes in the deep venous system and the development of the postthrombotic syndrome after an acute episode of lower limb deep vein thrombosis: a one- to six-year follow up. J Vasc Surg 1995; 21:307–12.

56. Kinmonth JB, Wolfe JH. Fibrosis in the lymph nodes in primary lymphoedema. Histological and clinical studies in 74 patients with lower limb oedema. Ann R Coll Surg Engl 1980; 62:344–54.

57. Browse NL, Stewart G. Lymphoedema: pathophysiology and classification. J Cardiovasc Surg (Torino) 1985; 26:91–106.

58. Browse NL. The diagnosis and management of primary lymphoedema. J Vasc Surg 1986; 3:181–4.

59. Wright NB, Carty HM. The swollen leg and primary lymphoedema. Arch Dis Child 1994; 71:44–9.

60. Chant ADB. Hypothesis: why venous oedema causes ulcers and lymphoedema does not. Eur J Vasc Surg 1992; 6:427–9.

61. The diagnosis and treatment of peripheral lymphedema: consensus document of the International Society of Lymphology. Lymphology 2003; 36:84–91.

62. Gloviczki P, Calcagno D, Schirger A et al. Noninvasive evaluation of the swollen extremity: experiences with 190 lymphoscintigraphic examinations. J Vasc Surg 1989; 9:683–98.

63. Collins CD, Mortimer PS, D'Ettorre H et al. Computed tomography in the assessment of response to limb compression in unilateral lymphoedema. Clin Radiol 1995; 50:541–4.

64. Haaverstad R, Nilsen G, Myhre HO et al. The use of MRI in the investigation of leg oedema. Eur J Vasc Surg 1992; 6:124–9.

65. Duewell S, Hagspiel KD, Zuber J et al. Swollen lower extremity: role of MR imaging. Radiology 1992; 184:227–31.

66. Case TC, Witte MH, Unger EC et al. Magnetic resonance imaging in human lymphoedema: comparison with lymphangioscintigraphy. Magn Reson Imaging 1992; 10:549–58.

67. Ruehm SG, Corot C, Debatin JF. Interstitial MR lymphangiography with a conventional extracellular gadolinium based agent: assessment in rabbits. Radiology 2001; 218:664–9.

68. Ruehm SG, Shroeder T, Debatin JF. Interstitial MR lymphangiography with gadoterate meglumine: experience in humans. Radiology 2001; 220:816–21.

69. Fink C, Bock M, Keissling F et al. Interstitial magnetic resonance lymphography with gadobuterol in rats: evaluation of contrast kinetics. Invest Radiol 2002; 37:655–62.

70. Lohrmann C, Foeldi E, Speck O et al. High resolution MR lymphangiography in patients with primary and secondary lymphedema. Am J Rad 2006; 187:556–61.

71. Lohrmann C, Foeldi E, Bartholoma JP et al. MR imaging of the lymphatic system: distribution and contrast enhancement of gadodiamide after intradermal injection. Lymphology 2006; 39:156–63.

72. Lohrmann C, Foeldi E, Bartholoma JP et al. Interstitial MR lymphangiography – a diagnostic imaging method in patients with clinically advanced stages of lymphedema. Acta Tropica 2007; 104:8–15.

73. Bollinger A, Amann-Vesti BR. Fluorescence microlymphography: diagnostic potential in lymphedema and basis for the measurement of lymphatic pressure and flow velocity. Lymphology 2007; 40:52–62.

74. Mortimer PS. Swollen lower limb. 2. Lymph oedema. Br Med J 2000; 320:1527–9.

75. Badger CM, Peacock JL, Mortimer PS. A randomised, controlled, parallel-group trial comparing multilayer bandaging followed by hosiery versus hosiery alone in the treatment of patients with lymphedema of the limb. Cancer 2000; 88:2832–7.

This is a randomised, controlled, parallel-group trial in which 90 women with unilateral lymphoedema (of the upper or lower limbs) underwent 18 days of multilayer bandaging followed by elastic hosiery or hosiery alone, each for a total period of 24 weeks. The reduction in limb volume due to multilayer bandaging followed by hosiery was approximately double that from hosiery alone and was sustained over the 24-week period. The mean overall percentage reduction at 24 weeks was 31% ($n$ = 32) for multilayer bandaging versus 15.8% ($n$ = 46) for hosiery alone, for a mean difference of 15.2% (95% CI 6.2–24.2, $P$ = 0.001). Level I evidence.

76. Pappas CJ, O'Donnell TF. Long-term results of compression treatment for lymphedema. J Vasc Surg 1992; 16:555–64.

77. Palmer A, Macchiaverna J, Braun A et al. Compression therapy of limb oedema using hydrostatic pressure of mercury. Angiology 1991; 42:533–42.

78. Liu NF, Olszewski W. The influence of local hyperthermia on lymphedematous skin of the human leg. Lymphology 1993; 26:28–37.

79. Cheville AL, McGarvey CL, Petrek JA et al. Lymphedema management. Semin Radiat Oncol 2003; 13:290–301.

80. Ko DS, Lerner R, Klose G et al. Effective treatment of lymphedema of the extremities. Arch Surg 1998; 133:452–8.

81. Weiss JM, Spray BJ. The effect of complete decongestive therapy on the quality of life of patients with peripheral lymphedema. Lymphology 2002; 35:46–58.

82. Badger C, Preston N, Seers K et al. Benzo-pyrones for reducing and controlling lymphoedema of the limbs. Cochrane Database Syst Rev 2004; 2:CD003140.

83. Szuba A, Skobe M, Karkkainen MJ et al. Therapeutic lymphangiogenesis with human recombinant VEGF-C. FASEB J 2002; 16:1985–7.

84. Yoon YS, Murayama T, Gravereaux E et al. VEGF-C gene therapy augments postnatal lymphangiogenesis and ameliorates secondary lymphedema. J Clin Invest 2003; 111:717–25.

85. Brorson H, Svenson H. Liposuction combined with controlled compression therapy reduces arm lymphedema more effectively than controlled compression therapy alone. Plast Reconstr Surg 1998; 102:1058–67.

86. Sando WC, Nah F. Suction lipectomy in the management of limb lymphedema. Clin Plast Surg 1989; 16:369–73.

87. Greene AK, Slavin SA, Borud L. Treatment of lower extremity lymphedema with suction-assisted lipectomy. Plast Reconstr Surg 2006; 118:118–21.

88. Kinmonth JB, Hurst PA, Edwards JM et al. Relief of lymph obstruction by use of a bridge of mesentery and ileum. Br J Surg 1978; 65:829–33.

89. Hurst PAE, Stewart G, Kinmonth JB et al. Long-term results of the enteromesenteric bridge operation in the treatment of primary lymphoedema. Br J Surg 1985; 72:272–4.

90. Weiss M, Baumeister RG, Hahn K. Post-therapeutic lymphedema: scintigraphy before and after autologous vessel transplantation: 8 years of long-term follow up. Clin Nucl Med 2002; 27:788–92.

91. Baumeister RG, Frick A. The microsurgical lymph vessel transplantation. Handchir Mikrochir Plast Chir 2003; 35:202–9.

92. Campisi C, Davini D, Bellini C et al. Lymphatic microsurgery for the treatment of lymphedema. Microsurgery 2006; 26:65–9.

93. Campisi C, Eretta C, Pertile D et al Microsurgery for the treatment of peripheral lymphedema: long term outcome and future perspectives. Microsurgery 2007; 27:333–8.

# 19

# The acutely swollen leg

Anthony J. Comerota
Faisal Aziz

## Introduction

Acute leg oedema is a major concern for the patient as well as the physician. Depending upon the aetiology, the oedema may be a manifestation of a chronic underlying disease which only recently became symptomatic or may represent an acute problem that may be life threatening and associated with lifestyle-changing long-term morbidity.

This chapter briefly reviews the underlying pathophysiology of acute limb oedema and a rational diagnostic approach to patients presenting with the acutely swollen leg. Treatment strategies are straightforward for most aetiologies; however, patients with extensive (iliofemoral) deep vein thrombosis (DVT) face substantial acute *and* chronic morbidity, which is avoidable if a strategy of thrombus removal is implemented early in the course of their disease.

The terms *acute* and *chronic*, as they relate to limb oedema, are arbitrary and depend upon when patients present, which is often a measure of the patient's tolerance of symptoms. Generally, if a patient can identify a specific day in the recent past when symptoms began or identify a potential inciting event, the patient's swollen leg can be viewed as acute, even if the patient presents 14 days or more after symptoms began.

## General pathophysiology

Tissue oedema is the cause of the acutely swollen leg. Oedema is the accumulation of excess water within the tissue spaces of the affected extremity. Total body water is distributed inside (intracellular) and outside (extracellular) of the cells. Acute oedema results from the rapid fluid expansion of the extracellular space. The extracellular space is comprised of the intravascular and extravascular (interstitial) spaces. Specifically, oedema is the result of water accumulation in the interstitial space. If the process includes salt (and water) retention by the kidneys, the patient will have generalised (not focal) oedema and most will be chronic.

The rapid expansion of the interstitial space is usually the result of one or more of four aetiologies:

1. **Increased hydrostatic pressure** forcing fluid out of the intravascular space. This is usually seen with any process that increases venous pressure. Central increases of hydrostatic pressure include congestive heart failure, right heart failure and tricuspid insufficiency. Focal or unilateral oedema is often the result of DVT causing main venous channel occlusion.
2. **Decreased oncotic pressure** allowing passive transfer of intravascular fluid to the interstitial compartment. This generally is the result of reduction of intravascular protein content (i.e. hypoalbuminaemia).
3. **Increased capillary permeability**, reducing the barrier to water moving from the intravascular space to the interstitial space. This is observed

with focal trauma, burns, infection, ischaemia and immunological injury.

4. **Lymphatic obstruction** resulting from hereditary hypoplasia, acute infection, or the consequence of lymphatic ablation following surgery, trauma or radiation.

# Clinical presentation and diagnosis

Typically, the patient's clinical presentation in addition to a careful history and physical examination will point to the likeliest aetiology, resulting in the most efficient diagnostic evaluation.

## Musculotendinous rupture

Sudden intense pain of the posterior lower leg usually suggests a musculoskeletal aetiology. If associated with sudden dorsiflexion of the foot, rupture of the musculotendinous portion of the medial head of the gastrocnemius muscle or the plantaris muscle (tendon) should be suspected. Localised pain in the medial or mid calf area and swelling at the ankle level is common. Ecchymotic discoloration at the ankle level often follows 2–5 days later due to blood tracking down the fascial planes when the leg is pendant. Excluding DVT with a venous duplex examination is appropriate.

Treatment consists of symptomatic and supportive care until symptoms resolve. Leg elevation, ice early followed by heat, analgesics and reduced weight bearing may be necessary until symptoms resolve, usually within a month.

## Popliteal cyst

Patients presenting with sudden, instantaneously severe calf pain and swelling are unlikely to have venous thrombosis. This clinical presentation is seen with musculotendinous aetiologies and is also consistent with rupture of a popliteal cyst.

Most popliteal cysts are found incidentally on venous duplex and may be related to more chronic symptoms of discomfort in the popliteal space and calf. Symptoms include posterior knee pain and swelling, and signs include tenderness to palpation, a palpable mass, leg oedema and occasionally calf tenderness. Popliteal cysts are generally composed of a fibrous wall, often communicating with the joint space of the knee and lined by synovium. It is usually the result of degenerative arthritis, but is also found and associated with meniscal tears, rheumatoid arthritis and gout. The diagnosis is uniformly made with a duplex ultrasound examination.

Treatment of a ruptured cyst is symptomatic, applying cold packs or ice, anti-inflammatory medications, reduced weight bearing and treatment directed at the underlying disease of the knee joint. Indications for operation, especially in patients with an intact cyst that is symptomatic, are best determined by orthopaedic surgeons.

## Cellulitis

Painful, erythematous, red unilateral leg oedema with increased warmth suggests cellulitis. A careful search often reveals a break in the skin integrity allowing bacterial ingress. Predisposing factors should be sought, such as foot blisters, skin excoriation, intertriginous fissures and prior episodes of cellulitis. Open wounds should be cultured. Venous thrombosis, though often suspected in this scenario, rarely exists. A venous duplex can be obtained as an elective, non-emergent examination. Antibiotics directed at the Gram-positive organisms of *Staphylococcus aureus* or group A streptococcus are appropriate in the majority of patients. Leg elevation and minimising/restricting ambulation will speed resolution.

## Lymphoedema

Although chronic lymphoedema is characterised by the accumulation of protein-rich fluid in the subcutaneous tissue, early- or new-onset lymphoedema can present with pitting oedema, although the distribution of oedema and the shape of the swollen leg suggest that the aetiology is lymphatic in origin.

The typical clinical picture is a young active woman who twists her ankle or sustains apparently minimal lower extremity trauma. Subsequently the leg swells and the oedema is persistent. This is often seen after girls reach puberty and is typical of lymphoedema praecox. This is one of the presentations of primary lymphoedema, inherited as an autosomal dominant disorder with variable penetrance. Although trauma often stimulates the presentation of unilateral oedema, with passage of time both legs become clinically affected. Lymphoscintigraphy is the diagnostic test of choice, although it is usually unnecessary.

Manual lymph drainage (lymphatic massage) and multilayered (inelastic) bandaging often result in the best long-term control of the lymphoedematous extremity. A small study showed benefit to coumarin reducing limb volume compared to a placebo control.[1] Confirmatory studies are required before oral anticoagulation can be generally recommended.

All patients with lymphoedema should be given a prescription for a broad-spectrum antibiotic to have available should they notice any evidence suggestive of early cellulitis. Infections sclerose existing lymphatics, exacerbating the severity of lymphoedema. Meticulous foot hygiene, preventing blisters and athlete's foot, is important in all patients, as even minor foot infections can have major deleterious consequences in patients with lymphoedema.

## Other aetiologies

A variety of other aetiologies are associated with acute unilateral limb swelling. Patients with chronic venous insufficiency may observe acute worsening of their chronic limb oedema, especially after more intense physical activity or from not wearing their compression garment. Patients suffering recent trauma may develop progressive oedema. Causes such as a ganglion cyst can rarely present as unilateral leg oedema.[2] The presence of venous thrombosis should always be excluded and is easily accomplished with a venous duplex ultrasound or negative D-dimer.[3,4] The true aetiology can then be identified with a careful history, physical examination and other suggestive findings on the duplex examination (i.e. identifying the ganglion cyst, venous valvular incompetence, etc.). Treatment is then directed at the underlying aetiology.

## Acute deep venous thrombosis

Acute DVT is the most worrisome of the aetiologies of acute limb oedema; untreated, it is potentially lethal and, if extensive, often associated with severe post-thrombotic morbidity.[5,6]

Diagnosis of acute DVT is most frequently made with venous duplex ultrasound (**Fig. 19.1**). In patients who present with unilateral leg symptoms but a low clinical probability of acute DVT, a negative D-dimer test reliably excludes DVT with a 99% negative predictive value.[4] Our diagnostic approach, integrating the patient's clinical probability of acute DVT with D-dimer and venous duplex ultrasound, is summarised in **Fig. 19.2**.

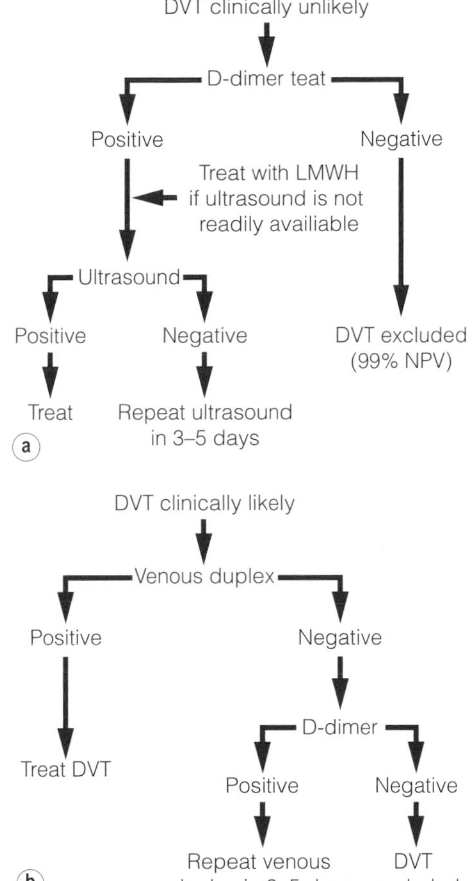


**Figure 19.2** • Illustration of a diagnostic approach that integrates the probability of acute DVT with D-dimer and venous duplex ultrasound. **(a)** DVT clinically unlikely. **(b)** DVT clinically likely.

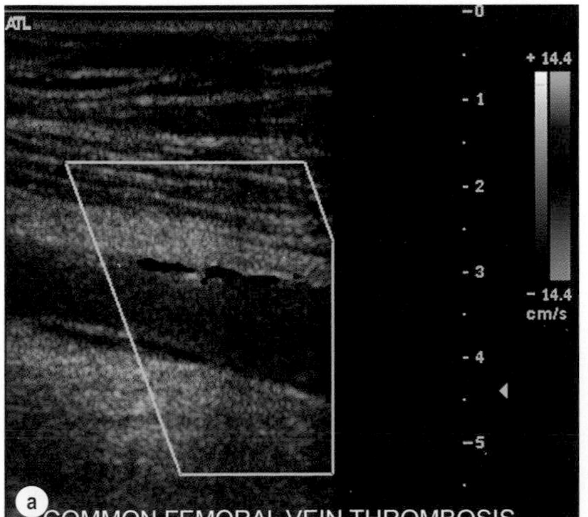


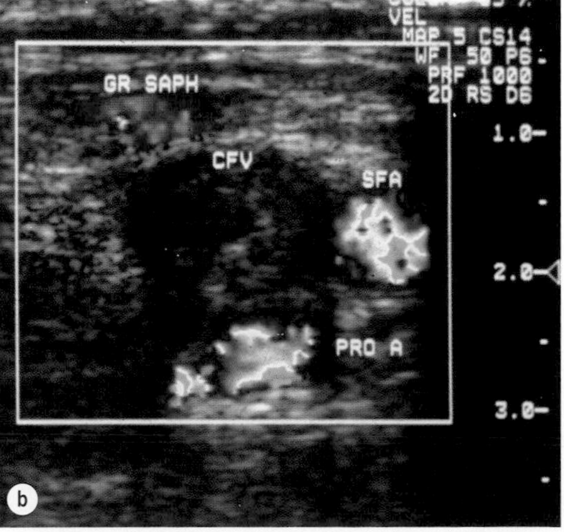


**Figure 19.1** • The diagnosis of acute DVT is most frequently made with venous duplex ultrasound.

Patients presenting with acute infrainguinal DVT are best treated with anticoagulation, ensuring that therapeutic anticoagulation is achieved from the time of diagnosis to reduce the risk of recurrence. Most physicians fail to recognise the 15-fold increased risk of recurrence if patients fall below therapeutic levels of anticoagulation early in their treatment with unfractionated heparin.[7] Low-molecular-weight heparin (enoxaparin) given subcutaneously at 1 mg/kg every 12 hours effectively treats the patient and offers benefits beyond unfractionated heparin, which include reduced risk of bleeding, more rapid thrombus resolution and decreased mortality, especially in patients with malignancy.[8] Conversion to oral anticoagulation, initiated immediately after the first dose of low-molecular-weight heparin, occurs during the next 5 days of therapy targeting an international normalised ratio (INR) of 2.0–3.0. The duration of oral anticoagulation depends upon patient presentation, history of prior venous thromboembolism and condition of the patient after 6–12 months of therapy.[9] Patients whose transient risk has resolved are best treated for 6 months. Patients suffering recurrent venous thrombosis and those who have antiphospholipid antibody are best treated indefinitely. Patients with malignancy are best treated with low-molecular-weight heparin for 3–6 months and then evaluated for conversion to oral anticoagulation. The American College of Chest Physicians' (ACCP) recommendations for the duration of anticoagulation are summarised in Table 19.1.[9]

Limb compression and ambulation are recommended for patients with acute DVT after the initiation of anticoagulation.[10] This reduces pain and swelling and is not associated with increased risk of pulmonary embolus. From the time of diagnosis, patients with acute DVT should have 30–40 mmHg ankle-gradient compression stockings applied and worn, which reduces post-thrombotic morbidity by 50%.[11,12]

## Iliofemoral deep venous thrombosis

Iliofemoral DVT, the most serious and extensive form of acute DVT, is associated with a 50% or more incidence of pulmonary embolism (most being asymptomatic) and results in the most severe post-thrombotic morbidity.[5,6] Thrombus occluding the outflow tract of the leg causes significant venous hypertension and, over the long term, results in venous claudication in 40–50% of individuals who are treated with anticoagulation alone.[5]

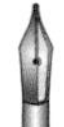

The majority of natural history studies that evaluate patients based upon the magnitude of acute thrombosis confirm that patients with extensive DVT have the worst post-thrombotic syndrome. This is especially true in patients with iliofemoral DVT.

Early internationally important guidelines on the management of acute DVT have failed to recognise the value of a strategy of thrombus removal;[9] therefore, the majority of physicians treat these patients with anticoagulation alone, without regard to the extent of thrombosis. A large body of evidence, however, supports treatment directed at clearing the venous system of thrombus, resulting in significantly reduced post-thrombotic morbidity. The eighth ACCP consensus

Table 19.1 • Current ACCP recommendations[9] for the duration of anticoagulation

| Patients | Modifier | Recommendation | Grade |
|---|---|---|---|
| First episode DVT<br>Calf<br>Proximal | Transient (reversible) risk factor | 3 months VKA | 1A |
| First episode DVT | Idiopathic | At least 6–12 months<br>**and**<br>consider indefinite | 1A<br><br>2A |
| VTE patients | Rx'ed with VKAs | INR 2.0–3.0<br>*Against* high intensity | 1A<br>1A |
| First episode DVT | Cancer | LMWH × 3–6 months<br>**and**<br>anticoagulation indefinitely (or cancer resolved) | 1A<br><br>1C |
| First episode DVT | Antiphospholipid antibody **or** ≥2 other thrombophilic conditions | Indefinite anticoagulation | 2A |
| Recurrent DVT | | Indefinite anticoagulation | 2A |
| VTE patients | Indefinite anticoagulation | Reassess risk/benefit | 1C |

LMWH, low-molecular-weight heparin; VKA, vitamin K antagonist; VTE, venous thromboembolism.

conference on antithrombotic therapy recognised the available evidence and supports a strategy of thrombus removal in patients with iliofemoral DVT.[13]

We have adopted such a strategy for these patients in order to offer them the best chance of continuing a normal lifestyle.

## Rationale

Patients with acute iliofemoral DVT are a clinically relevant subset of patients with acute venous thrombosis, since they suffer the most severe post-thrombotic morbidity and their risk of recurrence is 2.4-fold that of patients with femoropopliteal DVT.[14]

Studies of the pathophysiology of chronic venous insufficiency have clearly shown that residual luminal obstruction, in addition to venous valvular incompetence, causes the most severe post-thrombotic morbidity because it produces the highest ambulatory venous pressures.[15,16]

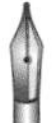

It is intuitive that treatment which successfully eliminates thrombus restores venous patency, thereby eliminating the obstructive component of the pathophysiology of post-thrombotic venous disease. Therefore, if the post-thrombotic syndrome occurs due to valvular incompetence alone (without obstruction), the severity should be considerably reduced and more easily controlled.

## Evidence for thrombus removal

Numerous data support the concept that early thrombus resolution after the onset of acute DVT results in improved outcomes. Animal experiments in the canine model have shown that thrombolysis for acute DVT preserves endothelial function, maintains venous valve competence and preserves structural integrity of the vein wall.[17,18]

A National Institutes of Health-sponsored long-term observational study of acute DVT patients treated with anticoagulation showed that patients demonstrating spontaneous clot lysis had a significantly better chance of preserving vein valve function, especially if lysis occurred early.[19–21] On the other hand, persisting proximal venous obstruction often produced distal valve incompetence, even in distal veins that were not initially thrombosed.[19]

Persistent thrombus at termination of anticoagulation is associated with an increased risk of recurrent DVT.[22,23] Patients with iliofemoral DVT have a large thrombus burden at the outset of therapy and therefore will likely have a larger residual thrombus burden at the completion of anticoagulation, if indeed anticoagulation alone is the chosen form of therapy. Douketis et al.[14] documented the anticipated observation that patients with iliofemoral DVT treated with anticoagulation alone had a significantly higher risk of recurrence compared to patients with infrainguinal DVT.

Persistent thrombus is likely to be associated with ongoing thrombus activity. Increased thrombus activity after termination of anticoagulation, manifested by elevated D-dimer levels, is associated with a threefold increased risk of recurrent venous thrombosis.[3] Therefore, the numerous clinical observations linking a large burden of venous thrombus with post-thrombotic morbidity and increased risk of recurrence suggest that initial treatment aimed at eliminating the thrombus burden is not only reasonable, but strongly recommended.

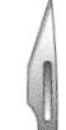

Recurrent DVT is an especially strong predictor of post-thrombotic syndrome. It is now recognised that iliofemoral DVT is associated with a significant increased risk of recurrent DVT compared to patients with thrombus limited to the infrainguinal veins.

Initial efforts to clear the thrombus using thrombolytic therapy for patients with acute DVT involved systemic, peripheral intravenous infusion of the plasminogen activators.[24] The overall results of these trials showed that approximately 45% of patients had substantial or complete lysis. Although this observation is significantly better than anticoagulation alone, the remaining 55% of patients had a large burden of residual thrombus following intravenous lytic therapy (Table 19.2).[25–39] In addition, during follow-up, those who successfully lysed had a significant reduction in post-thrombotic morbidity and preservation of venous valve function (Table 19.3).[34,35] Unfortunately early trials of streptokinase were complicated by a fourfold increased risk of major bleeding in lytic patients compared to those treated with anticoagulation alone.[40] This unquestionably dampened enthusiasm for systemic thrombolytic therapy.

## Venous thrombectomy

The Scandinavian investigators showed definitive benefit of mechanical thrombus removal by performing a randomised trial of iliofemoral venous

**Table 19.2** • Phlebographic results of anticoagulation versus lytic therapy for acute DVT (13 studies)[25–39]

| | Lysis | | |
|---|---|---|---|
| **Rx (no.)** | **None/worse** | **Partial** | **Significant/ complete** |
| Heparin (254) | 82% | 14% | 4% |
| Lytic therapy (337) | 37% | 18% | 45% |

Reproduced from Comerota AJ, Gravett MH. Iliofemoral venous thrombosis. J Vasc Surg 2007; 46(5):1065–76. With permission from Elsevier.

**Table 19.3** • Long-term, symptomatic results of heparin versus lytic therapy for DVT (two studies)[34,35]

| Rx | Points | Post-thrombotic symptoms Severe (%) | Moderate (%) | None (%) |
|---|---|---|---|---|
| Heparin | 39 | 8 (21) | 23 (59) | 8 (21) |
| Streptokinase | 39 | 2 (5) | 12 (31) | 25 (64) |

Reproduced from Comerota AJ, Gravett MH. Iliofemoral venous thrombosis. J Vasc Surg 2007; 46(5):1065–76. With permission from Elsevier.

thrombectomy versus anticoagulation alone.[41–43] Six-month, 5-year and 10-year follow-up consistently demonstrated that early thrombus removal was associated with better long-term venous function, improved patency of the deep venous system and fewer post-thrombotic symptoms.

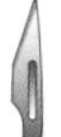

This multicentre randomised trial showed significant benefit of operative venous thrombectomy plus anticoagulation compared to anticoagulation alone in patients with iliofemoral DVT.

## Catheter-directed thrombolysis

The basic mechanism by which plasminogen activators dissolve clot is by activation of fibrin-bound plasminogen,[44] which produces the active enzyme plasmin. Intrathrombus delivery of plasminogen activators protects them from neutralisation by circulating plasminogen activator inhibitors (PAI-1 and PAI-2) and also protects the active enzyme plasmin from the otherwise instantaneous neutralisation by circulating $\alpha_2$-antiplasmins and $\alpha_2$-macroglobulin. Catheter-directed delivery of lytic agents into the thrombus accelerates thrombolysis, increasing the likelihood of a successful outcome. Accelerated clot lysis reduces the overall dose and duration of plasminogen activator infusion; therefore, one would reasonably expect that complications would also be reduced.

Although numerous reports of thrombolytic therapy have been published, three large series independently observed an approximately 80% success rate (Table 19.4).[45–47] Importantly, underlying iliac vein stenoses were treated with balloon angioplasty, stenting or both in order to provide unobstructed venous drainage into the vena cava, thereby reducing the risk of recurrent thrombosis.

Major bleeding complications occurred in 5–11% of patients, with the majority occurring at the puncture site. Fortunately, intracranial bleeding was rare, occurring in only two patients in the National Venous Registry.[46] Symptomatic pulmonary embolism occurred in 1% of patients in the series reported by Bjarnason et al.[45] and the National Venous Registry; however, fatal pulmonary embolism occurred in only one of the 422 patients. Therefore, death as a result of catheter-directed thrombolysis was rare.

In the National Venous Registry, in patients with acute, first-time iliofemoral DVT who had initially successful thrombolysis, 96% of the veins remained patent at 1 year. This is consistent with our observations. Sustained patency and early success directly correlated with valve function at 6 months. Only 38% of patients with minimal (<50%) lysis had normal venous valve function, whereas 72% of patients having complete lysis had normal valves ($P < 0.02$). A follow-up quality-of-life (QOL) study[44] documented that patients with iliofemoral DVT in the National Venous Registry had significantly better QOL than similar patients treated with anticoagulation alone.

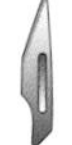

Patients receiving successful lysis for iliofemoral DVT had significantly better QOL at 16 and 22 months compared to those treated with anticoagulation alone or those who failed lysis.

A randomised trial[48] compared catheter-directed thrombolysis using streptokinase with anticoagulation alone. Results at 6 months demonstrated significantly better outcome in patients receiving catheter-directed thrombolysis. Assuming that anticoagulation is properly managed, the benefit achieved with thrombolysis at 6 months is likely to persist long term.

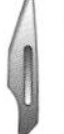

This small randomised trial demonstrated that successful lysis was associated with patency and preserved vein valve function at 6 months compared to anticoagulation alone. Observations made at 6 months appear to be indicative of long-term post-thrombotic sequelae.

## Pharmacomechanical thrombolysis

Mechanical techniques have been shown to fragment and accelerate lysis of intravascular thrombus. However, there appears to be a higher incidence of embolic complications if mechanical thrombectomy is used alone. An experimental model comparing mechanical, pharmacomechanical and

Table 19.4 • Efficacy and complications of catheter-directed thrombolysis in three series[45–47]

| | Bjarnason et al.[45] (*n* = 77) | Mewissen et al.[46] (*n* = 287) | Comerota et al.[47] (*n* = 58) |
|---|---|---|---|
| **Efficacy** | | | |
| Initial success | 79% | 83% | 84% |
| Iliac | 63% | 64% | 78% |
| Femoral | 40% | 47% | – |
| **Primary patency at 1 year** | | | |
| Iliac | 63% | 64% | 78% |
| Femoral | 40% | 47% | – |
| **Iliac stent: patency at 1 year** | | | |
| + stent | 54% | 74% | 89% |
| – stent | 75% | 53% | 71% |
| **Complications** | | | |
| Major bleed | 5% | 11% | 9% |
| Intracranial bleeding | 0% | <1% | 0% |
| Pulmonary embolism | 1% | 1% | 0% |
| Fatal pulmonary embolism | 0% | 0.2% | 0% |
| Death secondary to lysis | 0% | 0.4% | 0% (?2%)* |

*Death due to multiorgan system failure 30 days post-lysis, thought not related to lytic therapy.



pharmacological thrombolysis showed that pulse-spray mechanical thrombectomy was associated with the largest number and greatest size of distal emboli.[49] Embolic particles diminished in number and size and the speed of lysis increased when a plasminogen activator (urokinase) was added to the pulse-spray solution. Catheter-directed thrombolysis alone was associated with the slowest rate of reperfusion but also the fewest number of distal emboli. Our clinical experience indicates that pharmacomechanical thrombectomy alone most often is inadequate and thrombolysis is a necessary addition.

A number of percutaneous mechanical thrombectomy devices have been used either alone or in combination with thrombolytic agents for acute iliofemoral DVT. Assessment of the efficacy and safety of each device is somewhat difficult; however, we will review the most common devices and attempt to put available data into proper perspective.

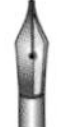

Observations show that combining mechanical techniques with pharmacological (intrathrombus) thrombolysis significantly accelerates a clearing of clot. The challenge is to quantify the benefits of pharmacomechanical techniques versus catheter-directed thrombolysis alone.

### Rotational thrombectomy devices

The Amplatz device utilises a rotational impeller design rotating at 100 000–150 000 rpm to macerate and recirculate the fragmented thrombus. Thrombus removal has been reported at 75–83% in lower-extremity acute DVT and a 6-month patency rate of 77%.[50] Transient procedural desaturation has been reported, although there is no record yet of a clinically significant pulmonary embolism.

The Arrow–Trerotola device also uses rotational design and consists of four helically arranged nitinol wires driven by a hand-held, battery-powered motor that rotates the catheter head at 3000 rpm. As with the Amplatz device, the thrombus is macerated and recirculated. Clinical use has incorporated thrombolytic therapy as well as necessary angioplasty and stenting. Technical and clinical successes have been reported in 100% of patients with a 16-month clinical success rate of 92%.[51,52]

### Rheolytic thrombectomy

The AngioJet device has a different design, using a high-velocity saline jet (350–450 km/h) to produce a zone of negative pressure (−760 mmHg) around the tip of the catheter. The theoretical advantages of this design include less vessel wall trauma and the capability of aspirating thrombus particles through the exhaust port. Kasirajan et al.[53] reported a small number of patients treated without adjunctive preprocedural thrombolytic therapy. Half of the patients treated had ≥50% of their thrombus removed. Patency was restored in 77% of those patients with ≥50% thrombus removal. Improved results are observed with the addition of thrombolytic therapy.

Lin et al.[54] reported their 8-year review of catheter-directed thrombolysis and of pharmacomechanical thrombolysis using the AngioJet device. They treated 93 patients who underwent 98 catheter-directed interventions for DVT. Their patient demographics and treatment outcomes are summarised in Table 19.5.[54] Significant reductions in the intensive care unit (ICU) and hospital length-of-stay (LOS) were observed in the AngioJet group (0.6 and 4.6 days) when compared with catheter-directed thrombolysis (2.4 and 8.4 days). There was no difference in primary patency rates at 1 year between the two groups. A hospital cost analysis showed significant reduction in the AngioJet-treated group compared with the catheter-directed thrombolysis group ($P < 0.01$). Unfortunately, no follow-up data regarding patients' QOL or vein function were reported.

### Isolated segmental pharmacomechanical thrombolysis

The Trellis® catheter (Bacchus Vascular, Santa Clara, CA) isolates a segment of the thrombosed venous system between two balloons (**Fig. 19.3**). This isolated segment is then infused with the plasminogen activator. The intervening catheter assumes a spiral configuration and rotates at 1500 rpm. After 15–20 minutes of maceration of the thrombus and mixing the plasminogen activator, the particulate and liquefied thrombus and residual plasminogen activator fluid are aspirated.

Martinez et al.[55] have reported their initial experience with isolated segmental pharmacomechanical thrombolysis ($n = 22$) compared with standard catheter-directed thrombolysis ($n = 21$). They attempted to quantitate the benefit of this new technique. They reported that treatment times were significantly shortened and the dose of lytic agent significantly reduced (Table 19.6).[55]

### Ultrasound-accelerated thrombolysis

A new and interesting adjunct to catheter-directed thrombolysis is the incorporation of ultrasound transducers into the infusion catheter. Ultrasound waves generated during plasminogen activator infusion increase the surface area of fibrin and speed lysis.

Parikh et al.[56] have reported 47 patients with 53 extremities treated with ultrasound-accelerated thrombolysis from eight centres in the USA. Both lower extremity (32/53) and upper extremity (19/53) were included as well as two hepatic vein thromboses. Patients were treated with urokinase, recombinant tissue plasminogen activator (rt-PA), recombinant plasminogen activator or tenecteplase. Complete clot lysis, defined as 90% or more resolution, was observed in 37/53 (70%) and overall lysis, which included complete plus partial lysis, was observed in 91% (48/53). Failure of lysis was observed in 9%, most of which were considered chronic occlusions. The median thrombolysis time was 22 hours. Major complications occurred in two patients (4%) with no reports of intracranial or retroperitoneal bleeding.

**Table 19.5** • Patient demographic and treatment outcome in the pharmacomechanical thrombolysis (PMT) and catheter-directed thrombolysis (CDT) treatment groups

| Variable | PMT therapy (rheolytic) | CDT therapy | *P* value |
|---|---|---|---|
| No. of patients | 49 | 44 | n/a |
| No. of treated limbs | 52 | 46 | n/a |
| Mean age (years) | 45 ± 12 | 49 ± 10 | NS |
| Male (%) | 22 (45%) | 19 (43%) | NS |
| Complete treatment success | 39 (75%) | 32 (70%) | NS |
| Partial treatment success | 13 (25%) | 14 (30%) | NS |
| Immediate clinical improvement | 42 (81%) | 33 (72%) | NS |
| No clinical improvement | 4 (8%) | 5 (11%) | NS |
| Adjuvant balloon angioplasty/iliac venous stenting | 43 (82%) | 36 (78%) | NS |
| No. of venograms (mean) | 0.4 ± 0.2 | 2.5 ± 0.7 | <0.001 |
| Mean ICU stay (days) | 0.6 ± 0.3 | 2.4 ± 1.2 | <0.04 |
| Overall LOS (days) | 4.6 ± 1.3 | 8.4 ± 2.3 | <0.02 |
| Haemorrhagic complication | 2 (4%) | 3 (6%) | NS |
| PRBC transfusion (U) | 0.2 ± 0.3 | 1.2 ± 0.7 | <0.05 |
| Total hospital cost ($) | 47742 ± 19247 | 85301 ±± 24823 | <0.05 |

PRBC, Packed red blood cells.

Reproduced from Lin PH, Zhou W, Dardik A et al. Catheter-direct thrombolysis versus pharmacomechanical thrombectomy for treatment of symptomatic lower extremity deep venous thrombosis. Am J Surg 2006; 192(6):782–8. With permission from Elsevier.

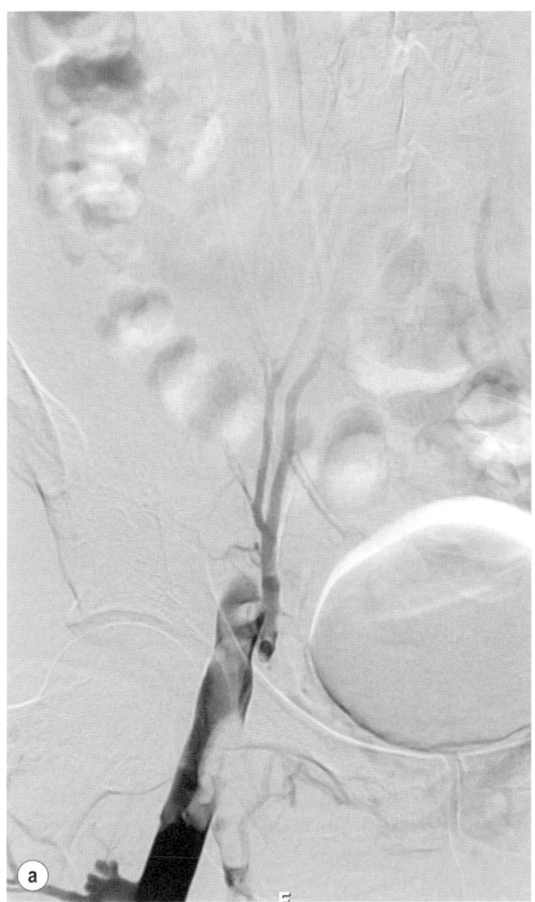


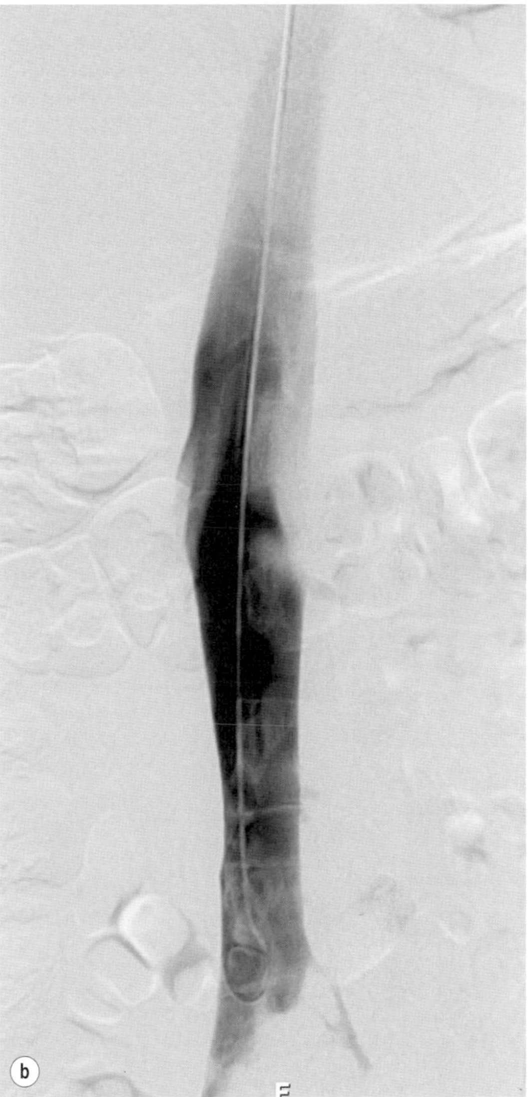


**Figure 19.3** • A 26-year-old woman was referred with a 2-day history of a swollen, painful left lower extremity. She had delivered her healthy second child 10 days earlier. Her past medical history was otherwise unremarkable. A venous duplex demonstrated thrombus in the distal external iliac vein. Iliofemoral venous thrombosis was confirmed with dye injection from the popliteal vein, which was entered with ultrasound guidance with the patient in the prone position **(a)**. The vena cava was patent and free of thrombus **(b)**. A Trellis® catheter was advanced through the thrombus and the proximal balloon placed above and the distal balloon below the thrombus. Isolated, segmental, pharmacomechanical thrombolysis (ISPMT) was performed using 3 mg of rt-PA **(c)**. After a 20-minute run, the thrombus was successfully lysed, revealing a tight stenosis of the left common iliac vein consistent with a May–Thurner type stenosis. A balloon venoplasty and stent was performed. The initial balloon inflation **(d)** shows the waist of the balloon at the site of stenosis. Successful balloon angioplasty and stenting **(e)** document thrombus resolution and correction of the iliac vein stenosis with unobstructed venous drainage into the vena cava. The treatment time of this patient was 20 minutes and she received a total dose of 3 mg of rt-PA. This represents the best-case scenario.

*(continued)*

## Treatment strategy for acute iliofemoral DVT

Our treatment strategy for patients with acute iliofemoral DVT is summarised in **Fig. 19.4.** Patients with acute iliofemoral DVT are often defined by painful leg swelling that involves the thigh and bluish discoloration otherwise known as phlegmasia coerulea dolens. Occlusive thrombus in the common femoral vein is frequently observed on venous duplex, and when these patients are evaluated as outpatients, hospitalisation is recommended.

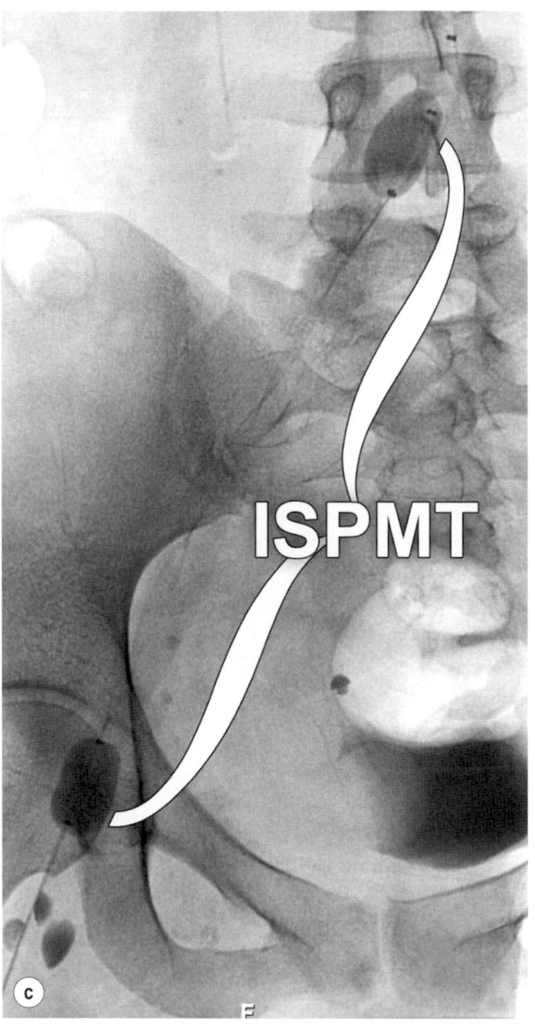


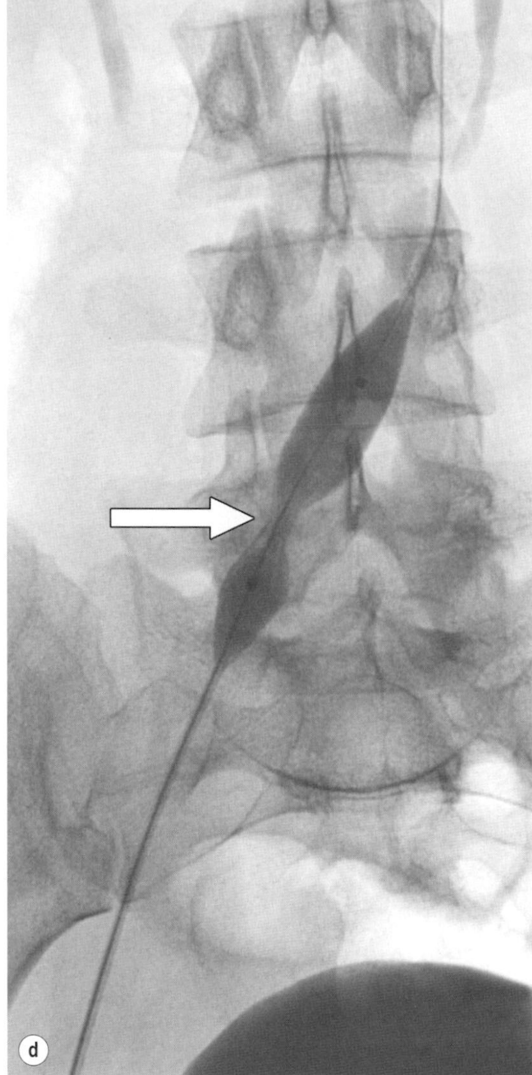


**Figure 19.3** • (*cont.*)

Patients are immediately anticoagulated, snug compression applied to the leg, and the leg elevated whenever they are not ambulating.

A rapid computed tomography scan with contrast of the chest, abdomen and pelvis is obtained to evaluate for asymptomatic pulmonary emboli (which is found in at least 50%) and examination for other underlying pathologies that might be associated with extensive venous thrombosis.

If the patient is physically active and has a reasonable survival (2 years or more), the patient is offered a strategy of thrombus removal. If the patient has a high risk of bleeding from thrombolysis, a contemporary venous thrombectomy or segmental, pharmacomechanical thrombolysis is recommended. If there is no contraindication to thrombolysis, pharmacomechanical thrombolysis with additional catheter-directed thrombolysis as needed is recommended. Following successful lysis, any underlying venous lesions are corrected and the patient is then therapeutically anticoagulated and placed in 30–40 mmHg ankle-gradient compression stockings.

If the patient is not physically active or if anticipated survival is less than 2 years, anticoagulation with good compression is the recommended therapy. This treatment algorithm is consistent with the most recent recommendations of the ACCP

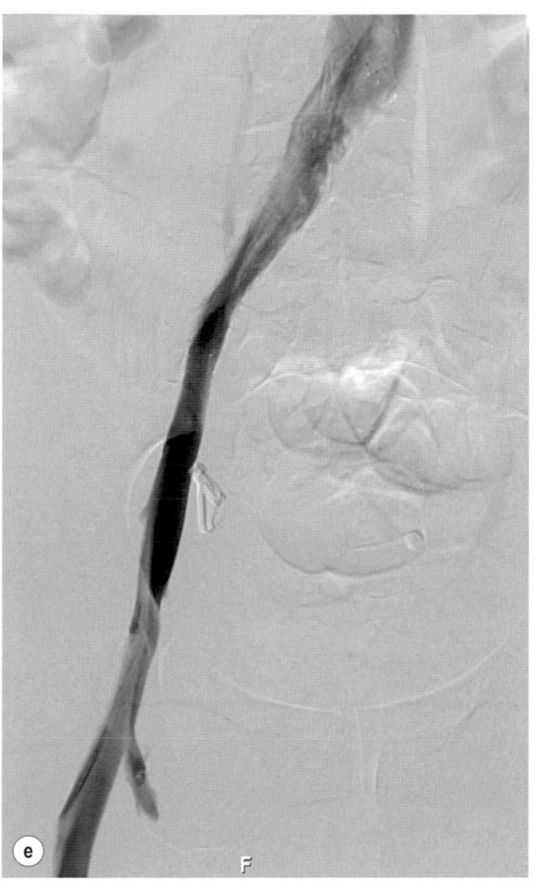


**Figure 19.3** • (*cont.*)

Table 19.6 • Quantitative benefit of isolated, segmental, pharmacomechanical thrombolysis for iliofemoral DVT[55]

| Outcome | CDT | ISPMT | *P* value |
|---|---|---|---|
| Complete lysis* (≥90) | 3/27 (11%) | 7/25 (28%) | 0.077 |
| Overall lytic success* | 60% | 80% | 0.0016 |
| Treatment time** | 55 hrs | 23 hrs | ≤0.0001 |
| rt-PA dose** | 55 mg | 33 mg | 0.007 |
| ICU LOS** | 2.89 ± 0.97 | 2.9 ± 1.24 | 0.92 |
| Hosp. LOS** | 7.8 ± 1.84 | 8.2 ± 4.7 | 0.69 |

CDT, catheter-directed thrombolysis; ISPMT, isolated, segmental, pharmacomechanical thrombolysis.
*per limb. ** per patient.

and should significantly improve long-term patient outcome.

Two large randomised trials are under way, one in Norway and one in the USA, which should definitively evaluate the quantitative risks and benefits of catheter-directed techniques versus anticoagulation for the management of extensive lower-extremity venous thrombosis.

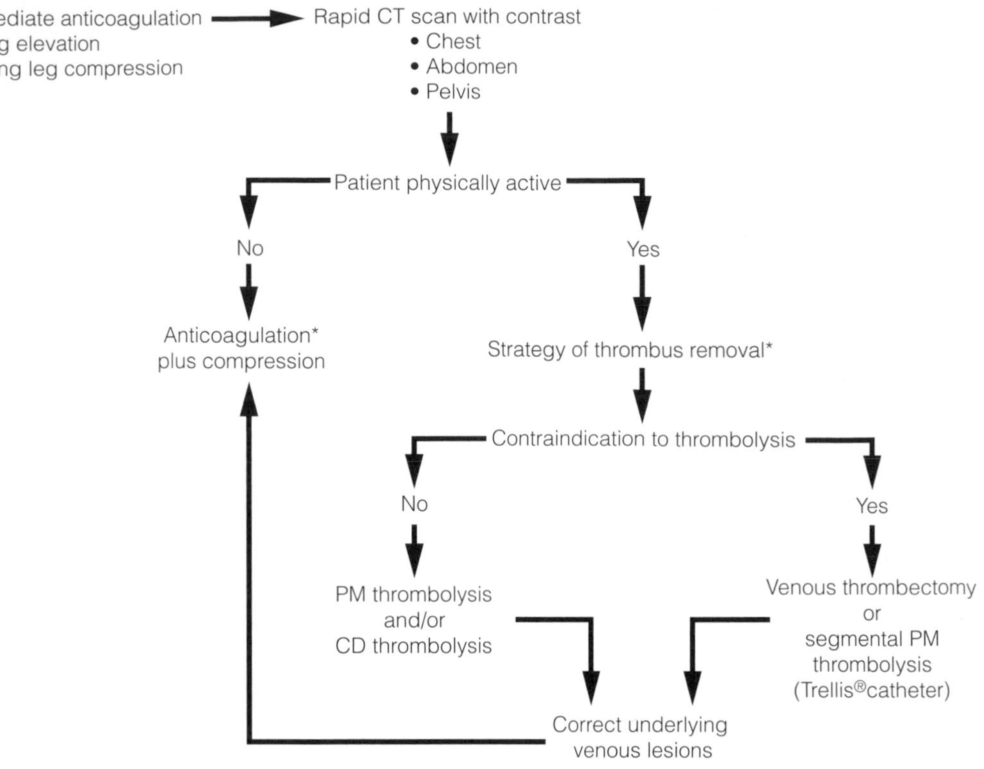


**Figure 19.4** • Algorithm illustrating the general treatment strategy for patients with iliofemoral DVT. Reproduced from Comerota AJ, Paolini D. Treatment of acute illiofemoral deep venous thrombosis: a strategy of thrombus removal. Eur J Vasc Endovasc Surg 2007; 33(3):10. With permission from Elsevier.

## Key points

- Acute leg oedema may indicate a chronic underlying disease or an acute life-threatening problem. The patient's clinical presentation and a careful history and physical examination usually point to the likely aetiology.
- Deep venous thrombosis is the most worrisome of aetiologies for acute limb oedema as it is potentially lethal and often associated with severe post-thrombotic morbidity.
- Patients with acute iliofemoral DVT are a clinically relevant subset of DVT patients as they suffer the most severe post-thrombotic morbidity and their risk of recurrent DVT is 2.4-fold that of patients with femoropopliteal DVT.
- Early thrombus removal after the onset of DVT results in improved outcomes.

## References

1. Casley-Smith JR, Morgan RG, Piller NB. Treatment of lymphoedema of the arms and legs with 5,6-benzo-α-pyrone. N Engl J Med 1993; 329(16):1158–63.
2. Bhan C, Corfield L. A case of unilateral lower limb swelling secondary to a ganglion cyst. Eur J Vasc Endovasc Surg 2007; 33(3):371–2.
3. Eichinger S, Minar E, Bialonczyk C et al. D-dimer levels and risk of recurrent venous thromboembolism. JAMA 2003; 290(8):1071–4.
4. Wells PS, Anderson DR, Rodger M et al. Evaluation of D-dimer in the diagnosis of suspected deep-vein thrombosis. N Engl J Med 2003; 349(13):1227–35.

5. Delis KT, Bountouroglou D, Mansfield AO. Venous claudication in iliofemoral thrombosis: long-term effects on venous hemodynamics, clinical status, and quality of life. Ann Surg 2004; 239(1):118–26.
6. Akesson H, Brudin L, Dahlstrom JA et al. Venous function assessed during a 5 year period after acute ilio-femoral venous thrombosis treated with anticoagulation. Eur J Vasc Surg 1990; 4(1):43–8.
7. Hull RD, Raskob GE, Hirsh J et al. Continuous intravenous heparin compared with intermittent subcutaneous heparin in the initial treatment of proximal-vein thrombosis. N Engl J Med 1986; 315(18):1109–14.
8. Lensing AW, Prins MH, Davidson BL et al. Treatment of deep venous thrombosis with low-molecular-weight heparins. A meta-analysis. Arch Intern Med 1995; 155(6):601–7.
9. Kearon C, Kahn SR, Agnelli G et al. Antithrombotic therapy for venous thromboembolic disease: American College of Chest Physicians evidence-based clinical practice guidelines (8th edition). Chest 2008; 133(6, Suppl):454S–545S.
10. Partsch H. Immediate ambulation and leg compression in the treatment of deep vein thrombosis. Dis Mon 2005; 51(2–3):135–40.
11. Brandjes DP, Buller HR, Heijboer H et al. Randomised trial of effect of compression stockings in patients with symptomatic proximal-vein thrombosis. Lancet 1997; 349(9054):759–62.
12. Prandoni P, Lensing AW, Prins MH et al. Below-knee elastic compression stockings to prevent the post-thrombotic syndrome: a randomized, controlled trial. Ann Intern Med 2004; 141(4):249–56.
13. Kearon C, Kahn SR, Agnelli G et-al. Antithrombotic therapy for venous thromboembolic disease: ACCP evidence-based clinical practice guidelines (8th edn). Chest 2008; 133:454S–545S.

    **These guidelines give a level IIb recommendation for adopting a strategy of thrombus removal in addition to anticoagulation in patients with iliofemoral DVT. These recommendations are based upon an exhaustive review of the literature and two randomised trials.**
14. Douketis JD, Crowther MA, Foster GA et al. Does the location of thrombosis determine the risk of disease recurrence in patients with proximal deep vein thrombosis? Am J Med 2001; 110(7):515–19.
15. Shull KC, Nicolaides AN, Fernandes e Fernandes J et al. Significance of popliteal reflux in relation to ambulatory venous pressure and ulceration. Arch Surg 1979; 114(11):1304–6.
16. Johnson BF, Manzo RA, Bergelin RO et al. Relationship between changes in the deep venous system and the development of the postthrombotic syndrome after an acute episode of lower limb deep vein thrombosis: a one- to six-year follow-up. J Vasc Surg 1995; 21(2):307–12.
17. Cho JS, Martelli E, Mozes G et al. Effects of thrombolysis and venous thrombectomy on valvular competence, thrombogenicity, venous wall morphology, and function. J Vasc Surg 1998; 28(5):787–99.
18. Rhodes JM, Cho JS, Gloviczki P et al. Thrombolysis for experimental deep venous thrombosis maintains valvular competence and vasoreactivity. J Vasc Surg 2000; 31(6):1193–205.
19. Killewich LA, Bedford GR, Beach KW et al. Spontaneous lysis of deep venous thrombi: rate and outcome. J Vasc Surg 1989; 9(1):89–97.
20. Markel A, Manzo RA, Bergelin RO et al. Valvular reflux after deep vein thrombosis: incidence and time of occurrence. J Vasc Surg 1992; 15(2):377–82.
21. Meissner MH, Manzo RA, Bergelin RO et al. Deep venous insufficiency: the relationship between lysis and subsequent reflux. J Vasc Surg 1993; 18(4):596–605.
22. Piovella F, Crippa L, Barone M et al. Normalization rates of compression ultrasonography in patients with a first episode of deep vein thrombosis of the lower limbs: association with recurrence and new thrombosis. Haematologica 2002; 87(5):515–22.
23. Prandoni P. Risk factors of recurrent venous thromboembolism: the role of residual vein thrombosis. Pathophysiol Haemost Thromb 2003; 33(5–6):351–3.
24. Comerota AJ, Gravett MH. Iliofemoral venous thrombosis. J Vasc Surg 2007; 46(5):1065–76.

    **This review article summarises the randomised trials of systemic thrombolytic therapy versus anticoagulation for acute DVT, in addition to other strategies of thrombus removal.**
25. Browse NL, Thomas ML, Pim HP. Streptokinase and deep vein thrombosis. Br Med J 1968; 3(5620):717–20.
26. Robertson BR, Nilsson IM, Nylander G. Value of streptokinase and heparin in treatment of acute deep venous thrombosis. A coded investigation. Acta Chir Scand 1968; 134(3):203–8.
27. Kakkar VV, Flanc C, Howe CT et al. Treatment of deep vein thrombosis. A trial of heparin, streptokinase, and arvin. Br Med J 1969; 1(5647):806–10.
28. Tsapogas MJ, Peabody RA, Wu KT et al. Controlled study of thrombolytic therapy in deep vein thrombosis. Surgery 1973; 74(6):973–84.
29. Duckert F, Muller G, Nyman D et al. Treatment of deep vein thrombosis with streptokinase. Br Med J 1975; 1(5956):479–81.
30. Porter JM, Seaman AJ, Common HH et al. Comparison of heparin and streptokinase in the treatment of venous thrombosis. Am Surg 1975; 41(9):511–19.
31. Seaman AJ, Common HH, Rosch J et al. Deep vein thrombosis treated with streptokinase or heparin. A randomized study. Angiology 1976; 27(10):549–56.
32. Rosch J, Dotter CT, Seaman AJ et al. Healing of deep venous thrombosis: venographic findings in a randomized study comparing streptokinase and heparin. Am J Roentgenol 1976; 127(4):553–8.
33. Marder VJ, Soulen RL, Atichartakarn V et al. Quantitative venographic assessment of deep vein thrombosis in the evaluation of streptokinase and heparin therapy. J Lab Clin Med 1977; 89(5):1018–29.

34. Arnesen H, Heilo A, Jakobsen E et al. A prospective study of streptokinase and heparin in the treatment of deep vein thrombosis. Acta Med Scand 1978; 203(6):457–63.
35. Elliot MS, Immelman EJ, Jeffery P et al. A comparative randomized trial of heparin versus streptokinase in the treatment of acute proximal venous thrombosis: an interim report of a prospective trial. Br J Surg 1979; 66(12):838–43.
36. Watz R, Savidge GF. Rapid thrombolysis and preservation of valvular venous function in high deep vein thrombosis. A comparative study between streptokinase and heparin therapy. Acta Med Scand 1979; 205(4):293–8.
37. Jeffery P, Immelman EJ, Amoore J. Treatment of deep vein thrombosis with heparin or streptokinase: long-term venous function assessment (Abstract No. S20.3). Proc 2nd Int Vasc Symp, 1989.
38. Turpie AG, Levine MN, Hirsh J et al. Tissue plasminogen activator (rt-PA) vs heparin in deep vein thrombosis. Results of a randomized trial. Chest 1990; 97(4, Suppl):172S–5S.
39. Goldhaber SZ, Meyerovitz MF, Green D et al. Randomized controlled trial of tissue plasminogen activator in proximal deep venous thrombosis. Am J Med 1990; 88(3):235–40.
40. Goldhaber SZ, Buring JE, Lipnick RJ et al. Pooled analyses of randomized trials of streptokinase and heparin in phlebographically documented acute deep venous thrombosis. Am J Med 1984; 76(3):393–7.
41. Plate G, Einarsson E, Ohlin P et al. Thrombectomy with temporary arteriovenous fistula: the treatment of choice in acute iliofemoral venous thrombosis. J Vasc Surg 1984; 1(6):867–76.
42. Plate G, Akesson H, Einarsson E et al. Long-term results of venous thrombectomy combined with a temporary arterio-venous fistula. Eur J Vasc Surg 1990; 4(5):483–9.
43. Plate G, Eklof B, Norgren L et-al. Venous thrombectomy for iliofemoral vein thrombosis – 10-year results of a prospective randomised study. Eur J Vasc Endovasc Surg 1997; 14(5):367–74.

Plate et al. reported 6-month, 5-year and 10-year follow-up of their randomised study of iliofemoral DVT treated with venous thrombectomy, arteriovenous fistula and anticoagulation versus anticoagulation alone. These outcomes resulted in the eighth ACCP consensus conference giving a level IIB recommendation for operative venous thrombectomy in patients with iliofemoral DVT who are good surgical candidates.

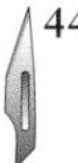

44. Comerota AJ, Throm RC, Mathias SD et al. Catheter-directed thrombolysis for iliofemoral deep venous thrombosis improves health-related quality of life. J Vasc Surg 2000; 32(1):130–7.

Although not a randomised trial, this case-controlled study demonstrated that successful catheter-directed thrombolysis offered significantly better long-term QOL than anticoagulation alone or failed thrombolysis for patients with iliofemoral DVT.

45. Bjarnason H, Kruse JR, Asinger DA et al. Iliofemoral deep venous thrombosis: safety and efficacy outcome during 5 years of catheter-directed thrombolytic therapy. J Vasc Interv Radiol 1997; 8(3):405–18.
46. Mewissen MW, Seabrook GR, Meissner MH et al. Catheter-directed thrombolysis for lower extremity deep venous thrombosis: report of a national multicenter registry. Radiology 1999; 211(1):39–49.
47. Comerota AJ, Kagan SA. Catheter-directed thrombolysis for the treatment of acute iliofemoral deep venous thrombosis. Phlebology 2000; 15:149–55.
48. Elsharawy M, Elzayat E. Early results of thrombolysis vs anticoagulation in iliofemoral venous thrombosis. A randomised clinical trial. Eur J Vasc Endovasc Surg 2002; 24(3):209–14.

This is the first randomised trial of catheter-directed thrombolysis versus anticoagulation for iliofemoral DVT. Although it was a small study, the benefits it demonstrated in patients treated with thrombolytic therapy were used to support the eighth ACCP consensus conference recommendation for catheter-directed thrombolysis for iliofemoral DVT.

49. Greenberg RK, Ouriel K, Srivastava S et al. Mechanical versus chemical thrombolysis: an in vitro differentiation of thrombolytic mechanisms. J Vasc Interv Radiol 2000; 11(2, Pt 1):199–205.
50. Gandini R, Maspes F, Sodani G et al. Percutaneous ilio-caval thrombectomy with the Amplatz device: preliminary results. Eur Radiol 1999; 9(5):951–8.
51. Lee KH, Han H, Lee KJ et al. Mechanical thrombectomy of acute iliofemoral deep vein thrombosis with use of an Arrow–Trerotola percutaneous thrombectomy device. J Vasc Interv Radiol 2006; 17(3):487–95.
52. Wildberger JE, Haage P, Bovelander J et al. Percutaneous venous thrombectomy using the Arrow–Trerotola percutaneous thrombolytic device (PTD) with temporary caval filtration: in vitro investigations. Cardiovasc Intervent Radiol 2005; 28(2):221–7.
53. Kasirajan K, Gray B, Ouriel K. Percutaneous AngioJet thrombectomy in the management of extensive deep venous thrombosis. J Vasc Interv Radiol 2001; 12(2):179–85.
54. Lin PH, Zhou W, Dardik A et al. Catheter-direct thrombolysis versus pharmacomechanical thrombectomy for treatment of symptomatic lower extremity deep venous thrombosis. Am J Surg 2006; 192(6):782–8.
55. Martinez J, Comerota AJ, Kazanjian S et al. The quantitative benefit of isolated, segmental, pharmacomechanical thrombolysis for iliofemoral DVT. J Vasc Surg 2008; 48(6):1532–7.
56. Parikh S, Motarjeme A, McNamara T et al. Ultrasound accelerated thrombolysis for the treatment of deep venous thrombosis: initial clinical experience. J Vasc Interv Radiol 2008; in press.

# 20

# Vascular anomalies

Brian Dillon
Ajmad Alomari
Patricia Burrows

## Introduction

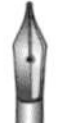

The most commonly used classification of vascular anomalies was proposed by Mulliken and Glowacki. In this classification based upon clinical, histological, histochemical and biochemical differences and supported by angiography and cross-sectional imaging, vascular anomalies are divided into two major categories: tumours (haemangiomas) and vascular malformations[1] (Box 20.1).

Infantile haemangiomas are proliferative endothelial cell tumours that present in infancy, undergo rapid growth in the first year of life and then involute. Other types of endothelial cell neoplasms include rapidly involuting and non-involuting congenital haemangiomas, haemangioendotheliomas and angiosarcoma. Vascular malformations, in contrast, are believed to result from disordered vascular morphogenesis. Vascular malformations are usually present at birth or noted shortly after birth and grow with the patient. Vascular malformations may be classified by flow characteristics as slow-flow and fast-flow lesions. Further subdivision by the type of channel abnormality is possible with slow-flow lesions consisting of venous malformations (VMs), lymphatic malformations (LMs) and capillary malformations (CMs), and fast-flow lesions consisting of arteriovenous malformations (AVMs) and arteriovenous fistulas (AVFs). Combined vascular malformations also occur.

Awareness of the clinical and imaging features that distinguish vascular anomalies is vital to arriving at the correct diagnosis, counselling regarding prognosis and planning the appropriate therapy.

## Clinical and imaging features of vascular anomalies

### Haemangiomas

Infantile haemangiomas (IHs) are the most common tumour of infancy. If present at birth, they are most often seen as a faint macular or telangiectatic stain. Typically, they appear within the first 3 months of life, undergo rapid growth related to endothelial cell proliferation, and then begin to involute at 9–10 months of age. They can involve any soft tissue, including the brain, but are most common in the head and neck and disproportionately affect female and premature infants.

IHs can be superficial, deep or combined. Cutaneous haemangiomas may have a characteristic ‘strawberry-like’ appearance (**Fig. 20.1**). The skin over deeper haemangiomas may have a bluish hue secondary to draining veins or appear completely normal. Haemangiomas are usually warm, can be pulsatile, and soften during involution due to endothelial cell dropout and fibrofatty replacement. The lesions may be single (focal) or multiple (multifocal).

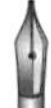

The association of facial haemangiomas with posterior fossa anomalies, arterial anomalies, cardiovascular defects and eye abnormalities has been termed PHACE association.[2]

Box 20.1 • Vascular anomalies

**Tumours**

Infantile haemangiomas
Congenital haemangiomas
RICH
NICH
Other vascular tumours
KHE
Epithelioid haemangioendothelioma
Angiosarcoma
Tufted angioma

**Malformations**

Slow flow
Venous
Lymphatic
Capillary
Combined
Fast flow
Arteriovenous malformations
Arteriovenous fistulas

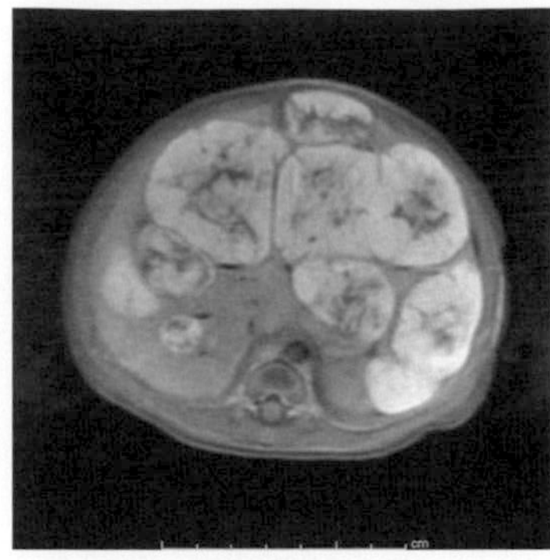

**Figure 20.2** • Axial T1-weighted postcontrast MRI image with fat suppression demonstrating multiple homogeneously enhancing liver masses consistent with haemangiomas. Multifocal liver lesions presenting in infancy tend to express GLUT1 and behave identical to cutaneous infantile haemangiomas.

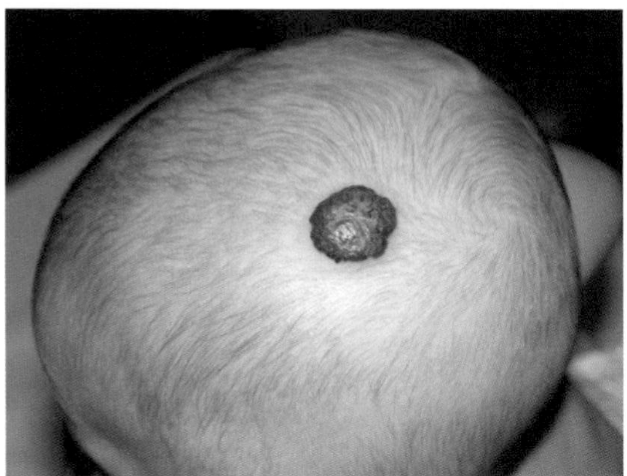

**Figure 20.1** • Typical 'strawberry-like' appearance of a cutaneous haemangioma.

Unlike the common IHs, congenital haemangiomas are present at birth and either undergo rapid involution in the first year of life (rapidly involuting congenital haemangioma, RICH) or persist (non-involuting congenital haemangioma, NICH). An erythrocyte-type glucose transporter protein, GLUT1, is expressed in endothelial cells of IH but is absent in congenital haemangiomas, other vascular tumours and vascular malformations. In vascular liver tumours of infancy, multifocal lesions tend to be GLUT1 positive and thus represent IH (**Fig. 20.2**). Solitary liver tumours present at birth tend to be GLUT1 negative and likely represent congenital haemangiomas.[3] Hepatic IHs almost always involute and are completely distinct from the so-called 'hepatic haemangiomas' in adults. While typically asymptomatic, liver IHs can be associated with severe high-output cardiac failure, hypothyroidism and liver dysfunction.

On magnetic resonance imaging (MRI), infantile haemangiomas appear as well-circumscribed, lobulated lesions that demonstrate homogeneous enhancement with the administration of contrast. Characteristically, there are dilated feeding arteries and draining veins within or at the periphery of the lesion as evidenced by flow voids on spin echo sequences or bright tubular structures on gradient recalled echo (GRE) sequences (**Fig. 20.3**). Ultrasonography will demonstrate a solid mass with evenly distributed fast-flow vessels that have low-resistance arterial waveforms and arterialised venous waveforms. Angiography, reserved for the rare haemangioma requiring embolisation, demonstrates dilated feeding arteries and draining veins and a mass with a dense, prolonged capillary blush.

IHs are distinct from kaposiform haemangioendothelioma (KHE). This lesion is characterised by rapid growth and a purple ecchymotic skin discoloration. On imaging studies, the underlying subcutaneous tissue demonstrates a reticular standing and confluent soft-tissue mass (best seen on T2-weighted images with fat saturation; **Fig. 20.4**). It is this lesion (not IH) that is associated with Kasabach–Merritt phenomenon (KMP). KMP is characterised by severe thrombocytopenia secondary to platelet entrapment within the lesion. Thrombocytopenia usually resolves with treatment, though the lesion itself is often highly refractory to therapy.

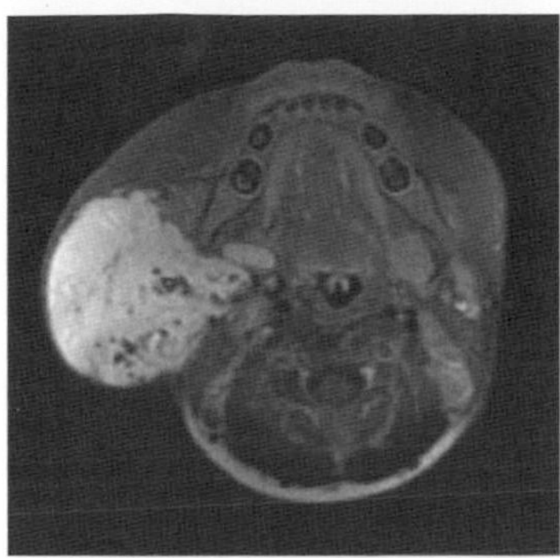

**Figure 20.3** • Axial T1-weighted postcontrast MRI image with fat suppression demonstrating a facial haemangioma. The lesion demonstrates homogeneous enhancement. Flow voids indicate fast-flow vessels.

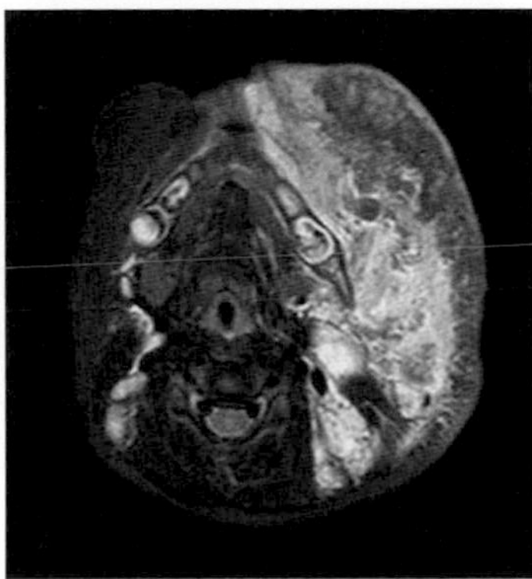

**Figure 20.4** • Axial T2-weighted MRI image with fat suppression demonstrating a kaposiform haemangioendothelioma (KHE) involving the face. The pattern of T2-hyperintense stranding in the surrounding subcutaneous tissues is characteristic of this lesion.

## Vascular malformations

### Venous malformations

Venous malformations consist of sinusoidal spaces lined by abnormal endothelial cells with variable communication with draining veins. Thinning and asymmetrical disruption of the smooth muscle and elastic layers of the channel walls, together with absence or insufficiency of valves within conducting veins, results in stasis of blood within the channels. Pooling of blood within the malformation and intralesional thrombosis result in pain and swelling. Some thrombi spontaneously lyse while others calcify and cause phleboliths, an imaging hallmark of VMs.

Venous malformations are usually soft and compressible, and the involved overlying skin is bluish or dark purplish. Lower-extremity VMs are most symptomatic after long periods of standing or activity.

Multifocal lesions may be seen in familial forms of VM, including mucocutaneous familial venous malformations, glomuvenous malformation, Maffucci syndrome and blue rubber bleb naevus syndrome. Blue rubber bleb naevus syndrome is a rare condition characterised by multiple cutaneous, musculoskeletal and gastrointestinal VMs resulting in gastrointestinal haemorrhage.

Venous malformations are hyperintense on T2-weighted MRI sequences and demonstrate diffuse, usually inhomogeneous enhancement following contrast administration. Phleboliths within the malformation may be apparent as signal voids on spin echo or GRE sequences, and are clearly visualised as lamellated calcifications on computed tomography (CT) and plain films. Compressible channels with venous flow may be visualised on ultrasonography, though the demonstration of flow can often be difficult secondary to the very low velocity of flow within the channels.

### Lymphatic malformations

Lymphatic malformations are generally classified as macrocystic, microcystic or combined. Macrocystic LMs contain large cysts (greater than 1–2 cm) and are located predominantly in sites of fetal lymphatic coalescence (neck, chest wall, axilla, pelvis). Microcystic LMs consist mainly of microscopic lymphatic spaces and present as diffuse soft-tissue swelling or overgrowth.[4] Combined macrocystic/microcystic LMs may have macrocysts, smaller cysts and true microcystic tissue. The overlying skin may have a CM, lymphatic vesicles, or appear normal. LMs swell intermittently related to viral illness and can enlarge acutely secondary to haemorrhage into the cysts or infection. Associated bony overgrowth can occur, particularly in lesions overlying the maxilla or mandible.

Gorham disease, a form of LM in which lymphatic channels diffusely replace normal bone, can result in severe bone weakening, poorly healing fractures, deformity, chylothorax or chylous ascites.

On MRI, macrocysts are evident as distinct cysts whereas microcystic disease usually appears as an infiltrating mass and/or sheets of T2-hyperintense signal, sometimes with a reticulated or stranded appearance (**Fig. 20.5**). Macrocysts may demonstrate enhancement of rims or septa following the administration of contrast but not of the fluid contents. Fluid–fluid levels may be present. Ultrasonography clearly demonstrates macrocysts. Microcystic components appear as an ill-defined soft-tissue thickening on sonography.

### Capillary malformations

Capillary malformations or 'port-wine stains' are present at birth and may be focal or extensive. Facial port-wine stain may have associated thickening of the skin and subcutaneous tissues and overgrowth of the underlying bone resulting in facial asymmetry or dental malocclusion.

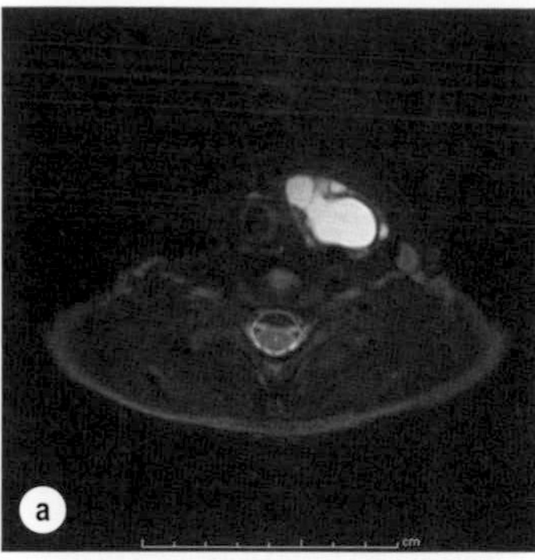

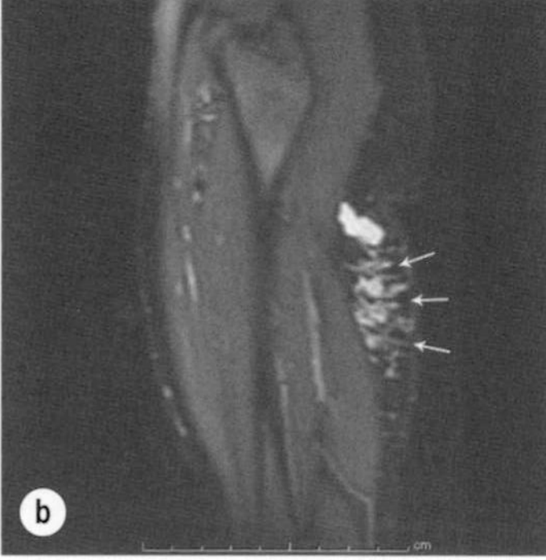

**Figure 20.5** • Inversion recovery images demonstrating a predominantly macrocystic lymphatic malformation of the neck **(a)** and a mixed macrocystic and microcystic lymphatic malformation of the posterior thigh **(b)**. The microcystic component appears as sheets of T2-hyperintense signal (arrows).

Capillary malformations are usually diagnosed clinically. Imaging is usually reserved for excluding a combined vascular malformation such as an AVM or LM or underlying neurological abnormality such as an encephalocele, spinal dysraphism or Sturge–Weber syndrome; 1–2% of patients with a facial port-wine stain will have Sturge–Weber syndrome.

## Arteriovenous malformations/ arteriovenous fistulas

In arteriovenous malformations, a plexiform collection of vessels forms a nidus between feeding arteries and draining veins, bypassing the capillary network. If extremely high flow, AVMs may present in infancy with congestive heart failure. Most often, however, AVMs are clinically inactive in the first one to two decades of life. AVMs are usually warm and have an associated cutaneous blush that intensifies with progression of the lesion. Affected tissues demonstrate accelerated growth. As an AVM evolves, shunting increases, causing swelling and venous engorgement. Shunting often increases during puberty, pregnancy, and following trauma or partial resection. With progressive arterial steal and venous hypertension, tense veins, pain, ulceration, heart failure and severe bleeding may develop.

Arteriovenous fistulas are direct non-nidal arteriovenous communications. They can be acquired, due to penetrating injury. Congenital AVFs may present in infancy with high-output heart failure or be diagnosed later in life with a bruit or pulsatile mass.

CT and MRI will demonstrate dilated feeding arteries and draining veins without a discrete mass. On MRI, signal abnormalities may be present in the region of the nidus representing fibrofatty matrix or oedema. Fatty overgrowth or muscle enlargement may be seen in affected soft tissues, and lytic or sclerotic changes or abnormal marrow signal on MRI may be seen in bone. Angiography demonstrates variable degrees of arterial dilatation and tortuosity, arteriovenous shunting and dilatation of draining veins. In a diffuse or early-stage AVM, a blush with early venous opacification may be seen rather than a discrete nidus.

## Combined malformations and complex syndromes

Klippel–Trenauney syndrome (KTS) or capillary–lymphatic–venous malformation may affect the extremities and/or trunk and consists of cutaneous capillary malformations, lymphatic malformations and venous anomalies with associated overgrowth. Varicosities of superficial veins are typically related to persistence of embryonic venous channels. The deep veins are often hypoplastic or discontinuous and can be dysfunctional. Orthopaedic sequelae include limb-length discrepancy, contracture and muscle atrophy. Dermal lymphatic vesicles may bleed or lead to infection. KTS is treated with a combination of compression stocking, physical therapy, sclerotherapy for lymphatic macrocysts, and surgical debulking. The importance of elastic compression stockings and physical therapy were underscored by Gloviczki's demonstration of severe venous incompetence with complex venous reflux patterns and venous hypertension in the affected limbs of KTS patients.[5] The deep venous system must be evaluated prior to venous surgery.

Maffucci syndrome is a rare anomaly characterised by multiple enchondromas with associated slow-flow vascular malformations similar to venous malformations. Malignant degeneration of the bone lesions to chondrosarcoma may occur 20–30% of the time.

Parkes–Weber syndrome is a diffuse fast-flow malformation of a limb with overgrowth and cutaneous capillary malformation. Focal AVM or AVF may be present but many patients have a diffuse microshunt involving the entire limb that cannot be effectively treated.

Hereditary haemorrhagic telangiectasia or Osler–Weber–Rendu syndrome is an autosomal dominant condition. Patients develop progressive cutaneous and mucosal telangiectasias, some with macroscopic AVMs. Typical lesions in the lung and brain manifest as AVF with a varix of the immediate draining vein or as complex AVMs. Cerebral AVMs may bleed. Pulmonary AVMs and AVF may result in cyanosis with clubbing, fatigability, or brain infarcts or abscesses. Lesions involving the nasal area result in recurrent epistaxis. Pulmonary and cerebral lesions are treated with trancatheter embolisation.

In Sturge–Weber syndrome, facial port-wine stains are associated with ophthalmic and leptomeningeal slow-flow vascular anomalies, typically with cerebral atrophy and cortical calcifications. Seizures, neurological deficits and cognitive impairment are classic presentations. Non-contrast CT and MRI of the brain may be normal in the first 1–2 years of life. Contrast-enhanced studies will demonstrate gyral enhancement with enlargement of the ipsalateral choroid plexus. Cortical atrophy and gyral calcifications develop later.

# Treatment of vascular anomalies

## Haemangiomas

Haemangiomas plateau in size at approximately 9–10 months, with most resolving spontaneously in the first few years of life. Treatment of haemangiomas is reserved for those in endangering forms associated with ulceration, congestive heart failure, obstruction of the orbit or airway, or other severe complications. Arterial embolisation may be helpful in hepatic lesions resulting in high-output heart failure or lesions resulting in bleeding refractory to medical management.

## Venous malformations

### Indications

Therapy for venous malformations may be performed to improve pain, appearance or functional problems related to the lesion. In small, localised lesions, eradication with surgery or sclerotherapy may be possible. For extensive lesions, repeated sclerotherapy and surgical procedures are required, and the goal is control of symptomotology rather than cure.

### Patient evaluation

Preprocedural clinical and laboratory assessment is absolutely necessary for planning safe and effective sclerotherapy. Features that are associated with increased risk of complications include: involvement of the skin, mucosa, airway or orbit; large conducting veins; proximity to major nerves; and extensive intramuscular VMs in the calf or forearm. The presence of superficial lesions increases the risk of skin necrosis following sclerotherapy. Treatment of lesions involving the airway requires intubation, careful intraoperative monitoring and occasionally prolonged postprocedural intubation secondary to the inflammatory response and swelling. Elective tracheostomy should be considered if a series of procedures is planned. Midline or diffuse hemifacial VMs may have associated calvarial involvement, intracranial venous anomalies and sinus pericranii.[6,7] Swelling of an intramuscular VM in the forearm or calf may lead to compartment syndrome following sclerotherapy, and early decompression is necessary should this complication develop. Neurophysiological monitoring can be used during treatment of a perineural VM.

Unless the lesion is small, patients undergoing treatment of a VM should have a full blood count and evaluation of clotting parameters, including fibrinogen and D-dimers. Patients with large lesions may have elevated D-dimers and depletion of platelets, fibrinogen and other clotting proteins within the lesion, a process termed localised intravascular consumption (LIC). LIC can rarely result in severe postprocedure coagulopathy.[8,9] As the clotting cascade is part of the mechanism of action of sclerotherapy, patients with LIC can also demonstrate a poorer response to treatment. Patients with reduced baseline fibrinogen levels should be treated with low-molecular-weight heparin for 2 weeks prior to sclerotherapy.[8]

### Techniques

Current management of venous malformations includes the use of compression garments, aspirin and/or anticoagulants, endovascular treatment, and excision.

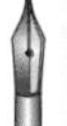

Percutaneous sclerotherapy is the primary treatment of venous malformations in most vascular anomalies centres.[10–17]

Excision is generally reserved for patients in whom the affected tissue can be removed without affecting function. Nevertheless, in delicate locations such as the hand and the orbit and in patients presenting with signs of nerve compression, swelling caused by sclerosant injection may be poorly tolerated and excision should be considered.[12]

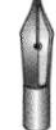

If intervention for a VM is required, the choice of resection vs. sclerotherapy is ultimately based upon the efficacy, morbidity and expected functional outcomes of each approach, and a combination of endovascular treatment and excision is often necessary.[4,10,18]

Sclerotherapy is the percutaneous injection of a sclerosing agent into the vascular malformation in order to damage the endothelium, incite inflammation and fibrosis, and ultimately obliterate the anomalous channels. Sclerotherapy of small lesions may be performed under sedation or even local anaesthesia. Sclerotherapy of large venous malformations and procedures utilising ethanol as the sclerosant are performed under general anaesthesia.

A channel within the VM is accessed with a needle, usually under ultrasound guidance. Contrast is injected with imaging by digital subtraction radiography or fluoroscopy to assess the character of the lesion and its drainage, how much of the lesion is accessed, and what volume of the sclerosant is necessary to displace the blood within the malformation. Sclerosant is injected until the lesion is completely opacified, increased resistance to injection is encountered, outflow veins are visualised, or imaging evidence of extravasation or changes in the overlying skin are seen.

Assessment of venous drainage is imperative. Focal venous malformations are usually 'sequestered', meaning that they drain to normal adjacent conducting veins via small channels. Diffuse venous malformations are often 'non-sequestered', meaning that they communicate directly with the main conducting veins, which are often abnormal.[19] Whereas sequestered venous malformations will usually respond well to sclerotherapy, non-sequestered venous malformation can be difficult to treat as sclerosant can enter the circulation leading to deep vein thrombosis, pulmonary embolism or (in the case of ethanol) pulmonary hypertension. Non-sequestered venous malformations are also more likely to recanalise following sclerotherapy.[11] In the presence of early draining veins, temporary control of the venous outflow during sclerosant injection may be accomplished in the head and neck by manual compression and in the limbs by the application of tourniquets. Alternatively, coils may be placed into the malformation, or at the junction of the malformation and the draining veins prior to sclerosant injection.[13] Dilute n-butyl-2-cyanoacrylate (NBCA) can also be injected to achieve outflow occlusion (**Fig. 20.6**).

Postprocedure, analgesia is often necessary. Unless contraindicated, intravenous fluids are administered at twice maintenance for several hours, and urine output is carefully monitored. Haemoglobinuria secondary to haemolysis occurs frequently after injection of large amounts of sclerosant and can be managed by aggressive hydration and urine alkalinisation. Swelling in extremities can be minimised by elevation of the treatment site and the application of ice packs. Swelling is maximum 24 hours after the procedure, so patients at risk of airway obstruction or compartment syndrome are observed overnight with consideration of prolonged intubation for airway lesions.[13] For lesions in which swelling would be poorly tolerated, systemic corticosteroids may be administered (0.1 mg/kg of dexamethasone every 8 hours with a tapering dose over the following week).

## Materials

Absolute ethanol (95–98%) is a potent sclerosant which causes instant precipitation of endothelial cell proteins and rapid thrombosis. While considered by many to be the most effective sclerosant, ethanol can also result in the most serious side-effects, including massive swelling (sometimes resulting in compartment syndrome), tissue necrosis, peripheral nerve injury, CNS depression, hypoglycaemia, hypertension and hyperthermia, haemolysis, pulmonary embolism, pulmonary vasospasm, cardiac arrhythmias and electromechanical dissociation.[13,16,17,20–22] Because of these potential side-effects, ethanol should be used only by experienced practitioners in a hospital setting with adequate anaesthesia and intensive care support.

Because of these potential adverse effects of ethanol, detergent sclerosants are often preferred, with ethanol reserved for large, deep VMs that are not in close proximity to major nerve trunks and have minimal venous drainage. Surfactant/detergent sclerosants include sodium tetradecyl sulphate,[12,23] polydocanol,[23] sodium morrhuate[24] and ethanolamine. Like ethanol, detergent sclerosants damage endothelial cells, resulting in thrombosis and fibrosis. In practice, detergent sclerosants are often opacified with oily contrast medium (Ethiodol or Lipiodol between a 1:10 and 3:10 concentration of contrast to sclerosant) and made into foam with an equal amount of air as the resulting 'microfoam' appears to result in a lower rate of recanalisation. Surfactant sclerosants have a lower rate of peripheral nerve injury and cardiovascular collapse compared with ethanol. However, sclerotherapy with detergent sclerosants can still cause severe adverse effects, such as skin and deep tissue necrosis, neuropathy, deep vein thrombosis and pulmonary embolism. In general, the quantity injected per session should not exceed 0.5 mL per kg or 20 mL.

## Outcome

The most commonly encountered complications of sclerotherapy are skin blistering and peripheral neuropathy. Blistering is common and usually heals uneventfully with appropriate supportive care. Full-thickness skin necrosis and scarring occurs in about 10–15% of patients undergoing ethanol sclerotherapy, usually at the site of cutaneous involvement of the malformation. Peripheral nerve injury with ethanol has been reported to occur in 1% of procedures and 10% of patients, and while it usually resolves at least partially, permanent injury can occur.[11] Neuropathy is less common with detergent sclerosants.

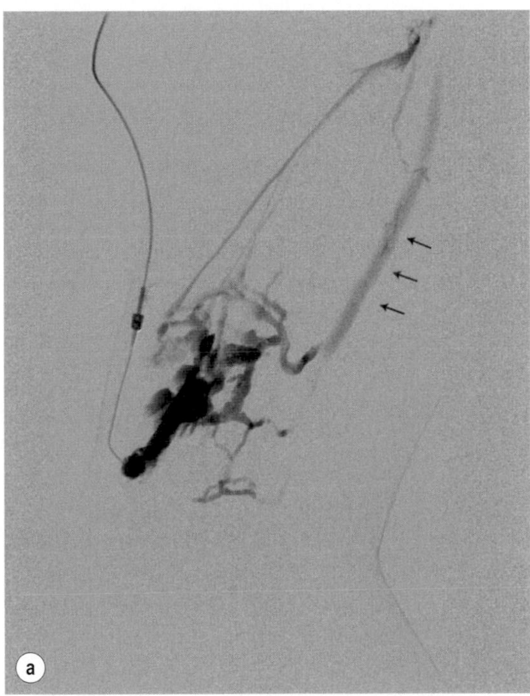

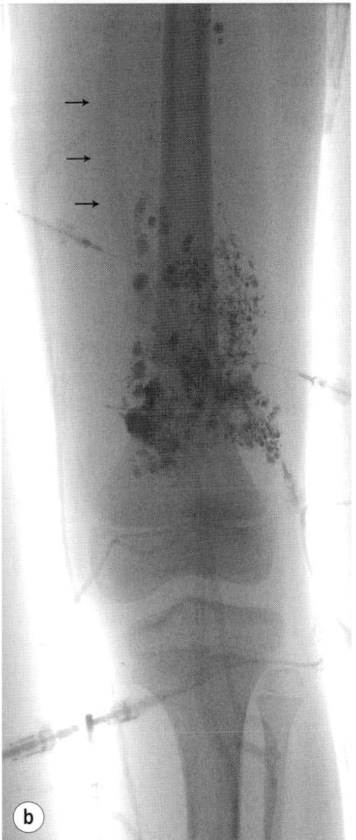

**Figure 20.6 • (a)** Following percutaneous access, contrast injection of an extensive venous malformation of the thigh demonstrates rapid opacification of the femoral vein (arrows). Before attempting sclerotherapy, the venous outflow could be controlled with tourniquets or occlusion of the communicating veins with coils or glue. Alternatively, the lesion could be accessed at another site with repeat contrast injection. **(b)** Final radiograph demonstrates alcohol opacified with Ethiodol within the lesion. Ascending venography via an angiocatheter placed in the foot demonstrates patency of the deep venous system following sclerotherapy (arrows indicate patent femoral vein).

Patients with painful, localised venous malformations are the best candidates for endovascular treatment. Focal, sequestered intramuscular or subcutaneous VMs can often be treated effectively with resolution or improvement in pain.[25,26]

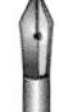

Most published series report successful outcome of sclerotherapy for relief of pain.[11,15,16,21,25,26]

With diffuse VMs, recurrence is common secondary to recanalisation and regeneration of anomalous venous channels, and the goal is not complete obliteration of the malformation but reduction of areas of maximum symptomatology. Long-term follow-up of extremity VMs has shown pain to be the most common problem cited on quality-of-life assessments.[15]

## Lymphatic malformations

### Indications

Sclerotherapy or surgery is useful for treatment of recurrent infection, functional complications and/or improvement of appearance.

### Patient evaluation

Ultrasound is usually performed to confirm the diagnosis of lymphatic malformation and to identify potential targets for therapy. For lesions in locations with complex anatomy, MRI is often helpful to evaluate the full extent of the lesion. In cervicofacial LMs, for example, MRI provides important information about airway and mediastinal involvement. Patients with lesions involving the airway will require intubation. If the lesion is extensive and multiple therapy sessions are planned, tracheostomy may be considered.

### Techniques

Macrocystic LMs were traditionally treated by resection.[4] Sclerotherapy of macrocystic lesions, however, has been shown to have a high rate of response with a lower risk of morbidity.[27,28] In centres where experienced practitioners are available, sclerotherapy should be the primary treatment of localised macrocystic LMs as well as recurrent cysts following resection.[29] Sclerotherapy of microcystic LMs is less successful. Microcystic LMs may be treated surgically provided that the benefits of excision outweigh the cosmetic and functional consequences.

The technique of sclerotherapy for LMs differs from that of VMs. Since LMs have a high rate of spontaneous infection, administration of prophylactic antibiotics is advisable. The lesions are accessed with sonographic guidance. Fluid is aspirated as completely as possible. The cysts can then be opacified with a small amount of contrast medium, which is then aspirated prior to sclerosant injection. Alternatively, needle position can be confirmed and sclerosant injected under sonographic monitoring. Regression of the macrocysts occurs slowly, and patients should be assessed at about 6 weeks following the procedure.

### Materials

Sclerotherapy agents for treating lymphatic malformations include doxycycline, ethanol, bleomycin, Ethibloc and OK-432.[27,30–32]

### Outcomes

Complications of sclerotherapy of LMs are uncommon but skin blistering or ulceration may occur if the lesions are overinjected. Lesions generally resolve with conservative treatment. Neuropathy is usually related to the use of ethanol. A questionnaire used to evaluate midterm results of sclerotherapy (mean time from first procedure 12 years, median 4 years) found that the response to treatment varied with the type of LM.

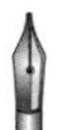

Patients with macrocystic, microcystic and combined-type LMs reported good to complete response to sclerotherapy 100%, 86% and 43% of the time respectively.[32]

## Arteriovenous malformations

### Indications

The evolution of an AVM can be documented by the Schobinger staging system (Table 20.1). Treatment is indicated in patients with significant symptoms or evidence of progression (Schobinger stage III). Specific indications for treatment of AVMs include cardiac volume overload, mass effect from dilatation of the draining veins, and tissue ischaemia or pain secondary to venous hypertension. Malformations composed of small vessels, such as Schobinger stage I AVMs and some diffuse AVMs seen in patients with Parkes–Weber syndrome, are not amenable to effective primary embolisation as the shunts are too small for direct cannulation and arteries supplying the AVM cannot be distinguished from the normal circulation.

**Table 20.1** • Schobinger clinical staging system for AVMs

| | |
|---|---|
| Stage I | Quiescence |
| Stage II | Expansion |
| Stage III | Destruction – pain, bleeding, ulceration |
| Stage IV | Decompensation |

### Patient evaluation

Clinical evaluation of a patient with an AVM should include a physical examination to document flow-related abnormalities (overgrowth, increased pulsations, thrill), identify complications of the lesion such as trophic cutaneous changes (pigmentation, pseudokaposiform change, ulceration, bleeding), and determine the cardiovascular effects of the shunt. A cardiac evaluation including an electrocardiogram and echocardiogram should be obtained if there is any evidence of cardiac volume overload. Delineation of the angioarchitecture of the AVM including feeding arteries and draining veins is important for treatment planning. In adults, this is often accomplished with a separate diagnostic angiogram, whereas non-invasive imaging such as magnetic resonance angiography is utilised in children.

While the terminology used is not anatomically precise and the system was originally applied to intracranial lesions, the angioarchitectural system of vascular lesions proposed by Houdart et al. is useful for understanding the decision process for approaching AVMs. The classification divides the fistulous communications in the lesions into arteriovenous, arteriolovenous and arteriolovenulous.[33]

Arteriovenous fistulas are direct arterial-to-venous communications. In arteriolovenous lesions, multiple (more than three) small arteries connect with one draining vein. Arteriolovenulous malformations represent the classic 'nidus' with multiple feeding arteries and multiple draining veins.

### Techniques

Endovascular techniques utilised in the treatment of fast-flow vascular malformations include arterial and venous embolisation and sclerotherapy. Arteriovenous fistulas and arteriolovenous lesions can be treated via either transarterial or transvenous embolisation, as occlusion of the draining vein can effectively close the shunt. Arteriolovenulous fistulas should be treated via transarterial embolisation only.

Arteries supplying the nidus must never be occluded proximally. Proximal occlusion, by either embolisation or ligation, produces a temporary decrease in flow through the malformation, followed by reperfusion of the nidus through collateral vessels and worsening of tissue ischaemia.

In preparation for endovascular treatment, the catheter access sites (usually the groins) and the area being treated are routinely prepped and draped so that either transcatheter embolisation or percutaneous sclerotherapy can be performed, so the skin overlying the AVM can be observed and cooled, and to facilitate application of a tourniquet or other compression device. After placing a vascular sheath in the access artery, a guiding catheter is used to study the vessels supplying the anatomical area involved. In most cases a microcatheter is introduced coaxially through a guiding catheter for superselective embolisation. For primary treatment, ablative permanent liquid embolic agents should be delivered directly into the nidus, preferably occluding the immediate draining vein. While NBCA and Onyx are administered as a single column, ethanol is delivered as series of boluses, separated by a time interval of at least 5 minutes, until the shunt is occluded. Primary treatment is usually staged to minimise the swelling and ischaemia from each procedure and to allow interval remodelling of the remaining arterial supply. Procedures are ideally spaced 4–8 weeks apart (**Fig. 20.7**).

Embolisation with particles is appropriate for preoperative devascularisation. The particles should be delivered as close as possible to the nidus.

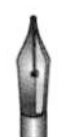

In extensive AVMs with numerous feeding arteries, direct percutaneous injection of particles (for preoperative embolisation) or NBCA or ethanol into the nidus can be more efficient and safer than individually catheterising and embolising each arterial feeding vessel, as the embolic agent is delivered only to the nidus and draining veins.[18,34–36]

In transvenous embolisation, the draining vein is catheterised and packed with coils. The coil mass may then be stabilised with a tissue adhesive such as NBCA, and the vessel may be sclerosed if necessary. The technique is suitable for AVMs with single outflow venous drainage.

## Materials

Embolic material used in embolisation of AVMs include liquid embolic agents such as NBCA and Onyx; particulate embolic agents such as polyvinyl alcohol particles and spheres, acrylic/gelatin microspheres and Gelfoam, and ethanol. Adhesive acrylic polymers such as NBCA have been used for decades to treat AVMs.[37] NBCA is injected as a liquid and polymerises instantly when it contacts ionic fluid, such as blood, saline or contrast medium. It results in permanent occlusion both via mechanical obstruction and secondary to an exothermic reaction that results in transmural necrosis. Precise placement of NBCA is difficult, and arterial rather than nidal occlusion can occur. Onyx is an ethylene vinyl alcohol copolymer dissolved in dimethyl sulphoxide which precipitates when the solvent dissolves in blood, forming a cast of the embolised vessels. Because the precipitation occurs centripetally from the vessel wall inward, the core of the Onyx column remains liquid and can be slowly pushed through the channels over minutes or even hours.[38] The use of Onyx in superficial vascular malformations is limited by its black colour secondary to the tantalum powder used to impart radio-opacity.[38]

Ethanol rapidly denatures endothelial proteins and, in stagnant channels, results in immediate thrombosis and destruction of the vessel wall. While ethanol is probably the most effective agent used to treat AVMs, it also has the highest rate of catastrophic, irreversible complications as discussed with its use in the treatment of VMs. Ethanol should never be injected into a proximal feeding artery, as penetration of the capillary bed will result in severe tissue necrosis. Even with appropriate catheter placement, if too much ethanol is delivered at once, nidal occlusion may occur during the injection with the possibility that ethanol injected subsequently with reflux into the normal arterial territory, causing severe tissue necrosis ('spill-over' effect). Particulate embolic materials mechanically obstruct blood flow to the lesion and incorporate thrombus in the occlusion. Recanalisation occurs as the thrombus is absorbed. These embolic agents are thus usually used for temporary preoperative embolisation of fast-flow vascular malformations and vascular tumours without macroshunts.[39]

## Outcomes

Symptomatic AVMs usually require serial embolisation (every 1–2 months) with liquid agents. The most symptomatic area and the largest shunts are targeted first, and embolisation is continued until as much shunting has been eliminated as possible. The patient is then followed clinically and if symptoms recur another embolisation is considered.

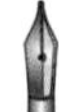

A review of patients who underwent ethanol embolisation for AVMs indicated that angioarchitecture was a good predictor of response, with arteriolovenous fistulas and arteriolovenulous fistulas with dilated fistulas having the best outcome.[40]

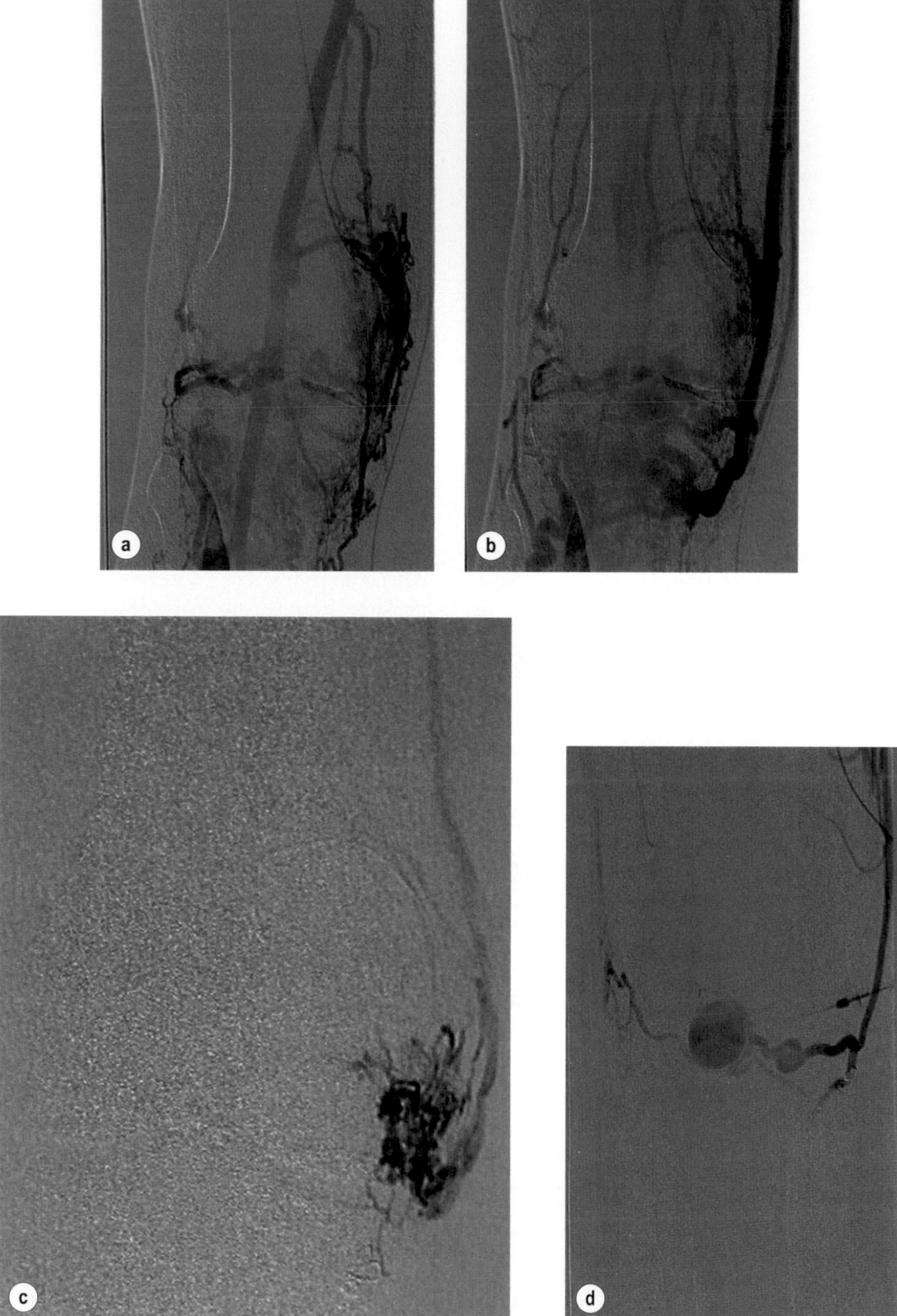

**Figure 20.7 • (a)** Arterial phase of a right superficial femoral artery arteriogram demonstrating an extensive AVM supplied predominantly by genicular branches of the poplital artery. **(b)** Venous phase demonstrating drainage predominantly to the greater saphenous vein with some drainage to the deep venous system. **(c)** Image taken following microcatheter injection of the nidus with ethanol opacified with Ethiodol. **(d)** Percutaneous access of a varix of a draining vein preceding direct injection of NBCA. **(e,f)** Arterial and venous phases of completion angiography demonstrating maintenance of patency of the major arteries of the lower extremity with minimal residual filling of the AVM.

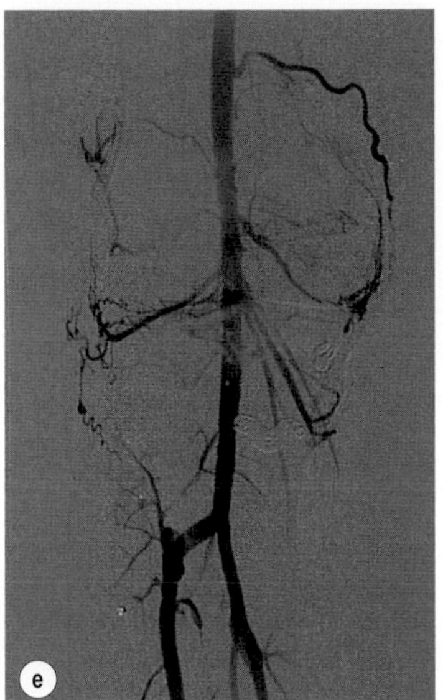

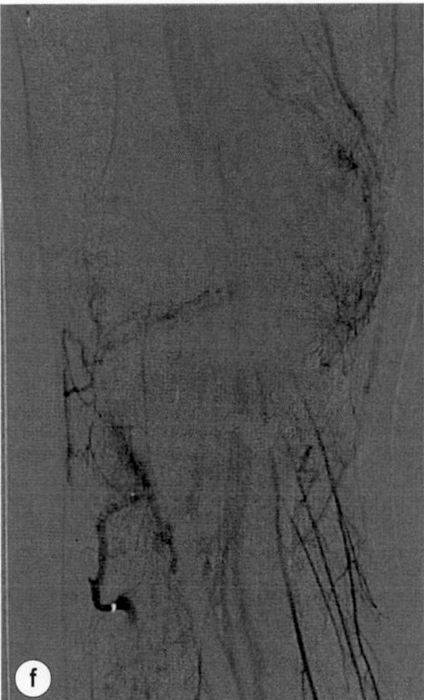

**Figure 20.7** • (*cont.*)

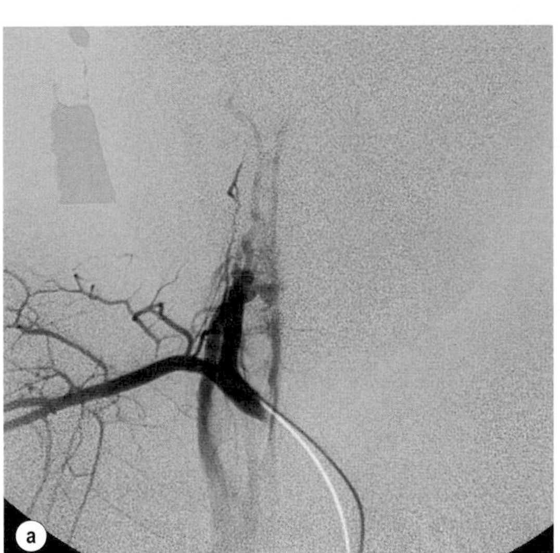

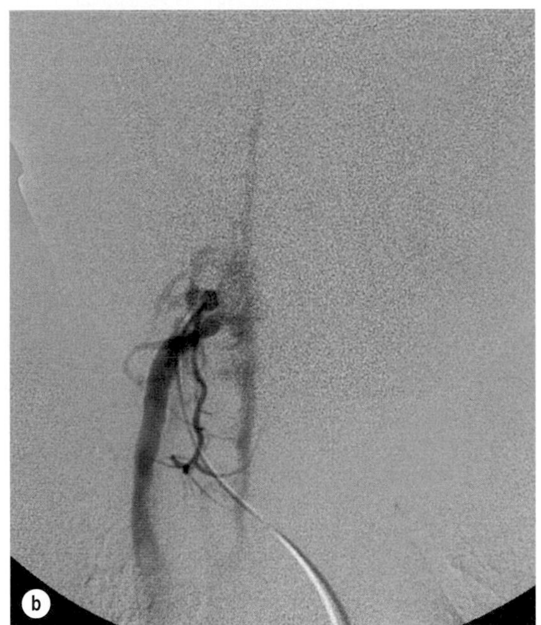

**Figure 20.8** • Embolisation of a right vertebral arteriovenous fistula. **(a)** Right subclavian arteriogram shows a direct shunt between the proximal right vertebral artery and the epidural and jugular veins. **(b)** Selective angiography with the microcatheter at the fistula site shows direct filling of the draining veins. **(c)** Radiograph showing the positioning of the coils in the fistula and immediate draining vein. **(d)** Right vertebral arteriogram performed 6 months after embolisation shows the right vertebral artery to be intact with permanent occlusion of the fistula.

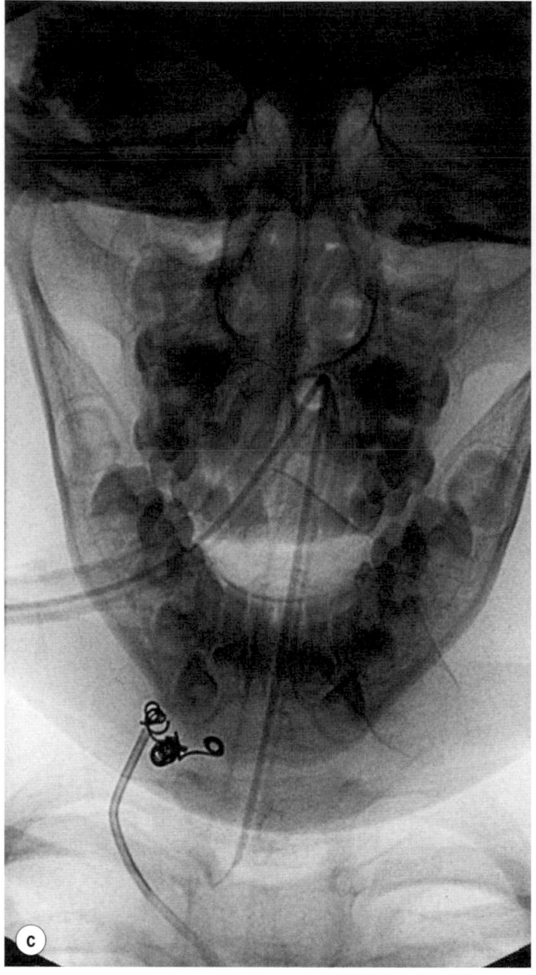


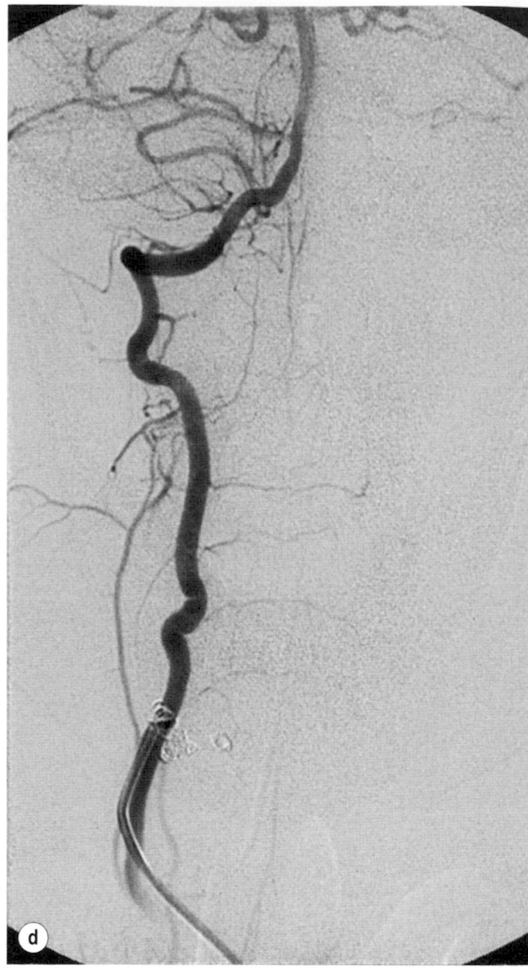


**Figure 20.8** • (*cont.*)

Effectiveness of embolisation was defined as complete resolution of signs and symptoms with 100% devascularisation (cure) or 50–99% devascularisation (partial remission) at angiography. By these definitions, ethanol embolisation was effective in 100% of arteriolovenous AVMs, 83% of arteriolovenulous AVMs with dilated fistulas and <50% of other types of AVMs.

## Arteriovenous fistulas

Simple AVFs can be cured by embolisation, and treatment is appropriate at the time of diagnosis in most cases. Most AVFs can be occluded with either NBCA or coils (**Fig. 20.8**). The Amplatzer occlusion device and covered stents/stentgrafts have also been used in older patients. The success of treatment depends on accurate placement of the occluding device at the site of the arteriovenous connection. Recurrence after technically successful occlusion is rare.

Congenital arterioportal fistulas are uncommon lesions that usually manifest in the first year of life, typically with signs of portal hypertension. If the ductus venosus is patent, cardiac failure may be seen in neonates, and gastrointestinal bleeding from portal varices can occur.

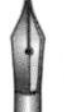
Treatment of congenital arterioportal fistulas should be undertaken soon after diagnosis in order to prevent portal vein thrombosis and other complications of portal hypertension.[41]

Serial ultrasound to assess portal vein patency should be performed following therapy, and anticoagulation should be considered subsequently to prevent portal vein thrombosis.

## Key points

- Vascular anomalies consist of two main categories, tumours (haemangiomas) and vascular malformations.
- Haemangiomas are only embolised for treatment of refractory high-output cardiac failure and bleeding, or to prepare for excision.
- Vascular anomalies can be distinguished by clinical and imaging features.
- MRI is the best imaging modality for the diagnosis of vascular anomalies.
- Symptomatic venous and lymphatic malformations are managed by serial sclerosant injection.
- Symptomatic arteriovenous malformations can be treated primarily by endovascular techniques using ablative liquid agents.
- Arteriovenous fistulas can be cured if the arteriovenous connection is occluded precisely.

# References


1. Mulliken JB, Glowacki J. Haemangiomas and vascular malformations in infants and children: a classification based on endothelial characteristics. Plast Reconstr Surg 1982; 69(3):412–22.
2. Frieden IJ, Reese V, Cohen D. PHACE syndrome. The association of posterior fossa brain malformations, hemangiomas, arterial anomalies, coarctation of the aorta and cardiac defects, and eye abnormalities. Arch Dermatol 1996; 132:307–11.
3. Hernandez F, Navarro M et al. The role of GLUT1 immunostaining in the diagnosis and classification of liver vascular tumors in children. J Pediatr Surg 2005; 40:801–4.
4. Mulliken JB, Fishman SJ, Burrow PE. Vascular anomalies. Curr Probl Surg 2000; 37(8):517–84.
5. Delis KT, Gloviczki P et al. Hemodynamic impairment, venous segmental disease, and clinical severity scoring in limbs with Klippel–Trenaunay syndrome. J Vasc Surg 2007; 45(3):561–7.
6. Burrows PE, Konez O et al. Venous variations of the brain and cranial vault. Neuroimaging Clin North Am 2003; 13(1):13–26.
7. Gandolfo C, Krings T et al. Sinus pericranii: diagnostic and therapeutic considerations in 15 patients. Neuroradiology 2007; 49(6):505–14.
8. Mazoyer E, Enjolras O et al. Coagulation abnormalities associated with extensive venous malformations of the limbs: differentiation from Kasabach–Merritt syndrome. Clin Lab Haematol 2002; 24(4):243–51.
9. Mason KP, Neufeld EJ et al. Coagulation abnormalities in pediatric and adult patients after sclerotherapy or embolization of vascular anomalies. Am J Roentgenol 2001; 177(6):1359–63.
10. Jackson IT, Carreno R et al. Hemangiomas, vascular malformations, and lymphovenous malformations: classification and methods of treatment. Plast Reconstr Surg 1993; 91(7):1216–30.
11. de Lorimier AA. Sclerotherapy for venous malformations. J Pediatr Surg 1995; 30:188–93.
12. Siniluoto TM, Svendsen PA et al. Percutaneous sclerotherapy of venous malformations of the head and neck using sodium tetradecyl sulphate (sotradecol). Scand J Plast Reconstruct Surg Hand Surg 1997; 31(2):145–50.
13. Burrows PE, Mason KP. Percutaneous treatment of low flow vascular malformations. J Vasc Interv Radiol 2004; 15(5):431–45.
14. Rautio R, Laranne J et al. Long-term results and quality of life after endovascular treatment of venous malformations in the face and neck. Acta Radiol 2004; 45(7):738–45.
15. Rautio R, Saarinen J et al. Endovascular treatment of venous malformations in extremities: results of sclerotherapy and the quality of life after treatment. Acta Radiol 2004; 45(4):397–403.
16. Rimon U, Garniek A et al. Ethanol sclerotherapy of peripheral venous malformations. Eur J Radiol 2004; 52(3):283–7.
17. Lee CH, Chen SG. Direct percutaneous ethanol instillation for treatment of venous malformation in the face and neck. Br J Plast Surg 2005; 58(8):1073–8.
18. Niimi Y, Song JK et al. Current endovascular management of maxillofacial vascular malformations. Neuroimaging Clin North Am 2007; 17(2):223–37.
19. Claudon M, Upton J et al. Diffuse venous malformations of the upper limb: morphologic characterization by MRI and venography. Pediatr Radiol 2001; 31(7):507–14.
20. Yakes WF, Luethke JM et al. Ethanol embolization of vascular malformations. Radiographics 1990; 10(5):787–96.
21. Lee BB, Do YS et al. Advanced management of venous malformation with ethanol sclerotherapy: mid-term results. J Vasc Surg 2003; 37(3):533–8.

22. Yakes WF, Rossi P et al. How I do it. Arteriovenous malformation management. Cardiovasc Interv Radiol 1996; 19(2):65–71.
23. Bhargava DK, Singh B et al. Prospective randomized comparison of sodium tetradecyl sulfate and polidocanol as variceal sclerosing agents. Am J Gastroenterol 1992; 87:182–6.
24. Yildirim I, Cinar C et al. Sclerotherapy to a large cervicofacial vascular malformation: a case report with 24 years' follow-up. Head Neck 2005; 27(7):639–43.
25. Suh JS, Shin KH et al. Venous malformations: sclerotherapy with a mixture of ethanol and lipiodol. Cardiovasc Interv Radiol 1997; 20(4):268–73.
26. Gorriz E, Carreira JM et al. Intramuscular low flow vascular malformations: treatment by means of direct percutaneous embolization. Eur J Radiol 1998; 27(2):161–5.
27. Sung MW, Lee DW et al. Sclerotherapy with picibanil (OK-432) for congenital lymphatic malformation in the head and neck. Laryngoscope 2001; 111(8):1430–3.
28. Bloom DC, Perkins JA et al. Management of lymphatic malformations. Curr Opin Otolaryngol Head Neck Surg 2004; 12(6):500–4.
29. Mikhail M, Kennedy R et al. Sclerosing of recurrent lymphangioma using OK-432. J Pediatr Surg 1995; 30:1159–60.
30. Molitch HI, Unger EC et al. Percutaneous sclerotherapy of lymphangiomas. Radiology 1995; 194(2):343–7.
31. Orford J, Barker A et al. Bleomycin therapy for cystic hygroma. J Pediatr Surg 1995; 30(9):1282–7.
32. Alomari AI, Karian VE et al. Percutaneous sclerotherapy for lymphatic malformations: a retrospective analysis of patient-evaluated improvement. J Vasc Interv Radiol 2006; 17(10):1639–48.
33. Houdart E, Gobin YP et al. A proposed angiographic classification of intracranial arteriovenous fistulae and malformations. Neuroradiology 1993; 35(5):381–5.
34. Gomes AS. Embolization therapy of congenital arteriovenous malformations: use of alternate approaches. Radiology 1994; 190:191–8.
35. Svendsen, PA, Wikholm G et al. Direct puncture of large arteriovenous malformations in head and neck for embolisation and subsequent reconstructive surgery. Scand J Plast Reconstr Surg Hand Surg 1994; 28(2):131–5.
36. Jackson JE, Mansfield AO et al. Treatment of high-flow vascular malformations by venous embolization aided by flow occlusion techniques. Cardiovasc Interv Radiol 1996; 19(5):323–8.
37. Pollak JS, White RI Jr. The use of cyanoacrylate adhesives in peripheral embolization. J Vasc Interv Radiol 2001; 12(8):907–13.
38. Arat A, Cil BE et al. Embolization of high-flow craniofacial vascular malformations with onyx. Am J Neuroradiol 2007; 28(7):1409–14.
39. Coldwell DM, Stokes KR et al. Embolotherapy: agents, clinical applications, and techniques. Radiographics 1994; 14(3):623–43; quiz 645–6.
40. Cho SK, Do YS et al. Arteriovenous malformations of the body and extremities: analysis of therapeutic outcomes and approaches according to a modified angiographic classification. J Endovasc Ther 2006; 13(4):527–38.
41. Burrows PE, Dubois J et al. Pediatric hepatic vascular anomalies. Pediatr Radiol 2001; 31(8):533–45.

# Index

Note: Page numbers in *italics* refer to figures and page numbers in **bold** refer to tables.

## A

## D

## E

## F

## G

## H



## I

## M

## Q



## R